Happy Nurses We
Michael Mayo & Nancy Simon
Frankfort Regional Medical Center

?

Public Health Nurse

Student Nurse

Modern Professional Nurse

Kaiserwerth Deaconess

Secular Servant Nurse

Sister of Charity

Brother of Mercy

Santo Spirito Sister

Franciscan Friar

Béquine

Knight Hospitaller

Barber Surgeon

9 10 11 12 13 14 15 16 17 18 19 20 21

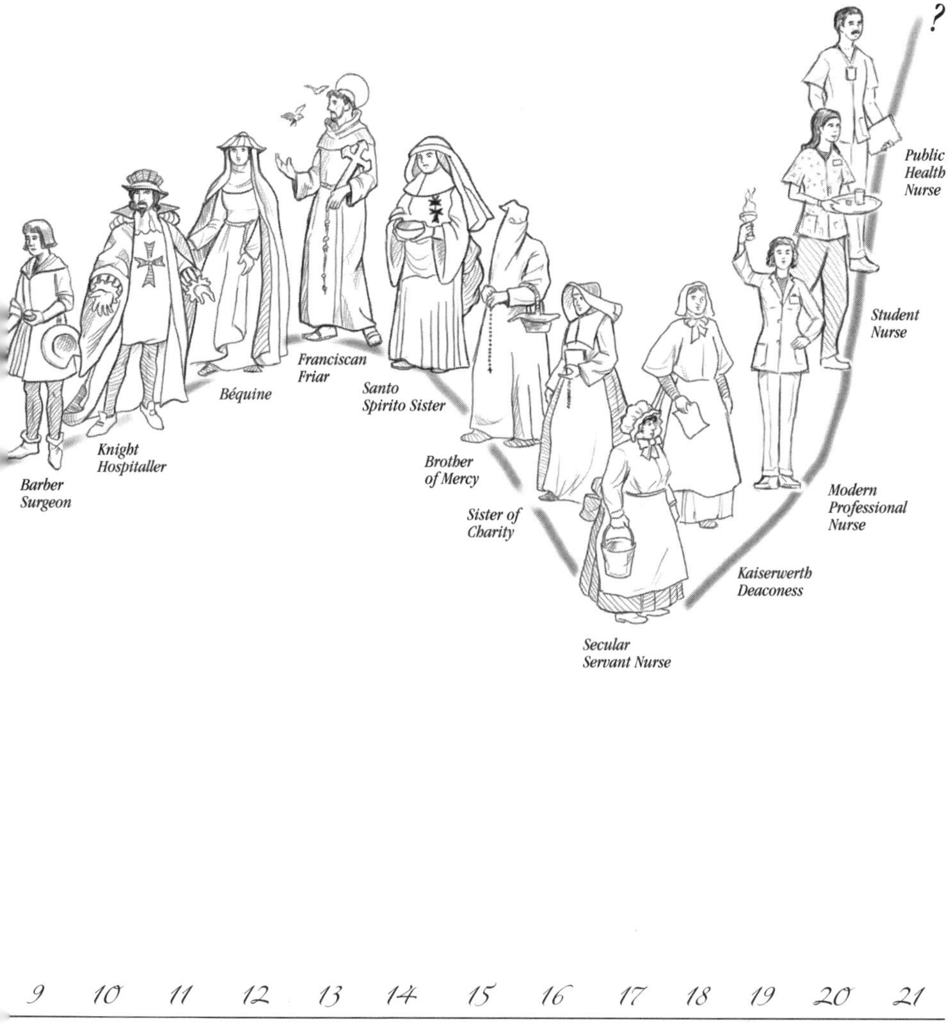

"The progressive world is necessarily divided into two classes—those who take the best of what there is and enjoy it—and those who wish for something better and try to create it."

FLORENCE NIGHTINGALE

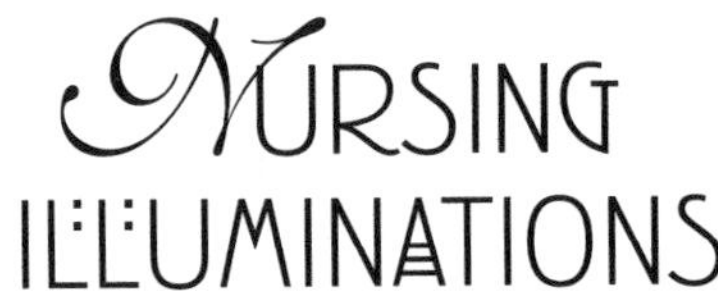

A BOOK OF DAYS

Daily inspirations, quotes, and insight into the lives of exceptional nurses, past and present

Depicting the similarities and bonds of nurses through their shared struggles and accomplishments, this unique daily reader rekindles the joy of nursing and illustrates the spirit of the profession.

Quotes and brief biographies draw on the life experience and dedication of influential nurses throughout history such as Lillian Bessie Carter, Barbara Montgomery Dossey, Isabel Adams Hampton Robb, Walt Whitman, Clara Barton, Florence Nightingale, and hundreds more.

With the many challenges that nurses face, including increased demands on the health care system and global nursing shortages, these stories of hope and inspiration help make every day of nursing brighter.

Nursing Illuminations takes a few minutes each day to reflect on nurses' special qualities and magnificent achievements, reminding us that all nurses make a difference in the lives of everyone around them!

NURSING ILLUMINATIONS

A BOOK OF DAYS

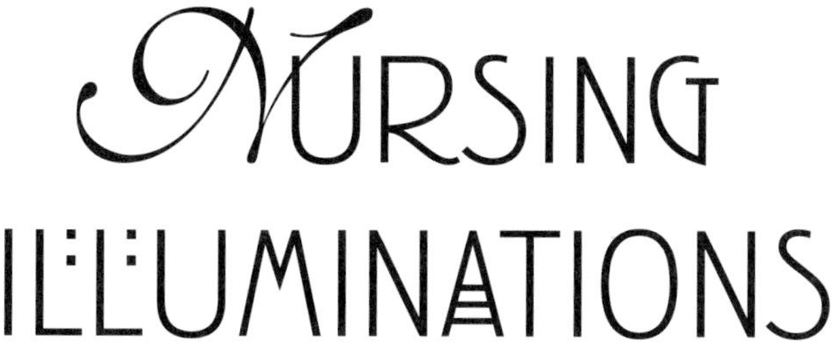

NURSING ILLUMINATIONS

A BOOK OF DAYS

PATRICIA T. VAN BETTEN, MEd, RN
Blue Diamond, Nevada

MELISA MORIARTY, BSN, RN
San Diego, California

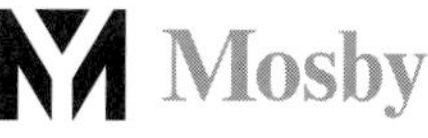

An Affiliate of Elsevier

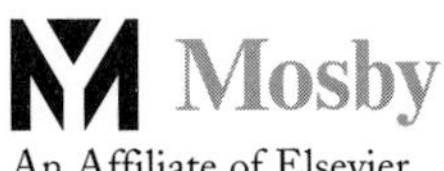

An Affiliate of Elsevier

11830 Westline Industrial Drive
St. Louis, Missouri 63146

NURSING ILLUMINATIONS: A BOOK OF DAYS

International Standard Book Number: 0-323-02584-6

Vice President and Publishing Director, Nursing: Sally Schrefer
Acquisitions Editor: Yvonne Alexopoulos
Developmental Editor: Danielle M. Frazier
Editorial Assistant: Julie Nebel
Publishing Services Manager: Melissa Lastarria
Designer: Amy Buxton

Printed in the United States of America

Last digit is the print number: 9 8 7 6 5 4 3 2

We dedicate this book to nurses everywhere,
but especially to Vern & Bonnie Bullough,
registered nurses whose vision, dedication, and resources
made our endeavor possible.

Acknowledgments

Pat would like to acknowledge the following:

I thank my family and friends, and my husband, Herman, in particular. Their wide circle of continual support and encouragement sustains me. I thank co-author and friend Melisa Moriarty for her continued enthusiasm, creativity, commitment, and dedication to this book project.

I thank these individuals and organizations who helped me locate nurses and/or information about nurses, which made it possible to complete book entries: Phoebe Letocha, Nursing Archives Project, Alan Mason Chesney Medical Archives, Johns Hopkins University; Taronda Spencer, Spelman College Archives, Spelman College, Atlanta, GA; Ben Hornsby, South Carolina Department of Archives and History, Columbia, SC; Aimee Brown, Archives specialist, Smith College Archives, Smith College, Northampton, MA; Alex Rankin, History of Nursing Archives, Boston University; Sister Betty Ann McNeal, archivist, and Tonya Crawford, assistant archivist, Daughters of Charity of St. Vincent de Paul, Archives and Mission Services, Daughters of Charity, Province of Emmitsburg, MD; Susan Osborn, librarian, archivist: Association of Perioperative Registered Nurses; Sister Mary Lonan Reilly, Congregation archivist, Sisters of St. Francis, Rochester, MN; Jennifer Peters, Archivist for Research and Public Service, The Archives of the Episcopal Church, Austin, TX; Sister Joan Brown, OSF, Sister of St. Francis; Sister Regina Bechtle, SC, Sister of Charity of St. Vincent de Paul of NY; Sister Teresa Marie OP and Sister DePaul OP, The Dominican Sisters of Hawthorne, Rosary Hill Home, Hawthorne, NY; Sister Mariah, University of Mary, Bismarck, ND; Major Jennifer L. Peterson and Major Constance Moore, Army Nurse Corps historians, Office of Medical

History, Falls Church, VA; Kazimiera Kozlowski, Curator, Prudence Crandell Museum, Canterbury, CT; Gail E. Farr, Curator, Center for the Study of the History of Nursing, University of Pennsylvania; Margaret A. Wilson, Library Coordinator, Sigma Theta Tau International, Indianapolis, IN; John White, Manuscripts Department, Wilson Library, University of North Carolina, Chapel Hill, NC; Janet L. Fickeissen, Executive Secretary, American Association for the History of Nursing; Eleanor Herrman, Past President, The American Association for the History of Nursing; Suzanne Hermann, Records Manager/Information Analyst, and Warren Hawkes, New York State Nurses Association; Nellie Powell, Librarian, Nursing/Biology Library, The Catholic University of America, Washington, DC; Angela Bellardini, Librarian, Nursing/Biology Library, The Catholic University of America, Washington, DC; Marian Taliaferro, Librarian, Nursing Biology Library, The Catholic University of America, Washington, DC; Chris Hollister, Librarian, and Jill Church, D'Youville College, Buffalo, NY; Fred Pond, Nursing Librarian, Dartmouth College/Dartmouth-Hitchcock Medical Center, Dartmouth, NH; Nancy Hall, Librarian, University of Texas at Austin School of Nursing, Austin, TX; Betty Skaggs, Director, Learning Center, University of Texas at Austin School of Nursing, Austin, TX; David McLellan, Librarian, Texas Department of Health, Austin, TX; Nina Mata, Librarian, Blue Diamond, NV; Beverly Colletti, Library, St. Rose Hospital, Henderson, NV; Florence Jacot, Librarian, West Charleston Health Sciences Library, Las Vegas, NV; Eunice Broadhead, Librarian, Reference/InterLibrary Loan, Clark County Library District, Las Vegas, NV; Patricia Labus, Medical Librarian, University Medical Center, Las Vegas, NV; Abigail Leah Plumb, Librarian, Sophie Palmer Library, The American Journal of Nursing; Lea Acord, Dean, Montana State University School of Nursing, Bozeman, MT; Rosemary Cox, Vietnam nurse "sister search" volunteer; Lisa Black, Executive director, Nevada Nurses Association; Robert Hirsch, South Carolina Hall of Fame, Myrtle Beach Convention Center, Myrtle Beach, SC; Kitty Manges, Programming Manager, South Carolina ETV Network; Ruth Annette Mills, Episcopal Church, Las Vegas, NV; Bill Lipson, Teachers College Columbia University Alumni office; Phyllis DiFilippo and Betty Jung, Office of Alumni Affairs, Columbia University; Nada DiFranco, Director of Alumni Relations, Case Western Reserve University; University of Minnesota Alumni Center; Jessica Emanuel, Administration Assistant, Catholic University of America Press, Washington, DC; Mara Reichman, American Academy of Family Physicians; Kimberly Hewitt, Catholic Health Association; Chandra Mays, Chandria Fulghum, and Terri Gaffney, staff, American Academy of Nursing, American Nurses Association; Kathy Apple, Executive Director, National Council of State Boards of Nursing; Illinois Nurses Association; Colorado State Board of Nursing; American Association of Nurse Attorneys; Janet Michael, RN, MS, JD; Amy Longo, BSN, JD; Pam Auchmuter, Associate Director, Health Sciences Publications, Emory University, Atlanta, GA; Gloria Smith, Congressional staff, Congresswoman Eddie Bernice Johnson; Robert Thompson, Records Technician, Hazel Braugh Records Center, American Red Cross, Falls Church, VA; American Nurses Association; National Park Service, Clara Barton National Historic Site; Ann Traub, RN, Connecticut; Karen Leary, Ohio and New York; Cecile B. Champagne, RN, East Stroudsburg University, PA; Sarah Ann Johnson RN, MSN, Medical College of South Carolina, College of Nursing; Elizabeth Bear CNM, PhD, Medical College of South Carolina, College of Nursing; Jackie Davis, Ida V. Moffett School of Nursing, Samford University, Birmingham, AL; Jackie Bush, RN, Nevada; Diane Millar; Carol Flack, University of Iowa.

The generous hospitality of these people made travel and research possible in different parts of the country: Mary Tringe, Lillian Tringe, Lorraine Kirkpatrick, Patricia Melady, Ann Berman, Ann and Charles Tartaglia, Linda and Randy Pearson, Clifton and Ann Sibley.

We are most grateful to the Sigma Theta Tau International Distinguished Writers Program, which allowed us the opportunity to work with Suzanne Beyea, our mentor for this project. Her encouragement, insights, support, and direction led to the successful completion and publication of our work.

I especially acknowledge and thank our editors, whose ongoing professional direction, support, expertise, and commitment to our book made it possible for us to do our very best.

Melisa would like to acknowledge the following:

I want to express my gratitude to my long time-friend and colleague Patricia van Betten, who invited me to share in the creation of this project. While reading daily meditation guides to learn more about ourselves and understand our actions, Pat saw the need to narrate nurses' great aptitude and their ability to steadfastly address the problems of the healthcare system.

Many others contributed directly and indirectly to the completion of this book. My 16-year-old grandson, Ryan Farrokhi, patiently tutored me in the use of the computer and the Internet. He was also very skilled in interpreting my ideas in artistic computer illustrations. My thanks go to my husband, John, who gave his undivided attention and sustenance during the seven years of our research. My good friend Cindy Bassuk helped me develop computer programs to manage the plethora of information we assembled. She also helped me devise a tracking list to facilitate the enormous job of seeking permission to reprint quotations from authors and publishers. Jacqueline Gervais, a friend for all seasons, helped me with the many days of tedious rewriting bibliographies. Vivian Martell, my friend and comrade, listened and encouraged me. I want to thank Suzanne Beyea for her patient consistent editing and support. Thanks to all of the nurses who allowed us to enter their lives and share their views about the meaning of health and how to attain and maintain it. I want to extend my thanks to the memory of Florence Nightingale, who defied her family and convention during a most repressive time for women. By her example and teachings she gave women courage and the beginning of a profession that allowed them to support themselves in a dignified way and simultaneously care for their fellows who were suffering. I am grateful to our editors, who have been supportive and constructive and given terrific direction. In conclusion, I want to say that to be researching, writing about, and sharing the lives of these outstanding individuals gave me a joyous sense of purpose, and I am most grateful for this opportunity.

Patricia T. van Betten, MEd, RN
Melisa Moriarty, BSN, RN

Note to Reader

When Pat and Melisa first contacted me, their idea of a daily reader for nurses about some of the greatest contributors to the nursing profession intrigued me. Each page that I reviewed enticed me to read more and to encourage these authors toward publication. In a few short months, I learned more about my profession than I ever had known and felt privileged to have walked among so many wonderful men and women who called themselves nurse.

The idea of a daily reader for nurses was not a new one, but this unique book provides a glimpse into many of the most significant contributions nurses have made toward the world's health. The vast majority of these nurses were unknown to me, despite my 30 years as a clinician, educator, and researcher. Yes, the most famous including Nightingale, Barton, and Whitman were well known to me. But each page revealed a treasure from the nursing profession's past generally forgotten by nursing textbooks. Each description of a nurse's work pushed me to stay with my own difficult and challenging work projects related to patient safety and the nursing shortage and brought encouragement to work harder.

Each morning I would read a page about a nurse to my husband, my adult children, or nurse colleagues. Those who listened were fascinated to hear about how nurses promoted health before there were modern hospitals or how nurses served in long forgotten wars to provide soldiers with the best of healthcare. There were stories of nurses working toward improving the work environment or educational process—always working to improve the profession and the health of those for whom nurses provided care.

This daily reader provides a brief but fairly comprehensive description of 366 nurses' biographies and a sampling of their lifetime contributions to the nursing profession. Starting with a quote of the nurse's own words, each page provides an opportunity for the reader to be inspired, encouraged, nurtured, or supported. It is remarkable how the comments of nurses, over time, address our current challenges, like the importance of quality patient care, the nursing shortage, healthcare reimbursement, and threats of bioterrorism. As one reads how nurses of the past prepared army nurses, faced gender and race discrimination, and addressed public health problems, one realizes that, as a profession, nursing can successfully address each of these many difficult challenges.

This unique reader makes nursing history accessible and readily available to any reader. The authors have compiled data from numerous sources and brought the past to the reader's hands without a trip to the library. These historical notes will hopefully stimulate some readers to pursue further research and study. But all readers will recognize the courage and abilities within themselves and within our profession as a collective whole.

On a personal note, it was a privilege to walk and work among these "greats in nursing." I enjoyed each story about many nurses I never knew. The contemporary nurses provide much delight, as some were known to me and I know more about their contributions. Working with Pat and Melisa provided me with great joy. After years of contributing to the profession—they know this book was important to their profession's future. They "came out of retirement" to make this contribution a reality and worked toward its completion with energy and love. This book, a significant contribution to nursing history and its future, should help every nurse know the work we do each day does make a difference to humanity and the future of the nursing profession.

My hope is that the reader will find great hope and inspiration in the words and stories of these nurses. Only 366 nurses are featured here, so there are many more stories that will never appear on paper. Those are the stories of nurses providing care in our inner cities, in third world countries, in our busy intensive care units, and in field hospitals across the world. Every nurse—famous or not—has made a difference in someone's life. Those contributions may vary from providing immunization to providing resuscitation to caring for a hospitalized patient or setting a health agenda for a nation. Regardless of the scope of the contribution, each act of caring provides comfort to those in need. This book should be a reminder that as a profession, nursing can make a difference one life at a time.

The authors' sincerest hope remains that this collection of inspiring stories will encourage non-nurses, nursing students, nurses—young and old—to find the vision and intensity within themselves to make a difference by being or becoming a nurse. This collection provides an exploration of the various pathways and diverse career opportunities for those considering nursing. Each page tells the reader a story of how one individual can make significant changes in the health of individuals, groups, or communities.

My instructions to the reader are to use this book as a daily reader. Each page will provide a quote from each nurse's own words which is intended to provide an opportunity for reflection about nursing leadership and scholarship. The story of each nurse's life that follows the quote provides a snapshot of each nurse's contributions. Finally, additional notations are made about each nurse's education, achievements, and honors. As one reads each page, the reader should consider his or her own contributions and their significance while gaining some perspective on the many other wonderful men and women who lead the way. Their work inspires me each day and makes me believe that nursing will continue to be a strong profession and one that is integral to solving today's heath care crisis.

I have told the authors that there is no doubt a second volume needs to be written. So if you do not find your name here or the name of another nurse who should have been included, remember that we must all work together to preserve the legacy of our profession.

Suzanne Cushman Beyea, RN, PhD, FAAN

Foreword

Pat and Melisa's *Book of Days* provides great insight into the lives and accomplishments of individual nurses, many of whom have been long been forgotten or seemingly neglected in the past. Yet, nurses across the centuries have been a significant part of health care in the United States and across the world. This day book recognizes many of the important nurses of the past and present and goes beyond a number of biographical dictionaries that have begun to include individual nurses.

This small but meaningful volume offers a unique exploration of nurses' contributions to health and society. Until this publication, there has not been a readily available source that describes in such detail the contributions of the 366 nurses included in this volume. This book brings these contributions to the public's attention and as well offers nurses' stories of hope and inspiration during a time of a serious nursing shortage and great demands on the healthcare system. Hopefully, it will arouse further interest of nurses and even the public to learn more about the history of a profession that has done so much to make this world a better place in which to live. I highly recommend this book. It is my sincerest hope that readers will be as inspired by nursing history as I have been.

Vern L. Bullough, PhD, RN

Preface

"Nursing is the conscience of the health care system."
—Dorothy Cornelius, 1970.

Our *Book of Days* illuminates the culture of nursing: its compassion, commitment, and connection. At one time or another, each person's life has been touched by a nurse. As nurses, we are excited to present this unique, new kind of book. A *Book of Days* is timeless and timely. Its appealing style nurtures and supports the reader with a daily opportunity to be enriched and inspired by a nurse. Readers will also see parallels between past and present concerns. We hope to stimulate an interest in nursing history, as readers discover and want to know more about those nurses with whom they feel a personal relationship.

The idea for this book came about after seeing the popularity and variety of daily readers, and realizing that nothing existed to tie today's nurse to the reinforcing words of nursing leaders, past and present. Contemporaries, and nurses long forgotten, have written words that are very relevant today, and we want everyone to know about them. We want to awaken, strengthen, and promote new interest in the diversity of nursing. Our book shows the bond between nurses from the past, contemporaries, volunteer nurses, and professionals. Although it gives a glimpse of background and achievements, it is not intended to be a comprehensive study of each nurse.

Our *Book of Days* dedicates each day of a nonspecific year to an individual nurse, on or near his or her birth date.* The combined

*A note about birth dates: If contemporary nurses share a birth date, the day is given to the nurse with the earlier birth year. When the page for a nurse is not on her actual birth date, the date is followed by a rose. The true birth date is in the biographical data. Also, if a nurse shares a birth date with a known nursing legend, the true date is given to the latter.

history and quotation tell of the rich traditions within nursing: its commitment to caring, its vision of equality, its dedication to the health of the world's citizens, and its willingness to take risks to improve conditions for many.

Our references include published nursing biographies, textbooks, journals, histories, archives, and personal correspondence.* We worked to contact contemporary nurses so that information would be correct. We are especially grateful to Vern and Bonnie Bullough, to whom this work is dedicated. Their extensive writings about nursing and nursing history were resources to us and inspired us. They invite each of us to do more, as they emphasize the importance of knowing and reflecting on our own history. We hope that we have built upon their strong base in a way that will encourage others to also explore and then share our professional heritage.

We urge each nurse who aspires to research, write, and publish to explore mentorship programs. We are immeasurably grateful to the Sigma Theta Tau Distinguished Writers Program, which made it possible for us to work with and benefit from the support, encouragement, direction, and expertise of our mentor, Suzanne Beyea. Suzanne made this book happen. In addition to her continual help with editing our work, she established a realistic timeline for completion and then successfully guided us through the process of preparing a proposal and applying for publication. We are privileged to have the opportunities to learn and grow in scholarship provided by this mentorship program.

Patricia T. van Betten, MEd, RN
Melisa Moriarty, BSN, RN

---

*In the References and Credits section, the symbol † appears next to the sources of the opening quotes, which have been used with permission. The order of the indicated references corresponds to the order of the quotes.

Santa Filomena

BY HENRY WADSWORTH LONGFELLOW

Whene'er a noble deed is wrought,
Whene'er is spoken a noble thought,
Our hearts, in glad surprise,
To higher levels rise.

The tidal wave of deeper souls
Into our inmost being rolls,
And lifts us unawares
Out of all meaner cares.

Honor to those whose words or deeds
Thus help us in our daily needs,
And by their overflow
Raise us from what is low!

Thus thought I, as by night I read
Of the great army of the dead,
The trenches cold and damp,
The starved and frozen camp,—

The wounded from the battle-plain,
In dreary hospitals of pain,
The cheerless corridors,
The cold and stony floors.

Lo! in that house of misery
A lady with a lamp I see
Pass through the glimmering gloom,
And flit from room to room.

And slow, as in a dream of bliss,
The speechless sufferer turns to kiss
Her shadow, as it falls
Upon the darkening walls.

As if a door in heaven should be
Opened, and then closed suddenly,
The vision came and went,
The light shone was spent.

On England's annals, through the long
Hereafter of her speech and song,
That light its rays shall cast
From portals of the past.

A lady with a lamp shall stand
In the great history of the land,
A noble type of good,
Heroic womanhood.

Nor even shall be wanting here
The palm, the lily, and the spear,
The symbols that of yore
Saint Filomena bore.

The Atlantic Monthly; November 1857; "Santa Filomena," by Henry Wadsworth Longfellow; Volume 1, No. 1; pages 22-23.

Nursing Illuminations

A Book of Days

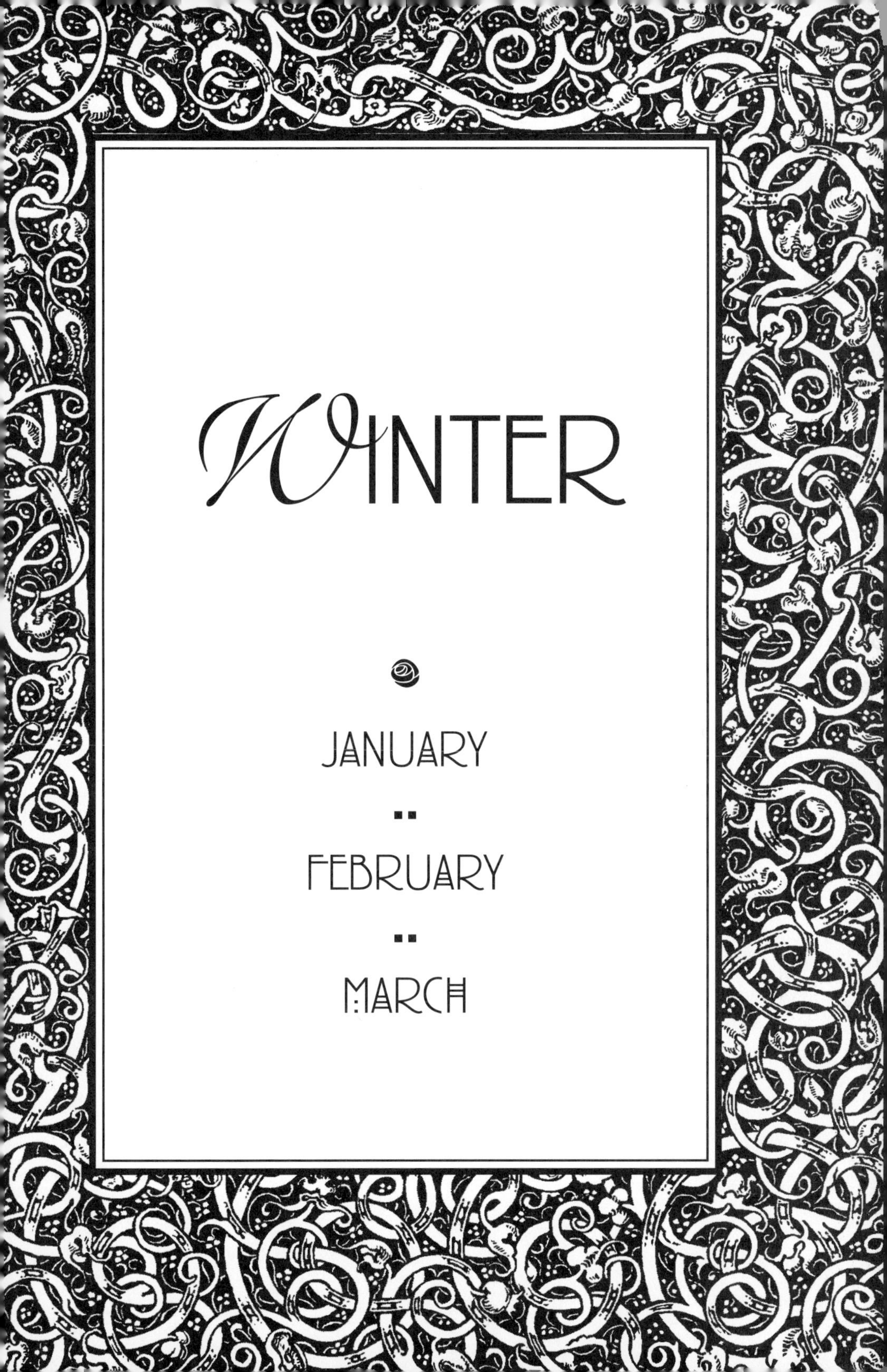

WINTER

JANUARY

FEBRUARY

MARCH

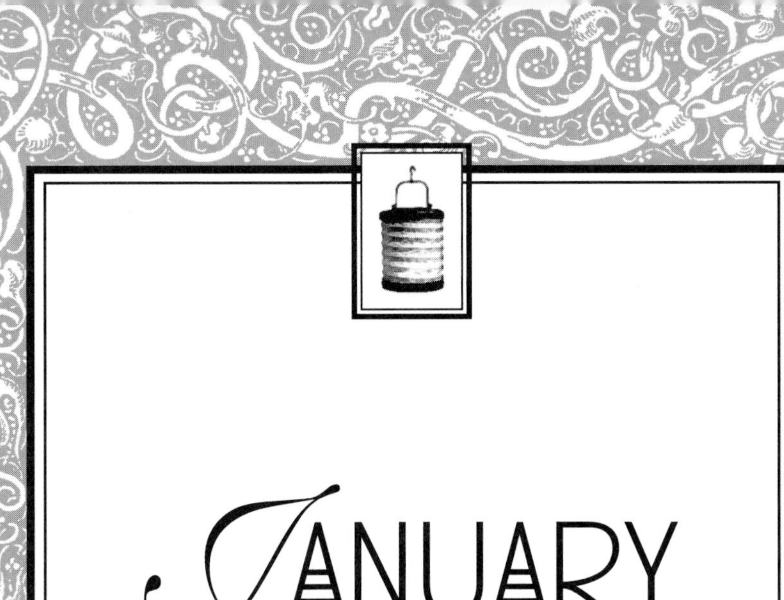

JANUARY

"The progressive world is necessarily divided into two classes—those who take the best of what there is and enjoy it—those who wish for something better and try to create it."

—Florence Nightingale
Nightingale, N.: Cassandra: An Essay. Introduction by Myra Stark. City University of New York, Feminist Press, 1979, p 29.

JANUARY 1

Margaret Anthony Tracy

1893–1959

"Ours is the fault if the student sees her patient as an 'acute appendix' or a 'fractured skull,' not as an individual with family and community relationships. As we help them acquire the very necessary skills which they need, to care for surgical patients, we must do so in a way which will also enable them to see those skills as a tool to help them in the role of teacher and promoter of the public health." (1926)

STANDARDS OF EXCELLENCE were part of Margaret Tracy's uncompromising vision for nursing's place in academia. When she replaced the three-year diploma program associated with the University of California Hospital with a five-year baccalaureate program, it became the first independent state-supported program of its kind. Tracy was a skilled problem solver, undaunted by the challenge of merging splintered nursing programs into one department to ensure a more uniform and standardized curriculum. Well informed and articulate, she collaborated with other nursing leaders to prepare and publish the text *Nursing, An Art and a Science.* She promoted nursing research and published her own research related to a time study of nursing procedures and care of surgical patients.

Biography

Born: Jan. 1, 1893, Danville, Ky. **Education:** Univ. of Cincinnati (AB); Army School of Nursing, Washington, D.C.; Yale (MS). **Work history:** Staff Nurse, then Adminstrator, Henry Street Visiting Nurse Service, N.Y.C.; Instructor, Administrator, Glens Falls (N.Y.) Hosp. School of Nursing; Instructor, Yale Univ. School of Nursing; Supervisor, New Haven (Conn.) Hosp.; Instructor, Rockefeller Foundation; Director, then Dean, Univ. of California School of Nursing, San Francisco and Berkeley; Nursing Education Advisory Committee of U.S. Public Health Service; member, editorial bd., *Nursing Research.* **Organizations:** unknown. **Awards:** Rockefeller Foundation Fellowship. **Died:** Mountain View, Calif.

References and Credits

†Tracy, MA: Supervision and teaching of surgical nursing. AJN 26:797, 1926.

Cooper SS: Margaret Tracy. In Bullough V, Sentz L, Stein AP (eds): American Nursing: A Biographical Dictionary, vol. 2. New York, Garland, 1992, pp 324–326.

JANUARY 2

Eleanor C. Lambertsen

1916 –1998

"The central concerns of nursing—care, comfort, guidance, and helping individuals cope with health problems—have not changed. However, the dimension and scope of practice of [their] components ... change along with social determinants for health care services. ... Social changes, attitudes and changing roles within the occupation are jeopardizing the nurse's role in the practice of nursing. *... The churning within the occupation can be a motivating force or could terminate in a period which might be labeled 'the great compromise.' As long as groups of nurses continue to curtail progress in clearly defining nursing functions of a professional nature and impede progress through advances in education because their 'status is showing,' the quality of nursing care will remain at an elementary and superficial level. Tradition rightfully belongs to history; complacency must be replaced by vigorous effort." (1988)*

WHEN ELEANOR LAMBERTSEN entered nursing, two-thirds of the nation's hospitals were staffed with students and did not hire graduate staff nurses. Much of the public regarded nursing as menial rather than intellectual work, and people tried to discourage her from going to nursing school. Education and work experience proved to her that nursing could be a rewarding career, and she recognized the importance of competent nursing interventions in patient outcomes. The post–World War II nursing shortage underscored the necessity of professional nursing for quality care. When nursing leaders and members of the President's Commission on Higher Education began speaking about professional and technical nursing, the concept of team nursing evolved. Lambertsen implemented this concept when she opened a new hospital in New York. The focus was always on the needs of the patient, and she required all team members to be involved with providing care. When she was invited to join the American Hospital Association to create a division of nursing, she became nursing's voice on policy and practice. As a member of a related committee for the Robert Wood Johnson Foundation, she helped strengthen the role of the nurse practitioner in primary care.

Biography

Born: Jan. 2, 1916, Westfield, N.J. **Education:** Overlook Hosp. School of Nursing, Summit, N.J.; Teachers College, Columbia Univ., bachelor's, master's, and doctoral degrees. **Work history:** various nursing positions, Overlook Hosp.; established then directed Nursing Division held other positions, American Hosp. Assoc.; various admin. positions, Teachers College, Columbia Univ.; Dean, Cornell Hosp. School of Nursing, N.Y.; Director of Nursing Services, New York Hosp.; member, bd. of directors, Kellogg Foundation; Adviser, Robert Wood Johnson Foundation and American Nurses Foundation. **Organizations:** N.Y. State Nurses Assoc., American Nurses Assoc. (ANA). **Awards:** McManus Award, Teachers College; awards from ANA, N.Y. State Nurses Assoc.; election to Institute of Medicine, National Academy of Sciences. **Died:** location unknown.

References and Credits

†Schorr T, Zimmerman A: Making Choices, Taking Chances: Nurse Leaders Tell Their Stories. St. Louis, CV Mosby, 1988, pp 176, 184.

Safier G: Contemporary American Leaders in Nursing: An Oral History. New York, McGraw-Hill, 1977.

January 3

Anne Hervey Strong
1876–1925

"Every thoughtful woman in public health work sees on the one hand enormous need of the work that nurses can do, not only to save life but to increase the physical efficiency of the nation; on the other hand, she sees the totally inadequate number of nurses already trained for public health nursing, the prospect of greatly increased need in the future, and the possibility of greatly decreased numbers of women preparing to meet it. ... Of all our national resources, human life is the most important. Public health nursing directly contributes toward the conservation of human life." (1917)

Described as scholarly, insightful, and visionary, Anne Strong is among those credited with the progress of public health nursing. She had a broad academic background and a college degree before entering the profession. After she was hospitalized for a back injury, she decided to study nursing instead of medicine. When she worked as a volunteer and then a staff nurse at the Henry Street Settlement, she was awakened to the importance of public health nursing. After teaching at Simmons College in a cooperative program of the college and the Boston Instructive District Nurses Association, she became the director of its school of public health nursing. She merged theory and practice through teaching and appropriate affiliations for nursing students. She saw college women as candidates for careers in public health and worked to recruit them to the profession.

Biography

Born: Jan. 1876, Wakefield, Mass. **Education:** Bryn Mawr College; Albany (N.Y.) Hosp. Training School for Nurses; Teachers College, Columbia Univ. **Work history:** Instructor, Albany Hosp. Training School; Math Instructor, Administrator, Mary C. Wheeler School Providence, R.I.; Staff Nurse, Henry Street Settlement N.Y.C.; Instructor, Teachers College, Columbia Univ.; Nursing Faculty, Simmons College; Consultant, Rockefeller Foundation. **Organizations:** National Organization for Public Health Nursing; National League for Nursing Education; American Child Health Assoc.; Mass. Nurses Assoc. **Awards:** American Nurses Assoc. Hall of Fame. **Died:** Boston.

References and Credits

†Strong AH: Teaching problems of public health instructors. AJN 17:1188–1192, 1917.

Stein AP: Anne Hervey Strong. In Bullough V, Sentz L, Stein AP (eds): American Nursing: A Biographical Dictionary, vol. 2. New York, Garland, 1992, pp 316–317.

ANA Hall of Fame 10/98 American Nurses Association, Washington, D.C. http://www.nursingworld.org/hof.

JANUARY 4

Edna Behrens

1897–1990

"Human beings should have a voice in determining the conditions under which they work." (Date unknown)

"You know, we too frequently elect officers because of their charm and personality. What we need now is not charm but achievement, not personality but perseverance, not glamour but gumption. ... Give us governing boards that are hard working, progressive, open and eager for new ideas, willing to try innovation ...and let them be characterized by originality and vision and courage." (Date unknown)

HER COLLEAGUES AGREED that when Edna Behrens described what nursing and its associations needed, she best described herself and her own vision for nursing. She was fired from one hospital job as a director of nursing, believing that she was dismissed because of her dedication to the Economic Security Program of collective bargaining. Starting at the district level with the California State Nurses Association (CSNA) and rising to president for a six-year term, Behrens demonstrated her negotiating skills as someone who understood and cared about nurses. She made certain that people knew that nurses needed living wages, good working conditions, a forty-hour week, health insurance, retirement, vacation leave, and to improve patient care. She did all her negotiating while the association's no-strike pledge remained in effect. Because she had to prove to a board that local nurses supported her demands, she met secretly with the hospital nurses in a linen closet to acquire their signatures to present to the board. Those nurses received their raises.

Biography

Born: Jan. 4, 1897, Petaluma, Calif. **Education:** School of Nursing, Franklin Hosp., San Francisco. **Work history:** OR Supervisor, Franklin Hosp., eighteen yrs.; Director of Nursing, three yrs.; helped organize nursing service in new hospital, Glenn County, Calif.; started her collective bargaining Economic Security Program. **Organizations:** member, bd. of directors; President (six yrs.), CSNA. **Awards:** Shirley C. Titus Award, American Nurses Assoc. **Died:** Mill Valley, Calif.

References and Credits

†Stanley J: Edna Behrens. In Bullough V, Sentz L, Stein AP (eds): American Nursing: A Biographical Dictionary, vol. 2. New York, Garland, 1992, pp 22–26.

JANUARY 5

Bonnie Bullough

1927–1996

"It has often been said that modern nursing could not have developed independently of modern medicine, but … modern medicine could not have developed without the emergence of modern nursing. This … has too often been overlooked. To explain the development of nursing it is necessary to consider a society's attitude toward its sick, its wounded, its mentally ill, toward its paupers and lepers, toward the crippled and malformed, toward the infant and the infirm. The historian of nursing must also consider the medical practices of the time, the place of the hospital, the economic and educational levels of society and the status of women in the society. … The history of nursing is … most rewarding … because it is basically concerned with man's humanity to his fellow man." (1964)

As a young child, Bonnie Bullough was eligible for the then-new provisions for disabled children under Social Security for Crippled Children. This provided for reconstructive surgeries for the extensive burns to her face, ear, and legs that she had suffered years earlier. While she endured these prolonged hospitalizations away from her family, she became determined to be a nurse. Her nursing career was full, creative, and versatile. A prolific writer and international lecturer, she was also a historian, sociologist, researcher, activist, educator, and nurse practitioner. She was instrumental in forming the national organization of nurse practitioners and was a founder of the American Association of the History of Nursing. She fought discrimination and helped to establish such organizations as the Medical Committee for Human Rights, Chicago, and the Fair Housing Council and Parents and Friends of Gays, both in Los Angeles; the last soon became a national organization. Her later research and publications focused on human sexuality and gender discrimination.

Biography

Born: Jan. 5, 1927, Delta, Utah. **Education:** U.S. Cadet Nurse Corps Program, Univ. of Utah and Salt Lake City General Hosp. (RN); Loyola Univ., Chicago; Youngstown (Ohio) Univ. (BS); Univ. of California, Los Angeles (UCLA) (MS, MA, PhD). **Work history:** Santa Rosa (Calif.) Hosp.; OR Nurse, Salt Lake General Hosp.; OR Nurse, Univ. of Chicago Hosp.; Chicago Public Health Dept.; St. Elizabeth Hosp., Ohio; Faculty, Youngstown Univ.; Northridge (Calif.) Hosp.; Faculty, UCLA School of Nursing; Fulbright Lecturer, Univ. of Cairo; Faculty, UCLA; Faculty, Administrator, nursing program, California State Univ., Long Beach; Director, Orange County (Calif.) Consortium; Dean, Faculty, State Univ. of New York, Buffalo; Faculty, Dept. of Nursing, Univ. of Southern Calif.; Consultant, Planned Parenthood. **Organizations:** numerous positions in American Nurses Assoc.; National League for Nursing; founder, first president, Coalition of Organized Nurse Practitioners; member, Calif. Bd. of Registered Nurses; Calif. State Nurses Assoc.; N.Y. Nurses Assoc., and others. **Awards:** Nurse Practitioner of the Year National Nurse Practitioner Groups; Alfred Kinsey Award for research into human sexuality. **Died:** Los Angeles.

References and Credits

†Bullough B, Bullough V: Preface to The Emergence of Modern Nursing. New York, Macmillan, 1964, p v.

Bullough V: Bonnie Bullough. In Bullough V, Sentz L (eds): American Nursing: A Biographical Dictionary, vol. 3. New York, Springer, 2000, pp 36–39.

January 6

Lydia Holman

1868–1960

"The distances are so great that one must waste much time on the road; often I ride from five to twenty-two miles to make a single visit, prolonging it several hours to give a 'while you wait nurses' course' to the family, lest I should not return again. At one time last winter with a bad pneumonia case at either end of a fifteen mile stretch, and numerous other patients scattered in between, I was in the saddle nearly all the time for three weeks and able to stop at home only long enough for baths and changes of clothing. ... There are compensations—the blue sky, the everlasting hills, exhilarating air, and the simplicity of the people. These all go to make my life here a happy one." (1907)

Lydia Holman moved to the North Carolina mountains and Mitchell County as a private duty nurse for a patient with typhoid fever and stayed for forty years. For twenty years she was physician, dentist, nurse, and the only caregiver in this remote, unserved area. She traveled by horseback to the mountain people, whose poverty and ignorance was worsened by isolation from supplies and services. A public health nurse and midwife, this "healing" nurse significantly improved maternity and newborn care. She charged people what they could afford to pay and was often compensated with crops and livestock. While living in Altapass, Holman taught classes in housework, cooking, and sewing. She also taught a kindergarten and gave parties for neighbors. Carolyn Conant Von Blarcom, an authority on obstetrical nursing, cited Holman as a special example of a public health nurse who worked to improve the conditions surrounding motherhood: "She alleviated distress and averted disaster in Altapass, North Carolina." Holman did her own housework and tended a garden that produced fresh vegetables to share with her visitors. State and federal agencies and the Red Cross have continued Holman's work in the North Carolina mountains.

Biography

Born: Jan. 5, 1868, Philadelphia. **Education:** Philadelphia General Hosp. School of Nursing; studied maternal care, child health, and midwifery for two additional years in Philadelphia. **Work history:** Charge Nurse, Mt. Carbon, Pa., 1894; Private Duty, Charge Nurse, Public Health Nurse, Henry Street Settlement, N.Y.C., with Lillian Wald; established Mountain Visiting Nurse Service, Ledger, N.C.,1902; established the Holman Assoc., 1911; raised money to promote "rural nursing, hygiene and social service"; established infirmary, Altapass, N.C. **Organizations:** member, first bd. of directors, National Organization for Public Health Nursing, 1912; elected to the Mitchell County (N.C.) Bd. of Health, 1936. **Awards:** unknown. **Died:** Osteen, N.C.

References and Credits

†Holman L: Visiting nursing in the mountains of western North Carolina. AJN 7:834, 1907.

Craft SN: Lydia Holman. In Bullough V, Sentz L, Stein AP (eds): American Nursing: A Biographical Dictionary, vol. 2. New York, Garland, 1992, pp 156–159.

JANUARY 7

Alice Griffith Carr

1887–1968

"To have a hospital with a high-class school for nurses had been their dearest wish for years and when at last these nurses stood in their uniforms at the dedication of this great institution, it was with tearful eyes that people looked on them, knowing that they were realizing what they had longed for and labored for during many years. No one else knew from such hard tragic experience how this great, shining, beautifully equipped hospital was needed, nor how much nurses were needed to carry on the work which nurses alone can do in the life of a nation." (1942)

ALICE CARR FIRST PREPARED and worked as a math teacher and then as a beautician. She later recognized that nursing could give her the financial independence that she sought. She was an outstanding and beloved Red Cross nurse who had a dramatic impact on public health in Europe and the Near East. Her life is a broad lesson of commitment and achievement. She drastically reduced the incidence of malaria and tuberculosis among the poor by teaching basic sanitation and disease prevention. In Turkey she worked with teenagers to literally drain swamps and kill mosquitoes to reduce the malaria epidemic. She helped rescue thousands of Russian orphans during the Bolshevik Revolution when she and other Red Cross nurses traveled with the children in boxcars to safety in Poland. She established centers for health care for children in Serbia and in Czechoslovakia. Many women refugees became economically self-sufficient because of Carr's encouragement and assistance. Upon her retirement to Florida she helped build her own home and enjoyed gardening.

Biography

Born: Jan. 7, 1887, Yellow Springs, Ohio. **Education:** Antioch College (BA); Beauty College; Johns Hopkins Hosp. Training School for Nurses. **Work history:** Private Duty Nurse;; army nurse with the Johns Hopkins Unit, France; Red Cross nurse, Poland, Czechoslovakia, Greece; Near East Relief, Greece, Turkey, Iraq, Syria, Kurdistan; Director of Public Health, Near East Foundation. **Organizations:** unknown. **Awards:** Order of the Phoenix, highest honor from Greece; honorary LLBs, Antioch College, Ohio State Univ.; other awards from American Red Cross, Veterans of Foreign Wars. **Died:** Melbourne, Fla.

References and Credits

†Carr AG: Nursing in pre-war Greece. AJN 42:371, 1942.

Thomas GM: Alice Carr. In Bullough V, Church OM, Stein, AP (eds): American Nursing: A Biographical Dictionary, vol. 1. New York, Garland, 1988, pp 58–61.

JANUARY 8

Agnes Hannah von Kurowsky Stanfield

1892–1984

"I am very happy indeed, because I feel I am doing some really worth while work, and my patients are so grateful, poor boys, for the slightest thing you do for them." (1918)

THE TWENTY-SIX-YEAR-OLD Agnes von Kurowsky was an American Red Cross nurse serving in Milan in July 1918, when a badly wounded Ernest Hemingway, then nineteen, was brought into the Ospedale Croce Rossa Americana for treatment of his leg wounds. He was a decorated war hero who had carried a wounded comrade to safety, ignoring his own wounds. He had survived a devastating blast, suffered machine gun injuries to his legs, and now knew that he was mortal. The pretty, accomplished nurse who spoke French, German, and Italian and answered to "Ag" was his first love and the model for the heroine of his best novel, *A Farewell to Arms*. Her effect on him was lasting. They corresponded while she was working in Treviso and Torre di Mosto. Henry Villard, also a patient and the coauthor of *The Lost Diary of Agnes von Kurowsky,* said, "When Agnes did appear, the entire place seemed to brighten because of her presence. Besides having what the boys called 'it' she was kind, quick, intelligent, and sensitive to the moods of a patient;

what's more, she was blessed with a sense of humor that verged on the mischievous. She was firm without being too strict, light-hearted yet professionally serious. Altogether the perfect temperament for a nurse." She continued her nursing career in the United States and abroad, satisfying her nature for adventure. Because of her fluent French, she was recruited to work in Haiti, and she was commended for setting high standards. As a result of "her gallant and commendable services" with the American Red Cross, Stanfield is buried alongside her parents and grandparents in Arlington National Cemetery in Virginia.

Biography

Born: Jan. 5, 1892, Germantown, Pa. **Education:** Bellevue Hosp., N.Y.C. **Work history:** Red Cross nurse (Italy, Romania, Haiti); Private Duty Nurse; tuberculosis sanitarium, Otisville, N.Y. **Organizations:** unknown. **Awards:** unknown. **Died:** Gulfport, Va.

References and Credits

†Villard HS, Nagel J: Hemingway in Love and War: The Lost Diary of Agnes von Kurowsky, Her Letters, and Correspondence of Ernest Hemingway. Boston, Northeastern University Press, 1989, p 132.

Kert B: The Hemingway Women. New York, WW Norton, 1983.

Brewer GW: Agnes Stanfield. In Bullough V, Sentz L (eds): American Nursing: A Biographical Dictionary, vol. 3. New York, Springer, 2000, pp 266–267.

January 9

Eleanor Lee

1896–1967

"During the last five years there has been an improvement in the candidates as a whole. Well-prepared nurses are joining our ranks, but unfortunately many candidates are handicapped by poor teaching and lack of experience in nursing practice. Surely the student is not to blame for this! Are not all nurses confronted by new situations almost daily and are not the schools of nursing responsible for preparing them to meet such situations? Isn't it good teaching that is going to be their salvation?" (1937)

Eleanor Lee was involved with the nursing programs at Columbia University and Presbyterian Hospital for four decades and was responsible for the affiliation agreement between the two institutions. She held positions at both locations and was Columbia University's first emeritus professor of nursing. She was a graduate of the Vassar Training Camp and, like several other graduates of that program, became an outstanding nursing leader. In addition to being actively involved in teaching, she coauthored major texts for nurses and wrote articles about nursing education. She was a successful nurse recruiter for the profession, especially through her work with the National Nursing Council. Then, during World War II, she left the university for a year to direct nurse recruitment for the military and the Red Cross. The curator of Columbia University's notable

Nightingale Collection, she was a widely regarded nurse historian as well.

Biography

Born: Jan. 5, 1896, Jamaica Plain (Boston), Mass. **Education:** Radcliffe College (AB); Vassar College Training Camp; Presbyterian Hosp. School of Nursing, N.Y. **Work history:** Head Nurse, Presbyterian Hosp.; Nursing Instructor, Peter Bent Brigham Hosp., Boston; Nursing Instructor, Presbyterian Hosp.; Education Director, Teachers College, Columbia Univ.; Nursing Faculty, Columbia Univ.; Director of Nursing, Presbyterian Hosp.; Assoc. Dean of Nursing, Columbia Univ. **Organizations:** various committees at Columbia Univ. and Presbyterian Hosp.; N.Y. Registered Nurses Assoc.; National League for Nursing; member, N.Y. Bd. of Nurse Examiners. **Awards:** Phi Beta Kappa; Columbia Univ. Bicentennial Medal; scholarship fund for nursing students established in her name at Columbia Univ. **Buried:** Mt. Auburn Cemetery, Boston.

References and Credits

†Lee E: Examinations in the nursing arts. AJN 37:1253–1256, 1937.

Downer JL: Eleanor Lee. In Bullough V, Church OM, Stein, AP: American Nursing: A Biographical Dictionary, vol. 1. New York, Garland, 1988, pp 209–211.

January 10

Lois Capps

1938–

"The shortfalls in [nursing] care currently being experienced by patients as a result of the growing shortage of nurses represent only a glimpse of horrors yet to come in the next decade if nothing is done now to prevent them. That is why we are working today—to provide immediate first aid to this caring, noble, yet ailing profession—to ensure that every American has access to the best possible health care available. A strong, well prepared nursing work force is essential to reach this goal." (2002)

Lois Capps is a Democratic member of Congress from Santa Barbara, California, who addressed the current nursing shortage by initiating the bipartisan and bicameral efforts in Congress to pass the Nurse Reinvestment Act, which was signed into law by President George W. Bush on August 1, 2002. In her twenty years as a nurse and health advocate for the Santa Barbara School District, Capps developed Santa Barbara County's Teenage Pregnancy and Parenting Project, and the Parent and Child Enrichment Center, which provided teens with support and the means to remain in school while preparing them to be parents and wage earners. Capps uses her broad health care background in her capacity as cochair of the Congressional Heart and Stroke Coalition and as cochair of the House Democratic Task Force on Health, where she continues her efforts to modernize Medicare. Accordingly, she is the founder and cochair of the bipartisan Congressional School Health and Safety Caucus, which educates House members about such important issues as school safety, nutrition, immunizations, and the role of the school nurse. She is also a member of the bipartisan Campaign Finance Reform Task Force; the Budget Task Force; the Congressional Task Force on Tobacco and Health; the Prescription Drug Task Force; the Diabetes Caucus; and the Congressional Caucus on the Arts. She serves on many powerful committees, including the subcommittees on Health; Commerce, Trade and Consumer Protection; and Environment and Hazardous Materials. Her focus remains on patients' rights, mental health, the environment, high technology, and telecommunications issues. She joined Congress in 1998 after winning a special election to succeed her late husband, U.S. Rep. Walter Capps.

Biography

Born: Jan. 10, 1938, Ladysmith, Wisc. **Education:** Pacific Lutheran Univ., Tacoma, Wash. (BSN); Yale Univ. (MA in religion); Univ. of California, Santa Barbara (MA in education). **Work history:** Nursing Instructor, Portland, Ore.; Head Nurse, Yale–New Haven Hosp.; School Nurse, Health Advocate, Santa Barbara School District (twenty yrs.); part-time instructor, early childhood education, Santa Barbara City College. **Organizations:** member, bds. of directors, American Red Cross, American Heart Assoc., Family Service Agency, Santa Barbara Women's Political Committee. **Awards:** unknown.

References and Credits

†Capps L, Fraley ME: Nursing shortage requires urgent first aid: Age, more career options, deteriorating working conditions contribute to crisis in care. Ventura County Star, May 28, 2002.

On-line biography of Capps posted at Congress on line, available at http://www.congress.org.

Catherine M. Kain

1909–1963

"The role played by American nursing advisors serving in the United States foreign aid program is as important to the security of the United States as it is to the social and economic growth of the countries in which they work. ...Participating in freeing these people from their basic problems so that they can both comprehend and engage in their own development is the basic aim of AID's [Agency for International Development] assistance to these countries. By helping in this way, the people gain full and sustaining membership in a world dedicated to peace and progress." (1963)

CATHERINE KAIN WAS the chief nursing adviser to the U.S. Agency for International Development. From 1947 to 1963 she was responsible for recruiting, educating, and dispatching most of the nurses who worked in nineteen countries throughout the world. She was known for her interpersonal skills, which fostered self-reliance in those she guided and taught. She believed that her mission was to free all people from their basic problems of illness and poverty. She knew that optimum health plays a major role in a country's strength and peaceful coexistence. Her work permeated other agencies that assisted underdeveloped nations. Her efforts were recognized by such international organizations as the World Health Organization,

United Nations Children's Fund, National Institutes of Health, Peace Corps, Defense Department, and U.S. Public Health Service. She is remembered for setting high standards for herself and her students.

Biography

Born: Jan. 11, 1909, Milwaukee, Wisc. **Education:** St. Mary's Hosp. School of Nursing, Milwaukee, 1928; Marquette Univ. (BS, 1931); Catholic Univ. of America (MS, 1953). **Work history:** Educational Director, St. Mary's School of Nursing, 1933–40; Instructor, Seattle College of Nursing, 1940–42; Lt. Cmdr., U.S. Navy Nurse Corps; Director, Navy Cadet Nurses, U.S. Naval Hosp., Portsmouth, Va.; Chief Nurse, U.S. Naval Operating Base Dispensary, Rio de Janeiro, Brazil; Supervisor of hospitalized navy men in American wing of the Brazilian Air Force Hosp.; Consultant Nurse, Health Sanitation Division, Institute of Inter-American Affairs; served in Point IV Program introduced by President Harry Truman after World War II; Chief Nursing Adviser, U.S. Agency for International Development, 1958–63. **Organizations:** Assistant Registrar, Milwaukee District Nurses Assoc.; bd. of directors, Wisc. League for Nurses, 1932–33; International Affairs Committee, American Nurses Assoc. (ANA); Secretary, National Committee, ANA; member, American Public Health Assoc.; Assoc. of Military Surgeons. **Awards:** commendation in Brazil, 1946; memorial fund, Catholic Univ.; Catherine Kain Memorial Library, St. Mary's School of Nursing Alumnae Assoc. **Died:** Milwaukee.

References and Credits

†Kain C: Nursing and the Agency for International Development. Nurs Outlook 11:902, 904, 1963.

Jones MVH: Catherine Kain. In Bullough V, Sentz L, Stein AP (eds): American Nursing: A Biographical Dictionary, vol 2. New York, Garland, 1992, pp 173–176.

JANUARY 12

Adah Belle Samuels Thoms (Smith)

CA. 1870–1943

"It is my unbiased conviction that nursing is the broadest professional field open to women today. Therefore I urge you to prepare yourselves to meet the present day needs and future demands. While we have faced these problems [state registration, postgraduate educational opportunities], they have been equally balanced with brighter outlooks for our future. ... The field for nurses today is very wide; it is no longer confined to the sickroom. It covers ... various avenues now open to the graduate nurse. And by the united effort of the members of this association, more of us shall engage in these activities. We as nurses should stand very close together, closer than any other women in public life; we should have deeper sympathies, more interests in common. ... In loyalty there is unity, in unity there must be strength. ... If we wish to succeed in this great work that we have undertaken, we must be earnest, we must be courageous, we must be imbued with absolute determination. Remember that every door of opportunity is open to women, and the professional nurse may find therein a place for herself. Let unity and service be our watchword, and may this association always stand for the highest standard of nursing, and for the purest ideals of true womanhood." (1916)

ADAH BELLE SAMUELS THOMS was a graduate of the outstanding Lincoln School for Nurses in New York City. Later, after she was appointed acting director of the school, she added a course in public health nursing. She then took the course with the students, because she realized it was an important new discipline for nursing. She actively crusaded for equal opportunities for black nurses throughout her career and worked with Martha Franklin to organize the National Association of Colored Graduate Nurses (NACGN). When Thoms had an opportunity to present a basket of roses to President and Mrs. Warren Harding, she let them know that two thousand nurses of color were ready to serve their nation during World War I. Thoms skillfully and successfully overcame discrimination against black nurses in the American Red Cross and in the U.S. Army Nurse Corps. She continued to study throughout her career and encouraged other nurses to do the same. She was one of the first black nurses to participate in the International Council of Nurses and in 1929 wrote the classic *Pathfinders: A History of the Progress of the Colored Graduate.*

BIOGRAPHY

Born: Jan. 12, 1870, Richmond, Va. **Education:** Richmond Normal School; Cooper Union, N.Y.; Woman's Infirmary and School of Therapeutic Massage, N.Y.; Lincoln Hosp., N.Y.C.; courses at New York School of Social Work, Hunter College, New School for Social Research. **Work history:** Nurse, N.Y.C.; St. Agnes Hosp., Raleigh, N.C.; Clinical Nurse, Assistant Superintendent of Nurses, Lincoln Hosp.; appointed to Woman's Advisory Council on Venereal Diseases, U.S. Public Health Service. **Organizations:** Lincoln Nurses Alumnae Assoc.; NACGN; National Urban League; NAACP; American Red Cross; American Nurses Assoc. (ANA); National Organization for Public Health Nursing; YWCA; N.Y. Urban League; National Health Circle for Colored People; Henry Street Nursing Committee. **Awards:** Mary Mahoney Medal, NACGN; ANA Hall of Fame. **Buried:** Woodlawn Cemetery, New York.

REFERENCES AND CREDITS

†Davis A: Early Black American Leaders in Nursing: Architects for Integration and Equality. National League for Nursing Series. Sudbury, Mass., Jones and Bartlett, 1999, pp 114–115.

Davis AT: Adah Belle Thoms. In Bullough V, Church OM, Stein, AP: American Nursing: A Biographical Dictionary, vol. 1. New York, Garland, 1988, pp 313–316.

ANA Hall of Fame 10/98 American Nurses Association, Washington, D.C. http://www.nursingworld.org/hof.

Kathy Lynn Batterman

1955–1999

"I don't think that there's that many people in the world that can say that they absolutely love their jobs to the point where they'd be willing to give their life for it, and I am. ...Every time I come back from a flight and I know I'm going back out again, it's a chance to save another life. ...You know the stress is there but the reward is the greatest feeling in the world." (1992)

"I try to remember the Golden Rule and treat others as I would like to be treated or have my family members treated. ...I feel I make a difference in my patient's lives from the moment I meet them. ...I try to be all that I can be for my patients. I have the best job in the world." (1997)

Kathy Batterman, one of America's premiere flight nurses, was one of the first certified flight nurses in the country. She was also a certified emergency nurse, a critical care nurse, an advanced trauma specialist, and Nevada's first prehospital nurse practitioner. A highly qualified and courageous professional, she was a strong leader of nursing. She was admired and loved by those who knew her, worked with her, and learned from her. A loving wife and mother, she was also a dedicated professional who loved flying and found it a spiritual experience. She had enjoyed helping people since she was four, and as a highly skilled professional she welcomed the challenge of rescue work because she saw it as a God-given opportunity to make a difference in this world. Friendly and supportive, she visited patients during their recovery, and coworkers could count on homebaked chocolate chip cookies in the pockets of her flight suit. She is credited with saving thousands of lives and flew more than three thousand flights during her nineteen-year career. Hundreds of first responders were her students, and she taught the importance of focusing on the patient. Her passion for excellence permeated her practice and her teaching and made her an excellent role model. Her contagious, energetic spirit, her smile, and her enthusiasm inspired many others to do their best. She died in a medical helicopter crash in bad weather after delivering a patient to a hospital in Las Vegas, Nevada.

Biography

Born: Jan. 13, 1955, Joliet, Ill. **Education:** St. Joseph School of Nursing, Ill.; Joliet Junior College; Northern Illinois Univ. **Work history:** Emergency Nurse, Joliet; Desert Springs Hosp., Las Vegas; Flight for Life, Valley Hosp., Las Vegas; Educator. **Organizations:** Emergency Nurses Assoc., National Flight Nurses Assoc., American Assoc. of Critical Care Nurses, Medical Explorers, Boy Scouts. **Awards:** March of Dimes Distinguished Nurse of the Year; Star of Excellence Award, Valley Hosp.; Clark County, Nev., has named a middle school in her honor. **Died:** near Indian Springs, Nev.

References and Credits

†Shields of honor, American Detective, television documentary, prod. P. Stanovitch, Warner Bros. Entertainment, Inc., May 11, 1992.

†Biographical form for March of Dimes Award that Batterman completed in 1997.

Schoenmann J: Nurse gave life to many. (Las Vegas) Review Journal, April 9, 1999.

Zekan K: Loved ones mourn loss of heroic nurse. Las Vegas Sun, April 9, 1999.

Batterman Kurt: personal communications, 2002, 2003.

Testimonials and eulogies at Batterman's memorial service.

JANUARY 14

Isabel Maitland Stewart

1878–1963

"When the mothers of the race made their first fumbling attempts to teach their daughters what they knew about the care of the young and the sick, and to pass on that part of their cultural heritage to the next generation, they were helping to lay the foundations of our modern system of nursing education. ...Probably we have been too much inclined in recent years to think that progress would come chiefly through intellectual effort and through technical improvements, forgetting that the dynamic drives in human beings are emotional and spiritual and that morale is as important as brains and techniques. ...Among those who have led nursing movements of the past were a number of great spiritual leaders who lifted nursing to a high spiritual plane and made it a vital part of the movement for human welfare and the advancement of civilization. We need such leaders at the present time to revive the spirit of nursing, to unite the whole body of nurses in a common purpose, and to give us a new vision of our part in the world of the future." (1943)

ISABEL STEWART WAS drawn to nursing from teaching because she believed that it would be a more challenging career. Her basic studies convinced her that nursing needed to be more standardized in both training programs and practice. She believed that the only way to achieve this goal was to have nursing become an independent discipline, in charge of its own education. Attracted to Teachers College by Adelaide Nutting, Stewart stayed to earn both a bachelor's and a master's degree. She later became a distinguished faculty member in nursing education for forty-five years. She was involved with nurse recruitment for both world wars, always stressing the importance of having qualified nurses serve. She was involved with the curriculum at the Vassar Training Camp, helped to form the National Nursing Council for National Defense, and assisted with the establishment of the U.S. Cadet Nurse Corps. A prolific writer, she was also known as "Miss Curriculum." Her involvement with curriculum standards effectively pulled together resources from professional organizations and the nursing community to produce the *Curriculum Guide for Schools of Nursing* in 1937. With Lavinia Dock she wrote *A Short History of Nursing.* Stewart also published nursing's first research journal.

Biography

Born: Jan. 14, 1878, Fletcher, Ontario, Can. **Education:** Manitoba Normal School (teaching certificate); Winnipeg General Hosp. Training School; Teachers College, Columbia Univ. (BS, MA, doctoral coursework). **Work history:** Private Duty, Clinical, and District Nurse in Canada; Faculty, Teachers College, Columbia Univ. (forty yrs.); Editor, *American Journal of Nursing.* **Organizations:** American Council on Education; Nurses Associated Alumnae of the United States; National League for Nursing Education; International Council of Nurses; Florence Nightingale International Foundation; Founder, Assoc. of Collegiate Schools of Nursing. **Awards:** honorary degrees, Western Reserve Univ., Columbia Univ., Univ. of Manitoba; Isabel Maitland Stewart Professional Chair in Nursing Research, Teachers College, Columbia Univ.; honorary member, History of Nursing Society, McGill Univ.; Adelaide Nutting Award, National League for Nursing; medal from Finland; Florence Nightingale Medal, International Committee, Red Cross; American Nurses Assoc. Hall of Fame.
Died: Chatham, N.J.

References and Credits

†Stewart IM: The Education of Nurses: Historical Foundations and Modern Trends. New York, Macmillan, 1943, pp 33, 381.

Donahue PM: Isabel Stewart. In Bullough V, Church OM, Stein AP (eds): American Nursing: A Biographical Dictionary, vol. 1. New York, Garland, 1988, pp 198–202.

ANA Hall of Fame 10/98 American Nurses Association, Washington, D.C. http://www.nursingworld.org/hof.

JANUARY 15

Hildegard of Bingen

1098–1179

"The more one learns about that which one knows nothing of, the more one gains in wisdom. One has, therefore, through science eyes with which it behooves us to pay attention." (Date unknown)

"Humanity finds itself in the midst of the world. In the midst of all other creatures humanity is the most significant and yet the most dependent upon the others." (Date unknown)

"All nature is at the disposal of humankind. We are to work with it. ... Without it we can not survive." (Date unknown)

HILDEGARD OF BINGEN was a twelfth-century abbess whose broad range of accomplishments make her one of the most outstanding women of the Middle Ages. She was known as a painter, playwright, prophet, poet, musician, mystic, social critic, scholar, scientist, theologian, abbess, healer, and writer. Her explanation of blood circulation preceded Harvey's by five centuries. In 1900 the French Academy reviewed her work in a University of Paris thesis and it received the first rank. She wrote three major works, *The Book of Life's Merits, The Book of Divine Works,* and *Know the Ways.* She wrote music for more than seventy chants, and she set her play, *Ritual of the Virtues,* to music. In her last years she continued to minister to patients, traveling with medical students and nuns by horse and boat along the rivers Rhine, Main, and Mosel. Her writing and music are available and enjoyed today.

Biography

Born: Jan. 15, 1098, Bückelhein, Germany. **Education:** studied at the Disibodenberg cloister under her aunt, Abbess Yutta (or Jutta) von Sponeim; made her vows at sixteen. **Work history:** compiled a reference book, *Book of Healing Herbs*; composed two-stage medical text, *Book of Medical Treatment and Causes and Cures*; wrote psychotherapy handbook, *Book of Life's Merits,* in 1163; spent eleven years recording visions for *That You May Know* (1152); supervised construction of facility for counseling patients, Rupertsberg, 1147; composed hymnal, *The Harmonic Symphony of Heavenly Revolutions;* estab. second priory at Eibingen, 1165. **Organizations:** unknown. **Awards:** Unknown. **Died:** Rupertsberg monastery near Bingen.

References and Credits

†Uhlein G: Meditations with Hildegard. Santa Fe, N. Mex., Bear, 1983, pp 66, 87, 71.

Achterberg J: Woman as Healer. Boston, Shambhala, 1990, pp 54–58.

Fox M: Hildegard of Bingen's Book of Divine Works with Letters and Songs. Santa Fe, N. Mex., Bear, 1987, p xi.

Snodgrass ME: Historical Encyclopedia of Nursing. Santa Barbara, Calif., ABC-CLIO, 1999, p 127.

Goodnow M: Outlines of Nursing History, 4th ed. Philadelphia, WB Saunders, 1931, p 35.

JANUARY 16

Carol A. Lindeman

1935–

"Knowledge... has value if it serves as a guide to effective action in day-to-day reality. Contemporary nursing practice requires the use of all sources of knowledge in the moment-to-moment reality of a patient care situation. ... The current world of nursing practice involves caring for individuals, families and communities where the health care problems are complex. There are few, if any, 'standard' patients. The nurse deals with uncertainty, uniqueness, instability, and value conflicts. Violence, substance abuse, stress, poverty and aging are examples of the complex social and health care issues that confront nurses today. ...In the process of providing care, the nurse must conceptualize and reconceptualize the patient's circumstances in light of available knowledge. If necessary, the nurse will have to create and test new theory." (1999)

CAROL LINDEMAN WAS attracted to nursing by the Cherry Ames series, because she enjoyed reading about the variety of choices and experiences open to nurses. She finds that nursing provides the opportunity to grow and develop personally and professionally through interactions with bright, caring peers. A highly honored nurse, Lindeman has had a versatile career that includes clinical nursing, teaching, research, writing, and consultation. She is known for her research on preoperative preparation. She calls nurses "knowledge workers." She believes that nursing practice depends on decision making by the nurse, who applies comprehensive knowledge to the unique needs of each patient and learns from each encounter. She defines nursing practice as necessarily complex and evolving. She writes that nurses need to remain "intellectually alive," guided by theory and research and open to opportunities for continued learning.

Biography

Born: Jan. 16, 1935, Racine, Wisc. **Education:** Evangelical Deaconess Hosp. School of Nursing, Milwaukee (RN); Univ. of Minnesota (BS, MEd); Univ. of Wisconsin, Madison (PhD). **Work history:** Staff Nurse, Wisc.; Private Duty Nurse, Minn. Instructor, Minn.; Faculty, Univ. of Wisconsin, Univ. of Minnesota; nursing research, Univ. of Wisconsin, Univ. of Minnesota; Administrator, Western Interstate Commission for Higher Education; Faculty, Univ. of Colorado, Oregon Health Sciences Univ.; Dean, School of Nursing, Oregon Health Sciences Univ.; Scholar in Residence, Duquesne Univ.; Editor, *Nursing and Health Care: Perspectives on Community;* Author; Consultant. **Organizations:** American Nurses Assoc. (ANA), American Assoc. of Colleges of Nursing, Sigma Theta Tau, Western Institute of Nursing, Ore. Nurses Assoc., National League for Nursing (NLN), National Advisory Council on Nurse Training (U.S. Dept. of Health and Human Services). **Awards:** honorary degrees from Univ. of Akron, Univ. of Colorado, Montana State Univ., Thomas Jefferson Univ., Duquesne Univ., Valparaiso Univ.; Distinguished Service Awards from Ore. Health Sciences Univ., Univ. of Minnesota, Ore. League of Women Voters, Evangelical Deaconess Hosp.; Brookdale Award, ANA; Linda Richards Award, NLN; Outstanding Achievement Award, Univ. of Minn.; Citation for Distinguished Achievement, Oregon Health Services Univ.; Special Achievement Award, Institute for Managerial and Professional Women. Fellow, American Academy of Nursing.

References and Credits

†Lindeman C, McAthie M: Fundamentals of Contemporary Nursing Practice. Philadelphia, WB Saunders, 1999, p 35.

Lindeman C: personal communication, 2002.

Carol Ann Lindeman. In Who's Who in American Nursing, 1996–97, 6th ed. New Providence, N.J., Reed Reference, p 375.

Angela Barron McBride

1941–

"If we wait to feel appreciated, nothing will change. The way to effect change... is to substitute a sense of ourselves as image makers in place of a preoccupation with our image... [and to] recognize that modern nursing is too complicated to be properly understood in terms of only one image. Our strength is in numbers and... variety. For too long we have been squelched by stereotype. We now have to address the fact that we are many types. We have to revel in the richness of our diversity. This richness is best exemplified in the many roles that nurses play, sometimes all at one time, but more often over the course of a career. ...Having a positive, vital image of the profession and being ready to be an image maker are predicated on having made a positive decision to have a career. ...If you do not see other nurses as projecting a positive image, then nursing can never succeed in projecting a positive image. (1983)

"The best way to improve the image of nursing is for all nurses to become image makers." (1988)

ANGELA BARRON MCBRIDE's feminist attitudes and life experiences as a new mother led her to write the highly acclaimed *Growth and Development of Mothers* in 1973. This was the first of many writings that explore women's issues and values. She sees common ground between nursing and feminism. She believes that it is important that both define options to encourage self-determination. A nurse researcher, teacher, and author, McBride recognizes nursing's important role in helping the public to become more self-reliant in matters related to health care. She was attracted to nursing by the range of career opportunities that it offers and believes that no part of her personality or abilities has not been fully realized in nursing. An outstanding nursing scholar and leader, she has published widely, including numerous books and articles for professionals and the public. She calls on nurses to take the initiative and inform the public about nursing's vital role in the multitude of positive health care outcomes that occur daily.

Biography

Born: Jan. 16, 1941, Baltimore. **Education:** Georgetown Univ. (BSN); Yale Univ. (MSN), Purdue Univ. (PhD). **Work history:** Distinguished Professor, University Dean, Indiana Univ. School of Nursing; Exec.Vice President, Clarian Health Partners; member, editorial bd., numerous professional journals; member, numerous nursing advisory councils. **Organizations:** Sigma Theta Tau International, American Nurses Assoc. **Awards:** Alumni awards from Yale, Purdue Univ.; Fellow, American Academy of Nursing; several awards for psychiatric nursing and women's health; numerous honorary degrees, incl. Georgetown, Purdue Univ.; election to Institute of Medicine, National Academy of Sciences; numerous Indiana awards.

References and Credits

†McBride AB: From being concerned about our image to becoming image makers. Keynote address to Sigma Theta Tau, 1983.

†Schorr T, Zimmerman A: Making Choices, Taking Chances: Nurse Leaders Tell Their Stories. St. Louis, CV Mosby, 1988, p 265.

McBride AB: personal communication, 2002.

January 18

Ruth Watson Lubic

1927–

"Let me set down some guiding principles that I believe will ensure a successful professional life:

1. *Begin with the needs of the people you serve.*
2. *Take care of all the people of a nation.*
3. *Trust your caring instincts.*
4. *Choose colleagues for their caring philosophy rather than professional orientation.*
5. *Beware the limits of the medical model.*
6. *Avoid anger. It consumes energy and clouds vision.*
7. *Avoid bitterness against political opponents.*
8. *Base your design on the best science possible; then test your performance.*
9. *Overcome the fear associated with leadership.*
10. *Remember—the people you serve are your strength.*
11. *Nursing prepares you for excellence. Be proud you are a nurse." (1988)*

RUTH WATSON LUBIC studied midwifery after completing her basic nursing program and became a proponent of family centered care. After completing advanced study, she became the director of the Maternity Center Association (MCA) in New York City.

She recognizes the great contributions possible for nurses involved in maternity care, the value of a nursing model, and the importance of considering cultural and belief systems. The only nurse in a 1973 delegation to China, Lubic returned committed to universal health care. Her 1979 dissertation, "Barriers and Conflict in Maternity Care Innovation," addresses political, bureaucratic, and vested interest obstacles to change in the health care delivery system in the United States. When she was sixty-seven, she initiated the District of Columbia Developing Families Center, an innovative collaboration with the D.C. Birth Center, the Healthy Babies Project, and the Nation's Capital Child and Family Development. Funded by grant money and donations, the Developing Families Center demonstrates a cost-effective way to reduce infant mortality and prevent complications during pregnancy. Lubic says the center's staff offers options to families, makes health care easier to obtain, and establishes a new community pattern for health and wellness. Certified nurse-midwives and nurse practitioners, with medical consultation and backup, help fulfill Lubic's dream of comprehensive family care from pregnancy through childhood. "When families are strengthened ... communities are strengthened," she says. Families Count: The National Honors Program selected the center as a 2003 honoree, with a $500,000 award from the Annie E. Casey Foundation.

Biography

Born: Jan. 18, 1927, Bucks County, Pa. **Education:** School of Nursing, Univ. of Pennsylvania Hosp. (diploma); Hunter College (BS); Columbia Univ. (MA, EdD); Maternity Center Assoc., Downstate Medical Center, Brooklyn (Certificate in Nurse Midwifery.) **Work history:** Staff Nurse, Head Nurse, Memorial Hosp. for Cancer and Allied Diseases, N.Y.C.; Clinical Associate, Graduate School of Nursing, New York Medical College; Parent Educator, Director, MCA; President, U.S. Committee for the World Health Organization; member, Committee on Graduates of Foreign Nursing Schools; bd. member, Frontier Nursing Service, Pan American Health and Education Foundation; Visiting Fellow, King Edward Memorial Hosp. for Women, Perth, Australia; Landsdowne Lecturer, Univ. of Victoria, B.C., Canada; Visiting Professor, Case Western Reserve. **Organizations:** American Nurses Assoc.; American Public Health Assoc.; American College of Nurse-Midwives; National Assoc. of Childbearing Centers; Sigma Theta Tau. **Awards:** R. Louise McManus Award, Teachers College, Columbia Univ.; election to Institute of Medicine, National Academy of Sciences; honorary degrees,

Biography continued on page 765

JANUARY 19

Carolyn Ladd Widmer

1902–1991

The greatest single help in reorienting the inactive nurse to her work is the refresher course. In this she not only has the opportunity to learn new procedures and regain her skill in old ones but she is a member of a group, all of whom feel as lost as she. Furthermore, she is more carefully supervised... and nothing can give more encouragement to the new "refreshee" than to see an efficient, competent nurse on duty and to learn that she was herself the graduate of a recent refresher course." (1943)

CAROLYN WIDMER ATTENDED the Yale nursing program when Annie Goodrich was dean and shortly after graduation helped organize a public health nursing program in Bogota, Colombia. Later, when she was dean of the School of Nursing at the American University in Beirut, Widmer upgraded the curriculum and widened the appeal of nursing to more Muslim women. Many of these women went on to become nursing leaders. Returning to the States at the start of World War II, Widmer started much-needed refresher courses to lure nurses back to the profession. Another career highlight was the nursing school that she established at the University of Connecticut. Under her leadership the school developed several different programs for nurses and arranged for clinical rotations at facilities throughout the state.

During her tenure the school ranked among the top quartile of schools in the country.

Biography

Born: Jan. 19, 1902, Randolph, Vt. **Education:** Wellesley College; Yale Univ. School of Nursing; Trinity College (MA). **Work history:** Biological research, Boston; Lab Instructor, Univ. of Vermont; Yale–New Haven Hosp.; Bogota, Colombia; School of Nursing, American Univ., Beirut (then Syria); Faculty, Yale–New Haven Hosp.; established Univ. of Connecticut School of Nursing. **Organizations:** Phi Beta Kappa; Sigma Theta Tau; Conn. Nurses Assoc. (CNA); Mansfield Historical Society; Conn. Heart Assoc.; Windham Hosp. Aux., Conn.; Storrs (Conn.) Golden Age Club. **Awards:** Honorary Recognition, CNA; Distinguished Alumna Award, Yale Univ. School of Nursing; scholarships in her name established by both Univ. of Connecticut Alumnae Assoc. and American Assoc. of Univ. Women; reading room in her name, Univ. of Connecticut School of Nursing. **Died:** Windham, Conn.

References and Credits

†Widmer C: The housewife re-enters nursing. AJN 43:10–14, 1943.

Cleveland S: Carolyn Ladd Widmer. In Bullough V, Sentz L, Stein AP (eds): American Nursing: A Biographical Dictionary, vol. 2. New York, Garland, 1992, pp 350.

Herrman E: personal communication, December 2002.

January 20

Sara Maiter Errickson

1905–2000

"Unless we unify, unless the nurses come together, unless we have unification of nurses in this country, we are not going anywhere." (1992)

SARA M. ERRICKSON has been called the "matriarch of New Jersey nurses." Several incidents in her childhood predisposed her to a career in nursing. She helped a friend comfort her mother, who was bedfast with advanced tuberculosis. Errickson spent time in the hospital after suffering a fractured leg, and she carried bandages around with her, seemingly prepared for anything. She joined the American Nurses Association (ANA) in 1926 and felt strongly about supporting one nursing organization that could speak on behalf of all nurses. Her career in public health included direct nursing service, organization, supervision, and teaching. She was instrumental in promoting and implementing high standards of nursing practice and good legislation for the health and welfare of the people of New Jersey. She also worked to protect the economic and general welfare of New Jersey's nurses. Her accomplishments include bringing civil service positions in line with nursing standards, functions, and qualifications; starting refresher courses at Rutgers University; lobbying for a state department of higher education; and participating in a study of nursing needs within New Jersey.

After employing agencies did not accept the plan of the New Jersey State Nurses Association to negotiate for nurses, she was instrumental in implementing the Economic and General Welfare Program of the ANA.

Biography

Born: Jan. 12, 1905, Long Branch, N.J. **Education:** Monmouth Memorial Hosp. School of Nursing, Long Beach, N.J., 1925; Univ. of Pennsylvania, 1942 (public health nursing certificate); Seton Hall Univ., 1946 (BSN). **Work history:** Long Branch Public Health Nursing Organization. **Organizations:** member, ANA, N.J. State Nurses Assoc., American Public Health Assoc., N.J. League for Nursing Education, N.J. Sanitary Assoc., American Assoc. for Science, and Sigma Theta Tau. **Awards:** Florence Nightingale Award, 1971; Dean Haley Award, Seton Hall, 1975. Seton Hall annually awards the Sara Errickson Medal for Outstanding Achievement to a graduate nursing student. **Died:** Bethesda, Md.

References and Credits

†Fickeissen JL: Sara Errickson. In Bullough V, Sentz L, Stein AP (eds): American Nursing: A Biographical Dictionary, vol. 2. New York, Garland, 1992, pp 101–102.

JANUARY 21

Alma Ham Scott

1885–1972

"The need for routine inspection of schools of nursing is ... the need for repeated analysis, evaluation, reorganization, and reconstruction. Outside inspection furnishes a stimulus for inspection from within and it is this stimulus that schools of nursing need. ... The purpose of routine inspection is ... to help schools meet their needs and ... to provide for their growth. ... The second inspection of a school indicates that the first inspection was most helpful. ... What is the ultimate aim of inspection of schools of nursing? It is inspection to prepare for the next inspection." (1925)

ALMA HAM SCOTT worked throughout her career to promote nursing. She served as a nurse in France during World War I, and upon her return to the States she worked to strengthen and unite nursing organizations and to build membership. She worked at all levels, from local to international. She helped standardize record keeping at nursing schools and created a nurse recruitment brochure for high school girls. When President Franklin Roosevelt introduced the New Deal in 1933 to counter unemployment during the depression, the many new jobs opened the possibility for unqualified persons to work in health care, prompting Scott to work with organized nursing to preserve the status and responsibilities of professional nursing. As World War II began to cut into the supply of available nurses, she called on nursing to help ensure adequate services in communities across the country. Her promotion of routine inspections of nursing schools resulted in better living and working conditions for students, curriculum improvements, and more qualified faculty.

Biography

Born: Jan. 21, 1885, Frankfort, Ind. **Education:** Presbyterian Hosp. School of Nursing, Chicago; coursework at Teachers College, Columbia Univ. **Work history:** Private Duty; Military Nurse, World War II; Night Supervisor, OR Nurse, Robert W. Long Hosp., Indiana Univ. School for Nurses; Educational Director, Indiana State Bd. of Examiners and Registration for Nurses; Exec. Secretary, Ind. State Nurses Assoc. (ISNA), administrative positions with Ind. League for Nursing Education (ILNE), American Nurses Assoc. (ANA). **Organizations:** ISNA, ILNE, ANA, International Council of Nursing. **Awards:** unknown. **Died:** Indiana.

References and Credits

†Scott A: Routine inspection of schools of nursing. AJN 25: 556, 557, 566, 1925.

Stein AP: Alma Ham Scott. In Bullough V, Church OM, Stein AP (eds): American Nursing: A Biographical Dictionary, vol. 1. New York, Garland, 1988, pp 285–286.

Flanagan L (ed): One Strong Voice: The Story of the American Nurses Association. Kansas City, Mo., Lowell Press, 1976.

Family Search, available on-line at http://www.familysearch.org.

January 22

Susan Edith Tracy

1864–1928

"Whoever succeeds in making an invalid happy and in maintaining the same state of happiness has gone a long way towards making him well. The secretory system has subtle connecting lines with his mental attitude, a temptingly arranged tray, a fine aroma, the sight of delicious fruit produce instant stimulation of digestive fluids: deeper breathing results from a sight of real grandeur, it is easy to take deep inspirations as we look out over a wide stretch of sea or up to towering mountains. May we not justly feel that wounds heal quicker where a tranquil mind exists, that the complex organism recognizes the atmosphere which dominates and settles down into comfort as naturally as a cat curls up before a fire on the hearth?" (1907)

Susan Tracy was an early believer in the connection between mind and body. She was the first person in the United States to incorporate systematic training in occupational therapy for nurses. Accordingly, she taught occupations as therapy to the sick. As a small child, she made her own toys from paper and scraps, a habit that may have prompted her to advise her clients to occupy themselves with a craft or a trade. She maintained that the goal of the project was to heal the patient, not to produce a product. Tracy was a prolific writer. Her *Studies in Invalid Occupations: A Manual for*

Nurse and Attendants (1910) is a classic. She expanded her teaching with a workshop that she gave to general and psychiatric hospitals, and to other organizations outside hospitals. Her aspiration was to create occupational therapy departments in health care settings, by setting up a model and training the personnel. Tracy's good friend and colleague Eleanor C. Slagel remarked that Tracy was dedicated to helping others and had an enthusiastic and magnetic personality.

Biography

Born: Jan. 22, 1864, Lynn, Mass. **Education:** Homeopathic Hosp. School of Nursing, Boston, 1895; Hosp. economics, Teachers College, Columbia Univ.; observer, Manual Arts Department College's kindergarten. **Work history:** Private Duty Nurse; Nursing Staff, Director, Adams Nervine Asylum, Jamaica Plain, Mass.; introduced occupational therapy in nursing curriculum, 1906; taught invalids, student nurses, graduate nurses; taught at School of Nursing, Teachers College, Columbia Univ., also Newton Hosp. and Children's Hosp., Boston, and Michael Reese Hosp. and Presbyterian Hosp., Chicago; set up model occupational therapy depts. at several hosps., trained personnel. **Organizations:** unknown. **Awards:** January 1917 issue of the *Maryland Psychiatric Quarterly* named in her honor. **Died:** Lynn, Mass.

References and Credits

†Tracy SE: Some profitable occupations for invalids. AJN 7:172–173, 1907.

Tao D: Susan E. Tracy. In Bullough V, Sentz, L, Stein AP (eds): American Nursing: A Biographical Dictionary, vol. 2. New York, Garland, 1992, pp 326–328.

JANUARY 23

Lucile Petry Leone

1902–1999

"I wanted to find opportunities in which science operated in human beings rather than in laboratories and nursing became my choice." (1977)

"The challenge to the college woman in the professions lies in something more than the urge to develop new technical knowledge and skill. The challenge lies in examining the values of what we do, in developing the human-relations potential in our fields, and in relating these larger goals of evolving the American culture." (1954)

"The horizon for nursing expands exhilaratingly. The depth has not been sounded. So we explore depths and distances. The nugget of truth lies in the nurse-patient relation. The distant star is the health of all people." (1977)

LUCILE LEONE WAS the first woman in the United States to serve as the chief nurse officer and assistant surgeon general. The rank of assistant surgeon general is equivalent to that of rear admiral in the navy or brigadier general in the army. She did not like the personal attention, but she was pleased that her rank elevated the stature of nursing. She served as director of nursing education for the U.S. Public Health Service (USPHS). She was the technical expert on nursing for the World Health Organization. She was appointed as the administrator of the Division of Nurse Education of the USPHS to oversee the Cadet Nurse Corps in World War II. She was responsible for developing a comprehensive recruitment program and educating 180,000 new nurses to provide nursing staffs for private hospitals and the military. The Bolton Act provided federal funds to subsidize nursing schools and all-expense scholarships to high school graduates. Her mantra was "keep it simple, keep it friendly," which she was remarkably skilled at doing. She strongly supported individualized nursing care and found it ironic that when the nurse-patient relationship was finally valued as therapeutic, nurses were spending less time with patients. Leone was active in planning statewide nursing education programs in Georgia and wrote extensively about the general upgrading of nursing education in the United States and internationally.

Biography

Born: Jan. 23, 1902, Lewisburg, Ohio. **Education:** Univ. of Delaware (BA in English and science); Johns Hopkins Hosp. School of Nursing, 1929; Teachers College, Columbia Univ., 1929 (MS); graduate work interrupted by appointment to USPHS. **Work history:** Clinical Instructor, Yale Univ.; Clinical Instructor, Associate Professor, Assistant Director, Univ. of Minnesota School of Nursing, 1929–40; Dean, New York Hosp. School of Nursing, Cornell Univ.; Nursing Administrator, USPHS; nurse recruiter, World War II; member, Expert Committee on Nursing, World Health Organization. **Organizations:** served many professional organizations as president, chair, member, and adviser; charter member, Bd. of Medicine, National Academy of Sciences; President, National League for Nursing (NLN); Editorial Adviser on nursing, McGraw-Hill. **Awards:** NLN established an award in her honor to be given to outstanding nurse-instructors; Distinguished Service Medal, USPHS; Florence Nightingale Medal, International Committee, Red Cross; honorary degrees from Univ. of Delaware, Boston Univ., Alfred Univ., Hood College, Adelphi College, Keuka College, and Wagner College; special citation from the Univ. of Buffalo. **Died:** San Francisco.

References and Credits

†Safier G: Contemporary American Leaders in Nursing: An Oral History. New York, McGraw-Hill, 1977, pp 164, 178.

Haritos DJ: Lucile Leone. In Bullough V, Sentz, L, Stein AP (eds): American Nursing: A Biographical Dictionary, vol. 2. New York, Garland, 1992, pp 190–193.

ANA on-line, available at htttp://www.ana.

Nursing pioneer dies. Nursing Insider on line. January 2000. http://www.nursingworld.org/news/nws01_00.htm.

January 24

Mary Ann Leonarda Garrigan

1914–2000

"The knowledge of our heritage brings a lift to the chin, a squaring of the shoulders, and a feeling of belonging. This … is a good time to bind together in our efforts, to negotiate our differences, and to keep nursing in its ascendancy." (1976)

"To work toward a goal when support is not forthcoming; to be willing to start again in a new direction; to believe in yourself and the worth of the work you are doing. … Yes, you have to have courage." (1986)

In the "Tribute to Mary Ann Garrigan" in the *Journal of Nursing History,* many of her peers express their sentiments about her courage in contributing her numerous talents to the nursing profession. She was described as a spark plug, someone with high ethical standards, personal integrity, self-respect, respect for others, deep inner resources, and as someone who enjoys hard work. She was a great fund raiser and was known for her sense of humor, fine mind, great capacity for sustained effort, great humanity, and the ability to identify and sympathize with others. Finally, she had a gift for friendship. With this abundance of talent and energy, Garrigan saw the need for and founded the Nursing Archives at Boston University in 1966. In 1971 it was named the official repository for the American Journal of Nursing Company and the American Nurses Association. She is also credited with being the initiator of the *Journal of Nursing History* in 1985. Anne G. Hargreaves, former director of the Massachusetts Nurses Association, told the *Journal of Nursing History* that "Mary Ann Garrigan believed history was best understood when viewed through the eyes of those who observed and experienced significant events in nursing."

Biography

Born: Jan. 24, 1914, New York City. **Education:** Westchester School of Nursing, Valhalla, N.Y., 1935; Women's Hosp. of New York, 1936 (certificate in maternity nursing); Teachers College, Columbia Univ. (BSN); Boston Univ., 1947 (MA in education). **Work history:** Instructor, Westchester School of Nursing; Staff Nurse, Adviser, Henry Street Visiting Nurse Service, N.Y.C.; Director, Precinct #43, New York Disaster Relief; managed and trained all nurse cadets in East as member of U.S. Army Nurse Corps at Halloran Hosp., Staten Island; Instructor, Assistant Professor, Associate Professor, and Professor, Boston Univ.; Director, four-yr. baccalaureate nursing education program, 1956–66, Boston Univ.; established the Nursing Archives, Boston Univ., March 1966; founded *Journal of Nursing History,* 1985. **Organizations:** Chair, Historical Resource Committee, Mass. League for Nursing. **Awards:** Curator Emerita, Nursing Archives; honorary degrees, Univ. of San Diego, Boston Univ., 1979; Edith More Copeland Founders Award, Sigma Theta Tau. **Buried:** Marblehead, Mass.

References and Credits

†Garrigan MA: In the spirit of '76. AJN 76:37, 1976.

†A tribute to Mary Ann Garrigan. Journal of Nursing History 2:6, 9, 1986.

Sentz, L., Mary Ann Garrigan. In Bullough V, Sentz, L, Stein AP (eds): American Nursing: A Biographical Dictionary, vol. 2. New York, Garland, 1992, p 131.

January 25

Lydia E. Anderson

1863–1939

"It is obvious to all that she [the teacher] must have the required education and mental grasp in order to undertake this work, but there is an equal, if not greater, necessity that she shall be possessed of a high moral character. The conscious influence exerted by what a woman says *and* does *cannot compare in power with that unconscious influence emanating from what she is. ...It is only as we set up high ideals, keeping them always in sight, and constantly endeavoring to approximate them, that we may have any ground for the hope of their ultimate realization. ...Then let us demand for our training schools that teaching, with its preparation, which we believe to be vital to the best interests of nurses and nursing." (1910)*

Lydia Anderson had a distinguished professional career as a nurse educator and administrator. She always worked to model the kind of ideals that she felt were necessary to promote the highest standards for nursing, and she inspired by example. She served as the president of the New York State Board of Nurse Examiners for several years. She held a special fondness for the New York Hospital School of Nursing, where she first studied, and she later compiled and published its history. Although she was primarily a nursing instructor for the Mt. Sinai School of Nursing and the New York Training School, she also lectured at numerous other schools in

New York and New Jersey. On one occasion, when she was honored by other nurses, the affair raised money to establish a loan program. It was named in her honor, and the money helped others prepare to become instructors. Bertha H. Lehmkuhl, a former student of Anderson's, wrote that "life itself speaks through her teaching. ...The mysteries of life are unfolded clearly and reverently... so humanly, that bodily weariness is forgotten and the ward work is resumed with keener interest, a brighter eye and a warmer smile."

Biography

Born: Jan. 16, 1863, New York City. **Education:** Rutgers Female College, N.J.; New York Hosp. Training School for Nurses; Teachers College, Columbia Univ. **Work history:** Homeopathic Hosp., Providence, R.I.; Sloane Maternity Hosp., N.Y.C.; private duty nursing; Long Island Hosp.; Mt. Sinai Hosp., N.Y.C.; taught nursing at thirty-two schools, primarily Mt. Sinai School of Nursing and New York Hosp. Training School. **Organizations:** New York Hosp. School of Nursing Alumni Assoc., American Red Cross; American Nurses Assoc.; National League for Nursing Education; History of Nursing Society. N.Y. State Bd. of Nurse Examiners. **Awards:** Lydia Anderson Loan Fund, N.Y. League for Nursing Education, for nurses studying to be instructors; library at New York Hosp. School of Nursing named in her honor. **Died:** location unknown.

References and Credits

†Birnbach N, Lewenson S: First Words: Selected Addresses from the National League for Nursing, 1894–1933. New York, National League for Nursing Press, 1991, p 29.

Falk G: Lydia Anderson. In Bullough V, Sentz, L, Stein AP (eds): American Nursing: A Biographical Dictionary, vol. 2. New York, Garland, 1992, pp 7–8.

Lehmkuhl BH: Eminent teachers: Lydia Anderson, An appreciation. AJN 29:201, 1929.

JANUARY 26

Hazel M. Avery

1906–1995

"Some procedures are peculiar to the gynecologic patient. [Their] performance ... may become commonplace to the nurse, but the patient may find them disturbing and difficult to accept unless handled with tact and understanding. ...Make the patient feel at ease. Good rapport is best accomplished by demonstrating a real interest in the patient and her problems. A patient who has been shown consideration and courtesy from the time of admittance, a patient who senses friendliness and respect for her personal feelings, will have much less difficulty in accepting necessary invasion of privacy. ...Too often we expect patients to fit promptly into hospital routine, something which may be difficult to do, especially today when so much of the hospital routine is geared to the convenience of the people who work there rather than to the patient. ...Gentleness is important. In few fields of nursing are so many nursing procedures carried out with the principal aim of providing comfort and pain relief for the patient." (1959)

HAZEL AVERY was nine when her mother died, and she was raised by her father, older sister, and paternal grandmother. When Hazel turned sixteen, she left home to earn room and board by working as a live-in babysitter while she completed high school. She earned a college degree that qualified her to teach history or sociology, but those jobs were hard to find during the depression. She accepted an offer of financial help to study nursing at the University of Michigan and remained in obstetrics at the university for four decades. In the early 1950s she introduced family-centered obstetrical nursing there, based on her observations at a Detroit hospital and a course at Yale. This was a welcome contrast to the traditional and common practices of parent-infant separation and rigid feeding schedules. The program encouraged fathers to be present during labor, delivery, and postpartum and allowed for sibling visits. The new maternity concept of rooming-in allowed mother and baby to share quality time together. Avery was an early leader in this now-common practice of family-centered obstetrical care. She and Dr. Norman Miller published a textbook about gynecologic nursing, and she published teaching booklets about mother and baby care.

Biography

Born: Jan. 16, 1906, Pittsburgh, Kans. **Education:** Intermountain Union College, Helena, Mt. (AB); Univ. of Michigan Hosp. School of Nursing. **Work history:** Staff Nurse, Supervisor, Instructor, OB Charge Nurse, Univ. of Michigan Hosp.; Faculty, School of Nursing, Univ. of Michigan. **Organizations:** OB and GYN Organization for Physicians and Nurses. **Awards:** unknown. **Died:** Bremerton, Wash.

References and Credits

†Miller N, Avery H: Nursing routine in the care and treatment of the gynecologic patient. In Gynecology and Gynecologic Nursing. Philadelphia, WB Saunders, 1959, pp 365–366.

Strodman LK: Hazel Avery. In Bullough V, Sentz L (eds): American Nursing: A Biographical Dictionary, vol. 3. New York, Springer, 2000, pp 6–8.

JANUARY 27

Mildred Irene Clark

1915–1994

Prayer of an Army Nurse

"Hear my prayer in silence before Thee as I ask for courage each day
Grant that I may be worthy of the sacred pledge of my profession.
And the lives of those entrusted to my care.
Help me to offer hope and cheer in the hearts of men and my country,
For their faith inspires me to give the world and nursing my best.
Instill in me the understanding and compassion of those who led the way,
For I am thankful to You for giving me this life to live." (1955)

MILDRED IRENE CLARK was inspired to pursue military nursing by a nursing instructor who had served in World War I. After Clark was accepted in the Army Nurse Corps, she prepared as an anesthetist. She worked at hospitals in Hawaii and stateside before being named director of a nurse corps, first in Korea, then in Japan. During the 1950s she worked as procurement officer in the Office of the Surgeon General and devised creative ways to recruit nurses despite a national shortage. One approach was the Army Student Nurse Program, and another was to encourage nurses to be reservists. Nurses were also inspired and drawn to serve by Clark's "Prayer of an Army Nurse," which was then set to music, recorded by the U.S. Army Band, and subsequently widely performed. She was chief of the Army Nurse Corps when she retired. Clark remained active in issues related to professional nursing and to veterans.

Biography

Born: Jan. 30, 1915, Elkton, N.C. **Education:** Baker Sanatorium Training School for Nurses, N.C.; Babies Hosp., N.C., and Jewish Hosp., Philadelphia (postgraduate coursework); Medical Field Service School; Univ. of Minnesota (BSNE). **Work history:** Chief Nurse, Schofield Barracks, Hawaii, and numerous Stateside facilities; Director of Nurses, Korea; Chief Nurse, Tokyo; Procurement Officer, Surgeon General's Office; Chief Nurse, Presidio, San Francisco; Chief, Army Nurse Corps. **Organizations:** professional nursing and veterans' organizations. **Awards:** Distinguished Service Medal; Army Commendation Medal; lifetime membership, Sigma Theta Tau; Outstanding Alumna, Univ. of Minnesota; Mich. Women's Hall of Fame; Clark Health Clinic, Ft. Bragg, N.C., named in her honor. **Buried:** Arlington National Cemetery.

References and Credits

†Office of Medical History, Army Nurse Corps.

Sarnecky MT: Mildred Clark. In Bullough V, Sentz, L (eds): American Nursing: A Biographical Dictionary, vol. 3. New York, Springer, 2000, pp 52–54.

January 28

Mary May Roberts

1877–1959

"The spirit of the true nurse is one of the most beautiful gifts of a bountiful Creator. ...The spirit of nursing is one of the most indestructible elements in the lives of those who possess it. Like fine steel, it gives form and substance but yet is flexible, it is shining but durable. It is made up of... courage, ... love of truth, with the accompanying characteristics of frankness, fidelity and sincerity; kindness, tolerance, courtesy, generosity, compassion, sympathy and benevolence. ...It is one of the things of which nurses rarely speak and of which the possessor is probably unaware. ...Nursing offers opportunities for self-expression of a high order." (1925)

MARY MAY ROBERTS worked tirelessly and successfully to raise the standards of nursing, most notably during her thirty years as the editor of the *American Journal of Nursing (AJN).* Early in her career she worked as a clinic nurse, a private duty nurse, and a superintendent of nursing. She organized and directed a school of nursing in Georgia. During World War I she was a Red Cross nurse, a nurse recruiter, and director of an army school of nursing. After the war she earned a degree at Columbia University, then started her work with *AJN.* She taught by example and encouraged nurses to use the *Journal* to help them network and to address nursing issues. She wrote about the essential relationship between quality patient care and the knowledge, skill, and dedication of the individual nurse. She recognized the nurse as patient advocate and helped define nursing as a profession. She addressed the importance of refining the selection process for nursing school admissions and the importance of including in the curriculum public health nursing and coursework in ethics. Circulation increased during her tenure from twenty thousand to 100,000. A prolific writer, she authored a classic on American nursing, *American Nursing: History and Interpretation.*

Biography

Born: Jan. 30, 1877, Duncan City, Mich. **Education:** Jewish Hosp. Training School for Nurses, Cincinnati, Ohio; Teachers College, Columbia Univ. (BS). **Work history:** Baroness Erlanger Hosp., Chattanooga, Tenn.; Superintendent., organizer of nursing school, Savannah Hosp., Ga.; Superintendent, Jewish Hosp., Cincinnati; Private Duty Nurse, Superintendent, Evanston Hosp., Ill.; Superintendent, C.R. Holmes Hosp., Cincinnati; nurse recruiter, American Red Cross, World War I; Director, Army School of Nursing, Ohio; Editor, *AJN;* helped develop, then served as Director, Nursing Information Bureau; represented nursing on numerous committees dealing with health care and nursing service, incl. the Examining Committee, Ohio State Medical Bd. **Organizations:** President, Ohio Nurses Assoc.; numerous committees of American Nurses Assoc. (ANA), National League for Nursing (NLN), National League for Nursing Education; American Red Cross; International Council of Nurses. **Awards:** Florence Nightingale Medal, International Committee, Red Cross; Adelaide Nutting Award for Leadership in Nursing; Bronze Medal, Ministry of Social Welfare, France; Army Certificate of Appreciation; honorary life membership, American Hosp. Assoc.; awards in her name established by N.Y. State Nurses Assoc. and *AJN;* member, ANA Hall of Fame. **Died:** New York, N.Y.

References and Credits

†Roberts MM: The spirit of nursing. AJN 25:734, 1925.

Donahue PM: Mary Roberts. In Bullough V, Church OM, Stein AP (eds): American Nursing: A Biographical Dictionary, vol. 1. New York, Garland, 1988, pp 277–279.

ANA Hall of Fame 10/98 American Nurses Association, Washington, D.C. http://www.nursingworld.org/hof.

January 29

Signe Skott Cooper

1921–

"A commitment to lifelong learning is the mark of the truly professional person. To this individual, learning is as essential as breathing. Early in his career, he accepts a personal responsibility for his own continued education, seeing it as closely related to his own continued practice, and he pursues it with enthusiasm and zest. ...He devotes time and attention to learning how to learn. ...He has... learned to be selective. ...He recognizes that learning requires work. ...I believe that the evolvement of nursing as a profession rests upon a commitment by nursing's practitioners to their own continued learning." (1972)

Signe Skott Cooper was attracted to nursing by a favorite aunt, who was her role model and inspiration. Cooper, an early advocate for continuing nursing education, is a pioneer in the field. She recognized its importance for nurses and that each nurse has something of value to share with colleagues. She initiated telephone conferencing for continuing education in Wisconsin. More than six hundred nurses benefited from the first class by accessing twenty-four listening centers that were known as "telephone bridges." Through her efforts the extension nursing program at the University of Wisconsin expanded and gained national and international recognition. She is an accomplished author of books and articles about continuing education. She has been a consultant to the Clinical Center at the National Institutes of Health (NIH), the World Health Organization (WHO), and to universities. She has had a major, continual influence on the evolution of nursing education. In addition, she has devoted decades to preserving the history of nursing in Wisconsin, saying that it is important to know our own history and that each nurse has a responsibility to help the next generation.

Biography

Born: Jan. 29, 1921, Clinton County, Iowa. **Education:** Univ. of Wisconsin, Madison (nursing certificate); Univ. of Wisconsin, Madison (BS); Teachers College, Columbia Univ.; Univ. of Minnesota (MEd). **Work history:** U.S. Army Nurse, China-Burma-India Theater; Head Nurse, OB Unit, Univ. Hosp., Madison, Wisc.; Faculty, Univ. Extension and School of Nursing, Univ. of Wisconsin, Madison; Principal Investigator, North Central State Planning Project for Continuing Education in Nursing; Professor of Nursing, Univ. of Wisconsin, Madison; Helen Denne Schulte Professor of Nursing, Univ. of Wisconsin; Consultant to numerous organizations, incl. NIH; WHO; International Research Development Center, Can.; PLATO Nursing Project (computer-assisted instruction). **Organizations:** American Nurses Assoc. (ANA); (Madison) Wisc. Nurses Assoc.; District Nurses Assoc.; National League for Nursing (NLN); Adult Education Assoc. of the USA (AEAUSA). **Awards:** Linda Richards Award, NLN; Distinguished Service Award, Univ. of Wisconsin; Wisc. Governor's Special Award; awards from Wisc. Nurses Assoc.; Wisc. Heart Assoc.; Honorary Recognition Award, ANA; Pioneer Award, AEAUSA; Legislative Citation, ANA Hall of Fame.

References and Credits

†Cooper SS: This I believe . . . about continuing education in nursing." Nurs Outlook 20:579–583, 1972.

Mirr M: Signe Cooper. In Bullough V, Sentz L (eds): American Nursing: A Biographical Dictionary, vol. 3. New York, Springer, 2000, pp 59–60.

Cooper S: personal communication, 2002.

ANA Hall of Fame 10/98 American Nurses Association, Washington, D.C. http://www.nursingworld.org/hof.

JANUARY 30

Mary Eugenie Hibbard

1856–1946

"Here we see in a war a calamity so awful in its results, holding human life and torture in its clutches, with the price of the bullet only, scattering and blasting hopes and breaking hearts. On the other hand, we see the magnificent height to which human nature aspires and here attains in the sacrifice of self for country, and often the proof 'That greater love hath no man than this, that a man lay down his life for his friend.'" (1901)

DURING HER NURSING career Mary Hibbard served in the Spanish-American War and worked in South Africa, the Philippines, Cuba, and Panama. She was appointed superintendent of a nursing school in Cuba after the Spanish-American War, and the high standards and regulations that were established under her leadership resulted in an outstanding program. It won legal recognition for nursing one year earlier than similar legislation in the United States. In addition, she prepared nurses for the control of tuberculosis in Cuba and was recognized for her work to control yellow fever in the Panama Canal Zone. Hibbard is cited on a monument in Arlington National Cemetery that recognizes the nurses who served in the Spanish-American War.

Biography

Born: 1856, near Montreal. **Education:** Mack Training School for Nurses, with General and Marine Hosp., St. Catharine's, Ontario, Can. **Work history:** administrative positions, Mack Training School; Grace Hosp., Detroit; Newberry Training School for Nurses, Homeopathic Hosp., Trenton, N.J.; Chief Nurse, U.S. General Hosp., Savannah, Ga.; General Hosp., Ft. Meyers, Va.; served on the hospital ship *Maine;* worked in South Africa and Philippines; Superintendent, Training School for Nurses, Santa Isabel Hosp., Mantanzas, Cuba; Chief Nurse, Ancon Hosp., Panama; Superintendent, Leonard Hosp., Landisburgh, N.Y.; Administrator, Dept. of Nursing, Tuberculosis Section, Cuba; Chief, Bureau of Nurses, Cuba. **Organizations:** unknown. **Awards:** listed on memorial at Arlington National Cemetery to nurses of Spanish-American War; plaque in Panama Canal Zone dedicated to her.
Died: Jamaica.

References and Credits

†Hibbard ME: With the *Maine* to South Africa. AJN 1:400, 1901.

Healey PF: Mary Hibbard. In Bullough V, Church OM, Stein AP (eds): American Nursing: A Biographical Dictionary, vol. 1. New York, Garland, 1988, pp 177–179.

Katharine Greenough

1920–1975

"Our greatest assets in attracting members seem to be those parts and programs of the organization that offer the member opportunity to take a personal part in the improvement of her professional and economic life. ... The programs that are more directly framed and carried by the members are those that have the greatest sales appeal." (1954)

KATHERINE GREENOUGH WAS known as a very serious nurse when working for her causes, but she worked most comfortably in the background, not receiving the accolades that she so justly deserved. Her greatest skills were in organizational management and clinical nursing research. She worked with Barbara Schutt in Pennsylvania to devise a structure of local units to facilitate collective bargaining by nurses. She was excited by labor relations activities but during the McCarthy years suffered the abuse of her colleagues, who called her a commie and red. When she was appointed director of the Educational Services Division of the American Journal of Nursing Company, part of her brief was to develop new educational materials for the continuing education of practicing nurses. While working on the Pre-Hospital Coronary Care Project, she analyzed the efficiency of the ambulance service calls of patients with myocardial infarction. She established a corollary between rapidity of response and positive outcome. This study resulted in improvements to ambulance service and eventually the installation of the national 911 system. Greenough planned to use the data that she collected as the basis for her doctoral dissertation, which she was working on when she died.

Biography

Born: Jan. 16, 1920, New York, N.Y. **Education:** Radcliffe College, 1941 (political science); Columbia-Presbyterian School of Nursing, 1944 (MS); Univ. of California, San Francisco, 1965 (coursework for PhD). **Work history:** Head Nurse, Presbyterian Hosp., N.Y.; Polio Nurse, Minneapolis; OR Nurse, St. Luke's Hosp., Bethlehem, Pa., 1947–49; Assistant Exec. Secretary, Pa. Nurses Assoc.; organized units for collective bargaining; Exec. Secretary, Texas (Graduate) Nurses Assoc., 1957–63; Calif. Nurses Assoc., 1966; Lecturer, Univ. of California, San Francisco School of Nursing; Nurse Specialist, coronary care, Veterans Administration Hosp., Ft. Miley, Calif.; Research Coordinator, Planned Parenthood of Calif.; Research Coordinator, San Francisco Pre-Hospital Coronary Care Project, San Francisco Heart Assoc.; Consultant to special committee, International Council of Nurses (ICN), 1971; committee staff member when report was presented at the ICN Congress, Mexico City, 1972; Director, Educational Services Division, American Journal of Nursing Co., 1973; President, American Nurses Foundation, 1970–72. **Organizations:** Bd. of directors, American Nurses Foundation, American Nurses Assoc. (ANA), 1962–70; ANA Nominating Committee; ANA Finance Committee; served on committee that designed and named the Congress on Nursing Practice; helped to create American Academy of Nursing and served on committee to draft criteria for membership. **Awards:** unknown. **Died:** New York City.

References and Credits

†Greenough K: Why do they join? AJN 54:816–818, 1954.

Cooper, SS: Katharine Greenough. In Bullough V, Sentz, L, Stein AP (eds): American Nursing: A Biographical Dictionary, vol. 2. New York, Garland, 1992, pp 140–142.

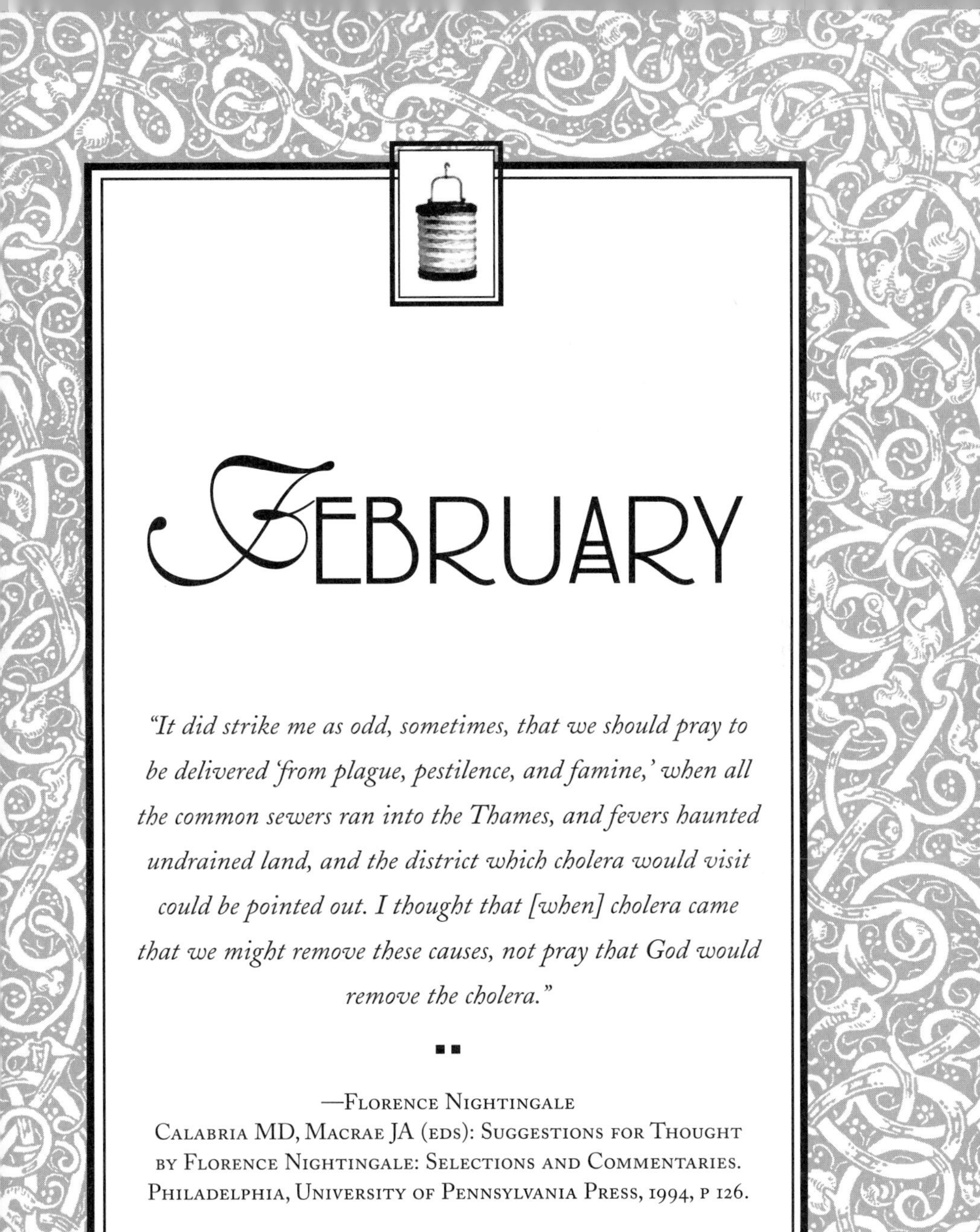

FEBRUARY

"It did strike me as odd, sometimes, that we should pray to be delivered 'from plague, pestilence, and famine,' when all the common sewers ran into the Thames, and fevers haunted undrained land, and the district which cholera would visit could be pointed out. I thought that [when] cholera came that we might remove these causes, not pray that God would remove the cholera."

—Florence Nightingale
Calabria MD, Macrae JA (eds): Suggestions for Thought by Florence Nightingale: Selections and Commentaries. Philadelphia, University of Pennsylvania Press, 1994, p 126.

February 1

Blanche Pfefferkorn
1884–1961

"A fundamental factor in the administration of a hospital nursing service is the bedside nursing personnel, or more accurately stated; the hours required to give the proper bedside nursing care to patients. Not infrequently a considerable discrepancy exists between the bedside nursing hours provided *and the bedside nursing hours* required. …*More emphasis is needed on the necessity of providing* enough *time to make possible a good quality of nursing." (1932)*

BLANCHE PFEFFERKORN HAD a professional career as an operating room nurse, a nurse supervisor, superintendent, instructor, and writer. She was also one of the very early nurse researchers. Her 1932 article, "Measuring Nursing, Quantitatively and Qualitatively," proposed time studies for hospital nursing and patient care. Although she acknowledged individual differences, she believed the research would give an idea of the average time needed to provide good nursing care under comparable conditions. In addition to its value as a source of information about adequate staffing, it showed nursing service administrators that insufficient staff *prevents* good nursing care. The culmination of her career was her effective leadership of the National League for Nursing, where she applied her findings and publications in ways that had a positive effect on both educational standards and standards of practice. Another of her interests was nursing history, reflected in her coauthorship of the early history (1907–1949) of the nursing school at Johns Hopkins.

Biography

Born: January 1884, Baltimore. **Education:** Johns Hopkins Hosp. Training School for Nurses; Columbia Univ. (BS, MA). **Work history:** Bellevue Hosp., Harlem Hosp., N.Y.C.; Faculty, Univ. of Cincinnati; Staff, Teachers College, Columbia Univ.; Director of Studies, National League for Nursing. **Organizations:** American Red Cross; Ohio State Assoc. of Graduate Nurses; Ohio State League for Nursing Education; American Nurses Assoc.; National League for Nursing Education. **Awards:** Isabel H. Robb Fellowship for Graduate Study at Teachers College, Columbia Univ. **Died:** Los Angeles.

References and Credits

†Pfefferkorn B: Measuring nursing, quantitatively and qualitatively. AJN 32:80–84, 1932.

Sentz L: Blanche Pfefferkorn. In Bullough V, Church OM, Stein AP (eds): American Nursing: A Biographical Dictionary, vol. 1. New York, Garland, 1988, pp 258–259.

February 2

Charlotte Albina Aikens

1868–1949

"It is not easy

To apologize	*To keep on trying*
To begin over	*To avoid mistakes*
To admit error	*To forgive and forget*
To be unselfish	*To keep out of the rut*
To take advice	*To make the most of a little*
To be charitable	*To maintain a high standard*
To be considerate	*To recognize the silver lining.*

But it always pays." (1935)

Charlotte Aikens wanted to be a missionary nurse in China but served in the Spanish-American War instead. Upon her return to the States, she served as director of Sibley Memorial Hospital in Washington, D.C., where she recognized the need for reform in hospital-based nurse-training programs. She observed that hospitals often used student nurses as a cheap labor pool instead of providing them with theoretical content and diverse clinical experience. She advocated a three-year curriculum in hospital training schools, and she combined her interest and skill in writing to author several textbooks for nurses. Her editorials for *the Trained Nurse and Hospital Review* focused on the need for a standardized curriculum as well as the need for an eight-hour day and nurse registration. Her studies of basic nursing skills, in 1916, started the ongoing debate about levels of preparation for nursing that continues today.

Biography

Born: 1868, Mitchell, Ontario, Can. **Education:** Alma College, Ontario; Stratford Hosp. School of Nursing, Ontario; New York Polyclinic Hosp.; **Work history:** Nurse, Spanish-American War; Director, Sibley Memorial Hosp., Washington, D.C.; Associate Editor, *Hospital Record;* Superintendent, Methodist Hosp., Des Moines, Iowa; Superintendent, Columbia Hosp., Pittsburgh, Pa.; Associate Editor, *Trained Nurse and Hospital Review;* Site Reviewer, Methodist Church Mission Bd. **Organizations:** Society of Superintendents of Training Schools (later the National League for Nursing); American Hosp. Assoc.; Detroit Nursing Home Assoc. **Awards:** unknown. **Died:** Detroit.

References and Credits

†Aiken C: A Study in Ethics for Nurses, 3d ed. Philadelphia, WB Saunders, 1935, cover.

Fulton J: Charlotte Aikens. In Bullough V, Church OM, Stein AP (eds): American Nursing: A Biographical Dictionary, vol. 1. New York, Garland, 1988, pp 1–3.

Helen Edith Browne

1911–1987

"Perhaps one of the most important aspects of this type of health care program is the manner in which it helps strengthen or maintain family ties and helps individual members assume greater responsibility for one another. In times of childbirth or illness, there is a natural pulling together of the family. If various members within the family are supported in their efforts to help one another and the necessary guidance is provided, much can be done to alleviate the stress and loneliness of illness and to increase the joy and satisfaction of parenthood. If the health care system is organized in a manner whereby primary care is readily accessible with good specialty care linkages, much can be done to lessen chronic disability and perhaps maintain and revive the community spirit that used to be so vital in the development of this country." (1976)

"BROWNIE," AS HELEN EDITH BROWNE was affectionately called, was fond of saying that "nurses care, doctors cure" to remind the nurses in her beloved Frontier Nursing Service (FNS) of their first obligation to their patients. She was an Englishwoman who responded to Mary Breckinridge's request for a midwife to come to rural Kentucky and work with her; Browne later was unanimously elected director of the FNS, where she remained for thirty-eight years.

Browne remained in the United States during World War II, although many other British nurses returned to England. She preferred to continue delivering babies, often at the point of a shotgun held by a distrustful husband, a man of the mountain culture. She often had to reach her patients under trying conditions, such as fording swollen streams on horseback. Her practice of midwifery brought maternal and infant mortality rates below the rates for modern facilities. She was a leader in midwifery and she is remembered, according to the writer Linda M. Calley, as "the ultimate midwife—strong, sure, sensitive."

Biography

Born: Feb. 3, 1911, Bury, St. Edmonds, England. **Education:** St. Bartholomews Hosp. School of Nursing, England, 1934; British Hosp. for Mothers and Babies, London (postgraduate work). **Work history:** Charge Nurse, St. Bartholomews Hosp.; Midwifery Supervisor, British Hosp. for Mothers and Babies, 1937; FNS, Ky., 1938–76; Supervisor, Superintendent, Hyden (Ky.) Hosp.; Director, fund raiser, speaker, Southeastern Kentucky Health Demonstration Corp.; integrated midwifery into educational curriculum, merged the American Assoc. of Midwives and American College of Nurses Midwifery to form American College of Nurse Midwives; worked with visitors from other nations to adapt midwifery practices of FNS to their cultures. **Organizations:** American Assoc. of Midwives, American College of Nurse Midwifery, American College of Nurse Midwives. **Awards:** Distinguished Service Award, Berea College; honorary doctorate, Eastern Kentucky University; Order of the British Empire, Commander of the Most Excellent Order of the British Empire. **Died:** Milford, Pa.

References and Credits

†Browne H, Isaacs G: Primary care nurse in community health. Am J Obstet Gynecol 124:14–17, 1976.

Calley LM: Helen Edith Browne. In Bullough V, Sentz L, Stein AP (eds): American Nursing: A Biographical Dictionary, vol. 2. New York, Garland, 1992, pp 46–48.

February 4

Mary Bristow Willeford

1900–1941

"The territory covered by the Service, comprising an area over seven hundred square miles in extent, is rugged and extreme. ... This topography has formed such barriers to outside influences that for generations people have been penalized by their geographic remoteness. The country is a real frontier, for there are no railroads, no bridges over the numerous streams, and only one highway 24 miles in length. In a country where horses furnish the ordinary mode of travel, it is necessary that nurses be not more than five or six miles from their more distant patients, as the usual speed on horseback is about four miles an hour. ... The midwifery supervisor ... literally lives in her saddle. She is on call for abnormal cases, which are reported to her first and through her to the medical director. ...At the close of the seventh fiscal year, 1,197 patients had been delivered, with 30 stillbirths and no maternal deaths due directly to obstetrical causes." (1933)

MARY WILLEFORD PREPARED as a nurse-midwife in London and later returned there to earn her midwifery teaching credentials. She practiced in Kentucky with what later became known as the Frontier Nursing Service (FNS). She was a nurse on horseback in rugged territory that allowed for no other means of travel. Her skilled horsemanship made it possible for her to move through challenging terrain to reach and provide care to women and families who lived in otherwise inaccessible areas. During her relatively short life she also focused on practical research issues. Her doctoral study with four hundred families in rural Kentucky demonstrated the relationship between income and health in remote, isolated areas. She earned one of the first doctoral degrees in nursing when she received hers in 1932. She helped establish schools of midwifery, including the school at the Tuskegee Institute in Alabama, with funding from the nursing education section of the Social Security Act.

Biography

Born: Feb. 4, 1900, Flatonia, Texas. **Education:** Univ. of Texas, Austin; Army School of Nursing, Walter Reed Hosp., Washington, D.C.; York Lying-in Hosp., London; Columbia Univ. (PhD). **Work history:** nurse-midwife, Ky.; Assistant Director, FNS; Consultant, California Health Dept.; Public Health Nurse Consultant, U.S. Children's Bureau. **Organizations:** charter member, Ky. State Assoc. of Nurse-Midwives and American Assoc. of Nurse-Midwives. **Awards:** unknown. **Died:** New York City.

References and Credits

†Willeford MB: The Frontier Nursing Service. Public Health Nursing 25:6, 7, 9, 1933.

Bullough V: Mary Bristow Willeford. In Bullough V, Sentz L, Stein AP (eds): American Nursing: A Biographical Dictionary, vol. 2. New York, Garland, 1992, pp 354–355.

FEBRUARY 5

Mary Sewall Gardner
1871–1961

"Everywhere the public health nurse stands as one of the most valuable co-operating agents of the community. This has, perhaps, been a rather unexpected development of her work, but had she failed to respond to this demand and confined her usefulness to the nursing care of her patients, public health nurses would hardly have been counted by thousands, as they are today. Co-operation has not only done much for the patient and his family, and much towards strengthening the hands of other agencies, but it has done more than many nurses realise [sic] *to relieve public health nursing of its most unbearable features. Many an early nurse remembers how constantly the misery she encountered haunted her off-duty hours. This was largely because she was helpless to deal with it herself and did not know how to get the assistance she needed." (1923)*

AFTER RECOVERING FROM TUBERCULOSIS as a teenager, Mary Gardner cared for her invalid stepmother, delaying her entrance into nursing school until she was thirty. She realized that her desire to do missionary nursing could be met in U.S. cities. She focused on improving the quality of public health nursing and broadening the scope of the nurse's involvement in community issues. Considered an international pioneer in public health nursing, she is ranked with Lillian Wald for laying the foundation on which this specialty flourished. Gardner's text, *Public Health Nursing,* is considered a classic and set the standard for practice at home and abroad. Her novel, *Katherine Kent,* is considered an autobiographical but idealized portrayal of the public health nurse. She helped establish the National Organization for Public Health Nursing (NOPHN), wrote often for its journal, and was a leader in the International Council of Nurses (ICN). Her papers are archived at the Schlesinger Library of Radcliffe College.

Biography

Born: Feb. 5, 1871, Newton, Mass. **Education:** Newton Hosp. Training School, Newport, R.I.; studied with Lillian Wald and others. **Work history:** Director, Providence District Nurses Assoc. (PDNA); helped establish NOPHN; helped found the journal *Public Health Nursing;* Temporary Director, American Red Cross Town and Country Nursing Service; Chief Nurse, American Red Cross Tuberculosis Commission for Italy; committee member, Bureau of Information for Nurses during World War I; Study Committee, Public Health/Europe. **Organizations:** NOPHN; American Red Cross; ICN. **Awards:** honorary director, PDNA; Walter Burns Saunders Medal, American Nurses Assoc. (ANA); honorary master's degree, Brown Univ.; ANA Hall of Fame. **Died:** Providence, R.I.

References and Credits

†Gardner MS: Public Health Nursing. New York, Macmillan, 1923, p 46.

Bullough V: Mary Sewell Gardner. In Bullough V, Church OM, Stein AP (eds): American Nursing: A Biographical Dictionary, vol. 1. New York, Garland, 1988, pp 130–132.

Sicherman B, Green C (eds): Notable American Women: The Modern Period. Cambridge, Mass., Belknap Press, 1980.

ANA Hall of Fame 10/98 American Nurses Association, Washington, D.C. http://www.nursingworld.org/hof.

February 6

Annie Warburton Goodrich

1866–1954

"How consistent [is] the history of nursing with the history of human progress... the gradual emergence into order, cleanliness, even beauty, through rigid and rigorous regimes zealously demanded... as a discipline imposed by the quite obvious necessity of stretching human capacity for a greatly needed service to the n*th degree. ...Through the nursing profession we have the opportunity of achieving in the community what was achieved by the pioneers of nursing for the hospitals. We should indeed consider the history of the hospital as a demonstration of the art and science of social betterment which could well be expanded... into every street of every town or city. Not to see this as the task imposed is to betray the high purpose, the far-reaching vision, the indomitable pride in their calling, the invincible spirit, of those who laid the foundation of a now world-wide social service." (1931)*

As a young adult, Annie Goodrich saw an untrained nurse attempt to care for her sick grandparents and realized how much more a nurse with education and skills could have done. When Goodrich became superintendent of nurses at New York hospitals, she worked continually to improve standards for nursing and patient care. She introduced the initial concept of primary care nursing and encouraged cooperative working relationships between nurses and doctors. She arranged daytime classes for students and affiliations with other hospitals to provide them with broader clinical experience. She tightened entrance requirements and started probationary periods. While a faculty member at Teachers College, Columbia University, she was also the director of nurses at the Henry Street Settlement, where she stressed the role of the public health nurse in prevention of disease. During World War I she worked to establish the Army School of Nursing and became its first dean. When the Rockefeller Foundation invited her to serve on a nursing education committee, she recommended that the foundation give money to universities to establish nursing schools. She viewed this as a way to achieve higher standards for nursing education and, subsequently, improve patient care. Yale University volunteered to have such an independent nursing school with Goodrich as dean and faculty member. Five years later the Rockefeller Foundation gave the nursing school at Yale a $1 million endowment as testament to her success.

Biography

Born: Feb. 6, 1866, New Brunswick, N.J. **Education:** New York Hosp. Training School for Nurses. **Work history:** Superintendent, New York Hosp., New York Postgraduate Hosp.; Superintendent of Nurses, St. Luke's Hosp., New York Hosp., and Bellevue Training School for Nurses; State Inspector of nurse training schools; Faculty, Teachers College, Columbia Univ.; Director of Nurses, Henry Street Settlement; Chief Inspecting Nurse, U.S. Army hospitals, World War I; Dean, Army School of Nursing; member, Rockefeller Commission; Dean, Faculty, Yale School of Nursing; Consultant, Rockefeller Foundation; Nursing Consultant, Institute of Living, Hartford, Conn.; Western Reserve Univ.; U.S. Public Health Service. **Organizations:** American Society of Superintendents of Training Schools for Nurses; numerous committees for different groups; American Federation of Nurses; International Council of Nurses (ICN); American Nurses Assoc. (ANA). **Awards:** Walter Burns Saunders Medal, ANA; citation from ICN; fellowship with American College of Hospital Administrators. Medals from US, France, Belgium; Adelaide Nutting Award, National League for Nursing; ANA Hall of Fame; honorary degrees from Mt. Holyoke, Yale Univ., Russell Sage. **Buried:** Cedar Hill Cemetery, Hartford, Conn.

References and Credits

†Goodrich AW: The past, present, and future of nursing. AJN 31:1385, 1388, 1389, 1931.

Gurney C: Annie Goodrich. In Bullough V, Church OM, Stein AP (eds): American Nursing: A Biographical Dictionary, vol. 1. New York, Garland, 1988, pp 145–149.

ANA Hall of Fame 10/98 American Nurses Association, Washington, D.C. http://www.nursingworld.org/hof.

FEBRUARY 7

Dorothy E. Reilly

1920–1996

"How did I become a master teacher? ... Teaching, like all helping professions, derives its art from caring, valuing, and continuing the search for self. ... On this teacher's odyssey towards mastery, one fact becomes evident: the events that are most influential are those that occur in the relational process of teaching, and not in those incidents where the teacher is the sole focus. Significant incidents in teaching, like those in nursing practice, should not remain ends in themselves, but rather they must be subjected to analysis of their meaning and their contribution to the achievement of professional mastery." (1996)

DOROTHY REILLY WAS an internationally renowned nursing scholar and educator. She was an award-winning author of numerous books about nursing and teaching. Her writings influenced those who teach nursing as well as the scope and manner of instruction. The *American Journal of Nursing* gave her Book of the Year Awards for *Behavioral Objectives in Nursing: Evaluation of Learner Attainment* (1976) and for *Clinical Teaching in Nursing Education* (1992). She was an outstanding master teacher who knew the importance of the interactive approach. A mentor and a valued consultant to nursing schools throughout the world, she devised new approaches to graduate nursing education that attracted numerous funding grants from the National Institutes of Health. She continued writing while recovering from a stroke, and the resulting insightful article reaffirmed her love for teaching. She recognized that the art of teaching, like nursing, can be enhanced by one's demeanor toward others as well as by the continuing quest for personal growth.

Biography

Born: Feb. 6, 1920, Holyoke, Mass. **Education:** Mt. Holyoke College (nursing diploma); Columbia Univ. Dept. of Nursing (BS); master's degree, Boston Univ.; Columbia Univ. (PhD). **Work history:** Head Nurse, Institute of Ophthalmology, Presbyterian Hosp., N.Y.C.; Nursing Instructor, Private Duty Nurse, Faculty, Boston Univ. School of Nursing; Faculty, nursing program, Columbia Univ.; Faculty, Wayne State Univ. College of Nursing. **Organizations:** Mich. Nurses Assoc.; American Nurses Assoc. (ANA); Sigma Theta Tau. **Awards:** Distinguished Alumni Award, Columbia Univ.–Presbyterian Hosp.; Sigma Theta Tau Award for Excellence in Education; Mt. Holyoke College Sesquicentennial Alumnae Award; American Academy of Nursing; ANA Hall of Fame. **Died:** Detroit.

References and Credits

†Reilly DE: A teacher looks back: The route to mastery. J Nurs Educ 35:131, 133, 1996.

Oermann M: Dorothy Reilly. In Bullough V, Sentz L (eds): American Nursing: A Biographical Dictionary, vol. 3. New York, Springer, 2000, pp 240–242.

ANA Hall of Fame 10/98 American Nurses Association, Washington, D.C. http://www.nursingworld.org/hof.

FEBRUARY 8

Katherine M. Olmsted

1888–1964

"It is true there is a shortage of nurses. ... We can ... get the finest and best things about our nursing profession before the public. ... If we are going to ... attract the finest type of young women ... we must portray our profession attractively and in a dignified manner. ... Publicity material must be prepared ... first to attract attention, secondly to interest the group that you want." (1920)

KATHERINE OLMSTED WAS a public health nurse with a versatile career. She worked as a rural public health nurse in Illinois, and then in 1916 she organized and taught a course in public health nursing for the Wisconsin Anti-Tuberculosis Association. It was one of the earliest such courses in the country, and it influenced the growth of public health nursing in that state. During World War I she worked in Europe with the Red Cross, part of a small group that faced adversity and challenge in Romania and Russia. After the war she did public health nursing among native Americans in Wyoming before she returned to Europe to help establish Red Cross schools of nursing. She also started an advanced nursing program in London and was highly decorated by many countries for her achievements. For reasons unknown, she left nursing. After graduating from the Cordon Bleu cooking school in Paris, she opened a French restaurant in New York in 1928 and was actively involved with it for the rest of her life.

Biography

Born: February 1888, Des Moines, Iowa. **Education:** Art Institute of Chicago; college in Wisconsin; Chicago School of Civics and Philanthropy; Johns Hopkins Hosp. School of Nursing; Univ. of the Sorbonne. **Work history:** Baltimore Instructive Visiting Nurse Assoc.; Johns Hopkins Hosp. Social Service Dept.; public health nursing, Ill.; Organizer, Instructor, course for public health nurses, Wisc.; Red Cross nurse, Romania; Public Health Nurse, Wyo.; Nurse-Director, nursing school organizer for Red Cross throughout Europe; Instructor, Red Cross (U.S.); French chef, restaurateur, Normandy Inn, Sodus, N.Y. **Organizations:** American Red Cross; N.Y. State Nursing Council for War Service. **Awards:** medals and awards from eleven countries for her work with Red Cross and in establishing nursing programs; all awards are housed at the Alumnae House of the Johns Hopkins Hosp. School of Nursing.
Died: Sodus, N.Y.

References and Credits

†Olmsted K: The recruiting of student nurses. AJN 20:974–976, 978, 1920.

Cooper SS: Katherine Olmsted. In Bullough V, Church OM, Stein AP (eds): American Nursing: A Biographical Dictionary, vol. 1. New York, Garland, 1988, pp 247–248.

Letocha P: personal communication, 2000.

February 9

Helen Winifred Kelly

1865–1956

"The great army of private duty nurses being made up chiefly of women who cheerfully face their responsibilities, and are prepared to take what comes so long as it offers an opportunity for service; who recognize the value of their work in relation to the great health movement of the day; who realize that a nurse does not live unto herself alone, but is one of a long line of descent; that she must be true to the women who have gone before, and have left to her a sacred heritage which she in turn must one day pass on to those who come after. They give thought to their obligation of adding to this treasured possession, and of passing it on a little greater and brighter than when they received it. True to the Past and the Future, they cannot go far astray in the Present." (1924)

Helen Kelly was a fearless Wisconsin leader who was determined to pave the road for registration and organization of nurses. She became the registrar of the Wisconsin Nurses Club and Registry in Milwaukee, and in that role she was influential in making nursing a powerful force. She served as the first president of the Wisconsin State Nurses Association (WSNA) and as president of several other important nursing organizations. She received the first Red Cross Badge, No. 2100, issued by the Wisconsin Red Cross Committee. She was a delegate to the International Council of

Nurses (ICN) in 1912 in Cologne, Germany. Kelly is remembered for the high standards she set and met herself. She was convinced that nurses must maintain high standards, a belief that was evident in her legislative efforts and her work as a registrar. She was always honest and respectful when confronted with opposition to her high standards. However, she never wavered.

Biography

Born: Feb. 9, 1865, Monches, Wisc. **Education:** Illinois Training School for Nurses/Cook County Hosp. School of Nursing, Chicago, 1895; attended Teachers College, Columbia Univ.; postgraduate courses at Chicago School of Civics and Philanthropy, School of Sociology of Loyola Univ., Chicago, and Univ. of Chicago. **Work history:** Private Duty Nurse; Assistant Superintendent, Illinois Training School; Superintendent of Nurses, Calif. Hosp., Los Angeles; Principal, Milwaukee County Training School, 1909; Superintendent, Mercy Hosp., Janesville, Wisc., 1928; Registrar, Wisc. Nurses Club and Registry, Milwaukee, 1924; Supervisor of Field Nurses, Chicago Health Dept.; public health worker, Red Cross; organized school health work. **Organizations:** first president, WSNA; President, School of Nursing Alumnae; President, First District Assoc. of Ill. **Awards:** featured in "Who's Who in the Nursing World," *American Journal of Nursing*, 1928. **Died:** Oconomowoc, Wisc.

References and Credits

†Kelly HW: The relation of the private duty nurse to the directory. AJN 24:963, 1924.

Mirr MP: Helen Kelly. In Bullough V, Sentz L, Stein AP (eds): American Nursing: A Biographical Dictionary, vol. 2. New York, Garland, 1992, pp 178–180.

FEBRUARY 19

Ludie Clay Andrews

1875–1969

"I worked unceasingly for almost ten years against tremendous odds to secure state registration for colored nurses in Georgia, and finally succeeded in 1920 with the result that all colored nurses graduating from certified training schools are permitted to take the examinations and register." (1926)

LUDIE CLAY ANDREWS is a notable woman in Georgia's history. Her successful struggle with the Georgia State Board of Nursing for equality took a decade. The battle was spurred and perpetuated by white nurses who feared that registration of black nurses would interfere with their own employment. Although Andrews met the state requirements, had the support of white physicians, and was offered job opportunities in other states, she was unable to convince the Board of Nursing to treat her fairly. She hired a lawyer and worked with him to prepare a brief that showed her nursing preparation at Spelman Seminary (now Spelman College) met Georgia's requirements. Before their court appearance, and at her request, she and her attorney presented the information to the white nurses association; that group then withdrew its opposition. This allowed Andrews and other Spelman Seminary graduates to have equal testing and registration in Georgia. Andrews had earlier refused a license that was offered only to her but not to other black nurses who were equally qualified. She once recalled, “I had decided while in training that I wanted to work for my people, how or where this was to be done I did not know.”

Biography

Born: 1875, Milledgeville, Ga. **Education:** Nursing program, Macaicar Hosp., Atlanta; Spelman Seminary Nurse Training Dept. **Work history:** Private Duty Nurse; Superintendent, Lula Grove Hosp. and Training School, Atlanta; Charge Nurse, colored ward, Grady Hosp., Atlanta; Founder, first director of nurses, Municipal Training School for Colored Nurses, Grady Hosp.; Charge Nurse, Morehouse College Infirmary; College Infirmary, at Atlanta Univ.; Faculty, Atlanta School of Social Work, Morehouse Summer School; Morehouse-Spelman Summer School; Organizer, Neighborhood Union and Preschool Clinic. **Organizations:** Atlanta Graduate Nurses Club; Ga. State Nurses Assoc. (GSNA); Neighborhood Union; Georgia Interracial Commission; Church Cooperation Committee; member, bd. of directors, Leonard Street Orphans Home. **Awards:** Mary Mahoney Award, National Assoc. of Colored Graduate Nurses; Ludie Andrews Award, established by GSNA; Ludie Andrews Distinguished Service Award, given annually by Ga. Nurses Conclave. **Died:** location unknown.

References and Credits

†Hine DC: Black Women in White: Racial Conflict and Cooperation in the Nursing Profession, 1890–1950. Bloomington, Indiana University Press, 1989, p xxi.

Deceased Alumnae Collection, Ludie Clay Andrews file, box 1, Spelman College Archives, Atlanta.

Spencer T: personal communication, January 2001.

Carnegie M: The Path We Tread: Blacks in Nursing, 1854–1984. Philadelphia, JB Lippincott, 1986.

FEBRUARY 11

Susie Walking Bear Yellowtail

1903–1981

"Before I left [nursing school] ...I had to take my state board examination. ...I was really scared. ...After it was all over I was amazed how easy the test was for me. ...Before graduation, I had reminded the school to use my full name at the ceremony. ...When I went up to receive my diploma it was the first time they used my full name, Susie Walking Bear. ...I was really proud. ...Everybody sat there wide-mouthed. ...It was a big deal in those days, seeing as how I was the first Native American lady R.N. ever." (1923)

SUSIE WALKING BEAR YELLOWTAIL, an orphan, was part Crow, part Oglala Sioux, and a descendent of Red Cloud. She became a traditional native American healer and was an activist, educator, dancer, humorist, and entertainer. She was a goodwill ambassador for the U.S. State Department and was dubbed "Queen Mother Susie" by Prince Charles of England. She and her husband, Tom, toured Europe and Israel with the Native American Indian Dance Troop in 1950; both were traditional healers among the Crow. President John F. Kennedy appointed her to the Public Health, Education and Welfare Board in 1961. She was a proponent of better health care and education for her people and believed in combining mainstream medicine with the traditional Crow Sun Dance healing ceremony.

Biography

Born: 1903, Crow Agency, Pryor Mountain, Montana. **Education:** Bacone College, Okla.; East Northville Hosp. Training School, Springfield, Mass.; internship, Boston City Hosp. School of Nursing, 1926. **Work history:** Public Health Nurse, U.S. Public Health Service (USPHS), reservations in Minnesota and Montana; Public Health Nurse, midwife, until 1960 at Crow Agency, Mt.; promoted scholarships to train native Americans to be nurses and doctors; promoted reform of USPHS treatment of native Americans on reservations. **Organizations:** helped found Native American Nurses Organization; member, U.S. Public Health, Education and Welfare Bd. **Awards:** President's Award for Outstanding Nursing and Health Care, 1962; American Nurses Assoc. Hall of Fame. **Buried:** Crow Agency, Mt.

References and Credits

†Weatherly MB: excerpted from unpublished manuscript about her graduation from Boston City Hosp. School of Nursing.

Weatherly MB: personal communication, 1996.

Davis SM: Susie Yellowtail. In Bullough V, Sentz L, Stein AP (eds): American Nursing: A Biographical Dictionary, vol. 2. New York, Garland, 1992, pp 367–369.

ANA Hall of Fame 10/98 American Nurses Association, Washington, D.C. http://www.nursingworld.org/hof.

February 12

Sojourner Truth
1797–1883

"I want to say a few words about this matter. I am a woman's rights [sic]. *I have as much muscle as any man, and can do as much work as any man. I have plowed and reaped and husked and chopped and mowed, and can any man do more than that? I have heard much about the sexes being equal; I can carry as much as any man, and can eat as much too, if I can get it. I am as strong as any man is now. As for intellect, all I can say is, if woman have a pint and man a quart—why can't she have her little pint full? You need not be afraid to give us our rights for fear we will take too much—for we won't take more than our pint'll hold. The poor men seem to be all in confusion and don't know what to do. Why children, if you have woman's rights give it to her and you will feel better. ...I can't read, but I can hear. I have heard the Bible and have learned that Eve caused man to sin. Well if woman upset the world, do give her a chance to set it right side up again. ...And how came Jesus into the world? Through God who created him and woman who bore him. Man, where is your part?" (1851)*

BORN A SLAVE and illiterate throughout her life, Sojourner Truth was a gifted speaker, women's rights advocate, and famous abolitionist. She chose her descriptive name because she traveled widely to share God's truth (her legal name was Isabella Van Wagener). To raise money for supplies for runaway slaves, she sold captioned pictures of herself at her free lectures. She also supported herself and her causes by selling her book, *Narrative of Sojourner Truth: A Bondswoman of Olden Time* (1850). More than one hundred years before the civil rights movement of the twentieth century, she brought three successful lawsuits. In one of the first victories for a black woman against a white man, she sued a New York slaveowner who had violated state law when he sold her child out of state. He then had to return the child to her. A second lawsuit involved slander against her, and the third involved a physical dispute and subsequent injury related to her demand for equal seating on public transportation, as protected by law. During the Civil War she collected food and clothing for black regiments in the Union Army, taught cleanliness and basic nursing skills to caretakers at the Freedman's Hospital in Washington, D.C., lobbied Congress for money to prepare nurses and doctors, and was received by President Abraham Lincoln.

Biography

Born: 1797, Hurley, N.Y. **Education:** none. **Work history:** Slave, Abolitionist, Lecturer; Civil War nurse, Activist for civil rights, women's rights; counseled ex-slaves on resettlement as appointee to National Freedmen's Relief Assoc. **Organizations:** unknown. **Awards:** Mich. Women's Hall of Fame; National Women's Hall of Fame; U.S. postage stamp in her honor, 1986. **Died:** Battle Creek, Mich.

References and Credits

†Mabee C, Newhouse SM: Sojourner Truth: Slave, Prophet, Legend. New York, New York University Press, 1993, pp 81–82.

Adler D: A Picture Book of Sojourner Truth. New York, Holiday House, 1994.

Hardy GJ: Sojourner Truth. In Bullough V, Sentz L, Stein AP (eds): American Nursing: A Biographical Dictionary, vol. 2. New York, Garland, 1992, pp 330–332.

Truth S: Narrative of Sojourner Truth: A Bondswoman of Olden Time. New York, Oxford University Press, 1991.

Louise Zabriskie

1887–1957

"The ... time allotted by ... schools of nursing for the study of obstetrics is only sufficient for a foundation or a brief survey. ...For the nurse this is a wholly new phase of nursing. Past teachings have been based on the 'curative' point of view. ...In this course there is ... the study of ... changes during pregnancy, the crisis during labor and delivery, and the adjustments involved during the return to normal in the postpartum period and the months following. The nurse's attitude should be to aid nature in carrying through this reproductive function in a normal way. She must be able, not only to observe and evaluate with some precision the functions of the physical organs of reproduction, but, also, to have some understanding of the emotional reactions which accompany pregnancy ... [the nurse's] responsibility begins early in the prenatal period and extends several weeks and sometimes months beyond the birth of the child." (1937)

LOUISE ZABRISKIE WAS an early advocate for prenatal care because she recognized its importance to the health of mother and child. Her professional publications, notably, the *Nurses Handbook of Obstetrics* and her columns in popular magazines, were resources for professionals and parents. The *Nurses Handbook,* first published in 1929, appeared in nine editions. Few people realized that she became a quadriplegic when she was thirty-five, after suffering a fractured neck in an auto accident. Called "an example of nursing courage," she would arrive in the classroom before the students, in time to establish herself behind the desk, with a chin brace as the only visible means of support. After the accident she became an author, established and directed the Maternity Consultant Service in New York City, and worked as a lecturer at the New York University School of Nursing. Her ability to synthesize detail for critical assessments made her a valued consultant as well. One of her students said, "She never failed to give you something—knowledge, courage, strength or renewed interest."

Biography

Born: 1887, Preston City, Conn. **Education:** Northfield Seminary, Mass.; Columbia Univ.; New York Hosp. School of Nursing. **Work history:** New York Lying-In Hosp.; Public Health Nurse, Nashville, Tenn.; New York Maternity Center Assoc.; Faculty, New York School of Nursing, New York Univ. **Organizations:** unknown. **Awards:** memorial scholarship for nurses, New York Hosp. **Died:** New York City.

References and Credits

†Zabriskie L: Nurses Handbook of Obstetrics. Philadelphia, JB Lippincott, 1937, pp 3, 6, unnumbered page in "Orientation."

DeVincenzo DK: Louise Zabriskie. In Bullough V, Church OM, Stein AP (eds): American Nursing: A Biographical Dictionary, vol. 1. New York, Garland, 1988, pp 344–345.

Obituary for Louise Zabriskie, AJN 58:802, 1958.

FEBRUARY 14

Franc Florence Henderson

1874–1956

"In the nursing profession, as in all other lines of work, the tendency… is towards specialism, and… more efficient work is being accomplished. …Each nurse can find the line of work which is particularly adapted to her abilities, and by concentrating her energies she will attain a degree of skill in one direction which it would be impossible to acquire in all. …One special work… which is being taken up by nurses… is the giving of anaesthetics. …More and more surgeons are coming to realize the importance of having a regular anaesthetist and… a competent one from a well-trained surgical nurse. …Her whole attention is concentrated upon the welfare of the patient. …The habits of observation, …instilled into the nurse's makeup during… training, will be of great advantage. …The patient's confidence in the anesthetist is most important. …Patients are apt to yield themselves much more readily to the suggestive influence of the nurse." (1909)

FLORENCE HENDERSON STUDIED at the Mayo Clinic in Minnesota with Alice Magaw (Kessel), the "Mother of Anesthesia," and was an anesthetist there for more than a decade. Henderson was in demand as a practitioner, teacher, and speaker. She stressed the importance of each nurse-patient relationship and gently used the power of suggestion while administering open-drop ether.

She based her individualized approach on her careful observation and assessment of the patient, the nature of the surgery, and good rapport and communication with the surgeon. Surgeons sought out nurses to be taught by Henderson and Magaw when the surgeons saw the contrast between the nurse-anesthetist's personalized technique and that of the interns, who did not use suggestion, used excessive anesthesia, and often had to physically restrain their patients. The surgeons preferred to use nurses as anesthetists because the nurses could give their full attention to the patient and could easily build on the confidence that patients have in them. Henderson worked for only a few years after she moved to California to care for her mother. Her early retirement was related to pressure from the medical community. Later when California physician-anesthetists filed an unsuccessful lawsuit against a nurse-anesthetist, Dagmar Nelson, they tried to implicate Henderson. Although the decision clearly established the role for the nurse-anesthetist, Henderson did not practice again.

Biography

Born: Feb. 14, 1874, Illinois. **Education:** Knox College, Galesburg, Ill.; Bishop Clarkson Memorial Hosp. Training School for Nurses, Omaha, Neb.; learned to administer anesthesia at Clarkson Hosp., then studied with Alice Magaw (Kessel) at Mayo Clinic. **Work history:** Superintendent of Nurses, Clarkson Hosp.; Anesthetist, Mayo Clinic and several Los Angeles hospitals; ran a boardinghouse for professional women, Los Angeles. **Organizations:** American Red Cross, Calif. State Nurses Assoc., Los Angeles Nurses Club. **Awards:** unknown. **Died:** Los Angeles.

References and Credits

†Henderson, FF: The nurse as an anaesthetist. AJN 9:947, 949, 1909.

Harris NA: Franc Florence Henderson. In Bullough V, Sentz L (eds): American Nursing: A Biographical Dictionary, vol. 3. New York, Springer, 2000, pp 132–134.

FEBRUARY 15

Frances V. Brink

1889–1978

"Do not diagnose, *do not use* curative *methods without a physician's orders and a parent's permission. Do not take children to clinics without parents' permission. Do not confide your difficulties and criticisms to the teachers and townspeople, take them to your nursing committee. Do not make of your office a reception room for teachers and friends, keep your office private for all patients, old and young. Attend as many nurses' district, state and national meetings, conventions and institutes as possible. Remember that one hour [of] home calling is worth more than four hours in the office. Do not give up your work in the community in a short time after entering because it seems discouraging—this is pioneer work." (1921)*

FRANCES BRINK BROADENED rural nursing services in Minnesota and helped define public health nursing across the country when she was doing fieldwork for the National Organization of Public Health Nursing (NOPHN). While at Milwaukee County Hospital during the depression, she worked successfully with professionals and the community to improve salaries and adopt the eight-hour workday for graduate nurses. She was noted for high standards; and while she was in charge of the school of nursing, it became one of the first hospitals in the country to earn national accreditation from the National League for Nursing Education. She also developed an effective canvas restraint for restless patients, the "Brinksides," to replace the commonly used and less humane wooden bed bars.

Biography

Born: Feb. 14, 1889, Goodwin, S.D. **Education:** Philadelphia Hosp. Training School for Nurses. **Work history:** Staff Nurse, Philadelphia General Hosp.; Superintendent of Nurses, Minnesota Health Dept.; Public Health Nursing Administrator, Red Cross, Minn.; Staff, NOPHN; Nursing Educator, Administrator, Bellevue Hosp., N.Y.C.; Superintendent of Nursing, Principal, School of Nursing, Milwaukee County Hosp.; Director of Nursing, Principal, School of Nursing, Children's Memorial Hosp., Chicago. Consultant, Fla. State Tuberculosis Dept.; Consultant, Morris Memorial Polio Hosp., W. Va.; Teacher, Administrator, St. Mary's School of Nursing, W. Va., and W. Va. State Mental Hosp. **Organizations:** unknown. **Awards:** unknown. **Died:** Milton, W. Va.

References and Credits

†Brink FV: Suggestions for the county nurse. Public Health Nursing 13:173, 1921.

Dickson GL: Frances Brink. In Bullough V, Church OM, Stein AP (eds): American Nursing: A Biographical Dictionary, vol. 1. New York, Garland, 1988, pp 48–50.

February 16

Eleanor Crowder Bjoring

1930–

"Not one to be easily deterred by barriers I persisted in the pursuit of history. The longer I was involved the more convinced I was that some basic knowledge of nursing history was not only interesting but vital, if nurses were to have some idea of their past so the same rocky roads would not be repeatedly trod. . . . I do not expect all nurses to be history enthusiasts. However, I do think that history can and should be made palatable enough that even the most ardent opponent of nursing history will take one small step into the arena to get a taste of it." (1980)

Eleanor Crowder Bjoring's first career goal was to become an engineer, and she claims she was forced into nursing by her father. After completing a diploma program, she enrolled in a required American history course while she was an undergraduate at the University of Texas. Her young enthusiastic professor made history so fascinating, alive, and relevant that she was hooked. When she learned of the need for nurse historians, she was determined to fill that void. What she found was that, despite the work of notable other nurse historians, such as Mildred Newton and Teresa Christy, the discipline was not highly regarded. As Bjoring pursued her interest, she became more convinced that nurses need to know their past if the profession is to move forward. Nursing stereotypes cannot persist, she said, in the face of history. An eminent nurse historian, she prepared a pictorial history of nursing in Texas and established the Southwest Center for Nursing History at the University of Texas, Austin. She was one of the early organizers of the American Association for the History of Nursing (AAHN), which hosts an annual national conference for sharing historical research in nursing. A past president of AAHN, she continues to be actively involved and serves on the editorial review board of its official journal, *Nursing History Review.* Her professional career also included decades in university-level nursing education, disaster relief nursing, and she established the School Health Program at the American International School in New Delhi, India.

Biography

Born: Feb. 16, 1930, Harrisburg, Pa. **Education:** Univ. of Pennsylvania Hosp. School of Nursing (diploma); Univ. of Texas (BSN, MSN, PhD). **Work history:** Staff Nurse; OR Superintendent, Air Force flight nurse; YMCA camp nurse; disaster relief during the 1952 polio epidemic; Professor, Univ. of Texas, Austin, and Pennsylvania State Univ. **Organizations:** AAHN, American Nurses Assoc., National League for Nursing. **Awards:** four Teaching Excellence Awards; Sigma Theta Tau; Phi Kappa Phi.

References and Credits

†Crowder EM: Nursing in Texas: A Pictorial History. Waco, Texas, Texian Press, 1980, p vii.

Bjoring E: personal communication, 2002, 2003.

FEBRUARY 17

Mary Breckinridge

1881–1965

"Our best preventive work has grown out of the actual bedside nursing we have given the sick in their homes. It is in times of anxiety and strain that one gets close to people and the help so sorely needed then lays the foundation of trust which makes all things possible afterwards. The family which sleeps with open windows now is the one whose three-year-old boy we nursed through pneumonia last winter, the mother who consults us about her daughter's baths is the one whose same little daughter hung between life and death with typhoid, for whom we did everything until we had taught the mother how to do it. The baby who never misses a consultation is the one over whose bedside we hung when it was a feeding case at the lowest ebb. After such hours lived together we are welcomed as friends and our counsels do not seem like an intrusion." (1921)

MARY BRECKINRIDGE WAS the founder of the first modern rural comprehensive health care system in the United States. She was a public health nurse and the first certified U.S. midwife; she cared deeply for the underserved residents of rural Kentucky. She grew up in an educated and privileged home. Breckinridge wanted to attend college, a desire her family thought beneath her station. She married, and her first husband died of appendicitis. After his death she entered St. Luke's Hospital School of Nursing in New York and graduated in 1910. During her second marriage she had two children, a son and a daughter, both of whom died. Then she divorced her husband, resumed her maiden name, and volunteered to serve as a nurse in 1918 during the influenza epidemic. She spent the rest of her life studying and teaching midwifery and raising money to support the concept of rural maternal and child nursing. She used her inheritance to establish her beloved Frontier Nursing Service (FNS). She divided more than seven hundred square miles into six outpost nursing centers that served ten thousand people. Traveling by horseback to their patients, Breckinridge and her nurses brought maternal and infant mortality rates below the national average. In 1930, during the depression, she and her staff cut their salaries and continued to raise money to keep FNS functioning. Her motto: "If the father can come for the nurse, no matter what the weather, the nurse will always get to the mother." Banners in memory of Mary Breckinridge hang in the National Cathedral in Washington, D.C.

Biography

Born: Feb. 17, 1881, Memphis, Tenn. **Education:** Rosemont-Dezaley School, Lausanne, Switzerland; Heywood School, Stamford, Conn.; St. Luke's Hosp. School of Nursing, N.Y., 1910; attended special course sponsored by the Visiting Nurse Assoc. in Boston; studied public health, Teachers College, Columbia Univ., 1923–24; British Hosp. for Mothers and Babies, Woolwich, London, 1923 (midwifery certificate); toured nursing stations of Scottish Highlands and Inner and Outer Hebrides to learn about rural nursing. **Work history:** Nurse, Nursing Instructor, 1918 flu epidemic, Washington, D.C.; volunteered to work in France on behalf of American Committee for Devastated France; organized Ky. Committee for Mothers and Babies, Wendover, Ky., 1925 (it became FNS in 1928); established medical, surgical, and dental clinics; provided nursing and midwifery services around the clock; formed American College of Nurse Midwives, 1929; developed hospital and health center, FNS headquarters, Hyden, Ky.; formed graduate school of midwifery, 1939. **Organizations:** unknown. **Awards:** honorary doctor of laws degree, Univ. of Kentucky; Medaille Reconnaissance Française, France; Eleanor Van Rensselaer Fairfax Medal, National Society of Colonial Dames; Distinguished Service Medal, National Federation of Business and Professional Women's Clubs; Adelaide Nutting Award, National League for Nursing; ANA Hall of Fame.
Died: Hyden, Ky.

References and Credits continued on page 765

Wilma Scott Heide

1921–1985

"Reconceptualizing power itself can mean the empowerment of us all so that the power of love (in the sense of caring for ourselves and each other) can exceed the love of power to control others." (Date unknown)

"War is the ultimate expression of the 'masculine' mystique of which the 'feminine' mystique has been conditioned to sustain and even glorify. Feminism advances the 'feminine' as the humane, the peaceful, the thinkable, be-able and do-able. World policy-makers ignore, devalue, and/or peripheralize feminist implications at enormous cost." (1985)

WILMA SCOTT HEIDE's lifelong endeavor was to educate those who live in androcentric cultures and to elevate women to a position of equality. She spent her life learning about poverty, with a focus on women and poverty, and educating others about peaceful ways to eradicate poverty and suffering. She was responsible for reversing the position of the American Nurses Association (ANA), which had opposed the Equal Rights Amendment (ERA). She was a nurse, educator, writer, administrator, dynamic speaker, and scholar. As the two-term president of the National Organization for Women (NOW), she worked to remove every aspect of discrimination against women. Among the subjects that she pursued were passage of the ERA, segregation of employment advertisements in newspapers, sexist language, equal pay for women in all fields, health care for women, child care, poverty, illiteracy, racism, and the strengthening of international women's movements. Heide was a driving force in the *Pittsburgh Press* case that ended sex-segregated help-wanted ads. As a result of her endeavors, the ANA later formed a political wing, Nurses' Coalition for Action in Politics (N-CAP). In 1964 she wrote a twelve-part series, "Poverty Is Expensive," that appeared in the *Valley Daily News, New Kensington Daily Dispatch,* and other area newspapers in April 1965. She described herself as a feminist and humorist-at-large.

Biography

Born: Feb. 16, 1921, Ferndale, Pa. **Education:** Brooklyn State Hospital, N.Y., 1945 (nursing diploma); Univ. of Pittsburgh, 1950 (BS in sociology); Univ. of Pittsburgh, 1955 (MS in nursing and sociology); Union Graduate School, 1975 (PhD in psychology). **Work history:** Attendant, Staff Nurse, Pennsylvania Mental Hosp., Torrance, Pa.; Nurse, Pennsylvania College for Women; Health Education Instructor, School Nurse, Oswego, N.Y.; Educational Director, School of Nursing, Orangeburg (S.C.) Regional Hosp. **Organizations:** president, National Organization for Women, 1971–74. **Awards:** unknown. **Died:** Norristown, Pa.

References and Credits

†Heide WS: Feminism for the Health of It. Buffalo, N.Y., Margaretdaughters, 1985, rear cover and p 137.

Symonds JM: Wilma Scott Heide. In Bullough V, Sentz L, Stein AP (eds): American Nursing: A Biographical Dictionary, vol. 2. New York, Garland, 1992, pp 146–148.

February 19

Yssabella Gertrude Waters

1862–1938

"Industrial nursing is one of the newest developments of the public health field, it is also one of the most rapidly growing groups. Business interests demand it because it insures the health of the workers, therefore greater efficiency and a larger output is assured. From the nurses' standpoint it is an important one. It must be treated seriously with due regard to its very complex demands. It is not merely a matter of technical knowledge and skill in surgical dressings; a nurse thoroughly trained in all that her profession calls for possesses a most necessary foundation for the work, but she must have far more than that. She must have an infinite amount of tact, and good will. She must love people—human beings of whom none finer or more interesting exist than those found among the workers. ...Home visiting and the methods of handling family problems are very important factors of the work ... and fortunate is the nurse who can be independent of an interpreter." (1919)

YSSABELLA WATERS WORKED with Lillian Wald and served as a nurse in the Spanish-American War, but Waters's major contributions to nursing were her research and publications. While working at the Henry Street Settlement, she pursued a personal interest and began gathering data about public health nursing. Her interest in statistics provided information about nursing activities distributed by the National Organization for Public Health Nursing (NOPHN). Although she did this work as a volunteer, her comprehensive and detailed findings provided annual data used by other agencies. She published reports on industrial nursing that addressed its history as well as nursing qualifications and responsibilities. Her book *Visiting Nursing* addressed principles, organization, and administration and was considered a major resource regarding public health.

Biography

Born: Feb. 22, 1862, Groton, Mass. **Education:** Johns Hopkins Hosp. Training School for Nurses. **Work history:** Statistician, Henry Street Settlement. **Organizations:** NOPHN; Endowment Committee, Johns Hopkins Training School for Nurses; Society of Spanish-American War Nurses; Nurses Club of N.Y.C.; American Red Cross; Committee on Labor. **Awards:** unknown. **Died:** Groton, Mass.

References and Credits

†Waters Y: Industrial nursing. Public Health Nursing 11:731, 1919.

Bullough V: Gertrude Waters Yssabella. In Bullough V, Sentz L, Stein AP (eds): American Nursing: A Biographical Dictionary, vol. 2. New York, Garland, 1992, pp 345–346.

Agnes K. Ohlson

1902–1991

"We must be our own severest critics. We must safeguard the public from unethical and unqualified practitioners. We must control the practice of our profession. We must set our own standards, publicize them widely, and then effectively implement ever-improved excellence of practice. We must continue to search for ways to recognize and reward members of our profession for outstanding competency and performance. No nurse alone can hope to achieve the improvements we have been discussing. It will require the power and force of a unified profession working through the professional nurses' associations in districts, in states, and on the national level." (1958)

AGNES OHLSON RESPONDED to the discrepancies in state licensing examinations by asking the American Nurses Association (ANA) to convene a meeting of state board representatives from across the country. They set up a committee that included members of the National League for Nursing Education. Ohlson played a central role in forming the coalition and developing the first national qualifying examination for nurse licensure in the United States. Between 1944 and 1950 the State Board Test Pool Examinations steadily became the accepted test for all states. Ohlson served as the permanent secretary and chief examiner for the Connecticut State

Board of Examiners for Nursing from 1936 until her retirement in 1963. She held high offices in many nursing organizations, including secretary and president of the ANA and president of the International Council of Nurses (ICN) in 1957. She was the first recipient of the Agnes K. Ohlson Award for Outstanding Contributions to Nursing through Political Action, which was established in her honor by the Connecticut Nurses Association (CNA).

Biography

Born: Feb. 20, 1902, New Britain, Conn. **Education:** Peter Bent Brigham Hosp. School of Nursing, Boston; Teachers College, Columbia Univ. (BSN); Trinity College, Hartford, Conn. (MA in government). **Work history:** Supervisor, Wesson Maternity Hosp., Springfield, Mass.; Assistant Superintendent of Nurses, Truesdale Hosp., Fall River, Mass.; Director of Nursing Service and School of Nursing, Waterbury (Conn.) Hosp.; Chief Examiner, Conn. State Bd. of Examiners for Nursing; Consultant, U.S. Cadet Nurse Corps, World War II. **Organizations:** worked with state boards of nurse examiners; Chair, ANA Bureau of State Boards of Nurse Examiners Committee on State Board Problems of the National League for Nursing Education; President, ANA; President, CNA; Conn. State League for Nursing Education; President, American Nurses Foundation; President, ICN. **Awards:** ANA Hall of Fame; Agnes K. Ohlson Award for Outstanding Contributions to Nursing through Political Action. **Died:** location unknown.

References and Credits

†Ohlson A: Toward better nursing in our world (1985). In Flanagan L (ed): One Strong Voice: The Story of the American Nurses Association. Kansas City, Mo., Lowell Press, 1976, pp 539–540.

ANA on-line, available at http://www.ana.org/hof/ohlsak.htm.

Daisy CA: Agnes Ohlson. In Bullough V, Sentz L, Stein AP (eds): American Nursing: A Biographical Dictionary, vol. 2. New York, Garland, 1992, pp 255–257.

ANA Hall of Fame 10/98 American Nurses Association, Washington, D.C. http://www.nursingworld.org/hof.

February 21

Ethel Gordon Fenwick

1857–1947

"I venture to contend that the work of nursing is one of humanity all the world over." (1899)

Ethel Fenwick's remark about the universality of nursing was emblematic of the woman who helped establish the International Council of Nurses (ICN) during a lifetime of service to professional nursing. When she was appointed matron of St. Bartholomew's Hospital in London, she was only twenty-four but had studied nursing at two hospitals and brought ideas for nurse preparation that countered then-current practice. She understood that replacing poorly trained patient attendants with professional nurses, carefully selected and educated, would protect the public. She advocated a three-year period of study, standardized curriculum and testing, and compulsory national registration. Fenwick wanted the term *nurse* protected by law, such that only those who met specifically defined criteria could use it. Strong willed and controversial, she also supported one entry level for nursing education. Fenwick worked as a nurse for six years before marrying and leaving nursing, but she and her physician-husband both remained active in their support of professional nursing. Florence Nightingale, who focused more on nursing as a vocation, did not support Fenwick's goal of national registration. Fenwick persisted and used her position as founder and editor of the

British Journal of Nursing to promote her ideas. Although the struggle took thirty years, in 1919 the Nurse Registration Act was passed in England. It protected the term *nurse* and called for national standards for nurse education, examination, and registration. Fenwick was awarded Registration No. 1 in recognition of her work. She founded the ICN with Lavinia Dock and others and served as its first honorary president. She proposed and helped establish the Florence Nightingale International Foundation, in recognition of Nightingale's work and achievements. Fenwick was also instrumental in forming the British Nurses Association (BNA; later the Royal British Nurses Association) and the British College of Nurses (BCN).

Biography

Born: 1857, Elgin, Scotland. **Education:** Children's Hospital, Nottingham, England; Royal Infirmary, Manchester, England. **Work history:** London Hospital; Matron, St. Bartholomew's Hospital; founder, national and international nursing organizations; journal editor. **Organizations:** BNA; ICN; BCN; International Congress of Women. **Awards:** State Nurse Registration No. 1; commemorative plaque on her home in England. **Died**: England.

References and Credits

†International Council of Nurses on-line, available at http://www.icn.ch/PR15_99.htm.

Goodnow M: Outlines of Nursing History, 4th ed. Philadelphia, W.B. Saunders, 1931, pp 108, 113, 114, 227, 445.

Flanagan L: One Strong Voice: The Story of the American Nurses Association. Kansas City, Mo., Lowell Press, 1976, p 28.

Archives: Ethel Gordon Fenwick collection, St. Bartholomew's Hospital, London, England, on-line, available at http://www.aim25.ac.uk/cgi-bin/search2?coll_id=5168&inst_id=51.

On-line biography for Fenwick available at http://www.nurses.info/personalities_ethel_fenwick.htm.

Librario Publishing Ltd. on-line, available at http://www.librario.com:8080/librario/item/2508.

FEBRUARY 22

Sister Agnes Mary Gonzaga Grace
1812–1897

"The work of these Sisters began in the hospitals June 10, 1862, as a result of a requisition made for Sisters of Charity by Surgeon General Hammond. The hospital grounds covered... fifteen acres. The buildings... contained thirty-three wards, each accommodating seventy-five patients. On August 16, 1862, over 1500 soldiers were brought in, most of them from the Battle of Bull Run. Besides the usual maladies... there were a number of cases of smallpox, and the patients afflicted with this disease were removed to the smallpox hospital several miles from the city. But... the surgeon in charge obtained permission to keep the smallpox cases in the camp some little distance from the hospital. ...During a period of seven months there were ninety cases of smallpox, and all of them... were under the care of the sisters." (1897)

SISTER AGNES MARY GONZAGA GRACE was a member of the religious order of the Sisters of Charity of St. Vincent de Paul. Before, during, and after the Civil War, Sister Gonzaga was the administrator of an orphanage in Philadelphia. During the war she also worked with the staff at Philadelphia's Saterlee Hospital. According to the writer Lillie Sentz, research shows that when the physicians were setting up Saterlee Hospital, they asked that "it be staffed with Catholic sisters, stating that the sisters had two qualities that the so-called Dix nurses, i.e., the army nurses under the direction of Dorothea Dix, lacked: silence and obedience." Sister Gonzaga was one of more than two hundred religious who ministered to the armies of both sides. They worked on the battlefields, in the prisons, and in the hospitals of Philadelphia, Washington, D.C., and Gettysburg. Her journal documents that ninety-one members of her order cared for more than sixty thousand soldiers at Saterlee. In 1924 a monument was placed at the corner of Rhode Island and Connecticut avenues in Washington, D.C., to commemorate the work of the various religious orders that ministered to those on both sides during the Civil War. This tribute, "The Nuns of the Battlefield," was the result of the fundraising and lobbying efforts of the Ancient Order of Hibernians and its Ladies Auxiliary.

Biography

Born: Feb. 22, 1812, Baltimore. **Education:** St. Joseph's Academy, Emmitsburg, Md. **Work history:** Teacher, Pennsylvania; Administrator, St. Joseph's Orphan Asylum, Philadelphia; Assistant, Religious Novitiate, La.; Nurse, Administrator, Saterlee Hosp., Philadelphia. **Organizations:** unknown. **Awards:** Gonzaga Memorial Asylum, Philadelphia, built in her honor. **Died:** Philadelphia.

References and Credits

†Jolly ER: Nuns of the Battlefield. Providence, R.I., Providence Visitor Press, 1927, pp 67, 68.

Sentz L: Sister Agnes Mary Gonzaga Grace. In Bullough V, Sentz L, Stein AP (eds): American Nursing: A Biographical Dictionary, vol. 2. New York, Garland, 1992, p 134.

FEBRUARY 23

Julia Charlotte Thompson

1907–1972

"Throughout its history the ANA [American Nurses Association] has consistently supported legislation which would provide a greater measure of health and security to the public. Nurses consistently have been social minded in their approach to legislation believing that the federal government should provide services for the public which could otherwise not be secured. ...Behind all the legislative activities of the ANA stands the premise that every nurse is a lobbyist, that representatives and senators will be attentive to the wishes of their own constituents, that laws passed and the conduct of government are the responsibility of every citizen." (1960)

JULIA THOMPSON WAS a schoolteacher before she studied nursing. After nursing school she worked as a staff nurse, supervisor, and instructor in obstetrical nursing at Cook County Hospital in Chicago. When she moved to Kansas and joined the state nurses association, she worked on local and state legislative issues. Hired as the executive director of the ANA in 1951, she opened its Washington, D.C., office. She broke new ground when she created and filled the position of full-time lobbyist for the ANA. Thompson continued in this position for the next two decades and set the example for effective political action on behalf of nursing. She often was at Congress to speak on behalf of nursing, women's issues, health care, and social issues, and she wrote regular articles for the *American Journal of Nursing* to inform nurses of legislative concerns. She was involved with the legislative successes of Social Security for the disabled, federal funding for nurse education, and appropriate rank for military nurses. As a result of her lobbying success for Medicare, she accompanied President Lyndon Johnson to Independence, Missouri, for the bill signing.

Biography

Born: Feb. 23, 1907, Marathon County, Wisc. **Education:** Marathon County (Wisc.) Normal School; Cook County School of Nursing, Chicago; Univ. of Michigan (BS). **Work history:** various positions in obstetrical nursing, Cook County Hosp.; Instructor, obstetrics, Cook County School of Nursing; Staff Nurse, Infant Welfare Society, Chicago; Staff County Nurse, Utah Health Dept.; Superintendent, Director, Topeka-Shawnee County (Kans.) Health Dept.; Exec. Secretary, Lobbyist, ANA; consultant, ANA. **Organizations:** local, state nursing associations, legislative committees, ANA Legislative Committee. **Awards:** ANA Hall of Fame. **Died:** location unknown.

References and Credits

†Thompson J, Gerds G, Conners H: Every nurse a lobbyist. AJN 60:1244, 1960.

Cooper SS: Julia Thompson. In Bullough V, Church OM, Stein AP (eds): American Nursing: A Biographical Dictionary, vol. 1. New York, Garland, 1988, pp 311–313.

ANA Hall of Fame 10/98 American Nurses Association, Washington, D.C. http://www.nursingworld.org/hof.

February 24

Mary Lewis Wyche

1858–1936

"A nurse needs an occasional snapshot of herself, for her own scrutiny, to see her manners or lack of manners, and phonographic record of her tone, which might force her to exclaim:

'Wad some power the giftie gie us.
To see oursels as ithers see us.'

In some pictures one cries, 'A saint I see with voice and touch that soothes and inspires with hope.' We need… 'that ingrained regard for standards and ideas, for special knowledge and special skill, which marks the professional… and readiness to put the claims of public service and of intrinsic excellence of performers above considerations of private or personal gain.'" (1907)

Mary Wyche prepared to be a teacher before entering nursing. She returned to North Carolina after finishing nursing studies to establish the state's first nursing school in Raleigh. She was inspired and motivated by the presentations of nursing leaders that she heard at a meeting of the International Council of Nurses. She returned home with a strong belief in the importance of unity to strengthen the profession, and she organized what became the North Carolina State Nurses Association (NCSNA). She knew that registration of nurses would improve standards. She lobbied several sessions of the state legislature, unsuccessfully, for mandatory registration for nurses. However, as a result of her efforts, North Carolina did pass a nurse registration law and was the first state to offer the RN credential. Wyche recognized the importance of university-level nursing programs and is credited with starting the program at Duke University. She was active in the Red Cross and worked with a colleague to provide residential and financial resources for nurses who needed assistance.

Biography

Born: Feb. 26, 1858, Henderson, N.C. **Education:** Henderson College; Philadelphia General Hosp. School for Nurses. **Work history:** Superintendent, Rex Hosp., Raleigh, N.C.; Watts Hosp., Durham, N.C.; Sarah Elizabeth Hosp., Henderson, N.C.; Private Duty Nurse, Infirmary Nurse, State College for Women, Greensboro, N.C.; Red Cross nurse. **Organizations:** Raleigh Nurses Assoc., NCSNA, Bd. of Examiners of Trained Nurses of N.C.; Nurses Associated Alumnae of the United States; Red Cross Nursing Committee. **Awards:** ANA Hall of Fame. **Died:** Henderson, N.C.

References and Credits

†Wyche ML: Nursing conditions in the South. AJN 7:868, 1907.

Birnbach N: Mary Wyche. In Bullough V, Sentz L, Stein AP (eds): American Nursing: A Biographical Dictionary, vol. 2. New York, Garland, 1992, pp 366–367.

ANA Hall of Fame 10/98 American Nurses Association, Washington, D.C. http://www.nursingworld.org/hof.

February 25

Lavinia Lloyd Dock

1858–1956

"No occupation can be quite intelligently followed or correctly understood unless it is at least to some extent illuminated by the light of history interpreted from the human standpoint. The origin of our various activities, the spirit animating the founders of a profession, and the long struggle toward an ideal as revealed by a search into the past,—these vivify and ennoble the most prosaic labors, clarify their relation to all else that humanity is doing, and give to workers an unfailing inspiration in the consciousness of being one part of a great whole." (1920)

LAVINIA DOCK WAS born into a family of well-educated, liberal thinking, religious, affluent people. She was an accomplished organist and pianist. She seemed to have the ability to make the right choice at the right moment to put her talents to the best use. When her mother died, she and an older sister cared for their younger siblings. Years later, after her father died, she returned home to help her family again while her older sister completed her university studies in horticulture. Lavinia Dock worked in public health and education and wrote about nursing history. She was also active in the labor movement. She was an outspoken suffragette, war protester, and political activist who was jailed three times at demonstrations. She helped elevate nursing to a profession. In 1890, with her father's financial assistance, she was able to write and publish the drug manual *Materia Medica for Nurses,* the first nurses' manual on drugs and one of the first textbooks for nurses. In 1907 she shocked everyone by writing about venereal disease in her book *Hygiene and Morality.* She wrote the first two volumes of *The History of Nursing* with Adelaide Nutting and completed the last two volumes herself in 1912. She served as foreign editor of the *American Journal of Nursing* and was secretary of the International Council of Nurses (ICN) for more than twenty years. She was one of nursing's most outstanding historians. She was inducted into the American Nurses Association (ANA) Hall of Fame in 1976.

Biography

Born: Feb. 26, 1858, Harrisburg, Pa. **Education:** Bellevue Hosp. School for Nurses, N.Y.C., 1886. **Work history:** Visiting Nurse, Woman's Mission of New York City and Tract Society; Night Supervisor, Bellevue Hosp.; Supervisor of ward in temporary hospital for yellow fever victims under Jane Delano, 1888; helped flood victims in Johnstown, Pa.; Staff, Assistant Superintendent of Nurses (1890), Johns Hopkins Hosp.; Instructor, first-year classes, under Isabel Hampton Robb at Hopkins; Superintendent, Ill. Training School; lived at Nurses Settlement, N.Y.C., for twenty years, cared for sick immigrant poor and taught prevention, health education, and school nursing; helped organize women's local of United Garment Workers of America; researched various women's organizations; provided research material to found Nurses Associated Alumnae of the United States (later ANA); volunteer faculty member, postgraduate course for nurses, Teachers College, Columbia Univ.; **Organizations:** founder, secretary, ICN, London, 1899; helped Adah Thoms establish national organization for black nurses; worked on behalf of the Equal Rights Amendment. **Writings:** Contributing Editor, *AJN,* from 1900 to promote birth control; *The History of the Red Cross Nursing Service* (1922). **Awards:** ANA Hall of Fame. **Died:** Chambersburg, Pa.

References and Credits

†Dock L, Stewart IM: A Short History of Nursing from the Earliest Times to the Present Day. New York, GP Putnam's Sons, 1920, p 1.

Wilson JJ: Lavinia Dock. In Bullough V, Church OM, Stein AP (eds): American Nursing: A Biographical Dictionary, vol. 1. New York, Garland, 1988, pp 91–94.

Donahue, PM: Nursing, The Finest Art: An Illustrated History. St. Louis, Mo., CV Mosby, 1985.

ANA Hall of Fame 10/98 American Nurses Association, Washington, D.C. http://www.nursingworld.org/hof.

FEBRUARY 26

Luther Christman

1915–

"All professions are tied to the extraordinary expansion of science and technology. ... There's no way to avoid it. ... You have to look at how nursing articulates with it. If nursing doesn't stay in step ... it's going to be passed by. ... Nursing will fade out, because others are moving steadily into a format that allows them to do those things for patient care that nurses are now unwilling to do. Some aggressive action has to occur to prod nurses to respond as all other professions are doing, to survive. ... Nursing is not an island. It is surrounded by all other kinds of phenomena. ... If apathy, as we now see it, keeps going, then nurses are subdued. ... We'll slide into oblivion with no status, and nurses have to make that choice." (2000)

LUTHER CHRISTMAN WAS determined to have a career in professional nursing. A renowned nursing pioneer, he has been visionary, prophetic, innovative, and patient. Very concerned about nursing's future, he urges the profession to move forward, like all other professions, with research, technology, affirmative action, and a standardized entry level. He cites studies that link errors of omission in patient care to academic preparation of nurses and deems it unethical to issue the same license for differing entry levels. He outlasted prejudice against male nurses in clinical rotations, nursing degree programs, in the armed forces during World War II, as well as in professional organizations. He sparked the debate about the government policy against male military nurses that was not changed until the Korean War. Christman effected positive changes in clinical practice, collective bargaining, and college nursing programs. When he was appointed dean of the Nursing School of Vanderbilt University, he was the first male nursing dean in the country. In the 1950s he increased the number of male nurses there by actively recruiting medics being discharged from the military. He was the first to propose the American Academy of Nursing (1964) and founded the American Assembly for Men in Nursing (1974). During his tenure as dean of nursing at Rush University in Chicago, his analysis of hospital nurse staffing, cost, and quality of care connected professional nurse staffing patterns to improved professional initiative, accountability, and patient safety. This set the foundation for what later became known as primary nursing. He cites the lack of enforcement of affirmative action as a major reason for the nursing shortage, and he sees men as both the untapped resource and the solution. His publications and personal papers are held at the Nursing Archives Association, Muger Library, Boston University.

Biography

Born: Feb. 26, 1915, Summit Hill, Pa. **Education:** Pennsylvania Hosp. School of Nursing for Men; Temple Univ. (BSN; MEd); Mich. State Univ. (PhD). **Work history:** Corpsman, World War II; Faculty, Cooper Hosp. School of Nursing, Camden, N.J.; Yankston State Hosp., S.D.; S.D. State Bd. of Nursing; Associate Professor, Univ. of Michigan; Director of Nursing, Mich. State Mental Health Dept.; Dean, Vanderbilt Univ.; Director of Nursing, Vanderbilt Hosp.; helped establish Rush model of nursing at Rush Univ. College of Nursing and Allied Health Sciences, Chicago. **Organizations:** National League for Nursing; American Nurses Assoc.; Mich. Nurses Assoc.; Chicago Institute of Medicine; Alpha Kappa Delta; American Sociological Assoc.; National Academies of Practice; helped establish AARP in Tennessee. **Awards:** Fellow, American Academy of Nursing (AAN); Living Legend, AAN, 1995; Fellow, American Assoc. for the Advancement of Science; election to Institute of Medicine, National Academy of Sciences; honorary member, Alpha Omega Alpha (physician honor society); Old Master, Purdue Univ.; honorary doctoral degree, Jefferson Univ.; Founder's Award for Creativity, Sigma Theta Tau.; Marguerite Rodgers Kinney Award for a Distinguished Career; Lifetime Achievement Award, Sigma Theta Tau International and Tenn. Nurses Assoc. (TNA); honorary doctoral degree, Grand Valley State Univ., Allendale, Mich.; Dean Emeritus, Rush Univ.; Distinguished Alumnus Awards, Rush Univ., Michigan State Univ.; subject of two filmographies.

References and Credits continued on page 765

FEBRUARY 27

Mabel Keaton Staupers

1890–1989

"The issues of segregation and discrimination in nursing cannot be looked at narrowly. These two practices, wherever found, are mutually sustaining. Both must be eliminated if individuals and the nation are to realize their health and welfare." (1961)

MABEL KEATON STAUPERS was determined to reverse the arbitrary exclusion of blacks from the mainstream of nursing practice and was tireless in her efforts. She successfully championed the cause for equal opportunities, particularly in the military and in professional organizations. She put the focus on the need for integration in all areas. She was a leader in the National Association of Colored Graduate Nurses (NACGN) when membership in the American Nurses Association (ANA) was denied to black nurses, when options for entrance into nursing schools were limited, and when salaries were unequal. In addition, the service of black nurses in the Army Nurse Corps was limited by quota; the navy banned black nurses. Politically astute, Staupers used the wartime nursing shortage to work for change. She initiated a meeting with Eleanor Roosevelt, who backed Staupers's efforts to gain fairness for military nurses. Roosevelt's influence resulted in the elimination of racial barriers by the Army and Navy Nurse Corps in 1945. Staupers's efforts led the ANA to open its professional membership and become an integrated national nursing organization in 1948. Members of the NACGN subsequently voted to disband.

Biography

Born: Feb. 27, 1890, Barbados, West Indies. **Education:** Freedmen's Hosp. School of Nursing, Washington, D.C.; Henry Phipps Institute for Tuberculosis, Philadelphia. **Work history:** Booker T. Washington Sanitarium, Harlem, N.Y.; Jefferson Hosp. Medical College, Philadelphia, Researcher, N.Y. Tuberculosis and Health Assoc. (NYTHA); Exec. Secretary, Harlem Committee, NYTHA; Exec. Secretary, NACGN. **Organizations:** NACGN. **Awards:** Spingarn Medal, NAACP; ANA Hall of Fame. **Died:** Washington, D.C.

References and Credits

†Staupers, Mabel. No Time for Prejudice: A Story of the Integration of Negroes in Nursing in the United States. New Jersey, Pearson Education, 1961, p 176.

Hine DC: Mabel Staupers. In Bullough V, Church OM, Stein AP (eds): American Nursing: A Biographical Dictionary, vol. 1. New York, Garland, 1988, pp 295–297.

ANA Hall of Fame 10/98 American Nurses Association, Washington, D.C. http://www.nursingworld.org/hof.

Genevieve Cooke

1869–1928

"Inadequate as the numbers of nurses may be to succor more than an infinitesimal fraction of the precious lives now being sacrificed in battle, it is some small consolation to realize that even the simple title Nurse *means one who protects, one who nourishes, never one who destroys." (1915)*

GENEVIEVE COOKE IS remembered for her commitment to nursing journals as a method of educating and communicating with nurses. Accordingly, she was the founder of the *Pacific Coast Journal of Nursing,* an outgrowth of the *Journal of the California State Nurses Association.* She was so dedicated to the publication that she saved its financial records and contracts after her home was destroyed by the 1906 San Francisco earthquake. Cooke's other major interest was the advancement of nurse registration and professional organizations for nurses. She held many offices in nursing organizations, including the American Nurses Association (ANA), served on the board of the American Journal of Nursing Company, and was an ANA president. As president she advocated the creation of a house of delegates as the ANA governing body, and this came to pass in 1917. She worked for women's suffrage in California, and she always backed measures to provide nurses with a living wage and to limit workdays to eight hours for both students and nurses.

Biography

Born: Feb. 26, 1869, Dutch Flat, Calif. **Education:** California Woman's Hosp. Nursing School, San Francisco, 1888; Cooper Union Medical College, San Francisco (completed courses in anatomy and dissection); Harvard Summer School of Physical Training. Boston, 1901–1903. **Work history:** Private Duty Nurse, thirteen yrs.; Visiting Instructor, massage, several San Francisco hospitals; Editor, *Journal of the California State Nurses Association,* 1904–1909, 1912–15. **Organizations:** charter member, Women's Athletic Club, Calif. State Nurses Assoc. (CSNA); member, CSNA Committee on Legislation (to promote nurse registration); first CSNA delegate to ANA convention, 1906; First Vice President, ANA, 1907–1909; attended International Council of Nurses, Paris, 1907; twice elected president, San Francisco County Nurses Assoc. **Awards:** unknown. **Buried:** Mountain View Cemetery, Oakland, Calif.

References and Credits

†Cooke G: Address of the president of the American Nurses Association. AJN 15:920, 1915.

Englander S: Genevieve Cooke. In Bullough V, Church OM, Stein AP (eds): American Nursing: A Biographical Dictionary, vol. 1. New York, Garland, 1988, pp 65–68.

LeRoy N. Craig

1887–1976

"To a limited number of well-qualified young men, nursing offers an interesting educational and professional program. …Success in nursing depends on a considerable endowment of character and ability with capacity for growth. …The prospective student needs to be versatile in his interests and to possess a considerable degree of leadership. There should be evidence of adequate social growth and adjustment for his age. Nursing is not a profession for a poorly adjusted or inadequate person to undertake. The young man who is well liked and respected by his fellows and by older men is the most likely to succeed." (1940)

"There is satisfaction in doing work for which one is prepared." (1940)

"The status of the graduate registered man nurse today is more satisfactory than it was twenty-five years ago. There is evidence of better understanding in working relationships between men and women nurses. This parallels the broader viewpoint in the relationships and attitudes of men and women physicians. The increased esteem in which men nurses are held is probably due to a broadened viewpoint in the professions and to the fact that better prepared and more representative men are entering nursing as a career." (1940)

LeRoy Craig spent his nursing career working as a political and educational activist to promote male nurses in the fields of psychiatry and urology. He spent fifteen years as a political activist to ensure that federal legislation, the Bolton Bill of 1955, was passed. This law enabled qualified male nurses to receive equal status and equal commissions in the Army-Navy Nurse Corps. Craig was especially concerned about the effect on patient care if a nursing shortage occurred. He felt his efforts to promote nursing as a profession for men could significantly reduce the shortage. During his forty-two-year tenure as director of nurses at the Pennsylvania School of Nursing for Men, he proposed the inclusion of psychiatric nursing courses. His was one of the few schools of nursing to provide an intensive twelve-week course in neuropsychiatry to navy corpsmen serving in naval hospitals during World War II. Craig recognized the value of psychiatric training in treating war casualties.

Biography

Born: 1887, Dixmont, Maine. **Education:** McLean Hosp. Training School for Nurses, Waverley, Mass. **Work history:** Private Duty Nurse, Head Nurse, McLean Hosp. Training School for Nurses; Founding Director, Superintendent, Men's Nursing Dept., Pennsylvania Hosp. for Mental and Nervous Diseases, Philadelphia, 1914–56. **Organizations:** unknown. **Awards:** commendation for his unceasing efforts to end discrimination against male nurses, Pa. State Nurses Assoc. **Died:** Pemberton, N.J.

References and Credits

†Craig L: Opportunities for men nurses. AJN 40:666, 667, 670, 1940.

Buchinger KL: LeRoy Craig. In Bullough V, Sentz L, Stein AP (eds): American Nursing: A Biographical Dictionary, vol. 2. New York, Garland, 1992, pp 70–71.

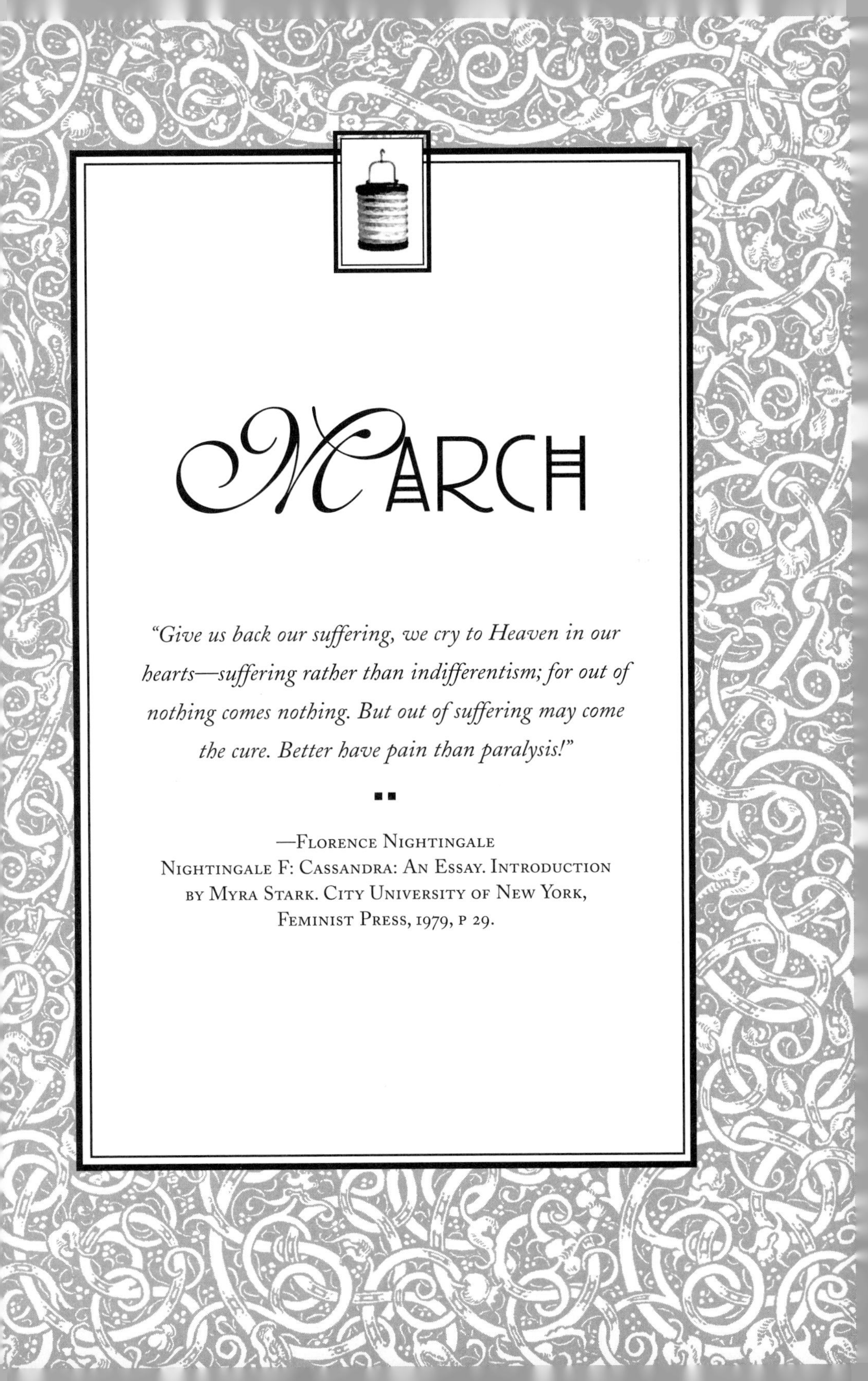

MARCH

"Give us back our suffering, we cry to Heaven in our hearts—suffering rather than indifferentism; for out of nothing comes nothing. But out of suffering may come the cure. Better have pain than paralysis!"

—Florence Nightingale
Nightingale F: Cassandra: An Essay. Introduction by Myra Stark. City University of New York, Feminist Press, 1979, p 29.

March 1

Harriet Bailey

1875–1953

"One of the most important nursing duties is to observe closely and record accurately the symptoms, often unexpected and transitory, which the patients disclose by changing moods; unusual, impulsive, or inhibited behavior; and the content of thought expressed spontaneously or in response to audible voices, or those of purely psychogenic origin. Many noted psychiatrists have acknowledged the help these notes may give in completing the social or medical history and supplying additional facts upon which to base diagnosis and treatment. To minimize the importance of or neglect instruction in this phase of nursing is to place a handicap upon the nurses' efficiency in the graduate nursing field." (1936)

Harriet Bailey was an educator, author, and dedicated advocate for mental health nursing. In 1935 the National League for Nursing Education (NLNE) and the American Psychiatric Association sponsored her to study state hospitals for the mentally ill and their nursing schools. Her findings were published in what became known as the Bailey Report. She referred to mental health nursing as the "unwelcome subject," and, while recognizing the need for nurses to learn psychiatric nursing, she addressed some of the limits on nursing schools in state hospitals. She addressed budget, the need for qualified faculty, opportunities for broad clinical experience for students, the availability of equipment, and the need for improved coursework and clinical practice for student nurses. She promoted the inclusion of psychiatric nursing in the general nursing school curriculum. Bailey proved to be both a pioneer and a catalyst for the recognition and growth of psychiatric nursing in the United States. Her textbook for psychiatric nursing, *Nursing Mental Diseases,* was the first of its kind by a nurse educator and was used by students for twenty years. Her persistence helped others to see the value and importance of this nursing specialty.

Biography

Born: 1875, location unknown. **Education:** Johns Hopkins Hosp. School of Nursing; Teachers College, Columbia Univ. **Work history:** Henry Phipps Psychiatric Clinic, Johns Hopkins Hosp., Baltimore; Manhattan State Hosp., N.Y.; Appointee, League of Red Cross Societies, Switzerland; Secretary, N.Y. State Bd. of Nurse Examiners; Associate Editor, *International Journal of Public Health.* **Organizations:** Accrediting team, NLNE. **Awards:** unknown. **Died:** Bangor, Me.

References and Credits

†Bailey H: Nursing schools in psychiatric hospitals: Report of a survey. AJN 36:504, 1936.

Church OM: Harriet Bailey. In Bullough V, Church OM, Stein AP (eds): American Nursing: A Biographical Dictionary, vol. 1. New York, Garland, 1988, pp 15–16.

Bertha Harmer

1885–1934

"What we learn from any one experience depends upon the amount of thought involved in it; that is, what we learn depends on the keenness with which we observe what goes on about us, upon the degree of thought such observations arouse, upon the degree in which our actions are controlled by such thoughts, and upon our ability to see the connections and relationships—that is, the how and the why—between what we and others do and what happens as a result of our doing. ... To learn or profit by experience, therefore, a student must learn to observe keenly, to think before she acts, and to learn from the results of her actions how to adjust, direct and control her future experience." (1925)

BERTHA HARMER SAID she entered nursing because she wanted a life of service. The writer Meta R. Pennock quotes Harmer as saying that she "found [nursing] satisfying from every standpoint, spiritual and intellectual. It satisfied my interest in human welfare, in science, philosophy, and administration." She excelled in nursing administration, teaching, research, and writing. When she was a faculty member at Yale's School of Nursing, she designed the curriculum so that theory correlated with practice. She put an emphasis on prevention as well as treatment. The *Textbook of the Principles and Practice of Nursing* (1922), which she completed in one year, was used throughout the world. It recognized the role of the nurse as health educator. The wide-ranging and comprehensive contents included hygiene, hospital admissions and discharge, and nutrition, as well as specialized information about medical and surgical conditions, their treatments, infectious diseases, and emergencies. Her text stressed the importance of observation in nursing and is still cited.

Biography

Born: March 2, 1885, Port Hope, Ontario, Can. **Education:** Jarvis Collegiate Institute, Toronto; Toronto General Hosp. School of Nursing (RN); Teachers College, Columbia Univ. (BS, MA). **Work history:** Instructor, Toronto General Hosp. School of Nursing; Instructor, St. Luke's Hosp., N.Y.; Instructor, Vassar Training Camp; Faculty, Yale School of Nursing; Assistant Superintendent of Nurses, New Haven (Conn.) Hosp.; Director, McGill Univ. Graduate Nursing Program. **Organizations:** unknown. **Awards:** unknown. **Died:** Toronto.

References and Credits

†Birnbach N, Lewenson S: First Words: Selected Addresses from the National League for Nursing, 1894–1933. New York, National League for Nursing Press, 1991, p 49.

Pennock MR (ed): Makers of Nursing History. New York, Lakeside, 1940, p 115.

Hermann EK: Bertha Harmer. In Bullough V, Church OM, Stein AP (eds): American Nursing: A Biographical Dictionary, vol. 1. New York, Garland, 1988, pp 164–166.

March 3

Esther Silverstein Blanc

1913–1997

"I developed the idea that if you created a therapeutic environment around yourself, you were the greatest beneficiary, because you lived in it. ...It worked in any place I ever worked. It worked in my house, in my marriage, and in my life. And it's so simple. There are eight rules. [They] have to do with how you deal with other people. You treat everyone you meet with respect and esteem and regard and normal affection. ...The next one has to do with genuineness. You definitely have to be real. ...The most important of all is egalitarianism. You really have to believe that all men are created equal. ...Next is empathy... [The] empathetic [person] says, 'I'm going to do my best to feel as you feel, and I will act accordingly.' The last one is desperately important too. It says that the only kind of love you're allowed is non-possessive. ...You can embody all these principles if you work at it—because they take work. ...This method keeps you from hurting other people. It keeps you looking at their insides instead of their outsides. And creating adequate responses from yourself, which produces adequate responses from the patients." (1992)

Esther Silverstein Blanc's parents were immigrant Jews from Romania, and she said they instilled in her a social consciousness. She inherited a gratitude for American ideals from them. This influenced her decision to go to Spain during the Spanish Civil War because she described herself as a stout antifascist and wanted to help. She was one of several nurses from the United States who volunteered in response to a call for help against the fascism threatening Spain in 1936. They carried their professional standards of practice across the Atlantic. In the face of very limited medical and financial resources, these women worked with physicians to use such life-saving approaches as "the mobile operating room, the triage concept…, refrigerated blood and transfusion procedures, and various techniques to treat major wounds and reduce gas gangrene infections," according to the historian Jim Fryth. The international nurse volunteers, he writes, "reduced mortality rates among the wounded to levels below that of any previous war." A film by Julia Newman, *Into the Fire: American Women in the Spanish Civil War,* documents the work of these volunteers and includes lengthy interviews with Blanc. Blanc also served as an army nurse during World War II and chronicled her nursing experiences in a three-act play, *Wars I Have Seen,* and in her published short stories. She also clearly described how the nurse can become a therapeutic tool by applying her eight rules to nursing practice, with subsequent increased trust on the part of the patient and increased insight on the part of the nurse. Blanc held a doctoral degree in the history of medicine, which she taught at the University of California, San Francisco. Dr. Helen Ference, director of the Nightingale Society, described Blanc's comfortable home in San Francisco as "reminiscent of Miss Nightingale's home … in London."

Biography

Born: 1913, Goshen County, Wyo. **Education:** Univ. of California, San Francisco and Berkeley; Univ. of Rochester; Univ. of Oklahoma; San Francisco State Univ. (master's); Univ. of California, San Francisco (PhD). **Work history:** Staff Nurse, Private Duty Nurse, Marine Hosp., San Francisco; (U.S. Public Health Service); Nurse, Spanish Civil War; Director, orphanage, San Francisco; ER Nurse, Berkeley (Calif.) General Hosp.; staff, Osborne Zoological Lab, New Haven, Conn.; Staff Nurse, Yale Hosp.; Staff Nurse, Visiting Nurse Assoc., Rochester, N.Y.; U.S. Army Nurse, World War II; staff, research,

Biography continued on page 766

March 4

R. Louise McManus

1896–1993

"Nursing... had not been able for some time to attract the numbers of high school graduates needed to fill... programs and meet health needs. ... Could preparation for registered nurses for practice under supervision be adapted to fit into the patterns of the technical programs of junior and community colleges? ...By qualifying for the registered nurse licensure in two academic years rather than three calendar years, the nurse would start earning a whole year earlier, and the community's supply of nurses would be built up more quickly. [Starting community college nursing programs] seemed worthy of experimentation." (1977)

LOUISE MCMANUS MARRIED a widower with six children and had one child of her own before her husband's death four years later. Her ability to combine single parenthood and a demanding career was exceptional. She was a creative thinker and a resourceful problem solver who is credited with envisioning the nursing team concept. A dedicated patient advocate and an internationally renowned resource on professional nursing, she held one of nursing's first earned doctoral degrees. She was one of nursing's innovative leaders. For example, she prepared a hospital-accepted Patient's Bill of Rights long before the twenty-first century debates. Among her many achievements are the Testing Service of the National League for Nursing (NLN) and the Institute for Nursing Research at Columbia University. She helped develop standardized testing and scoring with the State Board Test Pool Examinations, which made it easier for nurses to work in different states. In 1952 she initiated a research project, directed by Mildred Montag, to determine whether two-year nursing programs at community and junior colleges could prepare general duty nurses who would be clinically competent. The successful associate degree program for nursing addressed both the nursing shortage and advanced professionalism, by moving nursing to the college level.

Biography

Born: March 4, 1896, North Smithfield, R.I. **Education:** Pratt Institute, N.Y., Massachusetts General Hosp. School of Nursing (diplomas); Teachers College, Columbia Univ. (bachelor's, master's, PhD). **Work history:** Nursing Faculty, Administrator, Teachers College, Columbia Univ.; Author; Consultant to numerous federal agencies; Researcher; Nursing Education adviser, Turkey. **Organizations:** various Quaker organizations, Falmouth (Mass.) Family Planning Service, American Assoc. of Univ. Women, Cape Cod Community Health Council, various Cape Cod organizations. **Awards:** Columbia Univ. Bicentennial Award; Florence Nightingale Medal, International Committee, Red Cross; Adelaide Nutting Award, NLN; member, National Women's Hall of Fame; awards in her name given by Teachers College and National Council Boards of Nursing. **Died:** location unknown.

References and Credits

†Safier G: Contemporary American Leaders in Nursing: An Oral History. New York, McGraw-Hill, 1977, p 200.

National Women's Hall of Fame on-line, available at http://www.greatwomen.org.

Drusilla Rageu Poole

1921–1981

"In-service education . . . helps the nursing personnel to help themselves; it increases the availability of the educational opportunities present in every institution; it awakens the members of the staff to their own needs; it encourages them in their concern for nursing and their own professional growth." (1953)

Drusilla Poole's versatile career in nursing included clinical nursing, teaching, and leadership at home and abroad. She was an advanced medical-surgical nurse specialist and an advocate for in-service education. When she established one of the early in-service education departments at the Emory University Hospital in Georgia, her approach guaranteed success. After taking time to become oriented to the facility and its program in the school of nursing, she developed a survey questionnaire for the staff. She learned about educational and clinical backgrounds, concerns about clinical practice, and their interest in staff development programs. She established an advisory committee and a program committee, which ensured that the staff would participate in planning the programs. Poole also worked for the Yale-in-China program as an administrator and teacher, until escalating political interference resulted in her house arrest and forced her departure in 1950. Her interest in disaster nursing led to a leadership role at the University of

Minnesota School of Nursing. She served with the Army Nurse Corps in Korea, directed the Walter Reed Army Institute of Nursing, and was the speaker when the nursing memorial was dedicated at Arlington National Cemetery in 1972. She was buried with full military honors at Ft. Sam Houston, Texas.

Biography

Born: March 5, 1921, Cornersville, Tenn. **Education:** Martin Junior College, Pulaski, Tenn.; Scarritt College for Christian Workers, Nashville, Tenn. (AB); Yale School of Nursing (MN); Yale Institute of Far Eastern Languages; Univ. of Texas, Austin (PhD). **Work history:** Superintendent of Nurses, Instructor, Hsaing-Ya Hosp., Yale-in-China Program; Clinical Nurse, Grace–New Haven (Conn.) Hosp.; Instructor, Superintendent, Burbank Hosp., Fitchburg, Mass.; Director of In-Service Training, Emory Univ. Hosp., Atlanta; Army Nurse Corps; Head, Disaster Nurse Project, National League for Nursing; Univ. of Minnesota School of Nursing; Director, Walter Reed Army Institute of Nursing. **Organizations:** unknown. **Awards:** Dr. Anita Newcomb McGee Award; Distinguished Alumnae Award, Yale School of Nursing. **Buried:** Ft. Sam Houston, Texas.

References and Credits

†Poole D: In-service education reaches a milestone. AJN 53:1436, 1953.

Hays JC: Drusilla Poole. In Bullough V, Church OM, Stein AP (eds): American Nursing: A Biographical Dictionary, vol. 1. New York, Garland, 1988, pp 262–263.

March 6

Freddie Louise Powell Johnson

1931–1982

"Nurses also need to consider the influence of prescribed health practices on religious beliefs of the minority, to identify positive strategies, to explore the support systems utilized in gaining life satisfaction, and to determine the meaning of health or illness to the minority person." (1982)

"Ethnicity does influence life satisfaction and mental health. Influences of the norms and values of the predominate culture, whether favorable or unfavorable, cannot be discounted when assessing mental health and life satisfaction of minority groups. The uniqueness of each ethnic group must not be overlooked." (1982)

FREDDIE JOHNSON IS remembered for her many firsts—she was the first black graduate of the University of Nebraska School of Nursing and the first person to earn a doctoral degree through the American Nurses Association (ANA) Fellowship Award for Ethnic Minorities. Her major interests were nursing administration and the care of the elderly. She held positions that revealed her talents in such areas as research mentor, teacher, recruiter, and adviser to minority students, and through those positions she influenced the content of the health education programs. She served on many college, community, and nursing boards, and she was often recognized for her service and contributions to nursing. She founded and organized a health care clinic and, with the help of other like-minded and dedicated nurses, set an example by donating her time for health care screening. Her research thesis, about territoriality in the institutionalized elderly and the life of satisfaction of rural and urban elderly, started to attract national attention in the1980s. However, Johnson was diagnosed with pancreatic cancer and was unable to continue her work. Among the many tributes to her is a scholarship fund in her name at the University of Nebraska.

Biography

Born: March 6, 1931, Vicksburg, Miss. **Education:** Univ. of Nebraska School of Nursing, Omaha, 1952 (BSN); Margaret Hague Maternity Hosp., Jersey City, N.J., 1953 (postgraduate certificate); Univ. of Omaha (now Univ. of Nebraska) (MA in nursing education); Univ. of Nebraska, Lincoln, 1976 (PhD in adult and continuing education}. **Work history:** Staff Nurse, Assistant Head Nurse, Head Nurse for Obstetrics, Univ. of Nebraska Hosp.; Nursing Supervisor, Salvation Army's Booth Memorial Hosp.; Clinical Associate, Visiting Nurse Assoc.; Volunteer Primary Nurse, health maintenance clinic for elderly; Faculty, Assistant to the Director, Nursing Care Research Center College of Nursing, Univ. of Nebraska Medical Center, Omaha; Acting Director, Univ. of Nebraska Medical Center, 1981. **Organizations:** member, office holder in numerous professional and community organizations; ANA, National League for Nursing (NLN), Adult Education Assoc., American Heart Assoc., American Gerontological Assoc., Delta Sigma Theta Sorority, National Black Nurses Assoc.; President, Omaha Black Nurses Assoc.; Accreditation Visitor, NLN; member of review bd., Site Visitor, National Institutes of Mental Health, 1979–82; member, governing bd., Midwest Nursing Research Society, 1980–82; Girl Scout leader; President, Parent-Teacher Assoc.; Sunday School Teacher, Trinity United Methodist Church. **Awards:** Outstanding Teacher Award, 1982; recognized by College of Nursing Alumni Assoc., 1977; member, Sigma Theta Tau, 1978; listed in *Who's Who in Nebraska,* 1977, *Who's Who Among Notable Americans,* 1979. **Died:** Omaha.

References and Credits

†Johnson FLP et al.: Comparison of mental health and life satisfaction of five elderly ethnic groups. West J Nurs Res 10:626, 1988.

Schneckloth NW: Freddie Johnson. In Bullough V, Sentz L, Stein AP (eds): American Nursing: A Biographical Dictionary, vol. 2. New York, Garland, 1992, pp 166–168.

March 7

Emily Elizabeth Parsons

1824–1880

"My evening visits are important ones. One of the men who died here the other day interested me very much. I sat by him some time the evening he supposed would be his last; when I got up to go, he bade me good-by so touchingly, holding my hand in his poor trembling ones. I wonder whether I shall ever meet these dying ones again. I have watched by some I should like to see again bright and happy. This is a curious sort of life and there is one thing trying about it; every night when I review the day I see something which I could have done better, or ought to have done differently. It is rather discouraging to see one self so far from being just what one should be, or near it." (1863)

Despite serious health problems as a child, Emily Parsons was inspired by reports of Florence Nightingale's work in the Crimea. Parsons wanted to prepare herself to work as a nurse during the American Civil War. Family connections made it possible for her to study nursing with surgeons at the Massachusetts General Hospital for one and a half years. She learned about general hospital nursing care, diet, wound care, and organization. She then worked at the Ft. Schuler Hospital on Long Island Sound and Lawson Hospital in St. Louis, and was the head nurse on a hospital steamer that transported sick and wounded soldiers from Vicksburg,

Mississippi, to Memphis, Tennessee, for hospitalization. Her greatest contribution, however, was her service at the Benton Barracks Hospital near St. Louis. She was its superintendent of nurses for the male army nurses as well as the female nurses. Supported by the chief surgeon, she directed and guided her largely inexperienced staff to care for approximately two thousand patients. The hospital earned a reputation for excellent nursing care and patient recovery. She survived several bouts of malarial fever. Upon returning to Cambridge, Massachusetts, in 1864, she worked to establish a much-needed charity hospital there for women and children.

Biography

Born: March 8, 1824, Taunton, Mass. **Education:** Massachusetts General Hosp. **Work history:** Civil War Nurse, Ft. Schuyler Hosp., N.Y.; Lawson Hosp., St. Louis; *City of Alton* hosp. steamer, Benton Barricks Hosp., St. Louis; Western Sanitary Commission; Fundraiser, "Cambridge for Charity Hosp." **Organizations:** unknown. **Awards:** Office complex named in her honor at Mt. Auburn Hosp., Mass. **Died:** location unknown.

References and Credits

†Reverby S (ed.): Civil War Nursing: Hospital Sketches by Louisa May Alcott and Memoir of Emily Elizabeth Parsons, The History of American Nursing. New York, Garland, 1984, p 77.

Brockett LP: Women's Work in the Civil War. Computer program by H-Bar Enterprise, 1995.

James E, James J, Boyer P (eds): Notable American Women, 1607–1950: A Biographical Dictionary, vol. 3. Cambridge, Mass., Belknap Press, 1971.

Snodgrass ME: Historical Encyclopedia of Nursing. Santa Barbara, Calif., ABC-CLIO, 1999.

March 8

Leah Curtin

1942–

"We in nursing share a common cause and a common tradition. We ... have a tradition with a future. The tender loving care of human beings ... will never become obsolete. In today's strained world among tomorrow's strange machines, people more than ever *need to be touched to be restored, renewed, revived and redeemed. Today, technology has brought us closer than ever before to the pain of living, so finally we have learned that health really does lie in restoring independence, not merely ministering to illness. If we really believe this, then we know, as surely as anyone can know, that nurses' hands—helping hands—can also be used to help themselves." (1988)*

Leah Curtin is recognized as one of nursing's most widely read and articulate authors. She is known for her clear, sharp, concise writing style and her ability to cut to the core of the issue. A peer described her as "a national treasure." A knowledgeable resource on ethics and health care in the United States, she is the author of eight books, hundreds of articles, and even more editorials. Her factual and wide-ranging editorials address such topics as health care costs, patient safety, staffing ratios, leadership, ethical issues, and health care reform. She incorporates anecdotes, parables, and quotations from literature and history to make the point. The first virtual faculty member of the University of Colorado School of Nursing, Curtin also has been a scholar-in-residence in Australia and a visiting scholar at universities in Utah, Oklahoma, and Kentucky. She testified in Denmark, at the invitation of the Danish minister of health, about the effect on the safety of patient care of hospital restructuring in the United States. She has also been a distinguished lecturer for the Hong Kong Hospital Authority. A recent book, *Sunflowers in the Sand: Children's Stories of War*, was researched in the Balkans and written for a general audience. Its sale has raised nearly $100,000 for the care and treatment of children who suffered in that war.

Biography

Born: March 8, 1942, Chicago. **Education:** Good Samaritan Hosp. School of Nursing Cincinnati, Ohio (RN); Univ. of Cincinnati (BS, MS); Athenaeum of Ohio (MA). **Work history:** Staff Nurse; Visiting Nurse; Faculty, Univ. of Cincinnati College of Nursing and Health; Editor, *Nurse Management, Journal of Health Systems Management;* Virtual Faculty, Univ. of Colorado School of Nursing; Lecturer; Consultant; Author. **Organizations:** unknown. **Awards:** Fellow, American Academy of Nursing; honorary doctorates, State Univ. of New York, Medical College of Ohio; Businessman of the Year, Republican Congressional Committee; award from Ohio Nurses Assoc.; award from Franciscan Sisters of the Poor; listed in *Who's Who in America* since 1991, *Who's Who in the World* since 1992; *Who's Who in American Nursing.*

References and Credits

†Curtin L: Nursing: Why stay? In *Nursing into the Twenty-first Century*. Springhouse, Pa., Springhouse, 1996, pp 28, 29.

Curtin L: *Curtincalls*: available on-line at http://www.curtincalls.com.

Curtin L: resume.

Curtin L: personal correspondence, July, November 2002.

Who's Who in American Nursing, 1996–97, 6th ed. New Providence, N.J., Reed Reference, 1995, p 137.

March 9

Dorothy A. Cornelius
1918–1992

"There is great recognition of the need for nursing to speak with one voice on social issues in the areas of poverty, malnutrition, hunger and discrimination, all of which profoundly affect the health and well-being of the people of this country. ...The ANA [American Nurses Association] has a potential as a force in society which we have only begun to tap. Nursing is the conscience of the health care system. Through the years, nursing has taken leadership among the professions to secure the rights of human beings to receive adequate health care. Many times nursing has stood alone to support the principle that health care is a right, not a privilege. If we are to continue to advance the health care system and to fulfill our role as professionals, we must be prepared to stand alone again." (1970)

THE ANA HALL of Fame describes Dorothy Cornelius as "a charismatic leader, remarkable conciliator and expert strategist." Her professional leadership skills had a positive influence on both national and international nursing. When she was president of the ANA, she initiated an unprecedented meeting between nursing, the American Medical Association, and the American Hospital Association to define their common interests and concerns and identify approaches to working together. A testament to her expertise and professionalism was that four presidents—Dwight D. Eisenhower, John F. Kennedy, Lyndon B. Johnson, and Richard M. Nixon—called on her to serve on national committees. Another successful program during her tenure at ANA was the "BE-INvolved" search, which focused on the actions of individual nurses all over the country who were making a difference. She called on nursing to exercise its collective power to affect national policy, not only on health care but on social and environmental issues.

Biography

Born: March 9, 1918, Pennsylvania. **Education:** Conemaugh Valley Memorial Hosp. School of Nursing, Johnstown, Pa.; Univ. Pittsburgh School of Nursing (BSN). Work history: Public Health Nurse, Johnstown, Pa.; Nurse, American Red Cross; Exec. Director, Ohio Nurses Assoc. (ONA); member, Commission on Aging (Ohio); Chair, Ohio Women's Defense Council; national committee work as presidential appointee. **Organizations:** ONA, ANA, International Council of Nurses. **Awards:** Governor's Commendations, Ohio, Pa.; named one of Ohio's Top Ten Women; ANA Hall of Fame. **Died:** location unknown.

References and Credits

†Cornelius D: Is ANA relevant in the seventies? (1970). In Flanagan L (ed): One Strong Voice: The Story of the American Nurses Association. Kansas City, Mo., Lowell Press, 1976, pp 578, 579.

ANA Hall of Fame 10/98 American Nurses Association, Washington, D.C. http://www.nursingworld.org/hof.

March 10

Lillian D. Wald

1867–1940

"In the last two decades, coincident with a social unrest because of things detrimental to human happiness, the nurse has emerged into public movements. The appeal to her is the appeal of the community. And that is not at the cost of the single patient or the single mother, but because of the sanctity of life and motherhood and the conviction that the mother, as well as the unborn child and the infant newly born, have become the trust of society. These things challenge the attention of the educated nurse today. It has become her responsibility to make practical application in the homes of the people of the results of scientific thought and research." (ca.1906)

Lillian Wald was an activist and reformer in the fullest sense of those words. One of America's greatest humanitarians and most effective and influential women, she was attracted to nursing by the example of the nurse who provided care during her sister's difficult pregnancy. As a staff nurse in New York City's Juvenile Asylum, Lillian Wald was appalled by the conditions and lack of care. She entered medical school, thinking it the best way to become independent and effective in social reform. While teaching a home nursing class for immigrants on New York's Lower East Side, she was called to assist a hemorrhaging mother. This firsthand introduction to poverty and deprivation caused Wald to leave medical school and live among those who were in direct need of help. She found that the immigrants were "the most helpless of our population, and the most exploited." The settlement house on Henry Street was born. It attracted other pioneers, dynamic nurses who, while providing care in people's homes at little or no cost, did much to advance the profession of nursing and public health nursing in particular. Wald had a passion for reform in labor law as it applied to children and women, women's rights, world peace, and racial justice. Her lecture series on public health nursing at Teachers College, Columbia University, evolved into the nursing school. Her work to establish the Federal Children's Bureau demonstrated her belief that nurses have a responsibility to be effective agents for change in public policy. In 1902 she promoted the value of school nursing in a New York City demonstration project, starting the nationwide provision of what is now known to be an essential service.

Biography

Born: March 10, 1867, Cincinnati, Ohio. **Education:** New York Hosp. Nursing School; attended Women's Medical College of Pennsylvania. **Work history:** Staff Nurse, Juvenile Asylum, N.Y.C.; established Henry Street Settlement for public health nursing; pioneer activist in many social and political reform issues; Author; Lecturer. **Organizations:** Founder, Town and Country Nursing Service, American Red Cross (1912); founder, Women's Trade Union League (1903); Founder, Vocational Guidance Committee, Henry Street Settlement (1906); Cofounder, National Labor Committee (1924). **Awards:** Gold Medal, National Institute of Sciences; Rotary Club Medal; Better Times Medal; congressional and presidential recognitions; American Nurses Assoc. Hall of Fame. **Died:** Westport, Conn.

References and Credits

†Coss C: Lillian D. Wald: Progressive Activist. New York, Feminist Press, 1989, pp 67, 81.

Falk G: Lillian Wald. In Bullough V, Church OM, Stein AP (eds): American Nursing: A Biographical Dictionary, vol. 1. New York, Garland, 1988, pp 331–334.

March 11

Jean E. Johnson

1925–

"Patients scheduled for an endoscopic exam were subjects in the hospital experiments. ...In both experiments the patients who heard a description of the sensations frequently experienced during the examination required less tranquilizer to enable them to tolerate the tube than the patients who heard no taped message. Indications of emotional upset while the tube was in place were less for those patients who heard a description of sensations as compared to those who heard a description of the endoscopic procedure. ...The demonstration that the sensation and distress components of the pain experience can be rated separately and do not have a one-to-one relationship challenges the traditional method of measuring pain by determining thresholds." (1973)

Jean Johnson studied nursing because she wanted to earn a college degree, and she said she was allowed to go to college if she "studied a useful field for women, like nursing." Her distinguished career included staff nursing, teaching, and research. She writes that she did not appreciate the full value of nursing to society until she was introduced to the role of science in nursing. This helped her to realize the importance of evidence-based practice. Her doctoral dissertation addressed the effect of accurate expectations on the sensory and distress components of pain. Her findings demonstrated that the way that people are prepared for a health procedure affects their emotional response. This was defined as a separate consideration than the sensory response. She found that when people received an accurate description of the sensations that they would experience, they had realistic expectations and therefore less emotional distress. These findings had important implications for health care workers.

Biography

Born: March 11, 1925, Wilsey, Kans. **Education:** Kansas State Univ., Kansas Univ. Medical Center (BS in nursing and home economics); Yale Univ. (MS); Univ. of Wisconsin, Madison, (MS, PhD). **Work history:** Staff Nurse, Nursing Instructor, In-service Educator, Faculty, Director of Health Research, Wayne State Univ., Detroit; Faculty, Nursing and Cancer Center, Univ. of Rochester, N.Y. **Organizations:** American Nurses Assoc. (ANA); Oncology Nursing Society. **Awards:** election to Institute of Medicine, National Academy of Sciences; Fellow, American Academy of Nursing; awards, from ANA, American Nurses Foundation, Oncology Nursing Society, American Psychological Assoc.

References and Credits

†Johnson JE: Effects of accurate expectations about sensations on the sensory and distress components of pain. J Pers Soc Psychol 27:274, 1973.

Johnson JE: personal correspondence, 2002.

March 12

Louise Matilda Powell

1871–1943

"Not only the nurse, but every woman at the present time needs all the practice she can get in self government, as a means of preparation for intelligent, interested citizenship. Our educated, thinking women must be prepared to wield, through the franchise, an influence on political life that will be felt and will be acknowledged as worthwhile. In no better way can we give our nurses this practice than by allowing them a share in the government of one department of an institution which deals with human problems in infinite variety, a modern hospital." (1920)

Louise Powell first prepared to teach grade school but after working as a teacher decided that she would rather be a nurse. One deciding influence was thought to be her grandfather, a caring physician who was involved with the care of the mentally ill. When Louise Powell finished nursing school, Adelaide Nutting recommended her for the position of superintendent of nurses at the University of Minnesota. That school of nursing, established in 1909, had the distinction of being "the first university school of nursing in the world," according to the writer Brenda H. Caneday. Its admission requirements were the same as those for other university students. By 1919 Powell's pioneering achievements in curriculum changes and her "lionhearted courage" produced a five-year baccalaureate program for nurses. She was an advocate for student self-government, because she believed that it would promote personal responsibility, make the school attractive to thinking women, help develop the skills of good citizenship, and promote a sense of justice. Throughout her life she continued to study, remained active in professional organizations, and wrote for publication.

Biography

Born: March 12, 1871, Staunton, Va. **Education:** Stuart Hall, Staunton, Va.; St. Luke's Hosp., Staunton, Va.; Teachers College, Columbia Univ.; postgraduate clinical experience, Hosp. for Sick Children, Mt. Wilson, Md., and Municipal Hosp. for Contagious Diseases, Philadelphia; Teachers College, Columbia Univ. (education diploma); Smith College and Univ. of Virginia (bachelor's degree). **Work history:** Univ. of Minnesota School of Nursing; established Central School of Nursing, Univ. of Minnesota; Dean, Western Reserve Univ. School of Nursing. **Organizations:** Minn. League for Nursing Education; National League for Nursing Education; Minn. Nurses Assoc.; American Red Cross; Minn. Organization for Public Health Nursing. **Awards:** Univ. of Minnesota nursing residence named Louise M. Powell Hall. **Died:** Staunton, Va.

References and Credits

†Powell L: Student self government in schools of nursing. AJN 20:476, 1920.

Caneday BH: Louise Powell. In Bullough V, Church OM, Stein AP (eds): American Nursing: A Biographical Dictionary, vol. 1. New York, Garland, 1988, pp 265–266.

March 13

Faye Glenn Abdellah

1919–

"Professional nurses want to be able to do nursing. Poor utilization of nursing personnel, pressures of paper work, increased supervision of part-time employees and increased number of treatments requiring preparation away from the bedside are some of the barriers preventing nurses from nursing. ... The present hospital hierarchy has succeeded in taking the nurse away from the patient. The higher in the hierarchal structure she goes the less she sees of the patient. Education for improved practice is seldom utilized at the bedside. The bedside nurse is the low man on the totem pole. For economic reasons and for reasons of professional status, she must go up or out of the existing hierarchy. We must continuously ask, 'What reason can nursing have to exist as a profession without the patient?'" (1960)

Faye Glenn Abdellah made a career decision to enter nursing as a teenager, the day she had an opportunity to assist the victims of the *Hindenburg* dirigible explosion and fire. Her illustrious career of almost fifty years continued after her retirement with her work as founding dean and professor emerita at the Graduate School of Nursing at the Uniformed Services University of the Health Sciences in Bethesda, Maryland. When she retired as deputy surgeon general for the U.S. Public Health Service (USPHS) with the rank of two-star rear admiral, she left a legacy in nursing research, theory, and education that helped define progressive, patient-centered care, including the first federally tested coronary care unit. She called for changes in nursing school curricula that would broaden the concept of professional nursing and develop the abilities to define and address nursing problems as presented by the needs of each patient. This resulted in nursing theory based on science. She was part of the research effort that established Diagnostic-Related Groups and helped establish national health policy related to the AIDS epidemic as well as the needs of the elderly. She promoted the value of advanced nursing practice, particularly in school health, senior care, and the care of veterans. Her many publications include the classics *Patient-Centered Approaches to Nursing* (1960) and *Better Patient Care through Nursing Research* (1986). Her papers and publications are available at the National Library of Medicine in Bethesda.

Biography

Born: March 13, 1919, New York City. **Education:** Fitkin Memorial Hosp. School of Nursing (later Ann May School of Nursing), Neptune, N.J.; classes at Rutgers Univ.; Columbia Univ. (BS, MA, DEd). **Work history:** Director, Health Services, Child Education Foundation, N.Y.C.); Staff Nurse, Head Nurse, Columbia-Presbyterian Hosp., N.Y.C.; Faculty, Yale Univ. School of Nursing; Research Fellow, Teaching Assistant, Teachers College, Columbia Univ.; USPHS; Faculty, Univ. of Washington, Univ. of Colorado, Univ. of Minnesota; Author; Researcher; Consultant to World Health Organization, International Council of Nurses; founding dean, Graduate School of Nursing, Uniformed Services Univ. of the Health Sciences. **Organizations:** N.Y. Academy of Sciences; American Assoc. for the Advancement of Science; National League for Nursing; American Nurses Assoc. (ANA); American Nurses Foundation; Bd. of Regents, National Library of Medicine; Gerontological Society. **Awards:** twelve honorary degrees, more than eighty-eight awards, incl. Charter Fellow, American Academy of Nursing; Living Legend, American Academy of Nursing, 1994; awards from Sigma Theta Tau, ANA, USPHS, and military honors; Hall of Fame–Distinguished Graduates and Scholars, Columbia Univ.; National Women's Hall of Fame; G.V. "Sonny" Montgomery Award for Leadership in the Veterans Administration/Defense Dept. Distant Learning Program, 2002; election to Institute of Medicine, National Academy of Sciences.

References and Credits

†Abdellah FG: Rationale for patient-centered approaches to nursing. In Abdellah FG, Beland I, Martin A, Matheney R (eds): Patient-Centered Approaches to Nursing. New York, Macmillan, 1960, p 37.

References and Credits continued on page 766

March 14

Anna Caroline Maxwell

1851–1929

"The pioneers of nursing had to have courage, patience, and perseverance of rare quality. They had to convince the medical profession, the hospital management, and the public, of the value of instructed nurses, of the interdependence between medicine and nursing, and to gain the moral and financial support of our best people. ... To keep a true sense of proportion amid conflicting interests; to see the ebb and flow of events demolish our cherished hopes, or to wait years for results and then begin over again,—these require undaunted courage. A high privilege of service has been opened to the nursing profession. Let us prove worthy of the trust." (1921)

ANNA MAXWELL STUDIED with Linda Richards in Boston. Maxwell's commitment to high professional standards elevated both the status and dignity of nursing. She was a nursing leader with exceptional organizational skills, evidenced by her ability to establish schools of nursing and her outstanding work with nurses during the Spanish-American War. Her efforts to have nurses work in military hospitals during that war resulted in the historic decision to continue the practice. She is credited with envisioning and helping establish the Army Nurse Corps, and she lobbied for officer rank for nurses in the military. The eventual affiliation of Presbyterian

Hospital with Columbia University fulfilled her conviction that university-level education was essential for nurses. Called "the American Florence Nightingale" and "the dean of American Nurses," she was buried at Arlington National Cemetery with full military honors.

Biography

Born: March 14, 1851, Bristol, N.Y. **Education:** New England Hosp. for Women and Children; Boston Training School for Nurses, Massachusetts General Hosp. **Work history:** established school of nursing, Montreal; Superintendent, Boston Training School for Nurses; established Training School for Nurses, St. Luke's Hosp., N.Y.C.; established School of Nursing, Presbyterian Hosp., N.Y.C.; organized military nursing service, Spanish-American War; military nurse, World War I; worked to establish Army Nurse Corps.; worked to reorganize American Red Cross. **Organizations:** American Nurses Assoc. (ANA); American Red Cross; International Council of Nurses. **Awards:** Medaille d'Honneur de l'Hygiene Publique, France; honorary master of arts, Columbia Univ; nursing residence at Columbia named for her; member, ANA Hall of Fame. **Buried:** Arlington National Cemetery.

References and Credits

†Maxwell A: Struggles of the pioneers. AJN 21:321, 326, 329, 1921.

Downer JL: Anna Maxwell. In Bullough V, Church OM, Stein AP (eds): American Nursing: A Biographical Dictionary, vol. 1. New York, Garland, 1988, pp 232–236.

James ET et al. (eds): Notable American Women, vol. 2. Cambridge, Mass., Belknap Press, 1971.

ANA Hall of Fame 10/98 American Nurses Association, Washington, D.C. http://www.nursingworld.org/hof.

March 15

Sister Mary Olivia Gowan
1888–1977

"Nursing in its broadest sense may be defined as an art and a science which involves the whole patient—body, mind, and spirit; promotes his spiritual, mental, and physical health by teaching and by example; stresses health education and health preservation, as well as ministration to the sick; involves the care of the patients' environment—social and spiritual as well as physical; and gives health service to the family and community as well as to the individual." (1944)

When she was a young girl, Sister Mary Olivia Gowan heard stories about her Scottish great-grandmother's care of the sick. Gowan was the oldest child in her family and her own ill mother's caretaker. She completed nursing school before she entered a Benedictine convent. She had good teaching and administrative abilities, which led to opportunities to upgrade and standardize the hospital where she was superintendent. The hospital was placed on the prestigious list of hospitals approved by the American College of Surgeons upon its first review. The first nursing courses to be offered by a Catholic university or college were those that she established at the Catholic University of America, where she later served as dean of the School of Nursing.

Biography

Born: March 15, 1888, Stillwater, Minn. **Education:** St. Mary's School of Nurses, Duluth, Minn.; St. Scholastica College, Duluth, Minn. (BS); Teachers College, Columbia Univ. (master's degree). **Work history:** School Nurse, Faculty, College of St. Scholastica; OR Superintendent, St. Joseph's Hosp., Brainard, Minn.; Faculty, St. Mary's School of Nurses; Superintendent, St. Mary's Hosp.; Sister Superior, St. Gertrude's School of Arts and Crafts for Retarded Children, Washington, D.C.; Faculty, Catholic Univ. of America, Graduate School of Arts and Sciences, and later the School of Nursing Education; Consultant, U.S. Public Health Service; Adviser, Veterans Administration Nursing Service; Honorary Consultant, U.S. Navy Bureau of Medicine and Surgery; Honorary Fellow; American Hosp. Assoc. **Organizations:** National League for Nursing Education; Assoc. of Collegiate Schools of Nursing; Washington, D.C., League for Nursing Education; Council of National Defense; Nursing Council on National Defense; International Council of Nurses. **Awards:** unknown. **Died:** Duluth, Mich.

References and Credits

†Gowan MO: Aims of Nursing Administration: School of Nursing Education, Catholic University of America. Washington, D.C., Catholic University Press, 1947, p iii.

Stein AP: Sister Mary Olivia Gowan. In Bullough V, Church OM, Stein AP (eds): American Nursing: A Biographical Dictionary, vol. 1. New York, Garland, 1988, pp 152–159.

Bellardini A: personal communication, 2003.

March 16

Julia Otteson Flikke

1879–1965

"It is for the purpose of affording to each soldier the highest type of professional skill that nurses are asked to accept the responsibility of rendering professional care to the young defenders of their country, regardless of sacrifices which in many instances must be made." (1943)

COL. JULIA O. FLIKKE was the sixth superintendent of the Army Nurse Corps (1937–1943). At the convention of the American Nurses Association (ANA) in 1938, the corps announced that it would increase its strength from 600 to 675 nurses. By July 1941 the goal was four thousand nurses. On D-Day the U.S. Army had ten thousand nurses stationed in Great Britain alone. Flikke addressed the recruitment dilemma in all her writings and public statements. She wrote *Nurses in Action* to portray nurses' history in the corps and to encourage women to enlist. When she entered the service in 1918, she was assigned as a principal chief nurse in many hospitals around the world. She was the first woman to hold the rank of colonel in the U.S. Army. It was called a "relative rank"—she wore the insignia of her grade but was denied the pay of that grade because of a ruling from the comptroller general, who found that female army officers were not "persons" in the sense of the law under which they were promoted. In 1952 Congress passed a law that reversed the decision, and Flikke, then retired received the pay that had been withheld for ten years. She received an honorary doctor of science degree from Wittenberg University in Springfield, Ohio.

Biography

Born: March 16, 1879, Viroqua, Wisc. **Education:** Viroqua High School, 1899; Augusta Hosp. Training School, Chicago, 1915; studied administration and nursing education, Teachers College, Columbia Univ. 1915–16, 1925. **Work history:** Assistant Superintendent of Nurses, Augusta Hosp., Chicago, 1916; joined Army Nurse Corps, 1918; Chief Nurse, Base Hosp. No. 11, France; other overseas assignments; Principal Chief Nurse, Walter Reed General Hosp., 1922–34; Assistant Superintendent (1927), Superintendent (1937) with rank of major, Army Nurse Corps. **Organizations:** Lutheran Church; member, Twentieth Century Club, Washington, D.C.; American Legion. **Awards:** citation for "outstanding service and proficiency," Ft. Sam Houston, Texas. **Died:** location unknown.

References and Credits

†Flikke J: Nurses in Action: The Story of the Army Nurse Corps. Philadelphia, JB Lippincott, 1943, p 89.

Feller CM, Moore CJ (eds): Highlights in the History of the Army Nurse Corps. Washington, D.C., U.S. Army Center of Military History, 1995, pp 12–13.

Brook M: Julia Flikke. In Bullough V, Sentz L, Stein AP (eds): American Nursing: A Biographical Dictionary, vol. 2. New York, Garland, 1992, pp 116–117.

Margaret Baggett Dolan

1914–1974

"The skills of the professional nurse are needed throughout the world. The opportunity to travel, to learn of different cultures, to promote understanding among people of the world, to learn other languages, and to share knowledge and experiences with other nurses will appeal to more and more young nurses as they seize this opportunity for service and personal growth and enrichment. It is possible for the professional nurse to find employment in almost any part of the country she wishes to live. She can live, work, learn and earn as she travels in this country and throughout the world." (1961)

MARGARET DOLAN WAS a public health nurse whose career included stints as a visiting nurse, tuberculosis nurse-consultant, educator, and leader; she also worked in epidemiology. She was a knowledgeable advocate for quality health care, health care reform, and the versatility of professional nursing in primary care. For more than two decades she testified on health care legislation before Congress on behalf of the American Nurses Association (ANA). When she chaired a legislative committee for the ANA in 1960, she called for separate licensing exams for graduates of the two-, three-, and four-year basic nursing programs. In 1972 as president of the ANA, she worked to increase the organization's effectiveness by addressing its need to develop standards for clinical practice and education. She was a widely recognized leader in professional and governmental organizations. She emphasized the necessary role that the nursing profession plays in the health and social reform of communities. She also represented the ANA at several meetings of the International Council of Nurses.

Biography

Born: March 17, 1914, Lillington, N.C. **Education:** Anderson College Anderson, S.C. (AA); Georgetown Univ. (RN); Univ. of North Carolina, Chapel Hill, (BSPHN); Teachers College, Columbia Univ. (MA). **Work history:** Staff Nurse, Instructive Visiting Nurse Society, Washington, D.C.; Consultant, U.S. Public Health Service; Administrator, Greensboro (N.C.) Health Dept.; Administrator, Baltimore County (Md.) Health Dept.; Faculty, Univ. of North Carolina School of Public Health; Consultant to U.S. Army surgeon general and governments of Ghana and Thailand. **Organizations:** American Public Health Association (APHA); several national advisory councils on social policy, health, defense, insurance, and nursing education; President's Commission on the Status of Women, ANA, National League for Nursing, American Assoc. of Univ. Professors, Sigma Theta Tau, Phi Theta Kappa, Kappa Delta Pi, Delta Omega. **Awards:** John Carroll Alumni Award, Georgetown Univ.; Pearl McIver Award, honorary membership, ANA; APHA Centennial Award, memorial lectureship; honorary doctorates from Duke Univ., Univ. of Illinois; ANA Hall of Fame; memorial library fund at Univ. of North Carolina. **Died:** Cherry Hill, N.C.

References and Credits

†Dolan MB: Employment opportunities for nurses. Nurs Outlook 9:226, 1961.

Stein AP: Margaret Baggett Dolan. In Bullough V, Church OM, Stein AP (eds): American Nursing: A Biographical Dictionary, vol. 1. New York, Garland, 1988, pp 94–96.

Dolan M: Putting our own house in order. AJN 62:76–79, 1962.

Notes of March 10, 1960, ANA Committee on Legislation, ANA Archives, Boston University.

ANA Hall of Fame 10/98 American Nurses Association, Washington, D.C. http://www.nursingworld.org/hof.

Ellen Gertrude Ainsworth

1919–1944

"Second Lieutenant Ainsworth was on duty in a hospital ward while the area was being subjected to heavy enemy artillery shelling. One shell dropped within a few feet of the ward, its fragments piercing the tent in numerous places. Despite the extreme danger Second Lieutenant Ainsworth calmly directed the placing of surgical patients upon the ground to lessen the danger of further injury. By her disregard of her own safety and her calm assurance she instilled confidence in the assistants and her patients, thereby preventing serious panic and injury. Her courage under fire and her selfless devotion to duty was an inspiration to all who witnessed her actions, and reflect the highest traditions of the Army of the United States." (1946)

Ellen Ainsworth enjoyed having fun and engaging in antics with others. She was serious about her work, but she could always find the humor in serious situations. She had an enchanting sense of humor and was sensitive and kind. Her short life ended as a result of the wounds she sustained in the line of duty during the Battle of Anzio in Italy, just before her twenty-fifth birthday. She was the only nurse from Wisconsin to die from enemy fire in World War II. She was posthumously awarded the Silver Star, the nation's third-highest award for bravery; the Purple Heart; and the Red Cross

Bronze Medal. Ainsworth is buried at the U.S. Military Sicily-Rome Cemetery, in Nettuna, Italy. The inscription on the headstone reads, "She Lies Among the Men She Served." In 1980 the Ainsworth Conference Room in the Pentagon was dedicated to her.

Biography

Born: March 9, 1919, Downsville, Wisc. **Education:** Eitel Hosp. School of Nursing, Minneapolis, 1941. **Work history:** Assistant Supervisor, medical-surgical unit, Eitel Hosp.; Second Lieutenant, U.S. Army Nurse Corps, March 9, 1942, serving at Station Hosp., Camp Chaffee, Ark.; 56th Evacuation Hosp., Brooke General Hosp., Ft. Sam Houston, Texas, then was sent to Bizerte, Tunisia, and relocated to Anzio. **Organizations:** unknown. **Awards:** posthumous Silver Star, Red Cross Bronze Medal, Purple Heart; nursing care building at Wisconsin Veterans Home in King named Ainsworth Hall; dispensary at Ft. Hamilton, N.Y., named Ainsworth U.S. Army Health Clinic; conference room in Pentagon named for her. **Died:** Anzio, Italy.

References and Credits

†Cooper SS: Ellen G. Ainsworth. In Bullough V, Sentz L, Stein AP (eds): American Nursing: A Biographical Dictionary, vol. 2. New York, Garland, 1992, pp 3–4.

Red Cross Bronze Medal awarded posthumously. AJN 46:496, 1946.

March 19

Margretta Madden Styles

1930–

"I have encouraged nurses everywhere to
Think of a world in which nurses are a strong, vital, and dynamic social force.
Think of a world in which nursing is at the forefront of health care.
Think of a world in which the word 'nurse' has a singular, positive meaning and the image of nursing is sharp and distinct in the eyes of the public.
Think of a world in which nursing speaks with one voice.
Think of a world in which nurses bring honor and reward to themselves, to all women, and to all people.
Think of a world in which the words of Florence Nightingale, 'No system shall endure that does not march,' resound through our daily lives.
Think of a world in which the Director-General of the World Health Organization is a nurse. This, by the way, is my dream for nursing." (1985)

Margretta Styles, known as Gretta, personifies the global voice for nursing. Credentialing and the structure and governance of the profession are her foremost contributions to nursing. Styles is a nurse-scholar who has researched and synthesized nursing education and practice, and she has written extensively about her findings. Her career in academic nursing includes developing and harmonizing all three nursing programs (associate degree, baccalaureate, and higher-degree programs). She brought humility, devotion, and charismatic leadership to her positions when she served as professor and dean of various universities. She was a pioneer in defining nursing credentialing that recognized and differentiated quality in all aspects of nursing practice. She was the motivating force behind the creation of the American Nurses Credentialing Center (ANCC) as part of the ANA. This work expanded the services and programs in the United States and abroad, especially nursing specialty certification, magnet hospital recognition, and accreditation for providers of continuing education. She is a past president of the American Nurses Association (ANA), the International Council of Nurses (ICN), and the ANCC. Styles says, "Nursing is my identity, in fact, my obsession."

Biography

Born: March 19, 1930, Mt. Union, Pa. **Education:** Juniata College (BS in biology and chemistry); Yale Univ. (MN); Univ. of Florida (EdD). **Work history:** Management, Veterans Administration Hosp.; Faculty, diploma program, Brooklyn; Associate Director of Nursing, community hosp.; founding director, associate degree program, Florida; Assistant Dean, undergraduate studies, Duke Univ.; Founding dean, School of Nursing, Univ. of Texas Medical Center, San Antonio; Dean, Wayne State Univ., Detroit; Professor, Dean, Associate Director, nursing service, Univ. of California, San Francisco; President, ANA, 1986; President, ICN, 1993–97. **Organizations:** ANCC; Director, Credentialing International; Chair, World Health Organization committee studying regulatory standards, 1985. **Writings:** five books, incl. *On Nursing: Toward a New Endowment* and *On Nursing: A Literary Celebration.* **Awards:** nine honorary doctorates; awards from U.S. universities and abroad; Fellow, American Academy of Nursing; election to Institute of Medicine, National Academy of Sciences; ANA Hall of Fame, 2000; Magnet Nursing Services Recognition Award, ANCC; Gretta Styles Scholarship in Credentialing Research, ANCC; Fellow, Royal College of Nursing, U.K.; Living Legend, American Academy of Nursing, 1999.

References and Credits

†Schorr T, Zimmerman A: Making Choices, Taking Chances: Nurse Leaders Tell Their Stories. St. Louis, CV Mosby, 1988, pp 350–355.

ANA on line, available at http://www.ana.org.

CredentialingInternational, American Nurses Credentialing Center: Tribute to Greta Styles. July 2001. http://www.nursingworld.org/ancc/credsin.htm.

ANA Hall of Fame 10/98 American Nurses Association, Washington, D.C. http://www.nursingworld.org/hof.

March 29

Mary Patricia Donahue

1939–

"Nursing is not merely a technique but a process that incorporates the elements of soul, mind, and imagination. Its very essence lies in the creative imagination, the sensitive spirit, and the intelligent understanding that provide the very foundation for effective nursing care. These have been captured consistently in a wide range of illustrative material that can greatly enhance the study of nursing history through visual representation. Every art gallery has its nursing saints, nurturing mother, healing miracles, sick beds, and lying-in chambers. Many of the finest paintings and sculptures dealing with nursing objectives have been done by the 'great masters' and contemporary artists. All of these serve to capture the art of nursing." (1985)

M. Patricia Donahue's career reveals her deep commitment to preserving the heritage of nursing. She has worked and written extensively in the areas of oncology, terminal illness, patients' rights, and patient advocacy. She is a respected spokesperson for nursing history, issues, and ethics, and she has taught nursing history since 1973. She is researching a biography of Isabel Maitland Stewart. The second edition of her *Nursing: The Finest Art, An Illustrated History* strikingly portrays the nursing profession's past, present, and future by using the world's most beautiful paintings, objects of art, and photographs. This extraordinary work illustrates the social, political, and economic history of nursing. She is a professor and associate dean of academic affairs at the University of Iowa College of Nursing. She received the Hancher Finkbine Medallion in 1993, one of the highest awards given by the University of Iowa. It recognizes leadership, learning, and loyalty.

Biography

Born: March 19, 1939, Youngstown, Ohio. **Education:** St. Luke's Hosp. School of Nursing, Cleveland, Ohio, 1960 (RN diploma); Ohio State Univ. (BSN, MS); Univ. of Iowa (PhD in social foundations of education). **Work history:** Staff Nurse in variety of clinical areas; Staff Supervisor, Visiting Nurse Assoc., Dallas; Staff Nurse, Univ. of Iowa Hosps. and Clinics; presentation of programs on practice issues and trains hospice volunteers in community; Professor, Associate Dean of Academic Affairs, Univ. of Iowa College of Nursing. **Writings:** reviewer for several nursing journals; First Assistant Editor, "Inquiry, Insights, and History" column, *Journal of Professional Nursing;* Bd. of Advisors, Guest Editor, Contributor for issue of *Caduceus* devoted to nursing in wartime. **Organizations:** past president, director-at-large, American Assoc. for the History of Nursing. **Awards:** Teresa E. Christy Award; Sigma Theta Tau Award for special issue of *Caduceus;* two Book of the Year Awards for *Nursing: The Finest Art*; Distinguished Resident Scholar and Distinguished Professor, Westminster College, Salt Lake City, Utah; First Distinguished Visiting Professor, Univ. of Alberta, Edmonton, for Canada's first doctoral program in nursing.

References and Credits

†Donahue MP: Nursing: The Finest Art, An Illustrated History. St. Louis, CV Mosby, 1985, p ix; cover blurb from second edition (1996).

Donahue MP: resume.

MARCH 21

Alice Louise Fitzgerald

1874–1962

"I have come to the conclusion that even in the very small part I play, each day makes me a week older. I cannot quite explain it. It is not only the hard work, but the whole situation and atmosphere in which we live. At night the firing line is all lighted up by the star shells sent up to help locate positions. On a clear day, we can see much of the activities of the firing line: observation balloons, aeroplanes, shells bursting. ...It makes it all very vividly real that men are killing each other not so far away." (1916)

ALICE FITZGERALD'S CLINICAL and administrative experiences in the United States and her fluency in several languages contributed to a unique and versatile career in nursing. She introduced public health nursing in Indiana and is considered a nursing pioneer because of her nursing efforts during World War I. She did disaster relief nursing in Italy and worked with the British Red Cross as the first Edith Cavell Memorial Nurse in 1915. She provided direct care to the wounded in France during the war and facilitated cultural understanding with wartime health care workers. She held various positions with the Red Cross throughout Europe, and in the years following the war she was instrumental in establishing nursing programs abroad. In 1920 she established a course in public health nursing in London and helped make scholarship money available from the League of Red Cross Societies. By 1933 nurses were attending from forty-one countries. They brought a range of academic and cultural differences and found opportunities to learn about one another as they studied together. Many of these nurses returned to their own countries to become public health nursing pioneers. In Thailand (then called Siam) she gained the support of the royal family to establish a modern nursing school there.

Biography

Born: March 13, 1874, Florence, Italy. **Education:** France, Germany, Switzerland; Johns Hopkins Hosp. Training School for Nurses (RN). **Work history:** Johns Hopkins Hosp.; disaster nursing, Italy; Superintendent, Bellevue Hosp., N.Y.C.; Superintendent of Nurses, Wilkes-Barre (Pa.) General Hosp.; Superintendent of Nurses, Robert W. Long Hosp., Indiana; Head Nurse, student health, Wellesley College; Cavell Nurse with British Red Cross, nurse with American Red Cross (ARC), World War I; Director of Nurses, League of Red Cross Societies, Geneva; Rockefeller Foundation Nursing Adviser to Philippines and Thailand; Md. State Bd. of Nurse Examiners; Director of Nurses, Polyclinic Hosp., N.Y.C.; housemother, Sheppard Pratt Institute, Baltimore. **Organizations:** ARC. **Awards:** Edith Cavell Memorial Nurse; British Red Cross Medal, Campaign Medal, Victory Medal; French Campaign Medal and Victory Medal, Medaille d'Honneur with Rosette, France; Red Cross Medals of Poland, Serbia, Hungary, Russia, United States; Florence Nightingale Medal, International Committee, Red Cross. **Died:** Bronx, N.Y.

References and Credits

†Fitzgerald A: The Edith Cavell Nurse. Boston, Butterfield, 1917, pp 24–25.

Sabin LE: Alice Fitzgerald. In Bullough V, Church OM, Stein AP (eds): American Nursing: A Biographical Dictionary, vol. 1. New York, Garland, 1988, pp 113–115.

Roberts M: American Nursing History and Interpretation. New York: Macmillan, 1954.

MARCH 22

Annie M. Brainard

1864–1942

"At last we see the public nurse firmly established as one of the most important agents in the whole modern movement for the conservation of the public health. We have watched her slow evolution through the centuries; we have seen her as the deaconess of the early church; as the Lady Bountiful of the middle ages; as the district nurse of modern times; and, finally, as the highly trained public health nurse of today." (1922)

"Let her never forget her glorious past. The work of the public health nurse ... is not merely a profession; it is a vocation; not merely a gainful occupation, but a ministry. The truly great physician sees in his patient not only the case, but the human being. So with the nurse. The professional, the scientific, the purely business side of her work must never over-shadow the warm human side; she must still be not only a teacher, but a friend, so that those who are to benefit by her teaching and care will say, not "There goes the public health teacher,'—but, "There goes Our Nurse.'" *(1922)*

ANNIE BRAINARD WAS a renowned traveler and prolific writer. Little is known about her education. She was, however, interested in nursing education and public health nursing, and she wrote extensively about public health. She was the editor of *Visiting Nurse Quarterly* of Cleveland from 1911 to 1923. She was a founding member of the Cleveland Visiting Nurse Association (CVNA) and wrote *The Evolution of Public Health Nursing* in 1922. It traced the development of organized visiting of the sick in their homes from the time of early Christianity. Brainard was respected as a leader with a great sense of fairness. These qualities enabled her to promote the growth of public health nursing in Cleveland and throughout the country.

Biography

Born: March 14, 1864, Cleveland, Ohio. **Education:** unknown. **Work history:** member, Bd. of Trustees, CVNA under Isabel Hampton Robb and Mathilda Johnson, 1904; President, CVNA; Editor, first issue, *Visiting Nurse Quarterly,* 1909, which became official publication of the National Organization for Public Health Nursing in 1912 (it became *Public Health Nurse Quarterly,* then the monthly *Public Health Nurse* in 1918); Lecturer in administration of public health nursing, Case Western Reserve Univ., 1916–26; Advisory Committee for Univ. School of Nursing, Case Western Reserve, 1923–42; Committee on Nursing Education, Flora Stone Mather College, Cleveland; member, first bd. of governors, Nursing Center, Cleveland, an organization that promoted centralization of nursing in the city. **Organizations:** unknown. **Awards:** unknown. **Died:** Cleveland.

References and Credits

†Brainard AM: The Evolution of Public Health Nursing. Philadelphia, WB Saunders, 1922, pp 419–20.

Sentz L: Annie M. Brainard. In Bullough V, Sentz L, Stein AP (eds): American Nursing: A Biographical Dictionary, vol. 2. New York, Garland, 1992, pp 34–35.

Maude Blanche Muse

1879–1962

"Exercise that highest power of the mind—reasoning. ...Encourage that 'eternal why;' not always by direct answers, but always see that it reaches the 'therefore.' Then, 'dry bones' takes on new meaning, knowledge comes with new power and daily experiences are accompanied by a glow of understanding and resulting satisfaction even beyond all hopes." (1919)

MAUDE BLANCHE MUSE was a gifted nurse-educator and creative thinker who continually and successfully worked to integrate findings about the learning process into nursing programs. Orphaned before she was thirteen, she lived with various relatives, then entered nursing school after teaching for three years in a small country school. She was especially interested in nursing education, and she specifically wanted to help students learn study skills and develop the interpersonal skills necessary to become effective professionals. Her concerns that students be able to deal with the wide range of human behaviors as well as the duties and demands of the profession led her to write *A Textbook of Psychology for Nurses* in 1925. It had five editions; the last was published in 1945.

Biography

Born: March 9, 1879, Edinboro, Pa. **Education:** Lakeside Hosp. School of Nursing, Cleveland, Ohio (RN); Teachers College, Columbia Univ. (BS, master's). **Work history:** Private Duty Nurse; Instructor, St. Luke's Hosp., N.Y.C., and Stanford-Lane Hosp., San Francisco; Instructor, Vassar Training Camp; Faculty, Columbia Univ.; Associate Editor, *Physiotherapy Review.* **Organizations:** National League for Nursing Education; American Red Cross Nursing Service. **Awards:** unknown. **Died:** Savannah, Ga.

References and Credits

†Muse M: Teaching probationers how to study. AJN 20:220, 1919.

Sentz L: Maude Muse. In Bullough V, Church OM, Stein AP (eds): American Nursing: A Biographical Dictionary, vol. 1. New York, Garland, 1988, pp 239–240.

Cunningham BV, Stewart IM: Maude B. Muse—Nurse, educator, author and creative thinker. AJN 56:1434–36, 1956.

March 24

Sarah E. Sly

1870–1944

"We should not be frightened or discouraged by opposition, even if we must back water once in a while. No good thing is ever gained easily. The more vital the question, the greater the opposition. Any reform to be lasting must be brought about slowly. No one else will solve our problems for us. ...The greatest danger we have to face is failure to stand together for what we know is right. All our efforts lead to the more efficient care of the sick in the home, hospital, army, navy, and in every land. The gain is to come chiefly to those who follow us, not to ourselves, therefore we must build carefully on the foundation which was so securely laid by the pioneer nurses." (1912)

ALTHOUGH DIABETES, NEPHRITIS, and arteriosclerosis may have caused Sarah Sly to remove herself from active nursing early in her career, she continued to pursue a vigorous commitment to nursing. Her efforts helped the Nurses Associated Alumnae (NAA) of the United States evolve smoothly into the American Nurses Association (ANA). She spoke nationally of the responsibilities of professional organizations to not only advance nursing but also to find ways to provide quality health care for all people. As president of the American Journal of Nursing Company, she recognized its influence and called on nurses as individual shareholders to "help maintain and advance its high standard of excellence."

Biography

Born: March 24, 1870, Bloomfield Twp., Mich. **Education:** Farrand Training School, Harper Hosp., Detroit. **Work history:** Staff Nurse, Pennsylvania Hosp., Philadelphia; Private Duty Nurse; organizational work with NAA; bd. member, President, American Journal of Nursing Co. **Organizations:** NAA; ANA, Mich. State Nurses Assoc., International Council of Nurses. **Awards:** unknown. **Died:** Bloomfield, Mich.

References and Credits

†Sly S: Address to the Fifteenth Annual ANA Convention, 1912. In Flanagan L (ed): One Strong Voice, Kansas City, Mo., Lowell Press, 1976, p 392.

Stein AP: Sarah E. Sly. In Bullough V, Sentz L, Stein AP (eds): American Nursing: A Biographical Dictionary, vol. 2. New York, Garland, 1992, p 307.

MARCH 25

Barbara Gordon Schutt

1917–1986

"It has become apparent that the poor conditions under which nurses and others have been forced to work have been prodromal symptoms of a serious disease which affects everyone, whether giving, getting, or needing health care. The situation today demands that all *health workers become a knowledgeable and powerful force for the efficient extension of decent health services to the many people in this society." (1967)*

WHEN BARBARA GORDON SCHUTT was working as executive director of the Pennsylvania Nurses Association (PNA), her award-winning writing skills for the *Pennsylvania Nurse* earned her an invitation to serve as editor of the *American Journal of Nursing*. She held that position for more than ten years. During that period her forceful editorials influenced national thinking in support of economic and general welfare issues for nurses, particularly in support of their need to organize for collective bargaining. She also wrote about nursing's need to control its own practice. She applauded the advancement of nursing research because of the resulting improvements in patient care and stressed the importance of nursing to help patients maximize their potential. She believed it essential that all nurses understand health economics so they can be actively involved at every level of the discussion and decision making about health care.

Biography

Born: March 25, 1917, Ithaca, N.Y. **Education:** Jefferson Medical College Hosp. School of Nursing, Philadelphia; Bethany College, West Va., (BA); Univ. of Pennsylvania (MSNE). **Work history:** Staff Nurse; Student Health Nurse, Bethany College; camp nurse; Army Nurse Corps; Administrator, PNA; Administrator, Nursing Division, Mohegan (Conn.) Community College. **Organizations:** member, American Nurses Assoc. (ANA), PNA; Conn. Nurses Assoc. **Awards:** charter member, American Academy of Nursing; ANA Honorary Recognition Award; honorary doctorate, Bethany College; nursing scholarship in her name established by the Conn. Nurses Foundation. **Died:** Montville, Conn.

References and Credits

†Schutt BG: Editorial. AJN 67:1629, 1967.

Sentz L: Barbara Gordon Schutt. In Bullough V, Sentz L, Stein AP (eds): American Nursing: A Biographical Dictionary, vol. 2. New York, Garland, 1992, pp 294–296.

AJN editorials 1962, 1964.

March 26

Jane Arminda Delano

1858–1919

"Nursing is not alone caring for the sick, the prevention of infection *often constitutes as important a duty as the care of the patient. A woman who is without knowledge of the principles which should guide the performance of her work holds in her hands a capacity for doing infinite harm; she cannot avoid dangers she does not recognize." (1916)*

AFTER A BRIEF time as a teacher, Jane Arminda Delano entered nursing school following the death of an older sister. When she was quite young, her father died of yellow fever while in the Union Army, and as a young graduate she had an opportunity to effectively control an epidemic of yellow fever in Florida by having screens placed over the beds of patients. When she was the superintendent of the reorganized Army Nurse Corps, she fought to increase the pay and status for nurses and opposed the use of nurse's aides in the military. Her greatest joy, however, was her ability to organize and work with the Red Cross Nursing Service, establishing criteria for well-prepared professional nurses who could be available to serve. An inheritance allowed her to work with the American Red Cross for a decade as a volunteer. Described as thorough and modest, she was dedicated to her nurses and coordinated efforts with the Red Cross and the Nurses Associated Alumnae of the United States. As a result, more than eight thousand nurses were available before World War I, and she is credited with recruiting more than twenty thousand nurses for service during that war.

Biography

Born: March 26, 1858, Townsend, N.Y. **Education:** Bellevue Hosp. Training School for Nurses, N.Y.C. **Work history:** Head Nurse, Bellevue and Sands Hill Hosp., Fla.; Superintendent of Nurses, hosp. for Bizbee, Ariz., copper mines; Superintendent of Nurses, Univ. Hosp., Philadelphia; Administrator, House of Refuge, Randall's Island, N.Y.; Director, Bellevue Hosp. Training School for Nurses; Superintendent, Army Nurse Corps; chair, National Committee of American Red Cross Nursing Service. **Organizations:** American Nurses Assoc. (ANA); American Red Cross. **Awards:** ANA Hall of Fame; cited on nurse memorial at Arlington National Cemetery. **Buried:** Arlington National Cemetery.

References and Credits

†Delano J, McIsaac I: American Red Cross Textbook on Elementary Hygiene and Home Care of the Sick. Philadelphia, P. Blakiston's, 1916, p xiii.

Sabin L: Jane Delano. In Bullough V, Church OM, Stein AP (eds): American Nursing: A Biographical Dictionary, vol. 1. New York, Garland, 1988, pp 78–80.

ANA Hall of Fame 10/98 American Nurses Association, Washington, D.C. http://www.nursingworld.org/hof.

March 27

Eugenia Helma Waechter

1925–1982

"No one's emotions are left untouched by the death of a patient, but the death of the very young is particularly poignant because it speaks silently of unfulfilled promise and destroyed hopes. To defend ourselves, we may unconsciously avoid children with fatal illness and leave them largely alone to deal with their fears and anxieties at a time when comfort, nearness, and sympathetic understanding are most important to them ... questions and concerns which are conscious to the child threatened with death should be dealt with in such a way that the child does not feel further isolated and alienated from his parents and other meaningful adults. There should be no curtain of silence around his most intense fears. These feelings of isolation may also be relieved by efforts designed to keep the child closer, both spatially and emotionally, to others on pediatric wards." (1971)

THE DAUGHTER OF MISSIONARY PARENTS, Eugenia Waechter began her nursing career in public health and then settled into pediatrics. She had a specific interest in the problems faced by children with chronic or terminal illnesses, and their families. Her doctoral research focused on death anxiety in children with fatal illness and created a new awareness for pediatric nurses worldwide. She helped adults understand why children were not helped by "protective silence." Contrary to the thinking at that time, her findings showed that very young children also need opportunities to deal with fears and anxieties that are very real and that children benefit from opportunities to share their thoughts and feelings. She found that children need to know that they have permission to talk about their illness and that allowing for this decreases their feelings of isolation, alienation, and helplessness.

Biography

Born: March 29, 1925, Crespo, Argentina. **Education:** St. John's College, Kans. (AA); Lutheran Hosp. School of Nursing, St. Louis; Univ. of Chicago (bachelor's degree, MA); Univ. of California, San Francisco; Stanford Univ. (PhD). **Work history:** Public Health Nurse, Montgomery County (Ill.) Health Dept.; Nursing Consultant, Univ. of Illinois; Faculty, Univ. of California, San Francisco; Author; Researcher; Lecturer. **Organizations:** unknown. **Awards:** Fellow, American Academy of Nursing. **Died:** Redwood City, Calif.

References and Credits

†Waechter EH: Children's awareness of fatal illness. AJN 71:1168, 1172, 1971.

Bullough V: Eugenia Helma Waechter. In Bullough V, Sentz L, Stein AP (eds): American Nursing: A Biographical Dictionary, vol. 2. New York, Garland, 1992, pp 340–341.

March 28

Tim Porter-O'Grady

1941–

"The tragedy of our time would be for nurses to do nothing and simply wait for the changes to occur. The profession has too often in the past waited for the presumed appropriate time to respond and has, instead, had to react because it was too late with too little to affect the outcome. Because the script for the future of health care in America is not yet written, nursing leadership has a tremendous opportunity to share in its writing and to become its major advocate and provider. If nurses do their part and are positioned to manage the system and provide primary services, the American public gains, and the quality of health care is enhanced. There can be no greater benefit to either the public or the nurse. However, we must begin now." (1990)

Tim Porter-O'Grady wanted to be a nurse because his mother was a nurse and she inspired him to be a part of a profession that made a difference in people's lives. He has worked in hospitals as a clinical nurse specialist, an administrator, and as a consultant. He has a particular interest in conflict resolution and gerontology. He has written or cowritten thirteen books about nursing. His most recent publication, *A Textbook of New Leadership*, was published in 2002, and he has contributed more than 145 articles to professional journals. He offers his leadership abilities and his expertise to many local, state, and national organizations. He says that he has never regretted his decision to become a nurse.

Biography

Born: March 29, 1941, Edmonton, Alberta, Can. **Education:** Lower Columbia College, Longview, Wash. (AA in science); Seattle Univ. (BS); Univ. of Washington (MSN); Nova Southwestern Univ. (EdD). Georgia State Univ. (certification as clinical nurse specialist; gerontology); LaSalle Univ. (PhD); Georgia Supreme Court, Office of Dispute Resolution (registered mediation, arbitration, conflict resolution specialist); Harvard Univ. (advanced conflict resolution). **Work history:** Staff Nurse; Providence Medical Center, Seattle; Clinical Supervisor, Providence Medical Center; Patient Care Administrator, Allegheny Regional Hosp., Covington, Va.; Vice President, Patient Care Services, Doctors Memorial Hosp., Richmond, Va.; Nurse Administrator, St. Joseph's Hosp., Atlanta; President, bd. of directors, Affiliated Dynamics, Inc., Atlanta; Senior Partner, Tim Porter-O'Grady Associates, Inc., Atlanta **Organizations:** member, Governing Bd., Atlanta Community Health Program; Trustee, Ga. Nurses Foundation (GNF); member, advisory bd., Ga. State Dept. of Human Resources; Chair, AID Atlanta; Vice Chair, AID Atlanta; Chair, Ga. Health Reform Project; President, GNF, 2000–; recipient of Homeless Health Care grant, U.S. Dept. of Health and Human Services; Fellow, American Academy of Nursing, N.Y. Academy of Sciences; American Nurses Assoc.; National League for Nursing; American College of Health Executives; Gerontology Society of America; Amnesty International Health Care; Forum for Nurse Executives (bd. of directors); Sigma Theta Tau. **Awards:** National Commission on Nursing Service Award; National League for Nursing Community Award; Nursing Leader Award, Alumni 100 Award, Seattle Univ.; American Association of Critical Care Nurses Pioneer Award.

References and Credits

†Porter-O'Grady T: Reorganization of Nursing Practice: Creating the Corporate Venture. Rockville, Md., Aspen Publishing, 1990, p xiii.

Porter-O'Grady T: personal communication, August 13, 2002.

March 29

Lillian Sholtis Brunner

1918–

"The care of the patient in the operating room is just as important as his care at the site of an accident, in the emergency room, the surgical division, in anesthesia or the recovery room—only more so! Continuity of patient care is required from the time a person acquires the connotation of the word 'patient' until he leaves this classification. There can be no breaks, shortcuts, or elimination of links in the chain of care without the risk of undesirable effects. Of special concern to the physician, nurse, and patient are those times when the patient is unconscious, disassociated as a consequence of drugs or medications, or separated from reality as a result of anesthetic drugs. ... The broad umbrella of surgical nursing covers all phases of the patient's experience." (1968)

LILLIAN SHOLTIS BRUNNER excelled in and wanted to teach math and chemistry; she once said that she never considered nursing because the thought repelled her. This changed when she visited her hospitalized father, observed nursing, and saw it as the means to an end—a way to earn money for college so she could become a teacher. But the profession claimed her. During a fulfilling career that included surgical nursing, teaching, writing, and consulting, she helped alter the course of preparation and practice when she coauthored *Medical-Surgical Nursing* with Doris Suddarth.

Turning from the traditional practice of dealing with each aspect separately, this innovative text integrated the nursing process in all aspects of care. It proved popular and was used throughout the world. She defined surgical nursing as encompassing all aspects of care: pre- and postoperative, recovery, and convalescence. She viewed and saw the operating room as "the vital nerve center of the hospital," the place where the skills and knowledge of the professional nurse coalesce on behalf of the patient. The tenth edition of the Brunner-Suddarth textbook, now called the *Brunner Textbook of Medical-Surgical Nursing,* came out in 2000. Brunner has the distinction of being J.B. Lippincott's best-selling author. She also promotes nursing history. Her work for an artifact display during Philadelphia's bicentennial in 1976 led her to found the History of Nursing Museum at Pennsylvania Hospital, the oldest in the United States. Her primary interest, however, has always been students, and she has said that her greatest satisfaction was to know that she played a part in nurses' successful careers.

Biography

Born: March 29, 1918, Freeland, Pa. **Education:** School of Nursing, Univ. of Pennsylvania Hosp.; Univ. of Pennsylvania (BSN); Case Western Reserve Univ. (MSN). Univ. of Pennsylvania (postgraduate study). **Work history:** Head Nurse, Supervising OR nurse, Faculty, Univ. of Pennsylvania Hosp.; Faculty, Yale Univ. School of Nursing; Surgical Supervisor, Yale–New Haven Hosp.; Faculty, Bryn Mawr School of Nursing; Cofounder, Director, History of Nursing Museum, Pennsylvania Hosp., Philadelphia; Lecturer, Consultant, Bryn Mawr Hosp.; Trustee, Vice Chair, Presbyterian Medical Center, Philadelphia. **Organizations:** Presbyterian Foundation for Philadelphia; Hosp. Assoc. of Pa.; National League for Nursing; Assoc. of OR Nurses; American Nurses Assoc.; Assoc. of Critical Care Nurses; American Assoc. of the History of Nursing. **Awards:** Fellow, Living Legend, American Academy of Nursing, 2002; honorary doctorates from Univ. of Pennsylvania, Cedar Crest College, Pa.; Univ. of Pennsylvania has estab. scholarships, a chair in medical-surgical nursing, and an archives room in her name.

References and Credits

†Brunner L: Operating room nursing. In Brunner L (ed): The Nursing Clinics of North America. Philadelphia, WB Saunders, 1968, pp 557–558.

Dunphy LM: Lillian Brunner. In Bullough V, Sentz L (eds): American Nursing: A Biographical Dictionary, vol. 3. New York, Springer, 2000, pp 28–32.

MARCH 30

Frances Payne Bingham Bolton

1885–1977

"I am certain, that the nursing profession should be the hub of a wheel whose spokes are various grades of people trained in varying degrees—from those whose main occupation is keeping homes together and moving constructively while homemakers are ill or disabled to the most highly trained watchers and keepers of bodies, souls, hearts, and minds as well as teachers of health in all these levels of living, working side by side and in perfect understanding with the great profession we call medicine. All these workers would be dedicated to the service of humanity, and as such to the Infinite, in Whom all live and move and have their being." (1938)

FRANCES PAYNE BINGHAM BOLTON served briefly as a nurse's aide and spent the rest of her privileged upper-class life lobbying on behalf of nurses and improving nursing education. A descendent of two of the wealthiest families in Cleveland, she endowed a school of nursing at the Western Reserve University with $1.5 million from 1923 to 1928. Her husband, Chester Castle Bolton, was known as the "richest man in Congress" and when he died, she won the election for his seat in 1940. This started her political career as a champion of nurses. Her accomplishments include an appropriation of $1.25 million for nursing education in 1941, which was increased in 1942 to $3.5 million because of its success; and passage of the Nurse Training Act, later called the Bolton Act, of 1943, which created the U.S. Cadet Nurse Corps. The measure provided prospective nursing students with free schooling, uniforms, and a small stipend for thirty months in return for their commitment to enter the armed forces upon completion or to be a civilian nurse. The government gave participating universities subsidies to expand nursing facilities and hire more educators. This act was responsible for training 125,000 nurses in two years and enlisted the support of 1,125 nursing schools; it also prohibited any discrimination on the basis of race or marital status. Bolton worked tirelessly to commission male nurses in the military with equal military rank. In 1954 she promoted the congressional resolution that became the presidential proclamation for National Nurse Week. Because of her interest in foreign policy she was appointed to the United Nations as a delegate in 1953. She is remembered for her self-assurance, kindness, and instinct for personal relations. When she was defeated in her last election in 1968, she was eighty-three.

Biography

Born: March 29, 1885, Cleveland, Ohio. **Education:** private tutor, attended private girls' school. **Work history:** Created and supplied the Possum Bend (Ky.) Center of the Frontier Nursing Service; established two research institutions: the Payne Fund, which studied literature, film, and their effect on juveniles, and a center for studying parapsychology at Duke Univ. **Organizations:** member, Daughters of the American Revolution; League of Women Voters, Cleveland; Pen and Brush Club, N.Y.C. **Awards:** numerous honorary degrees; William Freeman Snow Award, American Social Hygiene Assoc.; Adelaide Nutting Award, National League for Nursing; Wings Award as an honorary flight nurse of U.S. Air Force. Case Western Reserve's School of Nursing was named for her. **Died:** Lyndhurst, Ohio.

References and Credits

†Pennock MR (ed): Makers of Nursing History: Portraits and Pen Sketches of Fifty-nine Prominent Women. New York, Lakeside, 1940, p 56.

Mernitz KS: Frances Bolton. In Bullough V, Church OM, Stein AP (eds): American Nursing: A Biographical Dictionary, vol. 1. New York, Garland, 1988, pp 42–46.

MARCH 31

Teresa Elizabeth Christy

1927–1982

"A study of the past points up the fact that things considered novel today are often new forms of old ideas. Certainly the present-day emphasis on research in nursing is thought to be a modern idea. Yet Miss [Adelaide] Nutting and Miss [Isabel] Stewart were advocating research more than forty years ago. Miss Stewart's concepts of pre-service and in-service education and the role of the clinical specialist fell on arid ground in the 1930's, only to spring up as a new idea three decades later. It would be interesting to conjecture upon how much further ahead the profession might be had there been nurses astute enough to recognize the value of these suggestions, and well enough prepared to pursue them." (1969)

TERESA CHRISTY WAS an outstanding, dedicated, enthusiastic nurse historian and researcher who promoted the importance of studying the history of nursing. As a member of the Commission on Nursing Research, she was able to expand its scope beyond clinical issues to include historical research. She was a widely recognized speaker, author, and educator who stressed the importance of the relevance of nursing's professional past to present concerns. Among her numerous publications are the biographical sketches in the "Portrait of a Leader" Series that she prepared for *Nursing Outlook* and her acclaimed dissertation, which traced the history of the nursing program at Teachers College, Columbia University. She was a high achiever who successfully combined teaching, writing, speaking, and organizational involvement in nursing. She was a primary organizer and first president of what is now known as the American Association for the History of Nursing.

Biography

Born: March 31, 1927, Brooklyn, N.Y. **Education:** Manhattan College of the Sacred Heart (BSN); brief convent enrollment; DePaul Univ., Chicago (MSN); Teachers College, Columbia Univ. (PhD); **Work history:** Nursing Instructor, St. Joseph's Hosp., Joliet, Ill.; Faculty, Molloy College, N.Y.; Research Assistant, Lecturer, Teachers College; Nursing Faculty, Teachers College, Adelphi Univ., Univ. of Iowa, Univ. of Illinois. **Organizations:** leadership positions in American Nurses Assoc., National League for Nursing, National Assoc. of Univ. Professors, American Public Health Assoc., American Historical Assoc., National Organization for Women; state nurses associations. **Awards:** Clara Hardin Fellowship, Nurses Educational Funds; numerous awards for outstanding scholarship and research, incl. Johns Hopkins, Teachers College, Sigma Theta Tau; DePaul Univ. Alumni Assoc.; member, American Academy of Nursing; honorary doctorate for public service, McKendree College, Ill. **Buried:** Thorn Rose Cemetery, Staunton, Va.

References and Credits

†Christy TE: Cornerstone for Nursing Education. New York, Teachers College Press, 1969, pp 110–111.

Donahue MP: Teresa Christy. In Bullough V, Church OM, Stein AP (eds): American Nursing: A Biographical Dictionary, vol. 1. New York, Garland, 1988, pp 61–64.

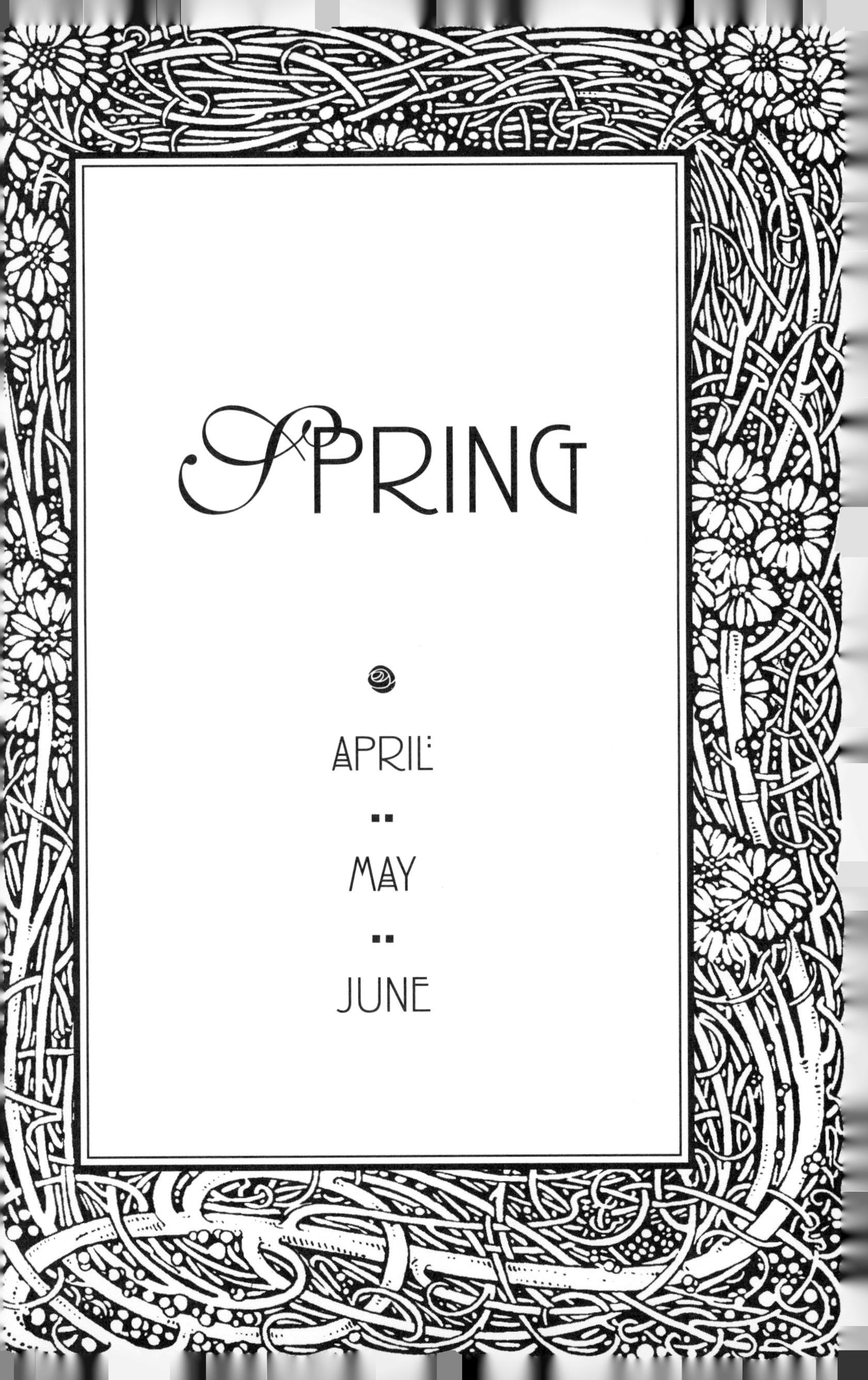

SPRING

APRIL

MAY

JUNE

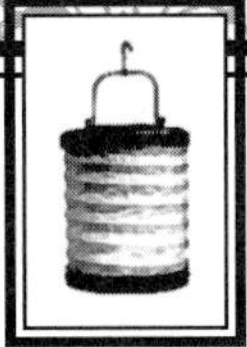

April

"It is the unqualified result of all my experience with the sick, that second only to their need of fresh air is their need of light; that, after a close room, what hurts them most is a dark room… .Who has not observed the purifying effects of light, … especially direct sunlight, upon the air of a room? …[The sick] should be able, without raising themselves or turning in bed, to see out of window from their beds, to see sky and sunlight at least."

—Florence Nightingale

Nightingale F: Notes on Nursing: What It Is, And What It Is Not. New York, D. Appleton, 1860, pp. 84–85.

Florence Aby Blanchfield

1882–1971

"The Army nurse plays a vital role in a proud and gallant service. Her patients are the men of the United States Army—the pick of the nation's manhood. She is a respected member of an important professional team, whether her assignment is hospital administration, operating room service, anesthesiology or neuropsychiatric nursing. Her sisters-in-service already have won the respect and affection of every American soldier. No more rewarding opportunity to serve mankind in a worthwhile and interesting career could be offered American women." (1947)

"THE LITTLE COLONEL" was the affectionate nickname given to Florence Blanchfield. She was the first woman to receive a regular army commission, and she was responsible for the equal pay received by army nurses who were commissioned officers. This achievement took ten years and a special act of Congress. In Washington, D.C., she filled key positions of nursing and assumed more and more responsibility. She eventually served as a colonel of the Army Nurse Corps (ANC), leading the largest military nursing organization in American history, a direct result of her recruitment efforts for World War II. She made certain that wounded soldiers received immediate surgical nursing care by getting nurses and evacuation hospitals to the front lines. She modernized nurses' uniforms by making them practical army fatigues. While managing fifty-seven thousand ANC members as acting superintendent of the corps, she never lost sight of the individual nurse's needs. She continued to be active in specialty training for nurses and believed that every superintendent of nurses should have a college degree. She was a woman with many interests, including tennis and other sports. She studied dressmaking, public speaking, commercial law, and auto shop. Blanchfield, who died on Florence Nightingale's birthday (May 12), was buried with full honors at Arlington National Cemetery.

Biography

Born: April 1, 1882, Shepherdstown, W. Va. **Education:** Southside Hosp. Training School for Nurses, Pittsburgh, Pa., 1906; postgraduate work at Dr. Howard Kelly's Sanitarium, Johns Hopkins Univ., Martin Business College. **Work history:** held many positions as Chief Nurse; General Duty Nurse, Washington, D.C.; Superintendent, ANC. **Organizations:** American Red Cross. **Awards:** ANA Hall of Fame; first nurse to receive Distinguished Service Medal; numerous military service awards; 1951 Florence Nightingale Medal, International Committee, Red Cross, for exceptional service on behalf of humanity. **Died:** Walter Reed Medical Center.

References and Credits

†Blanchfield F: New status in military nursing. AJN 47:604, 1947.

Gurney C: Florence Blanchfield. In Bullough V, Church OM, Stein AP (eds): American Nursing: A Biographical Dictionary, vol. 1. New York, Garland, 1988, pp 36–41.

ANA Hall of Fame 10/98 American Nurses Association, Washington, D.C. http://www.nursingworld.org/hof.

April 2

Edith Annette Aynes

1909–1980

"In my great wisdom and determination. . . .I committed the error that most young people do when they set out to reform the world: I failed to read history." (Date unknown)

". . .Help me to keep her safe, lest I should fail
That pledge I gave to Florence Nightingale,
If she must go, then I will know,
You called her Home 'cause you loved her so.
But, Father, e'er she goest to rest,
Help me to know I have done my best." (ca. 1932)

EDITH ANNETTE AYNES was born in Atwood, Kansas, and her father died when she was thirteen. Her mother was so opposed to her desire to be a nurse that she enrolled Edith in a business school where she perfected her clerical skills. She later used those skills throughout her nursing career, when she wrote books, and articles for many nursing journals. She felt strongly that nurses should have a well-rounded education, not just competency in nursing skills. She wrote many articles to enlighten the public about the health care system. She was proficient as a nurse-anesthetist, author, educator, and administrator. Early in her career she joined the Army Nurse Reserves. At the end of the Korean conflict Aynes, who had attained the rank of major, was assigned to Brooke Army Medical Center at Ft. Sam Houston, Texas, as an instructor at the Medical Field Service School. She also was creative in music and writing and excelled at entertaining armed forces personnel. When she was a student nurse, she wrote a poem, *Nurses Prayer,* after praying for the life of a child she was trying to save. She later set the poem to music and arranged it for the pop singer Jo Stafford to sing on a national radio program to recruit nurses for the army during World War II. In 1949 Aynes wrote the Nurse's Oath of Office to celebrate the forty-eighth birthday of the ANC, and Kate Smith read it on the radio.

Biography

Born: April 2, 1909, Atwood, Kans. **Education:** Presbyterian Hosp. School of Nursing, Denver, 1932; Philadelphia Jewish Hosp., 1939 (certification as nurse-anesthetist); Univ. of California, Berkeley, 1950 (BS in nursing education). **Work history:** Night Nurse, Surgical Nurse in rural hospital; Army Nurse Reserves; "Reserve" Nurse, Fitzsimmons General Hosp., Denver; OR Supervisor, Anesthetist, Ft. Bragg, N.C.; Chief Nurse, 148th General Hosp., San Francisco; 279th General Hosp., Osaka, Japan; Chief Nurse, Medical Section, HQ Japan Logistical Command; 5th Army Headquarters, Chicago; Instructor, Medical Field Service School, Brooke Army Medical Center, Ft. Sam Houston, Texas; Editor, *Army Nurse;* retired from army in 1956; Coordinator of Information and Public Education, National Foundation of the March of Dimes, N.Y.C.; Exec. Director, Cerebral Palsy School and Treatment Center, Belleville, N.J.; Administrator, Andrew Freedman Home, Bronx, N.Y. **Writings:** *From Nightingale to Eagle: An Army Nurse's History*. **Organizations:** member of twelve professional organizations, incl. those devoted to professional nursing, gerontology, music, and writing. **Awards:** Commendation Ribbon with Medal Pendant for recruitment and public relations work for ANC; Legion of Merit for service in Japan. **Died:** Bronx, N.Y.

References and Credits

†Aynes EA: From Nightingale to Eagle: An Army Nurse's History. Englewood Cliffs, N.J., Prentice-Hall, 1973, pp 16, 15.

Brook M: Edith Aynes. In Bullough V, Sentz L, Stein AP (eds): American Nursing: A Biographical Dictionary, vol. 2. New York, Garland, 1992, pp 14–16.

April 3

Barbara Montgomery Dossey

1943–

"In today's specialized world, we are often tempted to compartmentalize our lives, assigning our professional interests to one corner and our spiritual lives to another. To Nightingale, such fragmentation would have been unthinkable. As she put it, her work was her 'must'—her spiritual vision and her professional identity were seamlessly combined. Nightingale is therefore an icon of wholeness, an emblem of a united, integrated life. By her uncompromising, shining example, she invites each of us to find our meaning and purpose—our own 'must'—in our individual journey through life. May Florence Nightingale change your life, as she has mine." (2000)

Barbara Dossey is internationally recognized as a pioneer in the holistic nursing movement. She is respected for her abiding compassion and penetrating insights. With passion and a persuasive eloquence, she is expanding the domain of traditional nursing. She articulates how to promote healing by attending to the delicate interaction of body, mind, and spirit and how to successfully apply centuries-old concepts in the care of patients and in everyday living. She spans the full range of current nursing and health information with her inspired teachings. Her presentations provide challenging, practical, and innovative ways to combine holistic health care with high-level wellness. She has written or co-written nineteen books and is a seven-time recipient of the *American Journal of Nursing* Book of the Year Award. *Florence Nightingale: Mystic, Visionary, Healer*, published in 2000, is an example of her highly regarded research. As an educator, consultant, researcher, and author, Dossey profoundly alters perceptions about holistic nursing. According to Dossey, "Nursing is a wonderful healing journey; it is a gift to be able to participate and assist in this healing journey of others."

Biography

Born: April 3, 1943, Little Rock, Ark. **Education:** Baylor Univ. School of Nursing, Waco, Texas, 1965 (BSN); Texas Women's Univ. School of Nursing, Denton, 1975 (MS); Union Institute and Univ., Cincinnati, Ohio, 2002 (PhD). **Work history:** Critical Care Staff Nurse, Baylor Univ. Medical Center, Dallas, 1965–70; Clinical Instructor, El Centro Junior College, Dallas, 1970–72; Critical Care Staff Nurse, Memorial Hosp., Colorado Springs, Colo., 1973–74; Critical Care Staff Nurse (agency nurse part-time), Dallas, 1975–87; Clinical Instructor, Texas Woman's Univ., Dallas, 1976–79; Biofeedback Nurse, Dallas Diagnostic Assoc., 1982–87; Adjunct Nursing Faculty, Univ. of Texas School of Nursing, Arlington, 1988–90; Director, Holistic Nursing Consultants, Dallas, 1981–90; Director, Holistic Nursing Consultants, Santa Fe, N. Mex., 1990–; Teacher; Author, Coauthor of nineteen books; Consultant; Lecturer. **Organizations:** American Nurses Assoc.; N. Mex. Nurses Assoc.; Sigma Theta Tau International; American Holistic Nurses Assoc. (AHNA); International Assoc. of Human Caring; American Assoc. of the History of Nursing. **Awards:** Outstanding Baylor Univ. Alumni Award, 2002; Texas Women's Univ. 100 Great Nursing Alumni, 2001; seven-time recipient, *American Journal of Nursing* Book of the Year Award; Scientific and Medical Network, United Kingdom Book Prize, 1999; Pioneering Spirit Award, American Assoc. of Critical Care Nurses, 1999; Healer of the Year Award, Nurse Healers Professional Assoc. International, 1998; Fellow, American Academy of Nursing, 1992; Empathy Award, World Cultural Empathy International Alliance, Guadalajara, Mexico, 1989; Holistic Nurse of the Year, AHNA, 1985; Nursing 1984 Clinical Textbook Five-Star Award; American Medical Writers Award, 1982.

References and Credits

†Dossey BM: Florence Nightingale: Mystic Visionary, Healer. Springhouse, Pa., Springhouse, 2000, p vii.

Barbara Dossey on-line, available at http://www.dosseydossey.com.

Dossey BM: telephone conversation, July 17, 2002.

Dossey BM: written response to questionnaire interview, August 20, 2002.

Dorothea Lynde Dix

1802–1887

"What greater bliss than to look back on days spent in usefulness, in doing good to those around us. The duties of a teacher are neither few nor small but they elevate the mind and give energy to the character." (Date unknown)

"I proceed, gentlemen, briefly to call your attention to the present *state of insane persons confined within this Commonwealth, in cages, closets, cellars, and pens, chained naked, beaten with rods and lashed into obedience. . . . Gentlemen, I commit to you this sacred cause. Your action upon this subject will affect the present and future conditions of hundreds and thousands. In this legislation, as in all things, you may exercise that wisdom which is the breath of the power of God." (1843)*

Dorothea Dix is best known for her kind, courageous crusade on behalf of the mentally ill and disabled. In fact, her own mother may have been mentally retarded. Dorothea was shy and compulsive but always dedicated to the common good. She did the research and wrote about her findings, but left it to others to give the speeches. At fourteen she established her first school for small children and founded at least two more schools later in her life. When she arrived to teach a Sunday School class to women prisoners in the East

Cambridge jail, she knew her life's work would be as the advocate for these poor individuals. She referred to the first state mental hospital in Trenton, New Jersey, which she helped to establish, as her "first born child." During the Civil War she was appointed superintendent of army nurses, a position that she found difficult because she had no formal education in nursing or experience in hospital management. Upon her death Dr. Charles H. Nichols of the Bloomingdale Asylum in New York City wrote: "Thus has died and been laid to rest, in the most quiet, unostentatious way, the most useful and distinguished woman America has yet produced."

Biography

Born: April 4, 1802, Hampden, Maine. **Education:** used public library and public lectures to promote her education. **Work history:** opened three schools for girls; traveled to learn about European institutions humane in their treatment of mentally ill; surveyed hospitals, prisons, poorhouses, and asylums of Massachusetts and presented her findings to the Massachusetts Legislature; established funds and facilities for mentally ill in eastern states; Superintendent of Army Nurses, highest office held by a woman in Civil War; campaigned to finish the Washington Monument. **Writings:** *Conversations on Common Things, Hymns for Children, Evening Hours, Meditations for Private Hours, Garland of Flora, American Moral Tales for Young Persons; Remarks on Prisons and Prison Discipline in the U.S., Letter to Convicts in the Western State Penitentiary of Pennsylvania.* **Organizations:** unknown. **Awards:** U.S. Postal Service issued one-cent stamp in her honor; ANA Hall of Fame. **Buried:** Mt. Auburn Cemetery, Cambridge, Mass.

References and Credits

†Snyder CM: The Lady and the President. Lexington, University Press of Kentucky, 1975, pp 61, 68, 69.

Stein AP: Dorothea Lynde Dix. In Bullough V, Church OM, Stein AP (eds): American Nursing: A Biographical Dictionary, vol. 1. New York, Garland, 1988, pp 89–91.

ANA Hall of Fame 10/98 American Nurses Association, Washington, D.C. http://www.nursingworld.org/hof.

April 5

Alberta Hunter

1895–1984

"We sing the blues because our hearts have been hurt. Blues is when you're hungry and you don't have no money to buy food. Or you can't pay your rent at the end of the month. Blues is when you disappoint somebody else; if you owe some money to your best friend, and you know he needs it, but you don't have it to give to him. ...But just plain ol' ordinary 'I don't have some,'—that's not the blues. Most young people today don't have real needs. They just have a few worries. They have needs for things that maybe they could do without. That's not the blues." (Date unknown)

Born the daughter of a railway sleeping car porter and a bordello chambermaid, Alberta Hunter ran away from home when she was eleven to sing for prostitutes and pimps in a Southside Chicago club called Dago Frank's. She wanted to make money to help her mother. In the 1920s she was singing for many of the great vaudeville entertainers such as Bert Williams and Al Jolson when they visited Chicago. She was known as the "Southside's Sweetheart." In 1921 she began her recording career and later traveled throughout Europe, singing in musical productions, including *Show Boat* opposite Paul Robeson. She was the first singer to perform American blues in Europe. One of her compositions, "Downhearted Blues," was recorded by Bessie Smith around 1923 and became one of

Smith's biggest hits. Hunter returned to Paris in 1934 and replaced Josephine Baker at the Casino de Paris. Hunter performed for GIs when she entertained for the USO during World War II. She understudied Eartha Kitt in 1954. In 1956 she appeared in *Debut,* a play that flopped. Her mother died during this period, and Hunter was devastated. She did not want to sing and started a new career. She enrolled in a nursing program and worked in nursing for twenty years until she was forced to retire. Her employers thought she was sixty-five because she had lied about her age. She was eighty-two and started singing again at the Cookery in Greenwich Village.

Biography

Born: April 1, 1895, Memphis, Tenn. **Education:** YWCA, N.Y.C. (LPN), 1957. **Work history:** nursed in New York City hosps. until 1977. **Organizations:** unknown. **Awards:** sang at the White House for President Jimmy Carter; subject of two filmographies: *Jazz at the Smithsonian* and *Alberta Hunter: My Castle's Rockin'.* **Buried:** Ferncliff Cemetery, Hartsdale, N.Y.

References and Credits

†Johns RL: Alberta Hunter. In Smith JC (ed): Notable Black American Women. Detroit, Gale, 1992, p 525.

Gormick G: Liner notes for Alberta Hunter: Beale Street Blues, collectors' ed. (1921–40). Buckinghamshire, U.K., Magnum Music Group, 1996.

Taylor FC, Cook G: Alberta Hunter: A Celebration in Blues. New York, McGraw-Hill, 1987.

April 6

St. Catherine of Siena (Catherine Benincasa)

1347–1380

"If it seems very difficult for you to cope with your many trials, there are three things which I suggest may help you to endure more patiently. Firstly, I want you to think about the shortness of life, for you are not certain even of tomorrow. We can indeed say that we do not have our past troubles, nor those which are in the future; all we have is the moment of time in which we are now. Surely then we ought to endure patiently since time is short. Secondly, consider the benefit we gain from our troubles, for Saint Paul says there is no comparison between our difficulties and the fruit and reward of eternal glory. Thirdly, reflect on the evil consequences of indulging in anger and impatience. These evil consequences are with us both here and hereafter. So I beg you dearest brother to bear all your troubles patiently. ...Remain in the holy, gentle love of God." (Date unknown)

EARLY IN HER childhood Catherine dedicated herself to the will of God, and as a young woman she joined the lay order of Dominican sisters called the Mantellate. After three years of solitude and prayer, she felt called by God to a life of dedicated service. She was respected as a theologian and mystic; her writings focus on a merciful and loving God with a universality that still applies today. As she nursed and worked with the poor, she stressed that love of God cannot be separated from love of neighbor. In this essential connection, the increase in one results in an increase in the other. When Siena was stricken with plague, she and her followers walked through the streets with a lantern and a flask of disinfectant to care for the sick. In one instance, she is credited with the miracle of the full recovery of a friend who lay dying. Another story about Catherine deals with her care for a woman with advanced leprosy. Unaffected by the verbal abuse and insults that would greet her when she approached, Catherine reassured the woman, "I shall hasten to do anything that you need of me." She cared for the woman through death and burial, after which her own infected hands healed.

Biography

Born: March 25, 1347, Siena, Italy. **Education:** no formal education; learned through oral sources and spiritual insights; learned to read as a young adult and to write much later. **Work history:** served the sick and the poor; Theologian; Papal Adviser; worked as peacemaker and theologian during years of schism in the Roman Catholic Church; Author. **Organizations:** member, Mantellate religious order. **Awards:** Sainthood, 1461; first woman declared Doctor of the Church (1970). **Died:** Rome.

References and Credits

†O'Driscoll M: Catherine of Siena: Selected Spiritual Writings. New York, New City Press, 1993, p 21.

Giordani I: Catherine of Siena: Fire and Blood. Trans. Tobin B. Milwaukee, Wisc., Bruce Publishing, 1959.

Sister Bernadette Armiger

1915–1979

"Government priorities are an important determinant of demand as well as supply. …Extension of Medicare, emerging programs for the aged, plans for setting up clinics throughout the country for the early detection of breast cancer, opportunities for work in an increasingly wide range of treatment modalities in psychiatric—mental health nursing, and yet unforeseen options for nursing's 'fulfilled' role under national health insurance are among new perspectives in the use of nursing resources." (1973)

Sister Bernadette Armiger, a member of the Daughters of Charity of St. Vincent de Paul, was an innovative nursing leader, nursing educator, and qualified counselor. She published numerous articles about nursing care and nursing education. In the early 1950s she effected major changes in the baccalaureate nursing curriculum by having hospital affiliates stress education rather than service and with supervision by faculty instead of head nurses. During her years at Niagara (N.Y.) University she established a year-long health assessment class and promoted baccalaureate coursework to prepare nurse practitioners. Her combined fund-raising skills and design ideas resulted in federal appropriations for a new state-of-the-art, award-winning nursing education building at Niagara. The founder and first president of the American Association of Colleges of Nursing (AACSN), she was also active in professional counseling and nursing organizations. She served as a grant reviewer and adviser to the U.S. Bureau of Health Professional Education and Manpower Training. Armiger conceived and developed the Consultation Center for Priests and Religious in Baltimore. She surveyed needs and services, secured and furnished the site, recruited mental health professionals, and worked out financial arrangements for affordable service.

Biography

Born: April 7, 1915, Baltimore. **Education:** Catholic Univ. of America (BSN, MN); St. John's Univ., N.Y. (PhD); Univ. of Tel Aviv. **Work history:** Nursing Faculty, Catholic Univ. of America; Administrator, De Paul Hosp., Norfolk, Va.; Coordinator, Laboure School of Nursing, Mass.; Nursing Faculty, St. Joseph's College, Md.; Administrator, Niagara Univ.; Grant Reviewer for U.S. government; Consultation Center for Priests and Religious, Baltimore. **Organizations:** member and founder, AACSN; Counseling Center for Clergy and Religious of the Diocese of Buffalo; N.Y. Cancer Society; American Red Cross; American Nurses Assoc.; American Psychological Assoc.; Sigma Theta Tau; Psi Chi; Delta Epsilon Sigma. **Awards:** Armiger Award, established by the AACSN in her honor; Certificate of Recognition, U.S. Dept. of Health, Education, and Welfare. **Buried:** Albany, N.Y.

References and Credits

†Armiger B: Unemployment: Is there a nursing shortage? Nurs Outlook 21:316, 1973.

Sentz L: Sister Bernadette Armiger. In Bullough V, Church OM, Stein AP (eds): American Nursing: A Biographical Dictionary, vol. 1. New York, Garland, 1988, pp 5–8.

April 8

Euphemia Jane Taylor

1874–1970

"The real depths of nursing can only be made known through ideals, love, sympathy, knowledge, and culture, and expressed through the practice of artistic procedures and relationships. Nursing is 'a chapter in the book of life'—human, real, and akin to brotherly love. The nurse is in very truth her 'brother's keeper.' She knows his strengths and weaknesses. She shares his hopes and fears. She feels his elations and his depressions. She listens to the whisper from his innermost soul. Nursing shares in life's prosaic gloom, but also it shares in life's poetic beauty. Of such is the nature and spirit of nursing." (1934)

Euphemia Taylor was attracted to nursing by the example of nurses who were caring toward her and her father during his lengthy and terminal illness. She brought a liberal arts background to her nursing studies. This strengthened her belief in the value and importance of attracting people to nursing who had specialties in other fields. A psychiatric nurse, she promoted holistic nursing in her report as chair of the American Nurses Association (ANA) mental health section at the 1928 ANA convention. That report focused on using psychiatry and education in nursing to address the whole person, saying, "Nursing must change its viewpoint and embrace the idea that good nursing care of the physically ill patient involves a knowledge and an appreciation of the influences which the emotional and intellectual life bear on the physical well-being of the patient and *vice versa*." She was the second dean of the Yale School of Nursing, and her leadership furthered the distinction between nursing and medicine. Taylor refined the art of nursing through studies and teaching that focused on patient care and related to the patient's psychological as well as physical needs. During World War II she was president of the International Council of Nurses (ICN) and kept the group together by transferring the records to New Haven, Connecticut, and maintaining open communication with nurses around the world. Her nursing ideals stemmed from the dedication and service of Florence Nightingale.

Biography

Born: April 8, 1874, Hamilton, Ontario, Can. **Education:** Hamilton (Ontario) Collegiate Institute; Wesleyan Ladies College (Hamilton); Johns Hopkins Hosp. School of Nursing; Teachers College, Columbia Univ. (BS). **Work history:** Psychiatric Nurse, Henry Phipps Psychiatric Clinic, Johns Hopkins; Faculty, Dean, Yale School of Nursing. **Organizations:** National League for Nursing Education; ICN. **Awards:** ANA Hall of Fame; Medal for Humanitarian Work, Finland; honorary member, National Council of Nurses of Finland, Danish Nurses Assoc., and Norwegian Nurses Assoc.; Florence Nightingale Medal, International Committee, Red Cross; Adelaide Nutting Award, National League for Nursing; honorary master's, Yale Univ.; honorary doctorate, Keuka College, N.Y.
Died: Hamilton, Ontario.

References and Credits

†Taylor EJ: Of what is the nature of nursing. AJN 34:476, 1934.

ANA Hall of Fame 10/98 American Nurses Association, Washington, D.C. http://www.nursingworld.org/hof.

Church O: Euphemia Jane Taylor. In Bullough V, Church OM, Stein AP (eds): American Nursing: A Biographical Dictionary, vol. 1. New York, Garland, 1988, pp 304–305.

Roberts MM: American Nursing: History and Interpretation. New York: Macmillan, 1954, p 211.

April 9

Ida V. Moffett

1905–1996

"If I could give only one rule or piece of advice, it would be this: Allow yourself to care, really care for the people for whom you are responsible. Love them. Get involved in their struggle. Really care . . . patients are more concerned about the compassion, care, feeling and human interest shown them by the people of the hospital than they are about the technical skill demonstrated. . . . The desire for compassionate caring has never changed and it never will. . . . Caring is the shining thread of gold that holds together the tapestry of life." (1988)

Ida Moffett's seventy-year nursing career left a legacy beyond measure. Often described as the perfect nurse, she taught more than four thousand nurses by her example that the most important person in the hospital is the patient. Her reputation for knowing everyone by name began in her student days and continued throughout her career as she reviewed charts and made daily rounds. She defined compassionate care as active involvement to meet the needs of the patient. She would ask each of person, "Is there anything I can do for you?" Despite long hours of administrative and educational duties, she neither lost her bedside nursing skills nor missed an opportunity to give personal physical care. During her long tenure at Birmingham Baptist Hospital she held the dual positions for many years of director of nursing and director of the nursing school. She actively recruited nurses with academic credentials and encouraged nurses on her staff to seek further education. She stayed current with nursing techniques and procedures. According to her biographers Lee and Catherine Allen, Moffett could "turn red tape into red carpet." Among her many achievements, she was involved with federal funding for the first Cadet Nurse Corps in Alabama, the first practical nurse program in the state, the integration of black nurses into the state nurses association in 1949, Tuskegee Institute's School of Nursing, which was designated as Alabama's first four-year baccalaureate nursing program, nursing service at the Baptist Hospital (1952), nursing accreditation, and the start of the four-year degree program for nurses at the University of Alabama.

Biography

Born: April 9, 1905, Toadvine, Ala. **Education:** Birmingham Baptist Hospital (RN); postgraduate study: Univ. of Iowa Hosp. (Iowa City, Iowa) (orthopedic nursing); Univ. of Cincinnati General Hosp. (surgical nursing). **Work history:** private duty nursing, Atlanta; staff nursing, teaching, surgical nursing, administration, Birmingham Baptist Hosp.; Associate Director of Nursing, Highland Avenue Baptist Hosp., Birmingham, Ala.; Alabama State Board of Nursing and State Registration, League of Nursing Committees; Acting Director of Nursing, Birmingham Baptist Hosp.; Director, School of Nursing, Birmingham Baptist Hosp. **Organizations:** Ala. State Nurses Assoc. (ASNA); Baptist Hosp. School of Nursing Alumni; Ala. League for Nursing Education; **Awards:** Chief of Nursing Emeritus, Baptist Medical Centers; Nursing School at Samford Univ., Birmingham, named in her honor; Ala. Healthcare Hall of Fame; honorary doctorate, Judson College, Marion, Ala.; commemorative portrait, Samford University, Ida V. Moffett School of Nursing, Birmingham, Ala; honorary member, Sigma Theta Tau; lifetime member, ASNA; numerous testimonials. **Died:** Birmingham, Ala.

References and Credits

†Allen LN, Allen CB: Courage to Care: The Story of Ida V. Moffett. Birmingham, Ala., Samford University Press, 1988, pp 10, 182.

Computer printout Alabama Healthcare Hall of Fame. http://www.healthcarehof.org.

Allen, C., Ida V. Moffett. In Bullough V, Sentz L (eds): American Nursing: A Biographical Dictionary, vol. 3. New York, Springer, 2000, pp 208–211.

April 10

S. Lillian Clayton

1876–1930

"We must be actively interested, ourselves, in our profession. We must get a picture of the whole situation, nursing in relation to the past, present and future—our relation to the patient, to the doctor, and to the community. There has never been a time when it was so necessary for the individual nurse to be able to interpret her own profession, and her place in it, as at the present time. . . . Nursing was introduced in this country because patients needed nurses. Patients need nurses today. The need is not being met. What are the reasons? . . . The fundamental principles of a profession are the ability to assume individual responsibility, and . . . altruistic motives. If nurses met the needs of patients fifty years ago because they believed it their individual responsibility to do so, and if their altruistic motives led them to assume that responsibility, what [is] preventing our profession today from accepting these same fundamental principles?" (1928)

As a young girl, Lillian Clayton was attracted to both nursing and missionary work. She prepared academically for both, but the Boxer Rebellion cancelled her hopes of working in China. She joined her professional colleague Ella Phillips Crandell as a hospital administrator in Ohio before she returned to Teachers College at Columbia University for further study. Clayton subsequently assumed educational positions in nursing. Described as spiritual, inspirational, modest, and dedicated, she gave her gift of self to students, patients, and hospital workers. During her fifteen-year tenure as director of the training school at Philadelphia General Hospital, she focused on improving both health care and the educational program for nurses. She replaced volunteer help with paid employees, garnered public support for new hospital construction, and brought patient care under nurse supervision. She increased the number of graduate nurses on staff, improved their salaries, and provided residences for nurses. She improved the curriculum and instituted new coursework, including postgraduate classes, with additional, qualified faculty. She worked with the Rockefeller Foundation to visit European nursing programs, and her involvement attracted nurses to Philadelphia for work and study. Her work with the American Nurses Association (ANA) helped establish the ANA's first code of ethics.

Biography

Born: 1876, Kent County, Md. **Education:** Philadelphia General Hosp. (Blockley) School of Nursing (diploma); Baptist Institute for Christian Workers; Teachers College, Columbia Univ. **Work history:** Children's Hospital, Philadelphia; Philadelphia General Hosp.; Administrator, Miami Valley (Ohio) Hosp.; Teacher, Administrator, Minneapolis City Hosp.; Director, Illinois Training School for Nurses; Director, Philadelphia General Hosp.; Consultant, Rockefeller Foundation. **Organizations:** leadership roles in ANA, National League for Nursing, American Journal of Nursing Co., and Pa. State Bd. of Nurse Examiners. **Awards:** posthumous honorary MSN, Temple Univ. **Died:** Philadelphia.

References and Credits

†Clayton L: An Activity Update (1928). In Flanagan L: One Strong Voice: The Story of the American Nurses Association. Kansas City, Mo., Lowell Press, 1976, pp 448, 449.

Bullough V: S. Lillian Clayton. In Bullough V, Church OM, Stein AP (eds): American Nursing: A Biographical Dictionary, vol. 1. New York, Garland, 1988, pp 64–65.

Goodrich A: S. Lillian Clayton. AJN 30: 871–872, 1930.

Roberts MS: S. Lillian Clayton, 1876–1930, Educator, administrator, humanitarian, civic patriot. AJN 54:1360–1363, 1954.

In memoriam: S. Lillian Clayton. AJN 30:678–688, 1930.

APRIL 11

Mary Luciel McGorkey

1903–1990

"These ... forces [of change] ... made hospitals larger and larger until they aped the mammoth industrial corporations and even housed themselves in enormous skyscrapers. This ever-spreading complex ... magnified the pattern of life itself, and out of it all two far-reaching tidal waves emerged ... (1) work, including white collar work, became group activity on a scale so colossal that a single individual no longer had meaning: and (2) the employer ... was no longer a human being but an impersonal entity acting for unknown or absent human beings who did not own the enterprise. ... The first tidal wave made the white collar worker as insignificant individually as one of the laborers on an assembly line. The second tidal wave put the welfare of the white collar worker at the mercy of managers who did not own the enterprise." (1939)

MARY MCGORKEY WAS an advocate for professional nursing and quality patient care who saw unionization as critical to improving both. In 1937, when mainstream nursing leaders and organizations rejected union activity as inappropriate, she successfully organized more than three thousand nurses in New York State. Politically astute, she networked with elected officials to build support for nursing's issues. Her union leadership helped New York nurses replace the traditional ten-hour split shift with the eight-hour continuous shift. Some of her other successes included improved sanitation in the hospitals and keeping unqualified people from giving bedside care and administering medication. When the state legislature was revising the Nurse Practice Act, she lobbied against licensing for practical nurses, fearing it would tempt hospitals to replace RNs with "cheap labor." When organized nursing was touting the Harmon Retirement Plan as a smart investment, her study led to a scathing factual analysis that proved otherwise. In her support of unionization by white-collar hospital workers, she faulted the emerging impersonal, corporate hospital mentality and its focus on profit above all else. She referred to these forces of change as "tidal waves."

Biography

Born: April 11, 1903, Venice, Ohio. **Education:** Dixmont State Hosp., Pa. **Work history:** Private Duty; President, nurses' union, Hosp. Division of State, County, and Municipal Workers of America; Lobbyist. **Organizations:** Association of Hospital and Medical Professions. **Awards:** unknown. **Died:** San Francisco.

References and Credits

†McGorkey M: A red-head grows up. New Nurse 3:3–4, 1939.

Donahue MP: Mary Luciel McGorkey. In Bullough V, Sentz L (eds): American Nursing: A Biographical Dictionary, vol. 3. New York, Springer, 2000, pp 202–205.

McGorkey M: Pie-man, Pie-man, Let me taste your wares. New Nurse 12:6–9, 12, 1939.

April 12

Melanie Creagan Dreher

1943–

"Public health nurses have always been regarded as a bastion of liberal, futuristic, expansive thought for the larger nursing community. They are expected to perform as activists, change agents, planners, and social reformers. ...Does nursing possess the theoretical foundation for preparing nurses to care for the health of the public? ...Broader social issues are the essence of public health nursing. ...Opportunities to use political power for health legislation that could result in more far-reaching changes remain untapped. ...The realities of social conflict, vested interest, economic power, political sanctions, community factions, class struggles, and internecine competition that obstruct efforts to achieve consensus have not begun to be addressed. ...Nurses must be equipped to accomplish the far-reaching changes that will include the establishment of a comprehensive public health nursing system to which every individual will have equal access." (1982)

Melanie Creagan Dreher never really aspired to be a nurse. Because her family had no money for college tuition, she enrolled in a nursing school affiliated with a college, "but once I got into nursing, I was hooked." A distinguished anthropologist, researcher, writer, educator, administrator, and consultant, Dreher focuses on cultural influences in health care and public health nursing. She is also noted for her work and writings about applied anthropology in Jamaica. One of her early studies looked at marijuana use among fieldworkers, and her findings countered the then-popular "amotivational syndrome" believed to be associated with marijuana use. Her coworkers described her as "a superlative researcher" and "a field worker with few peers." She also studied prenatal marijuana use and neonatal outcomes in Jamaica. In a study of town nursing in a rural New England area, she found that health care at the community level meets all the criteria for good care. Her ongoing interest and studies in family and community health acknowledge the public health nurse's central role as caregiver, family advocate, and educator. However, she challenges the public health curriculum to move away from the narrow view of caring for individuals to the necessarily broader scope of socioeconomic and political issues that create barriers to care.

Biography

Born: April 12, 1943, Ft. Benning, Ga. **Education:** Long Island College Hosp. (RN); Long Island Univ. (BSN); Teachers College, Columbia Univ. (MA, PhD). **Work history:** Researcher, Writer, faculty positions at Columbia Univ., Univ. of Miami, Univ. of Massachusetts, Amherst, Univ. of the West Indies; member, numerous journal review boards. **Organizations:** President, Sigma Theta Tau International (STTI); Council of Nursing and Anthropology; charter member, National Institute for Nursing Research and the National Institutes of Health Council of Public Representatives. **Awards:** Chancellor's Medal, Univ. of Massachusetts; Leadership Award, STTI; citation for humanitarian work, Jamaica; Fogarty Senior International Fellowship; honorary member, Alpha Sigma Lambda; Fellow, American Academy of Nursing; Public Health Nurse Award, Fla.; Fellow, Society for Applied Anthropology; Univ. of Miami Award; Sigma XI Scientific Research Society; Sigma Theta Tau; Optimates Honor Society.

References and Credits

†Dreher MC: The conflict of conservatism in public health nursing education. Nurs Outlook (Nov.–Dec.): 505, 507, 509, 1982.

Dreher M: resume.

University of Iowa faculty website, available on-line at http://www.nursing.viowas.edu/faculty/dreher.htm.

Dreher M: District nursing: The cost benefits of a population-based practice. Am J Public Health 74:1107–1111, 1984.

References and Credits continued on page 766

April 13

Mabel Wandelt

1917–

"Nurses leave nursing and remain outside the work force because of conditions in the job setting that interfere with the practice of nursing. ... When overload reaches a point and continues for weeks with no support or relief, and nurses cannot give safe, adequate care, a nurse will leave. Her conscience will not allow her to remain in the situation. ... There is overwhelming evidence that what nurses complain about and report as reasons for leaving and staying out of nursing does exist; it is real. There is also evidence that distressful conditions need not exist. Where they do not exist, there is no shortage of nurses, and nurses judge the quality of care provided to patients to be good." (1981)

Mabel Wandelt sounded the wake-up call that resulted in the identification of the core characteristics of magnet hospitals. When she directed the Center for Health Care Research and Evaluation (CHCRE) at the School of Nursing at the University of Texas in Austin, she led research that examined the reasons that nurses leave hospital nursing. She found that nurses who left were those that could not control their own practice, had to increasingly or consistently compromise on patient care, and ultimately reached a dissatisfaction saturation point. When Wandelt's research explored the appeal of hospitals that did not experience problems recruiting and retaining nurses, she found similarities in administration, nursing leadership, and nursing practice. Common characteristics included knowledgeable and highly qualified nurse leadership that supported and valued a professional nursing staff that could control its practice and provide high-quality patient care. She later worked with the Task Force on Nursing Practice in Hospitals sponsored by the American Academy of Nursing (AAN). The task force designated as magnet hospitals those institutions with the power to attract and retain nurses. That study, published in 1983, resulted in a gold standard for hospitals that remains in use today. Her work, and that of subsequent scholars, resulted in the accreditation process for magnet hospitals by the American Nurses Credentialing Center (ANCC).

Biography

Born: April 13, 1917, Daggett, Mich. **Education:** Michael Reese Hosp. School of Nursing, Chicago (RN); Wayne State Univ., Detroit (BSPHN); Univ. of Michigan (MPH, PhD). **Work history:** tuberculosis and general staff nursing, Mich., Mass., N.Y.; Public Health Nurse, Detroit Dept. of Health; Army Nurse Corps; administration, Veterans Administration; Faculty, Wayne State Univ.; Assistant Dean, Univ. of Delaware; Director, CHCRE; volunteer, Southwest Center for Nursing History, Austin. Researcher; Author. **Organizations:** American Nurses Assoc.; Sigma Theta Tau International; National League for Nursing; American Public Health Assoc. **Awards:** Professor Emeritus, Univ. of Texas; Fellow, AAN; President's Award, AAN; Founders Award, Sigma Theta Tau; Living Legend, American Academy of Nursing, 1997.

References and Credits

†Wandelt M, Pierce P, Widdowson R: Why nurses leave nursing and what can be done about it. AJN 81:73, 74, 77, 1981.

American Academy of Nursing Task Force on Nursing Practice in Hospitals. St. Louis, American Nurses Association, 1983.

McClure M, Hinshaw A: Magnet Hospitals Revisited. Washington, D.C., American Academy of Nursing, 2002.

Crowder ELM: Mabel Wandelt. In Bullough V, Sentz L (eds): American Nursing: A Biographical Dictionary, vol. 3. New York, Springer, 2000, pp 279–282.

Who's Who in American Nursing, 1996–97, 6th ed. New Providence, N.J., Reed Reference, 1995.

Brown BJ: personal communication, 2002.

April 14

Maria Celina Phaneuf

1907–

"I learned more from the successes than I did from the failures. ...Never underestimate people's capacities. ...Never assume acceptance in the absence of evidence that it exists." (1936)

Maria Phaneuf was a researcher, teacher, and administrator who looked deeply into the tasks at hand to provide the leadership necessary to bring communities together for the benefit of all patients. She was asked to serve with a group that influenced the Medicare coverage for continued care outside acute-care hospitals during the Lyndon Johnson administration. She was knowledgeable in evaluating the quality of care. She believed that nurses should promulgate the standards that state insurance companies should meet in providing home care services. She worked closely with Blue Cross and the National League for Nursing to develop standards that were the precursor of today's Community Health Accreditation Program (CHAP) operated by the NLN. Phaneuf belonged to the Medical Committee for Human Rights, which provided medical support during civil rights demonstrations. Her careful reflection and guidance during and after the Detroit riots helped in the formation of an inner city health care clinic. She held faculty appointments in both the School of Medicine and Community Health at Wayne State University. She and a professor of medicine at Wayne State cochaired a committee that created a core curriculum for the Schools of Medicine, Nursing, Pharmacy, and Social Work. One course focuses on ethics. She received many honors and awards. She is professor emerita at Wayne State University. She is best known for her books *The Nursing Audit: Profile for Excellence* and *The Nursing Audit: Self Regulation in Nursing Practice.*

Biography

Born: April 14, 1907, Richford, Vt. **Education:** Richford (Vt.) High School, valedictorian, 1924; Grace Hosp. School of Nursing, New Haven, Conn., 1928; Teachers College, Columbia Univ., 1949, 1954 (BA, MA in nursing education); **Work history:** Head Nurse, Supervisor, Night Superintendent, Assistant Director of Nursing, Grace Hosp., 1928–35; established health program for students and faculty, Putney School, Putney, Vt.; Visiting Nurse Supervisor, New York; Henry Street Settlement House Nursing Service, ten yrs.; studied feasibility of providing Visiting Nurse Service to Blue Cross subscribers; Associated Hosp. Service; promoted development of NLN's Criteria for Evaluating the Administration of Public Health Nursing Service, 1961; Faculty, Wayne State Univ. College of Nursing; Chair, Public Health Nursing Dept., Wayne State; author of two books; Visiting Professor. **Organizations:** American Nurses Association, others. **Awards:** Award for Merit for Research in Medical Care Organization, Public Health Assoc. of N.Y.C., 1959; Wayne State Univ. Maria C. Phaneuf Quality Assurance Symposium Series, 1973; Award for Distinguished Achievement in Nursing Practice, the Nursing Education Assoc., Teachers College, Columbia Univ., 1977; Marie Hippensteel Lingeman Founder's Award for Excellence in Nursing Practice, Sigma Theta Tau International, 1987; Fellow, American Academy of Nursing, American Public Health Assoc.

References and Credits

†Redland A: Maria Phaneuf. In Bullough V, Sentz L, Stein AP (eds): American Nursing: A Biographical Dictionary, vol. 2. New York, Garland, 1992, pp 265–270.

Julia St. Lo Mellichamp

1877–1939

"To the community [the registry] affords ready access to all classes of nursing service and vouches for the moral and professional fitness of each of its members. By taking hourly visiting nurses and non-graduates, a registry will do much towards solving the problem of how to care for people of moderate means. Furthermore, it affords financial protection by its regular tariff on fees for various branches of work. In short, the nurse's registry should be the professional clearing-house for the community." (1916)

"State registration is meant to be the state's guarantee of efficiency and the registered nurse should be possessed of such dignity and knowledge as will enable her to be such a splendid exponent of registration that the public will easily discern the difference between the well-trained nurse and the non-graduate. Logically, then, the private duty nurse who is registered, coming as she does constantly in contact with people of means and influence, has a splendid opportunity to awaken public interest in nursing education." (1916)

JULIA ST. LO MELLICHAMP was an articulate advocate for the creation of a national registry for nurses. She devoted much of her career to improving nurses' working circumstances.

She started her career as a teacher, then became a legal secretary, and eventually graduated as a nurse. She worked as a private duty nurse until the lasting effects of infantile paralysis prevented her from continuing the demanding work. She became the first school nurse in Norfolk, Virginia, and it was then that she began to work in professional organizations. She served as the secretary-treasurer of the Virginia State Board of Examiners of Nurses for six years. She was an inspector of hospital training schools and advocated reforms that are now standard in the profession: the use of graduate nurses as night supervisors, a standard training program for student nurses, certification requirements for nursing teachers, and standard outlines for nursing courses. She is remembered for her "quiet understanding that created confidence everywhere," according to the writer Meta R. Pennock.

Biography

Born: April 13, 1877, Florence, S.C. **Education:** college graduate; Sarah Leigh Hosp. School of Nursing, Norfolk, Va., 1906, with honors. **Work history:** Private Duty Nurse, 1906–11; School Nurse, Norfolk, Va., 1911–17; Inspector, hosp. training schools, Norfolk, Va., 1917–20; member, bd. of directors, National Organization for Public Health Nursing, 1917; School Nurse, Social Worker, Greenbrier County, W. Va., 1920–27; Supervising Nurse, Social Worker, Dorchester County, S.C., 1927; Director, Bureau of Social Service, Jasper County, S.C., 1933–34; School Nurse, Jasper and Colleton Counties, S.C., 1934–35; Librarian, Charleston (S.C.) County Health Dept., 1935–39. **Organizations:** Treasurer, Va. State Nurses Assoc. (VSNA); State Chair, Red Cross Nursing Service, Va.; President, Sarah Leigh Alumnae Assoc.; President, Norfolk Division, VSNA; Exec. Secretary, Treasurer, Va. State Bd. of Examiners of Nurses, 1914–20; charter member, Va. State League for Nursing Education; Chair, Public Health Nursing Section, W. Va. Nursing Assoc. **Awards:** unknown. **Died:** Charleston, S.C.

References and Credits

†Mellichamp JSL: The development and value of a nurses' registry. AJN 16: 25, 27, 1916.

Pennock MR: Makers of Nursing History: Portraits and Pen Sketches of One-hundred and Nine Prominent Women. New York: Lakeside, 1940, pp 96–97.

Wells M: Julia Mellichamp. In Bullough V, Sentz L, Stein AP (eds): American Nursing: A Biographical Dictionary, vol. 2. New York, Garland, 1992, pp 223–224.

April 16

Hazel Corbin

1895–1988

"Rapid changes are taking place in maternity care across this country. ... Obstetrics is beginning to move out of the era of surgery, deep anesthesia, and forceps. Pregnancy is no longer considered a sickness of nine months' duration but a natural, common, normal function of the body. Hospital designs are being changed to place emphasis upon people and their personalities. Hospital administration policies are being altered to remove tensions and fears which can easily arise in the mind of a woman alone in labor, or in a delivery room where every professional is an impersonal masked automaton. Mothers are now getting the opportunity to cuddle and love their babies, and some fathers are no longer stopped by a cold pane of plate glass when they want to hold the new member of the family in their arms." (1952)

HAZEL CORBIN JOINED the organization known as the Women's City Club of New York and established the first maternity center in 1917. She became the first field nurse and trained other nurses. Certain parts of the city had very high rates of maternal and infant mortality, and Corbin became interested in doing something about it. In 1918, when the Maternity Nursing Center Association (MCA) was founded, Corbin joined the staff, becoming director in 1923. Corbin's creativity launched an exhibit at the

New York World's Fair of 1939 that depicted human reproduction and reached more than one million people. She was influential in developing the nurse-midwife certification programs. Accordingly, she assisted in founding the Association for the Promotion and Standardization of Midwifery in 1934. She recruited nurses for the American Red Cross during World War II. She held a special affection for a father's role, and in 1939 she wrote and published *Getting Ready to Be a Father.* She retired in 1965 to New Smyrna Beach, Florida.

Biography

Born: 1895, Nova Scotia, Can. **Education:** Brooklyn (N.Y.) Hosp. **Work history:** Field Nurse, trained nurses for Women's City Club, N.Y.C.; Charge Nurse, Brooklyn Maternity Center; Assistant Director, Director, MCA; developed nurse-midwife certification programs, Columbia Univ., Yale Univ., Johns Hopkins Univ., State University of New York, Downstate Medical Center; presented courses on maternal care programs, New York Hosp. and Teachers College, Columbia Univ.; promoted sculptures of developing fetus, 1939 World's Fair; developed book of photographs for publication by MCA. **Organizations:** unknown. **Awards:** The Hazel Corbin Fund, established by MCA, helps nurses to study midwifery; Martha May Eliot Award, American Public Health Association. 1966. **Died:** New Smyrna Beach, Fla.

References and Credits

†Corbin H: Nurse midwives: The torch bearers. AJN 52:499, 1952.

Stein AP: Hazel Corbin. In Bullough V, Sentz L, Stein AP (eds): American Nursing: A Biographical Dictionary, vol. 2. New York, Garland, 1992, pp 66–67.

Jessie Lulu Stevenson (West)

1891–1976

"Every nurse—institutional, private duty or public health—who gives bedside care or teaches the art of nursing to student nurses or families is responsible for making or preventing crippling. …Orthopedic nursing must be a part of all good nursing but the reverse is equally true, all good nursing is a part of orthopedic nursing." (1939)

"The nurse needs an appreciation of… the vital role she can play in promoting optimum health. …[She] has daily opportunities to apply the principles of protective body mechanics. …Teaching ways of preventing foot and back strain is a part of good prenatal instruction: helping the teacher see what adjustments are necessary to encourage good posture contributes to better health of the school child: demonstrating to an industrial worker correct method of lifting may prevent a serious disability." (1945)

JESSIE STEVENSON HAD studied at four universities, taught English, and was prepared in physical therapy before she entered nursing school. She was a catalyst for improving nursing service and patient care by demonstrating the value of networking with non-nurse specialties, such as physical therapy and social work. When funding came from the National Foundation for Infantile

Paralysis (NFIP) in 1939, the National Organization for Public Health Nursing (NOPHN) hired her to be the orthopedic consultant. She brought seventeen years' experience as director of orthopedic services for the Visiting Nurse Association (VNA) of Chicago and had supervised the orthopedic unit associated with Northwestern University's medical school. In addition, she had been the orthopedic director for NOPHN in New York State. Her work with NOPHN showed that nursing's cooperative efforts with other members of the health care team improved health services. Patients had reduced disability and faster recovery. Her goal was to see good nursing care facilitate recovery without complications or further disability. Her work in public health nursing, the exemplary programs that she established, and her many publications greatly enhanced nursing care of patients with poliomyelitis.

Biography

Born: 1891 (location unknown). **Education:** Univ. of South Dakota (BA); Harvard Medical School; Univ. of Chicago; Northwestern Medical School (physical therapy certificate); Presbyterian Hosp. School of Nursing, Chicago. **Work history:** Orthopedic Director, NOPHN; Orthopedic Director, VNA, Chicago; Supervisor, Orthopedic Unit, Northwestern Univ. Medical School; Author; established consulting services for NFIP. **Organizations:** American Nurses Assoc.; National League for Nursing Education; NOPHN; American Physiotherapy Assoc. **Awards:** unknown. **Died:** Santa Barbara, Calif.

References and Credits

†Roberts M: American Nursing: History and Interpretation. New York, Macmillan, 1954, p 276.

†Stevenson J: An orthopedic service for the community. Public Health Nurs 37:608, 1945.

Sentz L: Jesse Lulu Stevenson (West). In Bullough V, Church OM, Stein AP (eds): American Nursing: A Biographical Dictionary, vol. 1. New York, Garland, 1988, pp 297–298.

April 18

Florence Sophie Schorske Wald

1917–

"When hospice nurses were asked, in 1985, what their greatest difficulty was ... they said it was not knowing if they did the right thing. ...Managing symptoms of a hospice patient is a 'delicate titration.' Keeping a patient pain free, and comfortable enough to interact with the family requires expertise. Those who do this well are as skillful in their own way as a surgeon who repairs a delicate blood vessel." (1999)

FLORENCE WALD WAS hospitalized frequently as a child because of respiratory problems, and the nursing care that she received attracted her to the profession. A nursing leader, she changed the direction of health care in the United States. Death with dignity is a reality because of the concern, commitment, and dedication of Florence Wald. She recognized that, for the terminally ill patient, quality of life is more important than intensive clinical interventions. While at Yale, she was exploring new ways for nurses to deal more effectively with patient concerns when she met Dr. Cicely Saunders. When Wald learned of the hospice movement, she left her academic position to study and work with Saunders at St. Christopher's Hospice in London. Upon returning home Wald assembled a multidisciplinary team and successfully applied the concept in Connecticut. This gave birth to the hospice movement in the

United States. She later became involved with the prison hospice movement, which is concerned with inmates who are terminally ill and serving a life sentence.

Biography

Born: April 19, 1917, New York City. **Education:** Mt. Holyoke College (BA); Yale Univ. School of Nursing (MN). **Work history:** Research Technician, Army Signal Corps, World War II; Staff Nurse, New York Visiting Nurse Service; Research, College of Physicians and Surgeons; Instructor, Rutgers Univ. School of Nursing; Instructor, Research Associate, Professor, Dean, Yale Univ. School of Nursing; St. Christopher's Hospice, London; planning staff, Hospice, Inc., Conn.; Principal Investigator, National Prison Hospice Assoc. **Organizations:** unknown. **Awards:** Distinguished Alumna Award, Yale Univ.; Distinguished Woman of Conn. Award; Fellow, American Academy of Nursing; first recipient, Florence S. Wald Award for Contributions to Nursing Practice, Conn. Nursing Assoc.; Founder's Award, National Hospice Organization; Contribution to Hospice Award; American Nurses Assoc. Hall of Fame; National Women's Hall of Fame, Conn. Women's Hall of Fame; Living Legend, American Academy of Nursing, 2001.

References and Credits

†Friedrich MJ: Hospice care in the United States: A conversation with Florence S. Wald. JAMA 281:1684, 1999.

Wald F: personal communication, 2002.

Beaudoin C: Florence Wald. In Bullough V, Sentz L (eds): American Nursing: A Biographical Dictionary, vol. 3. New York, Springer, 2000, pp 276–279.

Announcement. Reflections on Nursing Leadership 28:45, 2002.

ANA Hall of Fame 10/98 American Nurses Association, Washington, D.C. http://www.nursingworld.org/hof.

Mary Elizabeth Carnegie

1916–

"The story of the achievements of black nurses in the United States has been one of faith, ambition, preparation, perseverance, aggressiveness, courage, conviction and the unwavering belief in the integrity of human beings. My story is of just one black nurse who managed to overcome many obstacles on the way to realizing her professional goals. . . . For 25 years as an editor of major nursing periodicals, I had noticed that black nurses had been left out of the history books in America, with the exception of one or two sentences alluding to the first black nurse, Mary Mahoney, and NACGN's [National Association for Colored Graduate Nurses'] existence from 1908 to 1951. I believed that it was up to me to fill this void with my book, The Path We Tread: Blacks in Nursing, 1854–1984 *(Carnegie, 1986). This, I think, has been my greatest contribution to nursing." (1988)*

Racial discrimination restricted Mary Elizabeth Carnegie's options to study nursing, to work in the profession, and to participate in nursing organizations. When she was a student nurse at Lincoln Hospital in New York City, she attended a meeting of the NACGN. There she became aware of the widespread prejudice, discrimination, and disregard for black nurses. She vowed that when she graduated she "would do all within my power to help change the system and break down the barriers that were keeping black nurses out of the mainstream of professional nursing." She never lost courage, even though the obstacles seemed to always be there. She faced rejection because of color when she tried to join the Navy Nurse Corps during World War II as well as discrimination against her student nurses when she was placing them on clinical rotation in the 1940s. Carnegie made a difference for black nurses because she was determined and she persevered. She taught by the courageous example of her professional practice. She is an internationally respected nursing leader who strengthens nursing with her written legacy.

Biography

Born: April 19, 1916, Baltimore. **Education:** Lincoln School for Nurses, N.Y.C.; West Virginia State College (BA); Univ. of Toronto (master's equivalent in Canada); Syracuse Univ. (master's); New York Univ. (PhD). **Work history:** Black Veterans Hosp., Tuskegee, Ala.; Freedmen's Hosp., Washington, D.C.; Nursing Faculty, Medical College of Virginia; Nursing Faculty, Hampton Institute; Dean, School of Nursing, Fla. A&M College, Tallahassee; editorial positions at *American Journal of Nursing, Nursing Outlook, Nursing Research;* Independent Consultant; Visiting Professor at numerous university schools of nursing; worldwide lecturer on behalf of nursing. **Organizations:** Fla. State Nurses Assoc., American Nurses Assoc. (ANA). **Awards:** honorary degrees, Hunter College; City College of New York; State Univ. of New York, Brooklyn; Marian College, Ind.; Thomas Jefferson Univ., Philadelphia; Virginia Commonwealth Univ.; Indiana Univ.; Syracuse Univ.; George Arents Pioneer Medal, Syracuse Univ.; Fellow, American Academy of Nursing; ANA Mary Mahoney Award; Lillian Wald Award, N.Y. Visiting Nurses Assoc.; Mable Staupers Award, Chi Eta Phi; endowed chair in her name, Howard Univ.; Carnegie Award for Excellence and Service to Others, established by Rutgers College of Nursing; ANA Hall of Fame; Living Legend, American Academy of Nursing, 1994.

References and Credits

†Schorr T, Zimmerman A: Making Choices, Taking Chances: Nurse Leaders Tell Their Stories. St. Louis, CV Mosby, 1988, pp 28, 30, 41.

Smalls SM: Elizabeth Carnegie. In Bullough V, Sentz L (eds): American Nursing: A Biographical Dictionary, vol. 3. New York, Springer, 2000, pp 44–47.

ANA Hall of Fame 10/98 American Nurses Association, Washington, D.C. http://www.nursingworld.org/hof.

April 29

Kate Cumming

1838–1909

"These notes of passing events often hurriedly penned amid the active duties of hospital life, but feebly indicate, and only faintly picture, the sad reality. I now pray, and will never cease to pray to the end of my days, that men may beat their swords into plowshares and their spears into pruning hooks, and that nation may not lift a sword against nation, nor learn war any more. It is with the hope that the same feeling may be aroused in every reader that I present this volume [The Journal of a Confederate Nurse] *to the public." (1866)*

KATE CUMMING WAS inspired by Florence Nightingale's work in the Crimea. Cumming, who was born in Scotland but raised in Mobile, Alabama, was politically committed to the cause of the Confederacy and began her war service as a volunteer untrained nurse caring for the wounded after the Battle of Shiloh. Her abilities with the care of the sick resulted in her promotion to hospital matron. Although she held the position of hospital matron in several Southern states, the prejudice of military leaders and doctors against physical nursing by women restricted her duties to housekeeping. According to the writer Marilyn M. Culpepper, this prompted Cumming to write in her journal that "a lady's respectibility [*sic*] must be at a low ebb when it can be endangered by going into a hospital." However, from 1862 until the end of the war she worked in field hospitals throughout Georgia after Union Gen. William T. Sherman's invasion. Her legacy is the diary she published with detailed information about hospital life during the war.

Biography

Born: 1838, Edinburgh, Scotland. **Education:** unknown. **Work history:** Volunteer Nurse, Hosp. Matron, Civil War; Teacher. **Organizations:** Episcopal Church, United Daughters of the Confederacy. **Awards:** unknown. **Buried:** Mobile, Ala.

References and Credits

†Harwell RB (ed): Kate: The Journal of a Confederate Nurse. Baton Rouge, Louisiana State University Press, 1959, p 3.

Sabin LE: Kate Cumming. In Bullough V, Church OM, Stein AP (eds): American Nursing: A Biographical Dictionary, vol. 1. New York, Garland, 1988, pp 72–73.

Culpepper MM: Trials and Triumphs: Women of the American Civil War. Lansing, Michigan State University Press, 1991, p 318.

Notable Women in Georgia's History: Pioneers in Health Care, 1998, available on-line at http://www.sos.state.ga.us/women's_history/_month/bio_health_care.htm.

April 21

Sara Elizabeth Parsons

1864–1949

"The nurse is the doctor's assistant, but her work is no less responsible than his; she has dozens of opportunities to make mistakes when he has one; his success often depends on her intelligent interpretation of his orders and she must not allow her work to be underestimated." (1916)

Sara Elizabeth Parsons interrupted her nursing studies for seven years to care for her sick mother and, after her mother's death, to raise two younger siblings. Her varied career included psychiatric nursing, military nursing, nursing education, and administration. She had an additional year of study at the McLean Hospital for the Mentally Ill after she completed nursing school, and she was always interested in promoting this nursing specialty. She served as a volunteer nurse during the Spanish-American War, working on a hospital ship that transported sick and wounded soldiers. She canceled plans to establish a nursing school at a state mental hospital in Massachusetts after she developed typhoid fever. Later, when she was superintendent of nurses at Massachusetts General Hospital (her alma mater), she hired full-time instructors, improved educational standards, started a library, and offered recreational programs. Parsons was known for using the case study method as a teaching tool, and she always worked to strengthen the educational programs in schools that she established or managed. She wrote *The History of the Massachusetts General School for Nurses, Nursing Problems and Obligations*, and a wide range of articles. She was active in lobbying for nursing legislation at the state and federal levels and helped to successfully lobby Congress for military rank for nurses in the armed services.

Biography

Born: April 21, 1864, Northboro, Mass. **Education:** Boston Training School for Nurses (later Massachusetts General Hosp.); advanced study, McLean Hosp.; Teacher's College, Columbia Univ.; Massachusetts General Hosp. (hosp. administration studies). **Work history:** Head Nurse, Massachusetts General Hosp.; Supervisor, McLean Hosp.; Superintendent of Nursing, Butler Hosp., R.I.; Volunteer, Spanish-American War; Superintendent of Nurses, Adams Nervine Hosp., Mass.; Sheppard and Pratt Hosp., Md.; Hosp. Administrator, Derby, Conn.; Superintendent of Nurses, Massachusetts General Hosp.; European military nursing service, World War I; Historian, Massachusetts General Hosp. School of Nursing; Registrar, Central Directory of Nurses, Boston. **Organizations:** Mass. General Hosp. Alumnae Assoc.; Mass. Nurses Assoc.; National League for Nursing Education. **Awards:** ANA Hall of Fame. **Died:** Jamaica Plain, Mass.

References and Credits

†Parsons S: The student nurse. AJN 16:1098, 1916.

Cooper SS: Sara Parsons. In Bullough V, Church OM, Stein AP (eds): American Nursing: A Biographical Dictionary, vol. 1. New York, Garland, 1988, pp 254–256.

ANA Hall of Fame 10/98 American Nurses Association, Washington, D.C. http://www.nursingworld.org/hof.

Emilie Gleason Sargent

1894–1977

"Does the reality of being a nurse compete successfully with the imaginary image of oneself in that capacity? I believe that it does. Looking back over my own experience as a professional nurse, I have found many personal and professional satisfactions. They spring primarily from the opportunity to fit knowledge and skills to an ever-appealing human need. To most of us who have the privilege of writing R.N. after our names, the nursing profession has given what more that 40,000 new students this year are hoping to discover." (1947)

EMILIE SARGENT ENTERED nursing after a brief career as a teacher, and public health nursing became her specialty. She worked for four decades with the Detroit Visiting Nurse Association, and her improvements in patient care became the standard adopted by other agencies across the country. She expanded services to include physical and occupational therapy, nutritional counseling, mental health screening, and industrial (occupational) health. In her program staff nurses worked with practical nurses and home health aides as part of the home care team. She was a forward thinker and a leader in innovative programs in home care for the chronically ill and aged. She promoted hospital discharge planning as a member of Detroit's Home Care Demonstration Project. Many of her ideas were incorporated into Medicare when it was established.

Biography

Born: April 26, 1894, St. Paul, Minn. **Education:** Univ. of Michigan (BA); Vassar Training Camp for Nurses; Mt. Sinai Hosp. School of Nursing, N.Y.C. **Work history:** Staff Member, Exec. Director, Visiting Nurse Assoc. of Detroit. **Organizations:** National Organization for Public Health Nursing (NOPHN); National League for Nursing; Michigan Public Health Assoc. (MPHA); member, bd. of directors, American. Journal of Nursing Co.; United Community Service of Detroit; American Red Cross; Michigan Crippled Children's Commission; White House Conference on Aging; Advisory Commission, U.S. Public Health Service. **Awards:** Life Member, NOPHN; honorary doctorate, Wayne State Univ.; Pearl McIver Award, American Nurses Assoc. (ANA); Outstanding Achievement Award, Univ. of Michigan; scholarship in her name, Univ. of Michigan School of Public Health; honorary membership, MPHA.; ANA Hall of Fame. **Died:** Detroit.

References and Credits

†Gleason E: Nursing: A service to humanity. School and College Placement 8:5, 1947.

Bullough V: Emilie Gleason Sargent. In Bullough V, Sentz L, Stein AP (eds): American Nursing: A Biographical Dictionary, vol. 2. New York, Garland, 1992, pp 288–289.

ANA Hall of Fame 10/98 American Nurses Association, Washington, D.C. http://www.nursingworld.org/hof.

Veronica Margaret Driscoll

1926–1994

"The evidence that nursing is a professional endeavor is far too overwhelming to refute. An examination of the nature of the nursing process reveals that it is founded on a body of knowledge which embodies an exquisite humanistic and intellectual mix, a process encompassing diagnosis, intervention, application, and caring skills and abilities of the highest order. The fact that this profession has not been so recognized, legally, is part of nursing's tragic history." (1972)

Veronica Margaret Driscoll was a determined and effective advocate for professional independence, high educational standards, and economic justice. She left a powerful legacy for nursing. The leader in collective bargaining efforts by the New York State Nurses Association (NYSNA) in the mid-1960s, she successfully negotiated for better working conditions and benefits. She also helped increase nurses' salaries above those of New York City sanitation workers at the time. She was lead author of the landmark, education-defining *Blueprint for the Education of Nurses in New York State,* which reinforced the position of the American Nurses Association (ANA) on education for nurses. Called a "skilled strategist and charismatic communicator," she was responsible for passage of the New York State Nurse Practice Act in 1972, which became a national model. A widely sought consultant and lecturer, she was committed to identifying the forces that suppress nursing so that nursing would recognize its value more fully, unify, and exert its independence.

Biography

Born: April 24, 1926, Brooklyn, NY. **Education:** St. Catherine's Hosp. School of Nursing, Brooklyn, N.Y.; St. John's Univ. (BS); Teachers College, Columbia Univ. (DEd).
Work history: Staff, Faculty, St. Catherine's Hosp.; Staff, Exec. Director, NYSNA; Chair, ANA Commission, Economic and General Welfare; Bd. of Director, American Journal of Nursing Co. **Organizations:** ANA; N.Y. State Hosp. Review and Planning Council.
Awards: NYSNA headquarters building named in her honor; Teachers College Nursing Alumni Assoc. Achievement Award; awards from NYSNA, ANA; ANA Hall of Fame.
Buried: Menands, NY.

References and Credits

†Driscoll VM: Liberating nursing practice. Nurs Outlook 20:26, 1972.

Birnbach N: Veronica Driscoll. In Bullough V, Sentz L (eds): American Nursing: A Biographical Dictionary, vol. 3. New York, Springer, 2000, pp 73–75.

ANA Hall of Fame 10/98 American Nurses Association, Washington, D.C. http://www.nursingworld.org/hof.

April 24

Sophie Gran Jevne Winton
1887–1989

"[I] gave anesthetics from the first of June [1918] to November after the Armistice. How many anesthetics I gave during the World War, I cannot determine, except that when the big drives were on, lasting from a week to ten days, I averaged twenty-five to thirty a day. The first three months I gave chloroform entirely, after which a ruling came that we were to use ether because there had been too many deaths from chloroform in inexperienced hands. Many a night I had to pour ether or chloroform on my finger to determine the amount I was giving, because we had no lights except the surgeon had a searchlight for his work, so the only sign I had to go by was respiration. …Patients came in so fast, that all the surgeons could do was remove bullets and shrapnel, stop hemorrhages, and put iodoform packs in the wound and bandage it. As soon as they were through operating on one patient, I would have to have the next patient anesthetized." (Date unknown)

"The most pitiful thing of the work overseas was to step outside the hospital tents and see hundreds of stretchers on the ground, each bearing a man who must wait probably for hours before he could be taken care of. We had 17 operating tables working day and night and yet we could not keep up with the work." (Date unknown)

SOPHIE WINTON WAS one of the first registered nurses in Minnesota. She then trained as an anesthetist, and when she join the Army Nurse Corps during World War I, she had already administered anesthesia more than ten thousand times without a fatality. While nursing in France, at the Mobile Hospital No. 1, she and her colleagues received numerous citations for bravery and dedication to the wounded. Their professional example prompted the British to instruct their army nurses in anesthesia as well. After the war she lived in California and was involved in a lawsuit filed by the California Medical Society against a nurse-anesthetist. The society claimed that it was a violation of the California Medical Practice Act to have anesthesia administered by anyone other than a physician or surgeon. Winton contributed financially and testified in the landmark case; the court ruled for the nurse-anesthetist, declaring that the administering of anesthesia is part of an "established and uniformly accepted practice followed by surgeons and nurses." Winton's active career spanned half a century. When she was ninety-seven, the American Association of Nurse Anesthetists (AANA) honored her with its Agatha Hodgkins Award for outstanding professional achievement.

BIOGRAPHY

Born: April 24, 1887, Minnesota. **Education:** Swedish Hosp., Minneapolis; Mayo Clinic, Rochester, Minn. **Work history:** demonstrated anesthesia machines for Dr. J. A. Heidbrink; Army Nurse Corps, France; Dental Clinic, Los Angeles; opened Jevne Memorial Surgical Hosp., Los Angeles. **Organizations:** Founder, Calif. Assoc. of Nurse Anesthetists; AANA. **Awards:** Croix de Guerre; six overseas service bars; honors from Overseas Nurses Assoc., American Legion, Veterans of Foreign Wars, Mexico Dental Society; Agatha Hodgkins Award for Outstanding Accomplishment, AANA. **Died:** Hollywood, Calif.

REFERENCES AND CREDITS

†Bankert M: Watchful Care: A History of America's Nurse Anesthetists. New York, Continuum, 1989, pp 47, 48.

†Bankert M: Sophie Gran Jevne Winton. In Bullough V, Sentz L, Stein AP (eds): American Nursing: A Biographical Dictionary, vol. 2. New York, Garland, 1992, pp 359–360.

April 25

Mary E. P. Davis

1840–1924

"Granted that the ideal woman is she who takes the correct attitude toward the issues of life, and regulates her conduct by her standard of character, and that the ideal nurse is but the ideal woman plus *her professional knowledge. ... Whether she stands, walks, sits or bends, let the body be so adjusted, the position so normal, that the least exhaustive demand be made on strength, power of endurance or the proper functioning of the body. This will produce correspondingly easy mental attitude, less friction, less fault-finding, fewer lions in the way. Teach her how to concentrate her whole attention to the thing in hand. 'This one thing I do,' and it is done well. One thing at a time. Don't let the mind get separated from the body, nor from bodily work, when the work is being performed. Teach her how to relax. We all know the recuperative power of a few minutes' sleep. A few minutes' relaxation is the best substitute when sleep is not possible. Drop everything, every tension, every care, and come as near the unconsciousness of sleep as possible. Let us hear the conclusion of the whole matter, with all our teaching let us endeavor to teach the pupil to get wisdom, which is to 'know herself.'" (1907)*

In 1897 Mary Davis remembered her alma mater, Massachusetts General Hospital, by organizing the School of Nursing Alumnae Association, which became one of the first associations to join the Nurses Associated Alumnae of the United States, later known as the American Nurses Association (ANA). Mary Davis's skills in organization and business, and her fervent belief that nurses must receive higher education, made her the powerful organizer that she was. She is credited with including a business course in nursing education by supporting a postgraduate course in hospital economics at Teachers College, Columbia University, in 1899. This was the first course for nurses at a school of higher education. She presented a paper at the 1893 World's Columbian Exposition in Chicago and described the role of superintendent of nurses as requiring advanced education, ethical precepts, flexibility, collegiality, and decision-making ability. She joined seventeen other superintendents to establish the American Society of Superintendents of Training Schools for Nurses (ASSTSN), later known as the National League for Nursing (NLN). In 1900 Davis served with Lavinia Dock, Anna Maxwell, Isabel Merritt, Sophia Palmer, and Isabel Hampton Robb on the Nurses Associated Alumnae Committee on Periodicals to establish the guidelines for development of the *American Journal of Nursing*. They knew nursing needed a voice that was prepared by nurses for nurses. A joint stock company was developed as the way to finance this project. The J.B. Lippincott Company of Philadelphia was selected as publisher. Davis was the president of the board of directors, and Palmer was the editor in chief. The journal became the official organ of the Nurses Associated Alumnae and set standards for nursing publications. Davis developed the book department of the *Journal* and was largely responsible for its financial solvency. She held many offices in many organizations and worked for the enactment of registration laws.

Biography

Born: 1840, New Brunswick, Can. **Education:** Massachusetts General Hosp. Training School for Nurses, 1878. **Work history:** Staff Nurse, Massachusetts General Hosp.; Private Duty Nurse, district nursing, Boston; Superintendent, Univ. of Pennsylvania Hosp. Training School

Biography continued on pages 766–67

April 26

Mary O'Neil Mundinger

1937–

"Autonomy is a concept about independence, identity, and authority. It is a necessary attribute of professional practice. Without autonomy nursing service can be limited according to the perspective and objectives of the one directing nursing. Only a nurse knows when nursing is needed, and without autonomy, the existence of that service is in jeopardy. ...Autonomous nursing care is a concept about theory-based practice and accountable, authoritative decision making. Autonomous practice happens whenever a nurse makes an independent judgment about the presence of a health problem and then provides the resolution through nursing care." (1980)

NURSING'S INDEPENDENCE IN caring attracted Mary O'Neil Mundinger, and she believes you will accomplish all that you believe you can if you share the credit. A nursing pioneer, leader, and visionary, she is a nurse practitioner and a noted expert on health policy. Widely published and highly honored, she helped define, establish, and promote autonomous nursing practice. This recognizes that nursing is essential, has its own unique expertise, and is accountable for delivering nursing care as an equal member of the health care team. She believes that nursing's knowledge is the basis for patient advocacy and for the nursing interventions that involve clients in addressing their health care needs. In the mid-1990s she initiated hospital admitting privileges for nurse practitioners at Columbia-Presbyterian Medical Center. At that time she was also an adviser to the Clinton administration on health care reform. Her voluminous publications reflect a career of interest and expertise on a range of issues, including evolution in nursing, primary care, advanced practice, health policy, and the future of health care. She challenges nurses to identify and remove the barriers to professional practice. She has called the nurse practitioner "the generic nurse of tomorrow" and identifies the four changes that have enhanced the development of professional nursing as physical assessment skills, history taking, illness management, and the comprehensive scope of primary nursing.

Biography

Born: April 26, 1937, Dunkirk, N.Y. **Education:** Univ. of Michigan (BS); Columbia Univ. (certificate as family nurse practitioner, MA, doctorate in public health). **Work history:** Faculty, Dean, Columbia Univ. School of Nursing; Faculty, Pace Univ.; Author; Consultant; Researcher; Consultant to Clinton administration on health care reform; member, Commonwealth Fund Commission on Women's Health. **Organizations:** Founder, first president, Friends on the National Institute for Nursing Research; Adviser, Consultant to numerous groups and organizations. **Awards:** Robert Wood Johnson Health Policy Fellowship; Nurse Practitioner of the Year from *Nurse Practitioner;* honorary doctorate, Hamilton College; Distinguished Alumni Award, Univ. of Michigan; election to Institute of Medicine, National Academy of Sciences; N.Y. Academy of Medicine; Fellow, American Academy of Nursing.

References and Credits

†Mundinger MO: Autonomy in Nursing. Germantown, Md., Aspen Systems, 1980, p 1.

Mundinger MO: resume.

Goldenberg G: Aches and pains? Call your primary care nurse. Columbia, winter, 1996.

Mary D. Osborne

1875–1946

Song of the Midwives (Tune: "As We Go Marching On")
"We aim to be good midwives of the state; we try hard to be up to date,
To be on time to meetings, and never be late, as we go marching on."
Chorus: "Glory, glory, hallelujah, Glory, glory, hallelujah, Glory, glory, hallelujah, As we go marching on."
"We tell our mothers they should breathe fresh air, we show them what they need to prepare,
We teach them what the baby should wear, as we go marching on.
We tell them plenty of water to drink, about good food we cause them to think,
We say, when tired, take of sleep a wink, as we go marching on."
"We put on water in a great big pot, we know of this we must have a lot,
We boil it all, use some cool, some hot, as we go marching on.
We put drops in the baby's eyes, whether the mother laughs or cries,
The State for us the eye drops buys, as we go marching on.
We report births and deaths of all, when anything is wrong, we the doctor call,
We hope we never from grace may fall, as we go marching on.
We wear clean dress, clean cap, clean gown, we have clean homes clean yards, clean town,

We'll make OUR COUNTY OF GOOD RENOWN, as we go marching on.
OUR COUNTY Midwives are the best in the state; they try hard to be up to date;
Are on time to meetings, and never are late, as they go marching on."
(Date unknown)

MARY OSBORNE MAY not have written the "Song for Midwives," which she included at the end of her *Manual for Midwives,* but it summarizes her instructions to midwives as they appear in the manual, which received international recognition. The report from the Mississippi Board of Health (1798–1937) noted that "the Mississippi midwife program attracted the attention of workers in other states and countries, and more requests have come from foreign countries for the midwife manual than all other public health bulletins combined." Osborne was the director of public health nursing for the Mississippi Department of Health from 1921 to 1946. She recruited public health nurses to teach and supervise midwives who would attend the very poor population. She believed in prevention, and she knew that instruction in the areas of home delivery, access to prenatal care, basic nutrition, and personal hygiene were paramount in reducing the country's highest maternal and infant mortality rates. Within two years Mississippi physicians recognized Osborne's efforts and supported the public health nurses and their supervising work with the lay midwives. According to the writer Margaret Morton, "While Osborne acknowledged working for and with physicians as a primary responsibility of public health nursing, she equally promoted public health nursing as a distinct and specialized art which required a higher degree of initiative and judgment by the nurse."

BIOGRAPHY

Born: April 27, 1875, Ohio. **Education:** Akron City Hosp. School of Nursing, 1902; six months' postgraduate work, Woman's Hosp., N.Y.C. **Work history:** Assistant Director of Nurses, Akron City Hosp., 1906; Assistant Director of Nurses, Woman's Hosp., N.Y.C.;

Biography continued on page 767

April 28

Frances Reed Elliot Davis

1882–1965

"Whatever you do—Whether it's weedin' the sweet potatoes or pickin' the black-eyed peas—always remember to do the best job you can. Get all the education you can—you'll have to work hard for it, maybe even fight for it—but an education is worth workin' and fightin' for." (Date unknown)

"A lot of the worthwhile jobs done in this world have been done by people who have been handicapped. I'm going to stick with this job." (Date unknown)

FRANCES DAVIS WAS the first black nurse to be officially enrolled by the Red Cross nursing service. She wanted to be a nurse so that she could take care of little children. Her white mother had fallen in love with a handsome laborer who was half Cherokee and half black and was banished from the plantation of her Methodist minister-father to have her child alone and in disgrace in another state. Davis was six when her mother died and for the next six years spent her childhood in many foster homes. When she was twelve, she started to work for a prominent family in Pittsburgh, the Joseph Reeds. The Reeds became her benefactors, paid for her to attend a boarding school, and remained close to her throughout her life. She continued to apply the standard of "excellence is its own reward" in her pursuit of a nursing education and throughout her work as a public health nurse. Her dignity was an example for student nurses when she stooped to do the most menial task. She was responsible for helping many jobless people during the Great Depression, working closely with Henry Ford to provide basic necessities for them. She enlisted First Lady Eleanor Roosevelt to help raise money to build a preschool child care project to help working mothers and give preschoolers a head start. Davis wanted nursing to transcend racial barriers, so that qualified black nurses could work in any community. She suffered from heart disease for almost her entire adult life, yet she managed to have high energy for giving of herself and her skills to others. She was to be honored for service by the Red Cross at its Detroit convention in May 1965, but she died shortly before receiving that honor. She is remembered for her excellence in giving.

Biography

Born: April 28, 1882, Shelby, N.C. **Education:** normal school, 1907; Knoxville (Tenn.) College; Freedman's Hosp., Washington, D.C., 1913; first black nurse to pass more difficult exam for white nurses in Washington, D.C.; American Red Cross; Teachers College, Columbia Univ., 1917. **Work history:** Housekeeper, helper as teen; Practical Nurse, Knoxville Hosp.; Teacher, third and fourth grades, Henderson (N.C.) Normal Institute; Private Duty Nurse, Washington, D.C.; Henry Street Settlement, N.Y.C.; worked in rural areas near Jackson, Tenn., 1917; application for Army Nurse Corps, World War I, rejected because of her race; worked with soldiers near Chickamunga, Tenn., 1918; Director of Nurses Training, John A. Andrew Memorial Hosp., Tuskegee, Ala., 1919; Director of Nurses Training, Dunbar Hosp., Detroit; secured appropriation from U.S. Sen. James Couzens (R-Mich.) to upgrade teaching facilities at nursing school; Child Welfare Division, Detroit Health Dept., 1927; worked primarily with blacks in Inkster, Mich.; Founder, Director, Commissary for the Unemployed at Ford plant in Inkster, Mich.; Visiting Nurse Assoc.; founded and directed nursery for Inkster residents; Eloise Hosp., Detroit, 1945–51. **Organizations:** American Red Cross. **Awards:** recognized by American Red Cross as first black person to be accepted in Red Cross training program for nurses. **Died:** Mt. Clement, Mich.

References and Credits

†Pitrone JM: Trailblazer Negro Nurse in the American Red Cross. New York, Harcourt, Brace and World, 1969, pp 26, 110.

DelBene SB: Frances Davis. In Bullough V, Church OM, Stein AP (eds): American Nursing: A Biographical Dictionary, vol. 1. New York, Garland, 1988, pp 76–77.

April 29

Shirley Carew Titus

1892–1967

"Should we not as a profession see to it that a system of nursing be established in our hospitals which will meet the actual needs of the hospital patient, and of the community at large, rather than ... a system which seems to meet only one need, namely the economic need of the hospital?" (1931)

Shirley Titus was a true visionary in quality care and hospital economics as well as an innovative leader in nursing education. In the 1920s she started one of the first college nursing programs, in Milwaukee, Wisconsin. Then, at the University of Michigan Hospital, she replaced student staffing with graduate nurses and argued that patients needed to be billed separately for nursing service. In the 1930s, when Vanderbilt University hired her to upgrade its nursing program, she increased admission requirements to two years of college, added public health to the curriculum, and hired full-time faculty. Despite criticism and opposition, she championed economic rights for nurses. She is probably the only nurse ever carried "on the shoulders of the delegates" at a convention of the American Nurses Association (ANA) in joyous celebration of passage of a collective bargaining initiative in 1946. Her determination and commitment led to successful negotiations for employee insurance plans, salary increases, and the forty-hour workweek in California hospitals.

She was a legislative activist who supported endorsement of candidates based on their positions on health issues.

Biography

Born: April 28, 1892, Alameda, Calif. **Education:** St. Luke's Hosp., San Francisco; Teacher's College, Columbia Univ. (bachelor's degree, diploma in administration); Univ. of Michigan (master's); advanced study, Univ. of Grenoble, France. **Work history:** U.S. Children's Bureau; Columbia Hosp., Milwaukee, Wisc.; Administration, Univ. of Michigan; Nursing Professor, Dean, Vanderbilt Univ.; **Organizations:** National League for Nursing Education; National Organization for Public Health Nursing; Assoc. of Collegiate Schools of Nursing; Mich. State Nurses Assoc.; Wisc. Bureau for Nurse Licensing; Exec. Director, Calif. State Nurses Assoc., American Nurses Assoc. (ANA); bd. member, American Journal of Nursing; International Council of Nurses. **Awards:** Shirley C. Titus Fellowship, Calif.; Shirley Titus Award, ANA; professorship in her name at Univ. of Michigan; ANA Hall of Fame. **Buried:** San Francisco.

References and Credits

†Titus S: Graduate nursing. AJN 31:203, 1931.

Lionne CA: Shirley Titus. In Bullough V, Church OM, Stein AP (eds): American Nursing: A Biographical Dictionary, vol. 1. New York, Garland, 1988, pp 316–319.

ANA Hall of Fame 10/98 American Nurses Association, Washington, D.C. http://www.nursingworld.org/hof.

April 30

Edith Augusta Draper

UNKNOWN–1941

"What we need is energy of purpose, enthusiasm, a spirit of philanthropy more developed, and ambition to lift our profession to a height to which the eyes of the nation shall look up and not down. Nothing is more conducive to the ruination of a project than lukewarmness and a conservatism which does not look beyond individual benefits. These are our main hindrances, but not insurmountable ones, for though acknowledging these faults, we are aware of counterbalancing virtues and know that the day will come when America will be justly proud of this association of her countrywomen." (1893)

EDITH DRAPER, SUPERINTENDENT of the Illinois Training School in Chicago, addressed the first national and international gathering of nurses at the World's Columbian Exposition in 1893. It included a special exhibit in the Women's Building that Draper supervised; it depicted a model emergency ward. This was one of the first occasions that nurses were able to show their effectiveness. She presented a paper that advocated creation of a national organization for nurses. As a result of her address, the American Society of Superintendents of Training Schools for Nurses in the United States and Canada was formed. This organization later became the National League for Nursing. Little is known of Draper's early life. She retired from nursing in 1896 and returned to Toronto.

Biography

Born: Date unknown, Canada. **Education:** Bellevue Hosp. Training School for Nurses, 1884. **Work history:** St. Paul's House, Rome; Assistant Superintendent of Nurses, St. Luke's Hosp., Chicago; Superintendent, Illinois Training School for Nurses, 1890–93; Supervisor, Royal Victoria Hosp., Montreal. **Organizations:** unknown. **Awards:** unknown. **Died:** Oakville, Can.

References and Credits

†Draper EA: Necessity of an American nurses' association. In Hampton I et al.: Nursing of the Sick (1893). Reprint, New York, McGraw-Hill, 1949, pp 150–151.

Church OM: Edith Agusta Draper. In Bullough V, Church OM, Stein AP (eds): American Nursing: A Biographical Dictionary, vol. 1. New York, Garland, 1988, pp 97–98.

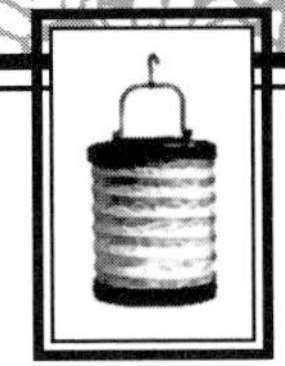

MAY

"Why have women passion, intellect, moral activity—these three—and a place in society where no one of the three can be exercised?"

■■

—FLORENCE NIGHTINGALE
NIGHTINGALE F: CASSANDRA: AN ESSAY. INTRODUCTION BY MYRA STARK. CITY UNIVERSITY OF NEW YORK, FEMINIST PRESS, 1979, P 25.

MAY 1

Mary Agnes McCarthy Hickey

1874–1954

"It might be justly asked why we, as nurses, join a veterans' organization. The answer is that we do so because there is among us a desire to perpetuate associations formed under the hardship of war. ... We can still continue to give service. ... The Jane A. Delano Post Number 6 was chartered July 9, 1919 in Washington, Department of the District of Columbia, American Legion. ... Each Memorial Day, exercises are held at the grave of Jane A. Delano in Arlington Cemetery. The post takes an active part in attendance at the funerals of nurses from all parts of the country who are buried in Arlington National Cemetery." (1928)

MARY HICKEY WAS one of the first school nurses in Massachusetts. She organized nutrition classes for children and did tuberculosis and public health nursing. She also served with the Army Nurse Corps at the front lines in France during World War I. She worked with the U.S. Public Health Service (USPHS) and later served for twenty years as superintendent of nurses for the forty-seven veterans hospitals now known as the Veterans Administration Program. She had a friendly and optimistic manner. During her tenure she actively supported high educational standards for nurses, particularly in tuberculosis and psychiatric nursing.

Biography

Born: Dec. 1, 1874, Ireland. **Education:** St. Mary's Hosp., Brooklyn, N.Y. (RN); Lying-In Hosp., N.Y.C. (postgraduate work). **Work history:** School Nurse, Springfield, Mass.; Supervisor, public health nursing, Mass.; American Red Cross nurse; member, Army Nurse Corps; Staff Nurse, Assistant Superintendent of Nurses, USPHS; Superintendent, Veterans Bureau; Volunteer, War Manpower Commission; Lecturer, Catholic Univ., Washington, D.C., and Columbia Univ. **Organizations:** American Nurses Assoc.; Washington, D.C., League for Nursing Education; Commander, Jane A. Delano American Legion Post. **Awards:** unknown. **Died:** Ft. Howard, Md.

References and Credits

†Hickey, MA: Nurses in the American Legion. AJN 28:590, 1928.

Sentz L: Mary Agnes Hickey. In Bullough V, Church OM, Stein AP (eds): American Nursing: A Biographical Dictionary, vol. 1. New York, Garland, 1988, pp 179–180.

May 2

Lucie S. Kelly

1925–

"The best image making is reality. If enough real nurses practice professionally with competence and caring, if they create, direct and/or practice in innovative settings that provide needed care to patients, if they are risk-takers not afraid to develop or assume 'different' roles in health care, if with research they find answers to better patient care, if they look beyond the crisis-centered here and now to anticipate and search out ways to meet the public's health care needs, if they simply demonstrate the existing diversity of nursing, there will be like-minded men and women who will see nursing as a worthwhile career opportunity. Do such creatures, such role models exist? Of course they do, but sometimes nurses themselves are not aware of all the creativity, the excitement, the variety out there in our profession." (1989)

Lucie Kelly, who has been called one of the fifty most influential nurses in the United States, has been a consistent articulate advocate for quality care, professional practice, and advanced practice. She willingly embraced new challenges and opportunities. She recognized mentoring as basic to nursing and relishes knowing that throughout her career she has been a positive influence on the careers and professional commitments of nurses. *The Nursing Experience* (now in its fourth edition) and *Dimensions of*

Professional Nursing (now in its ninth edition) are two of her major works. Her widely published writings seem timeless. Editorials that she wrote for *Nursing Outlook* during the 1980s and 1990s remain relevant and should be required reading today. Topics include nursing shortages, concerns about nurse administrators, educational funding, the importance of caring, nursing's image, unqualified personnel, and the need to celebrate nursing. When she was the director of nursing at a community hospital, she initiated positive and creative changes, such as a staff nursing council, admitting men and married students to the accredited diploma program, and replacing the diploma program with a community college affiliation. The nurse practitioner program that she established in California was one of the first in the nation. A popular speaker, she worked in clinical nursing, teaching, administration, and consultation. Her 1965 doctoral thesis envisioned two entry levels for nursing practice. While holding joint appointments to the Schools of Public Health and Nursing at Columbia University, she established a program for nurse administrators that included a paid one-year residency with top administrators.

Biography

Born: May 2, 1925, Stuttgart, Germany. **Education:** Univ. of Pittsburgh (BS, master's, PhD). **Work history:** Staff Nurse, McKeesport (Pa.) Hosp.; Faculty, Administration, Univ. of Pittsburgh; Director of Nursing, McKeesport Hosp.; Professor and Chair, Nursing Dept., California State College, Los Angeles; Faculty, Teachers College, Columbia Univ.; Administrator, Univ. of Medicine and Dentistry, N.J.; Faculty, Rutgers Medical School; Associate Dean, Academic Affairs, School of Public Health, Columbia Univ.; honorary professor of nursing education, Teachers College; editor, *Nursing Outlook* and *Image* (Sigma Theta Tau International); numerous editorial boards. **Organizations:** member, exec. committee, bd. of directors, Visiting Nurse Assoc. of N.Y.; member, bd. of directors, Palisades Medical Center; member, Health Professionals Advisory Panel, American Legacy Foundation; American Nurses Assoc. (ANA); National League for Nursing; various state nursing associations; Mid-Atlantic Regional Nursing Assoc.; President, Sigma Theta Tau. **Awards:** six honorary doctorates; Distinguished Alumna Award, Univ. of Pittsburgh; Bicentennial Medallion of Distinction, Univ. of Pittsburgh; numerous awards, Columbia Univ.; Fellow, American Academy of Nursing (AAN); ANA Honorary Recognition Award; Sigma Theta Tau International Mentor Award (now the Lucie S. Kelly Mentor Award); Living Legend, American Academy of Nursing, 2001.

References and Credits continued on page 767

May 3

Anne A. Williamson

1868–1955

"I... graduated in 1896. ...I remember how hard nurses worked at that time. People thought we were superior beings who could go on indefinitely, sometimes twenty-four hours out of the twenty-four. When we graduated, $25 a week for a private duty nurse was considered the height of affluence, and for the most part it was an all-night-and-day job. It took the greater part of fifty years to increase it to $11 for an eight-hour day. Now nurses can live a normal life like other professional women; most large hospitals have adopted the forty-hour week, salaries have certainly improved, and nurses no longer think it is unethical to consider the financial aspects of their professional work." (1950)

Anne Williamson was inspired by Clara Barton, whom she met when she was a teenager. After Williamson's fiancé died, Williamson dedicated herself to nursing. During her years in the profession she witnessed and experienced incredible changes. She served in the Spanish-American War and was with the California Hospital in Los Angeles for almost five decades. She preserved her experiences for nurses of today in the lively memoir *Fifty Years in Starch.* One of her vivid descriptions in "A Backward Glimpse" tells of a nurse's duties to prepare a home for surgery in 1896: removing carpets and wall hangings; scrubbing floors, walls, and windows the day before; assisting with the anesthetic by pouring chloroform on a wad of cotton in a newspaper cone and remaining to tend the patient toward a successful recovery.

Biography

Born: May 3, 1868, Palmyra, N.Y. **Education:** Mt. Holyoke College; Wilson College, Pa.; New York Hosp. School of Nursing. **Work history:** Private Duty Nurse; Red Cross nurse, Spanish-American War; various positions, California Hosp.; nurse recruiter, World War I. **Organizations:** American Red Cross; Calif. State Nurses Assoc. (CSNA); American Nurses Assoc. **Awards:** CSNA; numerous career-related testimonials; award from California Hosp. **Died:** South Pasadena, Calif.

References and Credits

†Williamson A: A backward glimpse. AJN 50: 637, 638, 1950.

Stein AP: Anne A. Williamson. In Bullough V, Sentz L, Stein AP (eds): American Nursing: A Biographical Dictionary, vol. 2. New York, Garland, 1992, pp 355–358.

May 4

May Shiga Hornback

1924–1976

"An unmistakable trend is in motion across the nation to look at continuing education as an important facet of professional life. ...A uniform system of measurement for continuing education in nursing adopted on a national basis would help nurses who are registered in more than one state. ...External uniformity in no way guarantees internal uniformity. We have individual interests, needs, and motives. We also practice nursing in different settings and with a variety of purposes. Indeed, our only commonality may be our desire to do the best possible nursing job. ...It may be that acknowledgment is long overdue for nurses who keep up through professional literature and independent study." (1973)

May Shiga Hornback was a Japanese American who was born in the United States and moved inland from Seattle to avoid being placed in the internment camps during World War II. Her nursing studies were interrupted when she married a soldier in 1944. At the time, nursing students were not allowed to be married. Her skills were so evident while she was working as an aide that she was encouraged to continue her studies. She completed her doctoral studies in nursing and joined the nursing faculty at the University of Wisconsin. She was a creative thinker and became a pioneer in the use of television and the telephone continuing education programs for distance learning. A national leader in this specialty, she produced videos about basic nursing, educational films, and a taped library for nursing. She served as a consultant on curriculum development and was also a consultant to other nurses, publishers, and the National Institutes of Health.

Biography

Born: May 4, 1924, Seattle. **Education:** St. Xavier's College, Chicago; Univ. of Wisconsin School of Nursing (BSN); Frances Payne Bolton School of Nursing; Case Western Reserve (MS); Univ. of Wisconsin, Madison (PhD). **Work history:** Nursing Aide, Lakeview Tuberculosis Sanitarium, Madison, Wisc.; Staff Nurse, Veterans Administration Hosp., Madison, Wisc.; Instructor, Univ. of Wisconsin (Madison) School of Nursing; Associate Professor, Professor of Nursing, Univ. of Wisconsin; Developer, Consultant, Project Director for numerous programs dealing with continuing education. **Organizations:** Wisc. Nurses Assoc. (WNA), American Nurses Assoc.; leadership positions, Continuing Education in Nursing, Pi Lambda Theta, Sigma Theta Tau. **Awards:** Service Award, WNA; May Shiga Hornback Scholarship. **Died:** Madison, Wisc.

References and Credits

†Hornback MS: Measuring continuing education. AJN 73: 1576, 1577, 1973.

Cooper SS: May Hornback. In Bullough V, Church OM, Stein AP (eds): American Nursing: A Biographical Dictionary, vol. 1. New York, Garland, 1988, pp 182–184.

May 5

Geneve Estelle Massey Riddle Osborne

1901–1981

"Too long the emphasis has been on racial differences. *We need a New Deal in approach to community problems in order that we may recognize* racial similarities. *Any group—white, black, or red—subjected to unhealthy environmental influences will present an unhealthy social picture." (1935)*

GENEVE ESTELLE OSBORNE was a pioneering black nurse who overcame racial discrimination and prejudice during a career of outstanding achievement. She was a spokesperson for both quality and equality in nursing. After she finished nursing school, she was awarded a scholarship for full-time study at Columbia University, where she earned a bachelor of science degree. She was the first black nurse in the country with a master's degree, which she completed the following year. Osborne worked as a researcher and consultant and helped improve opportunities for black nurses in the military. During World War II she worked with a unit of the National Nursing Council. It studied the status of black nurses and ways to promote professional growth. The council's history of involvement in helping to meet the demands for nurses in the military initially stood in stark contrast to the indifference of black nurses, who saw that the doors to military nursing were closed to them. In 1943, however, the council declared that all nurses who met the same professional requirements would have the same opportunities in the Army and Navy Nurse Corps. Osborne worked with organizations like the National Association of Colored Graduate Nurses (NACGN) and individuals to make that happen. In 1945 she was hired as New York University's first black instructor.

Biography

Born: May 3, 1901, Palestine, Texas. **Education:** Prairie View State College, Texas; St. Louis City Hosp. School of Nursing; Teachers College, Columbia Univ. (BS, MA). **Work history:** Head Nurse, St. Louis City Hosp.; Public Health Nurse, St. Louis; Faculty, Lincoln High School and Junior College, Kansas City; Instructor, Harlem Hosp. School of Nursing; Education Director, Freedman's Hosp. School of Nursing, Washington, D.C.; studied poverty and health problems in the South; Superintendent of Nursing, Director of Nursing School, Homer Phillips Hosp., St. Louis; Consultant, National Nursing Council for War Service; Advisory Commission to Surgeon General; Instructor, New York Univ.; Director, National League for Nursing. **Organizations:** President, NACGN; American Nurses Assoc. (ANA); International Council of Nurses; National Council of Negro Women; National Urban League; Legal Defense Fund of the NAACP. **Awards:** Estelle Massey Scholarship established by Fisk Univ.; honorary member, American Academy of Nursing and Chi Eta Phi Sorority; Mary Mahoney Award, ANA; New York Univ. Nurse of the Year; Estelle Massey Osborne Memorial Scholarship; ANA Hall of Fame. **Died:** California.

References and Credits

†Haupt A: A pioneer in negro nursing. AJN 35:859, 1935.

Sloan PE: Geneva Osborne. In Bullough V, Church OM, Stein AP (eds): American Nursing: A Biographical Dictionary, vol. 1. New York, Garland, 1988, pp 250–252.

Roberts M: American Nursing: History and Interpretation. New York, Macmillan, 1954.

ANA Hall of Fame 10/98 American Nurses Association, Washington, D.C. http://www.nursingworld.org/ hof.

Carnegie ME: The Path We Tread: Blacks in Nursing, 1854–1984. Philadelphia, JB Lippincott, 1986.

May 6

Gertrude LaBrake Fife

1902–1980

"Little has been said or written about the actual work of the nurse anesthetist. When lung surgery, heart surgery, and brain surgery were in their infancy, the nurse anesthetist was at the head of the table. When I left University Hospitals in 1946, we had performed so many heart operations that the anesthesia was a relatively simple procedure. At least we were past the pioneer stage. We, as nurse anesthetists, had been given a job to do, and we did it." (1956)

Gertrude Fife's dedication to the formation of the American Association of Nurse Anesthetists (AANA) was Herculean. Fife served as the second vice president, treasurer, and founder and editor of the *Bulletin of the National Association of Nurse Anesthetists* while teaching nurse-anesthetists full time. She eventually took over as director of the University Hospitals School of Anesthesia in Cleveland, Ohio. Concurrently, she made certain that the new association developed a program of certification for nurse-anesthetists through a national qualifying examination. She was an advocate for the accreditation for nurse-anesthetists schools. She believed that a nurse-anesthetist's work was neither medicine nor nursing. Therefore, she advocated separate legal status for them. Fife was the anesthetist for many outstanding surgeons, including George W. Crile, Elliot Cutler, and the ground-breaking heart surgeon Dr. Claude S. Beck. She and Beck perfected the anesthesia technique for pericardectomy and the use of the automatic respirator in open-chest surgery.

Biography

Born: 1902, Rutland, Vt. **Education:** Fanny Allen Hosp. School of Nursing, 1923, Winooski, Vt.; Lakeside Hosp. (University Hospitals) School of Anesthesia, Cleveland, Ohio, 1924. **Work history:** first assistant to Agatha C. Hodgkins, Lakeside Hosp., Cleveland; Nurse-Anesthetist, Director, University Hosps. School of Anesthesia. **Organizations:** founder, member of first bd. of directors, second president (1933–35), NANA; founding editor, *Bulletin of the NANA* (twelve yrs.). **Awards:** Agatha Hodgkins Award for Outstanding Accomplishment, 1978. **Died:** Cleveland.

References and Credits

†Fife, G: Speech at the 25th Anniversary, American Association of Nurse Anesthetists. J Am Assoc Nurse Anesthetists 26:4, 1956.

Bankert M: Gertrude Fife. In Bullough V, Sentz L, Stein AP (eds): American Nursing: A Biographical Dictionary, vol. 2. New York, Garland, 1992, pp 110–113.

Bankert M: Watchful Care: A History of America's Nurse Anesthetists. New York, Continuum, 1989.

MAY 7

Mary Eliza Mahoney

1845–1926

"A nurse who had made outstanding contributions to the nursing profession and to the community, and who also had worked to improve the professional status of the Negro nurse, thereby helping to improve intergroup and interpersonal relations within the nursing profession." (Staupers, 1936)

MARY MAHONEY WAS known as an excellent nurse and her references stated "high recommendation, no faults noticed, a good temper, discretion and loyalty." She graduated from nursing school in 1879 and was the first black professional nurse in the United States. Her nursing career spanned four decades. She was a strong backer of the women's suffrage movement, and she worked industriously to improve the progress of women as citizens. In 1921, when she was seventy-six, she was one of the first women in Boston to register to vote. Mahoney was thirty-three when she was accepted into the prestigious nursing program at the New England Hospital for Women and Children. The school admitted forty-two in 1878, and she was one of only four to complete the demanding program of sixteen-hour days plus night duty, and no days off. In the 1870s black women were not accepted into white schools of nursing, and no schools existed for black nurses. Mahoney became one of the first members of the American Nurses Association (ANA). A woman of small stature, pleasing personality, and enormous charm, she was an inspiration to all nurses. Her kindness, efficiency, and nursing skills surmounted the prejudice of her colleagues. Her dedication to give her best in nursing care and her intense efforts to create a strong body of organized nurses ready for world service were the hallmarks of her career. She is remembered as "Lady of Faith, Hope and Charity."

Biography

Born: May 7, 1845, Dorchester, Mass. **Education:** New England Hosp. for Women and Children, 1879. **Work history:** untrained nurse, 1863–78; Private Duty Nurse, hospital nursing; Administrator, Howard Orphan Asylum for black children, Kings Park, L.I. **Organizations:** gave welcoming address at first convention of National Assoc. of Colored Graduate Nurses (NACGN), Boston, 1909; worked for women's suffrage; early member, Nurses Associated Alumnae of United States and Canada (forerunner of ANA). **Awards:** NACGN established award in her name to honor her participation in nursing organizations and her efforts to raise status of black nurses, 1936; numerous local affiliates of NACGN named in her honor; honored by ANA in 1954 on 75th anniversary of her graduation; national pilgrimage to her grave organized by nursing sorority Chi Eta Phi and ANA, 1984; ANA Hall of Fame. **Buried:** Woodlawn Cemetery, Everett, Mass.

References and Credits

†Staupers M: No Time for Prejudice: A Story of the Integration of Negroes in Nursing in the United States. New Jersey, Pearson Education, 1961, p 35.

Davis AT: Mary Mahoney. In Bullough V, Church OM, Stein AP (eds): American Nursing: A Biographical Dictionary, vol. 1. New York, Garland, 1988, pp 226–229.

Dolan J, Fitzpatrick ML, Herrman EK: Nursing in Society: A Historical Perspective, 15th ed. Philadelphia: WB Saunders, 1978.

Salem DC (ed): African American Women: A Biographical Dictionary. New York, Garland, 1993, p 347.

Miller HS: Mary Eliza Mahoney, 1845–1926: American's First Black Professional Nurse, A Historical Perspective. Atlanta, Wright Publishing, 1986, p 42.

ANA Hall of Fame 10/98 American Nurses Association, Washington, D.C. http://www.nursingworld.org/hof.

May 8

Henri Dunant

1828–1910

"The moral sense of the importance of human life; the humane desire to lighten a little the torments of all these poor wretches; the furious and relentless activity which a man summons up at such moments: all these create a kind of energy which gives one a positive craving to relieve as many as one can." (1862)

"Would it not be possible, in time of peace and quiet, to form relief societies for the purpose of having care given to the wounded in wartime by zealous, devoted and thoroughly qualified volunteers?" (1862)

Henri Dunant, of Swiss heritage, visited Paris and gave assistance and support to the wounded and dying during the Franco-Prussian War of 1870. Earlier, in 1859, during a business pursuit, he stumbled upon the horror of the Battle of Solferino, where the French and Italians killed and maimed forty thousand men. Dunant was moved as he observed women tending to wounded men, regardless of their nationality. This compelled him to write *A Memory of Solferino,* which led to the creation of the International Committee for the Relief to the Wounded, which later became the International Committee of the Red Cross. Dunant was a member and acted as secretary, but he was not known as an organizer, which meant that he was unable to develop his ideas, but others did. He was instrumental in promoting the "complete and final abolition of the traffic in Negroes and the slave trade" at an international congress of abolitionists when it opened in London in 1875. He was also the initiator of the Geneva Convention. After he went bankrupt because he had neglected his business, he wandered about Europe in abject poverty. A journalist found him in a Swiss hospice and wrote an article about him that appeared in European papers and once again brought him to prominence. As the founder of the International Committee of the Red Cross, and the initiator of the Geneva Convention, he and the French economist Frederic Passy were the first to receive the Nobel Peace Prize, in 1901. Dunant's mantra was "Tutti Fratelli" ("All men are brothers")!

Biography

Born: May 8, 1828, Geneva. **Education:** received incomplete secondary schooling, apprenticed in Geneva bank. **Work history:** Banker; Founder, International Committee of the Red Cross; helped found World's Young Men's Christian Assoc. **Organizations:** unknown. **Award:** cowinner of first Nobel Peace Prize, 1901. **Died:** Heiden, Switzerland.

References and Credits

†Dunant H: A Memory of Solferino (Un Souvenier de Solferino). Geneva, 1862, available on-line at http://www.icrc.org./icrceng.nsf/c.

International Red Cross on-line, available at http://www.icrc.org.

Henri Dunant. Britannica CD 98. Chicago, Encyclopedia Britannica, 1998.

May 9

Elizabeth Freeman

ca. 1744–1829

"I heard that paper read yesterday, that says, 'all men are born equal, and that every man has a right to freedom.' I am not a dumb critter; won't the law give me my freedom?" (1781)

"Anytime, anytime while I was a slave, if one minute's freedom had been offered to me, and I must die at the end of that minute, I would have taken it–just to stand one minute on God's earth a free woman—I would." (Date unknown, probably ca. 1820)

Born into slavery and illiterate, Elizabeth Freeman was a slave for the Ashley family in Massachusetts when she overheard talk about the state constitution and the Bill of Rights. After being physically injured by her mistress in an act of violence intended for her own sister, Freeman successfully sued for freedom in 1781. She was the first to declare that slavery violated the constitutional provision that "all men are born free and equal" and then took the surname *Freeman.* According to the author Robert L. Johns, Freeman was also known as "Mum Bett," a diminutive of *Elizabeth* (Johns also reports that the spelling on Freeman's gravestone is "Mumbet"). Theodore Sedgwick was Freeman's attorney, and after her victory she worked for many years as a paid servant for his family. She nursed his wife through bouts of severe depression. The Sedgwicks loved her and highly valued her nursing skills. Around 1807 one of the Sedgwick children wrote of her: "Elizabeth Freeman was the only person who could tranquilize my mother when her mind was disordered. ...She treated her with the same respect she did when she was sane. ...Her superior instincts hit upon the mode of treatment that has since been adopted."

Biography

Born: ca. 1744, Claverack, N.Y. **Education:** Self-taught. **Work history:** slave to the Ashley family, Mass.; paid servant for the Sedgwick family. **Organizations:** unknown. **Awards:** unknown. **Died:** Stockbridge, Mass.; buried in the Sedgwick family plot, Stockbridge, Mass.

References and Credits

†Banks TL: Elizabeth "Mum Bett" Freeman. In Hine DC (ed): Black Women in America: An Historical Encyclopedia. Brooklyn, N.Y., Carlson, 1993, p 469.

Johns RL: Elizabeth Freeman "Mum Bett" "Mumbet" (c. 1744–1829), servant, nurse. In Smith JC (ed): Notable Black American Women. Detroit, Gale, 1992, pp 372, 373.

MAY 10

Peter Buerhaus

1954–

"There is a current shortage of hospital RNs and a much larger shortage is expected over the next ten to twenty years. Policy makers must make sure hospitals and nurses have the resources that will allow nurse staffing at levels that protect patient safety and reduce adverse outcomes. Nurses are the glue that holds the health care system together, and it is time that we invest more resources in the nursing profession." (2002)

"Nursing *leadership must get this issue out of the* nursing *sphere and into the larger social agenda. . . . We need our leaders to approach the public and say, 'We have really important problems. We cannot fix them in* nursing. *The health care industry cannot fix them. We're going to need societal and government help.' . . . The public can play a strong role in helping policy makers realize that the public needs and wants plenty of good nurses in the future." (2000)*

PETER BUERHAUS WAS "talked into" nursing by his sister, a registered nurse who was satisfied and happy with her profession. He has never regretted his decision to become a nurse and, other than being a husband and father, says that it is the most satisfying part of his life. A distinguished professor of nursing at

Vanderbilt University, he is also a renowned researcher, writer, speaker, and consultant on health care issues. Buerhaus places a strong economic value on quality nursing care and on improved patient outcomes related to RN staffing. This leads to an increased demand for nurses, which he believes can help draw people to the profession. He is an expert on all aspects of the nursing shortage. In 1998 he predicted the crisis of the early twenty-first century, which he sees as long term, worsening, and different from any earlier shortages. According to Buerhaus, contributing factors include the widespread misperception of the effect of managed care on hospitalizations in the 1990s, the subsequent hospital restructuring, and the recommended closure of some nursing schools. He calls on every nurse to promote nursing's image, recruit others to nursing, and to involve the public in addressing the problems that nursing faces.

Biography

Born: May 10, 1954, Zanesville, Ohio. **Education:** Mankato State Univ., Minn., (BSN); Univ. of Michigan (MS); Wayne State Univ. (PhD); Johns Hopkins Univ. (postdoctoral studies in health care finance). **Work history:** Staff Nurse, Ohio; health center administration, Mich.; health policy development; Editor of professional journals; Faculty, College of Nursing, Iowa; Director, Harvard Univ. Research Institute; Faculty, Harvard School of Public Health; Associate Dean, Research, Vanderbilt Univ.; Author, Researcher; Consultant, Adviser to federal policy makers and numerous organizations, incl. National Institute of Nursing Research, National Institutes of Health; Univ. of Texas, San Antonio; Joint Commission on Accreditation of Health Care Organizations; American Academy of Nursing; American Organization of Nurse Executives (AONE); Pew Health Commission Center for the Health Professions; election to Institute of Medicine, National Academy of Sciences; American Nurses Assoc. (ANA); Agency for Health Care Policy and Research, U.S. Dept. of Health and Human Services; U.S. Public Health Service. **Organizations:** bd. of directors, Sigma Theta Tau International, AONE, ANA, American Economics Assoc., Academy for Health Services Research and Policy, Southern Nursing Research Society. **Awards:** Robert Wood Johnson Fellowship for postdoctoral studies at Johns Hopkins; Fellow, American Academy of Nursing; Valere Potter Distinguished Professor, Vanderbilt Univ.; awards from Vanderbilt Univ. Medical Center, Sigma Theta Tau, AONE, Mankato State Univ.; member, International Council of Nurses Expert Bank; Thomas Jefferson Univ. Distinguished Scholar, College of Allied Health Sciences, Philadelphia; traineeship, scholarship, research awards, and T.C. Rumble Univ. Fellowship, Wayne State Univ.; nursing grant, Univ. of Michigan, Ann Arbor; *Who's Who in American Colleges and Universities.*

References and Credits continued on page 767

May 11

Martha Elizabeth Rogers

1914–1994

"Nursing exists to serve society, and nurses are directly responsible to the people they purport to serve. The nursing profession does not *exist to serve the ends of any other profession, nor does any one profession delegate anything to another profession. Each profession must determine its own boundaries within the context of social need. As a learned profession nursing has* no *dependent functions but, like all other professions, has many collaborative functions that are indispensable to providing society with a higher order of service than any one profession can offer. Only professionally educated nurses are safe or competent to guide nursing practice and to make the complex judgments that require substantive knowledge and a high degree of intellectual skill. ...It is nursing knowledge that adds new dimensions to human safety and human service; and it is nursing's body of scientific knowledge that guides nursing practice." (1972)*

Martha Rogers was an articulate, controversial, original thinker and theorist who promoted her revolutionary visions for professional nursing through her writings, lectures, and leadership. A voracious reader since childhood, she built on a broad base of synthesized knowledge when she defined professional nursing as a theory-based humanitarian science. She was a catalyst for dramatic changes in nursing education, insisting that professional nursing practice must emanate from a knowledge base of nursing science. She recognized professional nursing as a dynamic and learned profession with origins in vocational practice. She believed it was essential that vocational, technical, and professional nursing, each with necessary but different purposes, have different levels of preparation. Her ideas of nursing as a science evolved into what she defined as the "Science of Unitary Human Beings," which sees the synergism of human beings in their environment as central to nursing theory and practice.

Biography

Born: May 12, 1914, Dallas. **Education:** Univ. of Knoxville, Tenn.; Knoxville General Hosp. School of Nursing; George Peabody College, Nashville, Tenn. (BSN); Teachers College, Columbia Univ. (MA); Johns Hopkins Univ. (MPH; ScD). **Work history:** Staff Public Health Nurse, Michigan; various positions, Visiting Nurse Assoc. (VNA), Hartford, Conn.; Administrator, VNA, Phoenix, Ariz.; Lecturer, Catholic Univ. of America; Research Associate, Johns Hopkins Univ.; Faculty, administration, Nursing Education, New York Univ.; Editor, *Journal of Nursing Science;* Consultant, U.S. surgeon general, U.S. Air Force. **Organizations:** N.Y. State League for Nursing; National League for Nursing; American Nurses Assoc.; Society for Advancement in Nursing; American Assoc. for Higher Education; American Assoc. of Univ. Professors; Sigma Theta Tau; Kappa Delta Phi; American Academy of Nursing. **Awards:** numerous honorary degrees; Mary Tolle Wright Leadership Award; Leadership Award, Chi Eta Phi; awards from New York Univ., Division of Nursing Education; ANA Hall of Fame. **Died:** location unknown.

References and Credits

†Rogers M: Nursing: To be or not to be? Nurs Outlook 20:43, 44, 1972.

Malinski V, Barrett E, Phillips J: Martha E. Rogers: Her Life and Her Work. Philadelphia, FA Davis, 1994.

Buchinger KL: Martha Rogers. In Bullough V, Sentz L, Stein AP (eds): American Nursing: A Biographical Dictionary, vol. 2. New York, Garland, 1992, pp 278–280.

ANA Hall of Fame 10/98 American Nurses Association, Washington, D.C. http://www.nursingworld.org/hof.

Florence Nightingale
1820–1910

"Nursing is an art, and, if it is to be made an art, requires as exclusive a devotion, as hard a preparation, as any painter's or sculptor's work; for what is the having to do with dead canvas or cold marble, compared with having to do with the living body—the temple of God's spirit? It is one of the fine Arts; I had almost said, the finest of the Fine Arts." (1868)

THE MOTHER OF modern secular nursing, Florence Nightingale is remembered for her humanitarian concerns, social reform efforts, political activism, and her knowledge of statistics and sanitation. Throughout her life she networked skillfully and used her political savvy to advantage. Despite the chronic Crimean fever (brucellosis) that severely limited her physically, she made dramatic and universal changes in health care. The medical writer Roxanne Nelson reports that Nightingale also campaigned for the rights of prostitutes and the property rights of married women. She is said to have spent all but three years of her nursing career in bed, using the power of the pen to persuade powerful people to change care for the sick and promote the public health. A mystic, visionary, and healer, she had a concern for the poor from early childhood. She continued her studies and discussions of religion, theology, and philosophy throughout her life. In the Crimea Nightingale was responsible for caring for ten thousand wounded. She penetrated the bureaucracy at the Barrack Hospital in Scutari, Turkey, and fashioned a well-ordered system. Her statistical data regarding death, disease and sanitary deficiencies contributed to hospital and military reform, standardizations regarding hygiene and data collection, military nursing and the establishment of a Sanitary Commission. The knowledge-based Nightingale School of Nursing was free of church influence, focused on patient care, and had a system to monitor student performance. Nightingale laid the foundation for public health services and established the administrative framework for what eventually became England's National Health Service.

Biography

Born: May 12, 1820, Florence, Italy. **Education:** Educated at home and abroad, with contacts with social reformers, women achievers, scholars, philosophers, political leaders; Institution of Deaconesses, Kaiserwerth, Germany; nursing, Sisters of Charity, Paris. **Work history:** Superintendent, Institution for the Care of Sick Gentlewomen in Distressed Circumstances, London; Superintendent, Middlesex Hosp., England; Superintendent of Nurses, Barrack Hosp., Scutari, Turkey; Statistician; political strategist; designer of nurse training program; Author; Consultant. **Organizations:** unknown. **Awards:** Nightingale Fund for Nurses' Training; Bronze Cross, France; Prussian Cross of Merit; title of Lady of Grace of the Order of St. John of Jerusalem and Order of Merit, from King Edward VII of England; Order of Merit; Scroll of Freedom of the City of London. **Buried:** St. Margaret's Church, East Wellow, Hampshire, England.

References and Credits

†Dossey BM: Florence Nightingale: Mystic, Visionary, Healer. Springhouse, Pa., Springhouse Corp., 2000, p 294.

Nelson R: Good night, Florence. With nursing in crisis, some say it's time to retire Nightingale as a symbol. Washington Post, April 29, 2003: F1.

Achterburg J: Woman as Healer. Boston, Shambala, 1990, p 160.

MAY 13

Helen Wood

1882–1974

"We have ... a problem which is ever open for discussion and which we are earnestly trying to meet. ... It is the problem of 'How Shall We Take Care of Our Patients?' and is the vital factor in the very existence of hospitals. Before there were schools of nursing to teach women the theory and practice of the care of the sick, the problem was met in ways we shudder to recall. The first result of the establishment of schools was to attract to the field of hospital nursing a more cultured and better educated class of women; and upon their shoulders was placed this ever increasing burden." (1925)

HELEN WOOD WAS well qualified for her varied career in nursing education, administration, and regulation. In addition, she was involved with mission work in Labrador. She worked to improve and upgrade nursing education programs in New York, Massachusetts, and Missouri. During her leadership at Simmons College, the baccalaureate program widened its focus to more liberal coursework, and public health nursing was seen as a focus for graduate study. Her lifetime of service to nursing included active involvement with state boards of nurse examiners, professional organizations, and work with the Rockefeller Foundation's Winslow-Goldmark Committee. The committee did a comprehensive survey for nursing and nursing education in the United States, identified weakness, and in 1923 recommended the establishment of educational standards for nurse preparation, state licensure, and funding for university schools of nursing.

Biography

Born: May 13, 1882, Newton, Mass. **Education:** Mt. Holyoke College (AB); Massachusetts General Hosp. Training School for Nurses; Columbia Univ. (MA). **Work history:** Nursing Superintendent, Faulkner Hosp., Children's Hosp., Boston; Staff Nurse, Grenfell Mission, Labrador; Director, School of Nursing, Washington Univ., St. Louis; Nurse Administrator, Stanford Univ; Director, Strong Memorial Hosp. School of Nursing, Univ. of Rochester (N.Y.) Medical Center; Superintendent of Nurses, Massachusetts General Hosp.; Faculty, Brown Univ., Simmons College; Bd. of Nurse Examiners, Mass. and Mo. **Organizations:** American Nurses Assoc., National League for Nursing Education. **Awards:** recipient, Isabel Hampton Robb Scholarship; Phi Beta Kappa; residence hall named in her honor, award honoring her service to nursing, Strong Memorial Hosp. School of Nursing. **Died:** Newton, Mass.

References and Credits

†Wood H: The place of the student nurse in the nursing service of the hospital. AJN 25:183, 1925.

Stein AP: Helen Wood. In Bullough V, Sentz L, Stein AP (eds): American Nursing: A Biographical Dictionary, vol. 2. New York, Garland, 1992, pp 362–363.

Jamieson E, Sewall M: Trends in Nursing History: Their Relationship to World Events. Philadelphia, WB Saunders, 1949.

May 14

Sister Mary Joseph Dempsey
1856–1939

"It is economy to judiciously select our employees. An injustice is done to an institution by keeping unqualified help. They are a burden; they are to an institution what dead timber is to a forest. The best help we can get is the most profitable. They should be treated as members of the household and should be paid a living wage." (1923)

Sister Mary Joseph Dempsey was a Franciscan Sister whose order built St. Mary's Hospital in Rochester, Minnesota, now the world-famous Mayo Clinic. She served as superintendent there for more than four decades. Although her own nursing preparation was informal and very limited, she was a strong and effective advocate for excellence in nursing education. The Doctors Mayo loaned their office nurse, Edith Graham, to teach nursing basics to Sister Dempsey. The town's first trained nurse, Graham had Dempsey ready to assume the position of head nurse in the hospital six weeks later. Sister Dempsey was the first to recognize a specific nodule associated with umbilical cancer; it was named Sister Mary Joseph's Nodule to acknowledge her astute observation. She was the surgical assistant to Dr. William Mayo for more than twenty years. Mayo said of her: "Her surgical judgment as to the condition of the patient before, during and after operation was equal to that of any medical man of whom I have knowledge. Of all the splendid surgical assistants I have had, she easily ranked first."

Biography

Born: May 14, 1856, Salamanca, N.Y. **Education:** joined Sisters of St. Francis, 1878. **Work history:** Staff Nurse, Superintendent, Surgical Assistant to Dr. Mayo, St. Mary's Hosp., Rochester, Minn.; worked to establish nursing school at St. Mary's, then arranged cooperative education agreements with neighboring colleges; facilitated advanced degree study for colleagues; catalyst for hospital building programs. **Organizations:** Catholic Hospital Assoc. **Awards:** honored by Mayo Clinic on Golden Jubilee of St. Mary's, 1928. **Buried:** St. John's Cemetery, Rochester, N.Y.

References and Credits

†Dempsey MJ: The practice of economy in our hospitals. Hospital Progress, July 1923, pp 275–276.

In James ET (ed): Notable American Women, 1607–1950, vol. 1. Cambridge, Mass., Belknap Press, 1971, p 461.

Smyth K: Sister Mary Dempsey. In Bullough V, Church OM, Stein AP (eds): American Nursing: A Biographical Dictionary, vol. 1. New York, Garland, 1988, pp 82–84.

Reilly ML: personal correspondence, September 1999.

Harriet Fulmer

1877–1952

"The sooner we eliminate commercialism from the medical and nursing profession, the more rapidly will we accomplish our real service to mankind." (Date unknown)

HARRIET FULMER WAS an outstanding educator, leader, innovator, and organizer in the early days of the Visiting Nurse Association (VNA) of Chicago. Her leadership created the foundation for a profession to emerge. She advocated nurse registration and higher academic standards. In 1905 she published and edited her own professional journal, *Visiting Nurse Quarterly,* which preceded *Public Health Nursing.* Her scientific and professional approach at the VNA initiated programs of industrial nursing, home visiting for insurance-policy holders, and baby-welfare work. She was professionally modest and often gave credit to others for her achievements. A strong proponent of prevention, she developed tent colonies for the isolation and treatment of tubercular patients.

BIOGRAPHY

Born: ca. 1877, Fulmerville, Pa. **Education:** St. Luke's Hosp. Training School for Nurses, Chicago. **Work history:** Private Duty Nurse, 1897; Staff Nurse, Head Nurse/Superintendent, VNA, Chicago, 1898–1912; Supervisor, rural nursing services, Cook County, Ill., 1917–40. **Organizations:** Founder, first president, Graduate Nurses Assoc. of the State of Illinois (later, Illinois Nurses Assoc.); attended and addressed International Congress of Women, Berlin, 1901; International Congress of Nurses, Paris, 1906; Jubilee Congress of District

Nursing, the celebration of the fortieth anniversary of district nursing, Liverpool, England, 1907; member, Committee on Periodicals of the Nurses Associated Alumnae of the United States and Canada (later the American Nurses Assoc.); Editor, public health nursing reports for *American Journal of Nursing,* 1908; Secretary, Ill. State Assoc. for the Prevention of Tuberculosis. **Awards:** unknown. **Died:** Chicago.

References and Credits

†Burgess WK: Harriet Fulmer. In Bullough V, Sentz L, Stein AP (eds): American Nursing: A Biographical Dictionary, vol. 2. New York, Garland, 1992, pp 124–126.

May 16

Emma Louise Warr

1847–1937

"The work of nursing is difficult and exacting, and demands much practical knowledge. The almost lack of such knowledge or home training of any kind... renders it impossible for us to teach them in two years all that they should know." (1897)

Emma Warr was the sole survivor of a shipwreck that claimed both of her parents. Her spirited determination permeated a career in nursing that stressed exacting preparation, welcomed challenge, and resulted in her affectionate nickname: "The Florence Nightingale of Missouri." After the Civil War, Missouri state officials became interested in opening nursing schools. In 1884 she was hired to be the director of the first school of nursing in St. Louis. She was also the sole instructor and worked from a single textbook to teach nursing methods and ethics while making immediate plans for a three-year curriculum, which was finally implemented in 1907. According to the writer Mary K. Delmont, Warr's annual report in 1898 said, "In 1897, 30 nurses, including 6 in the nurses training program, and 5 night nurses, took care of 570 patients." Warr set the highest standards for patient care and ward management, a boost to both the profession and the movement for standardization and nurse registration. She was one of the U.S. nursing pioneers who helped make nursing a profession.

Biography

Born: 1847, location unknown. **Education:** New York Hosp. School of Nursing. **Work history:** Superintendent of Nurses, Hamat Hosp., Erie, Pa., and School of Nursing, St. Louis. **Organizations:** founded Mo. nurses assoc.; American Red Cross; St. Louis Training School; Nurses Associated Alumnae of the United States. **Awards:** *Alumnae Bulletin* of the St. Louis Training School named *The Warr-ior* in her honor; bronze plaque, Society of St. Louis Training School. **Died:** St. Louis.

References and Credits

†Delmont MK: Emma Louise Warr. In Bullough V, Sentz L, Stein AP (eds): American Nursing: A Biographical Dictionary, vol. 2. New York, Garland, 1992, pp 342–345.

Janet M. Geister

1885–1964

"There is no need for eulogy. The record of my life is written in the lives of the people I've loved, walked with, and touched on the long path of my years. I do not know of course how much I've helped nor how often I've harmed. I only feel certain that God has always understood that more than anything else on earth I've wanted to help—never to harm. I believe that we are measured, not by the fruits of our acts, but by the quality of the spirit that inspires them." (1963)

JANET GEISTER PREPARED as a social worker after nursing school, and the combined skills and knowledge of both professions were reflected in her work. She teamed with visiting nurse associations to conduct research that showed that babies were not getting enough milk, resulting in the "Save 100,000 Babies" campaign of the Children's Bureau in 1918. She helped design a mobile clinic, the "Child Welfare Special," which delivered health care to children in rural areas. She was involved in research studies about nursing education, outpatient services, and private duty nursing. She was very active in professional organizations and often spoke and wrote about the need for change in both the structure of nursing organization and nursing practice. She was influenced by her daily readings of Emerson, and, according to Virginia Deforge, saw nursing as "a reverential calling, and of nursing practice as idealism in action."

Biography

Born: 1885, Elgin, Ill. **Education:** Sherman Hosp. School of Nursing, Elgin, Ill. (RN); Chicago School of Civics and Philanthropy. **Work history:** Private Duty Nurse; Infant Welfare Nurse, Michael Reese Hosp., Chicago; Medical Social Worker, Cook County Hosp., Chicago; Supervisor, Visiting Nurse Assoc. (VNA), Chicago; Researcher, Planner, U.S. Children's Bureau; staff, National Organization for Public Health Nursing; Committee on Dispensary Development, New York; Exec. Director, ANA; Editor, *Trained Nurse and Hospital Review.* **Organizations:** National Organization for Public Health Nursing; American Nurses Assoc. (ANA); Ill. League for Nursing (ILN). **Awards:** Gold Medal for journalism, *Modern Hospital;* life member, ILN; honorary member, Ill. Student Nurse Assoc.; ANA Hall of Fame. **Died:** Evanston, Ill.

References and Credits

†Geister JM: To my dear ones. 1963 holograph. Nursing Biology Library, Catholic University of America, Washington, D.C., copy in author's collection.

Stein AP: Janet M. Geister. In Bullough V, Church OM, Stein AP (eds): American Nursing: A Biographical Dictionary, vol. 1. New York, Garland, 1988, pp 134–135.

ANA Hall of Fame 10/98 American Nurses Association, Washington, D.C. http://www.nursingworld.org/ hof.

Deforge V: Janet Marie Louise Sophie Geister, 1885–1964, Health Care Revolutionary [thesis] Boston University School of Nursing, 1986, p 3.

MAY 18

Lenah Sutcliff Higbee

1874–1941

"The greatest need... is the true spirit of service, that ideal of service for which our Lady of the Lamp pleaded in a time when training schools were not existing. ...The character and the ideals which the individual bring to labor and to the profession alone make possible... dignifying the laborer and ennobling the profession." (1918)

"More and more it is recognized that we must look to education to destroy irrational suspicion and to restore health and sanity. Reconstruction and rehabilitation of the ex-service men cannot be an affair of merely rearranging tangible elements, such as food, money and clothes. It is by example, by encouragement to make an effort to overcome helplessness, by explanations of the reasons for necessary treatment and restrictions, that the nurse will succeed in helping to replace quiescent independence with the unsleeping desire and motive of service as active citizens." (1922)

LENAH HIGBEE WAS one of the "sacred twenty," the first twenty nurses selected for formal training and service as navy nurses. After she became the second superintendent of the Navy Nurse Corps, in January 1911, she guided the development of the corps through World War I. President Woodrow Wilson presented the Navy Cross to Higbee "in recognition of her distinguished service in the line of her profession and devotion to duty." She was the first woman to receive the Navy Cross in her lifetime. In 1944 the destroyer USS *Higbee* was named for her, the first U.S. Navy combat ship to bear the name of a female member of the service. She retired from the navy in 1922 and lived in Winter Park, Florida. She is buried in Arlington National Cemetery next to her husband, Lt. Col. John Henley Higbee, USMC.

Biography

Born: May 18, 1874, Chatham, New Brunswick, Can. **Education:** Mt. Alison Seminary, Sackville, New Brunswick; Hamilton College, Ontario (MA); Science Univ. of Toronto; New York Post-Graduate Hosp. School of Nursing, 1899; postgraduate work, Fordham Hosp., N.Y.C., and Naval Medical School, Washington, D.C. **Work history:** appointed to Navy Nurse Corps, 1908; Chief Nurse, Naval Hosp., Norfolk, Va.,1909–11; Superintendent, Navy Nurse Corps, 1911–22. **Organizations:** unknown. **Awards:** Navy Cross, 1920; destroyer USS *Higbee* launched by Bath Iron Works, Maine, 1944. **Buried:** Arlington National Cemetery.

References and Credits

†Higbee L: Nursing as it related to war—The navy. AJN 18:1061–1064, 1918.

†Higbee L: Nursing in government service: Second paper. AJN 18:526, 1922.

Sentz L: Lenah Sutcliff Higbee. In Bullough V, Sentz L, Stein AP (eds): American Nursing: A Biographical Dictionary, vol. 2. New York, Garland, 1992, pp 152–153.

Online Library of Selected Images: People—United States, available at http://www.history.navy.mil/photos/pers-us/uspers-h/l-higbee.htm.

May 19

Carolyn E. Gray

1873–1938

"Every bill introduced by nurses in every one of the states that has nursing laws has had for its purpose:

1. *Improvement of the care of the sick.*
2. *Better education for the nurse so as to fit her to give this care.*
3. *Protection of the public by making it possible for them to differentiate between the nurses who have qualified themselves and those who have not.*

Not until public opinion has been educated to realize that the legislation for which we are working will really benefit the public, even more than the nurse, will the opposition be overcome. Perhaps when each and every private nurse makes it her special business to know all about proposed nursing legislation and is able to meet the arguments for and against it intelligently, so that each one does her share to educate public opinion, we shall find we have more friends than we need." (1917)

Carolyn Gray was one of the early dedicated nurses who focused on innovations, raising standards, improving nursing education, and advocating college nursing programs. She was the first to recommend the eight-hour day for student nurses. She established scholarships for nurses and promoted nursing as a profession to young women. One of her innovations, recommended to reduce the fatigue suffered by overworked nurses, was a rollerskate that made no noise. She rewrote *Anatomy and Physiology for Nurses* with Diane E. Clifford Kimber and later Carolyn E. Stackpole. Gray's heroines were Edith Cavell, Florence Nightingale, and Adelaide Nutting.

Biography

Born: 1873, New York City. **Education:** City Hosp. School of Nursing, Welfare Island, N.Y., 1893; Teachers College, Columbia Univ., 1917, 1920 (BS, MS). **Work history:** Superintendent of Nurses, Governeur Hosp., N.Y., where she was the only graduate nurse, 1893–95; Fordham Hosp., Bronx, N.Y., 1895–1907; taught undergraduate, postgraduate nursing; taught science, City Hosp., 1907–11; Superintendent of Nurses, Pittsburgh Homeopathic Hosp., 1911–13; Principal, New York City Hosp., 1914–19; first dean, Western Reserve Univ. School of Nursing, Cleveland, 1923; Associate Professor, nursing education, College for Women, Western Reserve Univ.; Instructor, Teachers College, Columbia Univ.; College of St. Teresa, Winona, Minn.; Univ. of California, Berkeley. **Writings:** revised *Anatomy and Physiology for Nurses* with Kimber and Stackpole; wrote for *Modern Hospital,* 1918–25. **Organizations:** Secretary, Board of Nurse Examiners, state unknown, 1919–20; Assistant Secretary, Committee of the Rockefeller Foundation for the Study of Nursing Education, 1920–21; Chair, National League for Nursing Education Committee for the Study of Nursing Education in Colleges and Universities, 1923–33; President, N.Y.C. National League for Nursing (NLN), N.Y. State NLN; Vice President, NLN. **Awards:** unknown. **Died:** Miami.

References and Credits

†Gray C: The relation of the private duty nurse to the public as an educator (1917). In Birnbach N and Lewenson S (eds). New York, NLN Press, 1991, p 123.

Thom LM: Carolyn Gray. In Bullough V, Sentz L, Stein AP (eds): American Nursing: A Biographical Dictionary, vol. 2. New York, Garland, 1992, pp 137–140.

Rose Hawthorne Lathrop (Mother Alphonsa)

1851–1926

"The poor are ... like a long dusty road with no tree or hill. They are the human race devoid of illusions, bare of superficial attractions, standing as sinners imprisoned by circumstances before the tribunal of spiritual and intellectual joy. ... They are ourselves in a different guise. If we, the fortunate, did not neglect the unfortunate, they would not be walled in behind circumstances over which they are powerless or imprisoned in ignorance and sin. And then, too, suddenly, ... there will spring up some flower of loveliness. The poor, I have learned, can feel and do heroic things. The difference between the rich and the poor, is that the lives of the poor are an open book while the sins of the rich are done in hiding." (ca. 1902)

ROSE HAWTHORNE LATHROP wrote, "My father [Nathaniel Hawthorne] made me see the inner beauty of serving others." After the death of her child and the failure of her marriage, she worked as a nurse in the New York Cancer Hospital. The course of her life changed when she saw the contrast between the death of her dear friend, the poet Emma Lazarus, and that of a seamstress. Both were diagnosed with incurable cancer. While Lazarus died at home, surrounded by the loving care of family, the seamstress was banished to the poorhouse on Blackwell's Island, because cancer was considered a contagious disease. The terminally ill poor were simply discharged with no further care, and many were sent to die at the poorhouse. Lathrop wanted to alleviate the suffering of the sick poor and dedicated her life to the care of the poor and homeless with terminal cancer. "A fire was then lighted in my heart where it still burns, to do something toward preventing such inhuman regulations for those who are too forlorn to protest." She first provided care at her home. Then, with royalties from her writings, she bought properties to provide hospice care in a patient-centered home setting. A convert to Catholicism, she founded a religious order, now called the Hawthorne Dominican Sisters. Their humanitarian mission continues to provide care and comfort to cancer patients with six homes in five states. They collect no fees and are supported by voluntary contributions.

Biography

Born: May 20, 1851, near Lenox, Mass. **Education:** home schooled, with a few months as a nurse at New York Cancer Hosp. **Work history:** Trainee, New York Cancer Hosp.; cancer care in the community and in homes operated by the Servants of Relief for Incurable Cancer, St. Rose's Free Home and Rosary Hill Home. **Organizations:** unknown. **Awards:** medal from National Institute of Social Science; honorary master's degree, Bowdoin College; Gold Medal for outstanding service to humanity, N.Y. Rotary Club; Lifetime Achievement Award (posthumously), Oncology Nursing Society; Mayor Rudolph Giuliani of New York City declared Oct. 11, 1996, "Rose Hawthorne Lathrop Day" to commemorate the hundredth anniversary of her work on the Lower East Side. **Died:** Rosary Hill Home, Westchester County, N.Y.

References and Credits

†Myers R: American Women of Faith. Huntington, Ind., Our Sunday.

Visitor Publication Division, 1989, pp 107–108, 110.

Jones MVH: Rose Lathrop. In Bullough V, Church OM, Stein AP (eds): American Nursing: A Biographical Dictionary, vol. 1. New York, Garland, 1988, pp 206–208.

May 21

Elinor Delight Gregg
1889–1979

"The nurses themselves created the nursing service [above the Arctic Circle]. ... What I would like to convey to you is the unchanging spirit of nursing. In a world of snow and ice with the fierce intensity of cold, in the bleakness of a land either without trees or unfriendly with impenetrable scraggly forests, in the appalling winter strain of darkness for twenty hours out of twenty-four, the essential spirit of nursing has made life not only possible but enhanced it, has nurtured the growth and protected the future of these people. Among the Indians and Eskimos of Alaska, nurses ... are bringing more fullness of life through their knowledge. They are conveying this knowledge slowly but surely to a people who have had no leisure from the hard struggle for mere existence ... to improve their physical well-being." (1936)

Elinor Delight Gregg was the Red Cross recruiting-poster nurse during the First World War, and she served as a Red Cross nurse in France. Upon her return home, she worked as a Chautauqua lecturer, touring the country to tell of her experiences during the war and to speak about public health. (Begun as an assembly for training Sunday school teachers at Chautauqua Lake, New York, the Chautauqua movement became a popular movement in adult education and entertainment.) After doing postgraduate work in public health in Boston, she again worked for the Red Cross, this time on Indian reservations in South Dakota. That was when her contributions to the health of native Americans began. She taught basic health and hygiene, established diagnostic and treatment clinics on the Rosebud and Pine Ridge reservations, and converted part of her home there into a public health clinic. She continually surveyed health care needs so that services would be provided, constantly worked to recruit nurses, and visited nurses and patients at all locations, including Alaska. The first nurse supervisor for the Bureau of Indian Affairs, she was always respectful of the native Americans' culture and was adopted as "Helper Woman" by the Sioux.

Biography

Born: 1889, Colorado Springs, Colo. **Education:** Colorado College; Waltham (Mass.) Training School for Nurses; postgraduate study, Massachusetts General Hosp., Boston; Simmons College, Boston. **Work history:** industrial nursing; Administrator, City Hosp., Cleveland; Supervisor, Infants Hosp., Boston; Red Cross nurse, World War I; Chautauqua lecturer; rural nursing, N.H.; Red Cross/public health nursing, Indian reservations; Bureau of Indian Affairs. **Organizations:** Fellow, American Public Health Assoc. **Awards:** unknown. **Died:** Santa Fe, N. Mex.

References and Credits

†Gregg E: A federal nursing service above the Arctic Circle. AJN 36:128–129, 1936.

Early JO: Elinor Gregg. In Bullough V, Church OM, Stein AP (eds): American Nursing: A Biographical Dictionary, vol. 1. New York, Garland, 1988, pp 154–156.

Harris W, Levey J (eds): The New Columbia Encyclopedia. New York, Columbia University Press, 1975.

MAY 22

Katherine Tucker

1885–1957

"The keynote of our health work today is the cause and prevention of disease. This at once implies a consideration of social problems because of their close interdependent relation to disease. ... To be able at the very start to visualize the homes from which the patients come, something of the forces at work that brought the patient to the hospital should, and does where tried, vivify and humanize all that otherwise might be impersonal and detached technic." (1916)

KATHERINE TUCKER INFLUENCED public health for four decades. In 1916 she was invited to head the fast-growing Visiting Nurse Society (VNS) of Philadelphia. She brought experience in nursing, social work, and administration. Her ideas and her skillful administrative abilities resulted in a restructured and highly effective agency that had more staff, more services, and an increased commitment to prevention of disease. By 1926 the agency nurses had more than doubled their number of patients and visits. She broadened the base of nursing education when she promoted public health nursing as essential in nursing school curricula. She brought a new direction and a new vision to the National Organization for Public Health Nursing (NOPHN) when she was its general director. During the depression she successfully lobbied for funding for nursing care through the Federal Emergency Relief Act of 1933. This resulted in more direct home health care, as well as community nursing for maternity care, communicable diseases, and schools. Besides expanding health care for the poor, her efforts also provided employment for public health nurses.

Biography

Born: 1885, location unknown. **Education:** Vassar College; Newton (Mass.) Hosp. **Work history:** Univ. of Pennsylvania Hosp., Philadelphia.; State Charities Aid Assoc. of N.Y.C.; New York Dispensary; N.Y. State Committee on Mental Hygiene; Visiting Nurse Society, Philadelphia; Director, NOPHN; Professor, Univ. of Pennsylvania. **Organizations:** Pa. State Organization for Public Health Nursing; NOPHN. **Awards:** unknown. **Died:** Philadelphia.

References and Credits

†Tucker K: The training school's responsibility in public health nursing education. In Birnbach N, Lewenson S (eds): First Words: Selected Addresses from the National League for Nursing, 1894–1933. New York, National League for Nursing Press, 1991, pp 44–45.

Buhler-Wilkerson K: Katherine Tucker. In Bullough V, Church OM, Stein AP (eds): American Nursing: A Biographical Dictionary, vol. 1. New York, Garland, 1988, pp 322–323.

May 23

Phyllis Jean Verhonick

1922–1977

"In all research as new insights are gained the researcher builds on the work of others—he stands on the shoulders of the giants who preceded him. It is the giants and leaders of the past who have given him direction. Hopefully, good teacher-researchers of nursing can provide shoulders for the future researchers in nursing. There is no place for narrow views or the occupational disease of intellectual myopia. The stimulation and motivation provided by combined research and teaching should ultimately have an impact on the care of patients." (1971)

Phyllis Verhonick was a nationally and internationally respected nurse-researcher who promoted nursing research by students at the baccalaureate level. After teaching the basics of research, she would then guide students as they applied the information to complete a study project. This practice increased students' awareness of the value of research and clinical studies and was reflected in the continuing work of her former students. She published numerous works related to nursing research. Her own area of concentration was decubitus ulcers and skin care, and her findings were internationally recognized. A dedicated professional, she was sent to study at Columbia University when she was serving in the Army Nurse Corps. After completing her doctoral degree, she worked with Harriet Werley at the Walter Reed Army Institute, Department of Nursing, where their work firmly established the facility as a leader in nursing research.

Biography

Born: May 26, 1922, Enumclaw, Wash. **Education:** College of Nursing, Univ. of Portland, Ore. (BSN); Teachers College, Columbia Univ. (MA, EdD). **Work history:** Instructor, Columbus Hosp., Great Falls, Mont.; Instructor, Seattle, Wash.; numerous positions in Army Nurse Corps., with service in the U.S. and Japan; Administrator, Walter Reed Army Institute for Research; member of review groups or committees, National Institutes of Health, U.S. Dept. of Health, Education and Welfare; reviewer for professional journals; Consultant, Veterans Administration, Pan American Health Organization, World Health Organization; Faculty, School of Nursing, Univ. of Virginia. **Organizations:** American Nurses Foundation; American Nurses Assoc. **Awards:** charter member, American Academy of Nursing; Legion of Merit; a facility at Walter Reed Army Med. Center is named after her, as were the Phyllis J. Verhonick Nursing Research Courses/Conferences, established. by Army Nurse Corps and Univ. of Virginia; Verhonick Research Award, established by the Univ. of Va. **Died:** location unknown.

References and Credits

†Verhonick P. Research awareness at the undergraduate level. Nurs Res 20:262, 1971.

McCarthy RT: Phyllis Jean Verhonick. In Bullough V, Sentz L, Stein AP (eds): American Nursing: A Biographical Dictionary, vol. 2. New York, Garland, 1992, pp 337–340.

May 24

Nellie Xenia Hawkinson

1886–1971

"I recall to your minds Cassius' classic reply to Brutus, 'The fault, dear Brutus, is not in our stars, but in ourselves that we are underlings.' We, as a professional group, have been far too reticent about bringing to the attention of the public our professional needs. This responsibility is one which we must be ready to assume and, if we will to do so, I believe we can become as potent a social force in the life of our nation as is any other professional group and can claim the attention and financial support of the community. ... We [are] a group which is vitally concerned with the health of the nation." (1938)

When Nellie Hawkinson was appointed professor of nursing at the University of Chicago, she was part of the dedicated efforts to establish nursing as a profession. The focus was broadening and building on an essential knowledge base of scientific facts in an academic rather than a hospital setting. The goal of the program in Chicago was to prepare nurses who would be nursing school instructors or nursing administrators. In addition, Hawkinson encouraged schools to write curricula that provided nurses with greater opportunities for community service. Issues that nursing leaders dealt with in the 1930s sound familiar today: curriculum, faculty qualifications, accreditation, staff nurse availability, and the functions of ancillary personnel. Under Hawkinson's leadership the National League for Nursing Education (NLNE) took responsibility for the accreditation of nursing schools.

Biography

Born: May 29, 1886, Webster, Mass. **Education:** Framington (Mass.) Hosp. School of Nursing (basic nursing); Teachers College, Columbia Univ. (BS, MA); European study of nursing schools for Rockefeller Foundation; postgraduate studies, Columbia Univ. **Work history:** bedside nursing, Framington Hosp.; Instructor, Vassar Training Camp for Nurses, Teachers College, Massachusetts General Hosp.; Faculty, Dean, nursing school, Western Reserve Univ., Cleveland, Ohio; Professor, nursing education, Univ. of Chicago. **Organizations:** NLNE, Assoc. of Collegiate Schools of Nursing. **Awards:** honorary member, Sigma Theta Tau; named one of Chicago's 100 Outstanding Citizens, 1957; first edition, *Who's Who of American Women*; Professor Emeritus, Univ. of Chicago. **Buried:** Webster, Mass.

References and Credits

†Hawkinson NX: The outlook in nursing education. AJN 38: 578, 1938.

Dixon GL: Nellie Hawkinson. In Bullough V, Church OM, Stein AP (eds): American Nursing: A Biographical Dictionary, vol. 1. New York, Garland, 1988, pp 172–174.

MAY 25

Julia Catherine Stimson

1881–1948

"Preparedness for all kinds of emergencies and disasters is a sign of the highest type of intelligence. As people learn the lessons of history and experience they become more conscious of the need of preventing calamities and of being ready to meet them. The American Red Cross has long led the way in teaching how to prevent emergencies and also in readiness to deal with them. ...One of its basic duties is to have qualified nurses ready. ...It is certain that they [nurses] can always be counted on when the country needs them. ...Experience has shown that the medical and nursing professions may be counted on to work together not only in attempting to prevent catastrophes but also in relieving the suffering caused by them." (1936)

JULIA STIMSON'S CAREER reflected her upbringing in a family that valued education and service to others. Although she had an undergraduate degree and was doing postgraduate study with intentions to go to medical school, a meeting with nursing's dynamic Annie Goodrich drew her to nursing. Stimson used every opportunity to encourage women who had completed college to consider nursing as a career. Her outstanding leadership in the military paved the way for the eventual equitable treatment of nurses in the armed forces. She was involved with the Red Cross and Army Nurse

Corps during World War I in Rouen, France. In a book called *Finding Themselves* her family printed letters that she wrote about the difficulties that the nurses faced there. Her efforts to obtain rank for nurses in the military started with World War I, and she worked with Congress and nursing organizations to achieve this goal. Success finally came in 1947, when nurses received full commissions rather than relative rank.

Biography

Born: May 26, 1881, Worcester, Mass. **Education:** Vassar College (BA); graduate work, Columbia Univ.; New York Hosp. Training School; Washington Univ. (AM). **Work history:** Superintendent of Nurses, Harlem Hosp., N.Y.C.; Superintendent of Nurses, Washington Univ. Hosp., St. Louis; Red Cross volunteer reserve nurse; Army Nurse Corps, Rouen, France; Chief, Red Cross nurses, France; Director of Nursing Services, American Expeditionary Forces; Dean, Army School of Nursing; Superintendent, Army Nurse Corps. **Organizations:** American Red Cross, American Nurses Assoc. (ANA). **Awards:** Distinguished Service Medal; British Royal Red Cross; several medals from France; honorary doctorate, Mt. Holyoke College; Florence Nightingale Medal, International Committee, Red Cross; ANA Hall of Fame. **Died:** Poughkeepsie, N.Y.

References and Credits

†Stimson J: Preparedness: Red Cross nurses and reserve medical units. AJN 36: 135–136, 1936.

Sabin LE: Julia Stimson. In Bullough V, Church OM, Stein AP (eds): American Nursing: A Biographical Dictionary, vol. 1. New York, Garland, 1988, pp 302–304.

ANA Hall of Fame 10/98 American Nurses Association, Washington, D.C. http://www.nursingworld.org/hof.

May 26

Sophia French Palmer

1853–1920

"In appointing a legislative committee the State Association should be careful to select women with marked leadership qualities, who, through the positions they occupy, whether social or professional, command some political influence. The chair... should be a woman who speaks readily and clearly and whose bearing is one of womanliness and dignity. To her should be intrusted [sic] *the planning of the campaign, the distribution of the work either of individuals or of committees, and she must be given the unqualified support of her associates. There must be absolute harmony in the ranks, and the women who are put forward to lead the movement must possess those qualities which quickly command confidence and respect." (1907)*

SOPHIE PALMER WAS the first editor of the *American Journal of Nursing*. She strengthened the nursing press and nursing organizations during her twenty-year tenure. She saw nursing organizations as "the power of the day," or the means by which education about nursing concerns would bring about change. She was involved in the establishment of both the American Society of Superintendents of Training Schools for Nurses and the Nurses Associated Alumnae of the United States and Canada. Her editorials were the forum for addressing critical issues, because she realized that information and organization could lead to reform. Among those issues were the nursing curriculum, the need for standardization in nursing preparation, the exploitation of nurses by hospital programs, the need for state laws for nursing registration, and the need for nursing to oversee the regulations for training schools. Palmer proposed that *Journal* subscriptions be included in organizational memberships. Although various subscription plans were made available to members over time, her dream was not realized until 1996, when a sales agreement made it possible to give a subscription to the *Journal* to each member of a state nurses association as a benefit.

Biography

Born: May 26, 1853, Milton, Mass. **Education:** Boston Training School for Nurses; journalism course. **Work history:** Nurse, Philadelphia; Private Duty Nurse; Superintendent, St. Luke's Hosp., New Bedford, Mass..; Charge Nurse, Massachusetts General Hosp.; Superintendent of Nurses, founder of training school for nurses, Garfield Memorial Hosp., Washington, D.C.; editor, *Trained Nurse and Hospital Review*; Director, Rochester City Hosp., N.Y.; helped establish, edited *American Journal of Nursing*. **Organizations:** founding member, American Society of Superintendents of Training Schools for Nurses; organizer, Associated Alumnae of the United States and Canada; first chair, Delano Memorial Fund. **Awards:** Sophia F. Palmer Library of *American Journal of Nursing*; Palmer-Davis Library, Massachusetts General Hosp. School of Nursing; ANA Hall of Fame. **Buried:** Forest Hills Cemetery, near Boston.

References and Credits

†Palmer SF: The essential features of a bill for the registration of nurses, and how to pass it. AJN 7:432, 1907.

Donahue PM: Sophia French Palmer. In Bullough V, Church OM, Stein AP (eds): American Nursing: A Biographical Dictionary, vol. 1. New York, Garland, 1988, pp 252–254.

Lewenson S: Of logical necessity... they hang together: Nursing and the women's movement, 1901–1912. Nurs Hist Rev 2:99–117, 1994.

ANA Hall of Fame 10/98 American Nurses Association, Washington, D.C. http://www.nursingworld.org/ hof.

Plumb A: personal communication, 2003.

May 27

Lynda Van Devanter Buckley

1947–2002

"The tears from our separate souls of old pain
Mingle and become the same
As they roll from the eyes of our souls
Merging on our embracing cheekbones
Flowing over and under our lips and chins
Landing drop by measured drop
Upon our hearts
Watering our freeze-dried memories
And washing them clean." (2000)

LYNDA VAN DEVANTER BUCKLEY wrote and dedicated her poem, "An Introduction in Many Languages to Bach Diep," part of which is quoted here, after meeting Bach, a former member of the Viet Cong, at a commemoration marking the twenty-fifth anniversary of the end of the Vietnam War. Buckley, a first lieutenant in the Army Nurse Corps, was an operating room nurse at both the 71st Evacuation Hospital at Pleiku and the 67th Evacuation Hospital at Qui Nhon. In 1983 she published *Home before Morning,* her personal account of service as an army nurse in Vietnam. She said that she started writing it "as a form of therapy... to exorcise the Vietnam War from my mind and heart" but found "my feelings about the war will never go away. I don't want them to. For if I forget entirely,

I may be passively willing to see it happen again." The television series *China Beach* was inspired by this book. Later, she coedited *Visions of War, Dreams of Peace,* a collection of heart-wrenching poetry by forty Vietnamese and American women who served in Vietnam, to benefit the Vietnam Women's Memorial project. She was an activist for the rights of women veterans. When the government ignored female Vietnam veterans returning from the war, Buckley worked to have them represented in the national salute to Vietnam veterans. She traveled extensively to speak about the war and the women who served. Her work helped convince Congress to extend veterans' benefits to women, including access to research studies and health care, Veterans Administration (VA) loans, and educational assistance. Her child's birth defects were connected to her own chemical exposures in Vietnam, and she again lobbied Congress for inclusion of these children in VA services. She served as the national women's director of the Vietnam Veterans of America (VVA). After attending a commemoration of the twenty-fifth anniversary of the end of the war, she wrote of her powerful realization of and experience with that necessary part of healing, the forgiveness of others and the forgiveness of self. Buckley had service-related posttraumatic stress disorder and later developed a progressively debilitating, then fatal, autoimmune collagen vascular disease, as a result of her chemical exposure in Vietnam.

BIOGRAPHY

Born: May 27, 1947, Arlington, Va. **Education:** Mercy Hosp. School of Nursing, Baltimore (RN); Antioch Univ. (BA). **Work history:** OR Nurse, Army Nurse Corps, Vietnam; Poet; Author; national speaker; Consultant, Office of Technology Assessment, U.S. Congress; National Women's Director, VVA; advocate for benefits to women Vietnam Veterans; trained counselors for the VA's Vietnam Veterans Readjustment Center. **Organizations:** VVA; American Nephrology Nurses Assoc.; National Kidney Foundation; member, bd. of directors, Council of Nephrology Nurses and Technicians. **Awards:** Outstanding Woman of America; Woman of the Year, American Assoc. of Minority Veterans Program Administrators; National Vietnam Veterans Award, American G.I. Forum; American Culture Contribution Award, VVA; Foremost Woman of the 20th Century; Nurse of the Year, National Assoc. of Kidney Patients Organization. **Died:** Herndon, Va.

References and Credits continued on page 768

May 28

Walt Whitman

1819–1892

"An old man bending I come among new faces,...
Bearing the bandages, water and sponge,
Straight and swift to my wounded I go,
Where they lie on the ground after the battle brought in,
Where their priceless blood reddens the grass the ground,
Or to the rows of the hospital tent, or under the roof'd hospital,
To the long row of cots up and down each side I return,
To each and all, one after another I draw near, not one do I miss,
An attendant follows holding a tray, he carries a refuse pail,
Soon to be fill'd with clotted rags and blood, emptied, and fill'd again.
I onward go, I stop,
With hinged knees and steady hand to dress wounds;
I am firm with each, the pangs are sharp, yet unavoidable,
One turns to me his appealing eyes—poor boy! I never knew you,
Yet I think I could not refuse this moment to die for you, if that would save you." (ca. 1891)

Walt Whitman is considered America's greatest poet. He went to Virginia to nurse his brother George, who had been wounded in the Civil War, and stayed on as a nonpartisan volunteer nurse in Washington, D.C., hospitals. He estimated that he visited as many as eighty thousand wounded and dying men during his five years of service. With income from part-time jobs he would buy small gifts, such as fruit, tobacco, writing paper, and pencils, to give to the soldiers. Yet he knew that his gift of self was the most meaningful. Before his hospital visits he ensured a pleasant appearance by being well groomed, well rested, and well nourished. "In my visits to the hospitals, I found it was the simple matter of personal presence and emanating ordinary good cheer ... that succeeded and helped more ... than anything else. ...Behold, I do not give lectures or a little charity, when I give, I give myself." His prose work, *Specimen Days,* shares his personal observations and thoughts about the sorrows and human costs of war. Compassionate and tender, he identified with the soldiers and worked to reduce their pain and suffering. He would sit and hold the hand of the lonely and the frightened, sometimes for hours. His hospital visits were expressions of his very nature: "Agonies are one of my changes of garments, I do not ask the wounded person how he feels, I myself become the wounded person."

Biography

Born: May 31, 1819, Huntington, L.I. **Education:** unknown; avid reader. **Work history:** Printer's Helper, Schoolteacher, Journalist, Carpenter, War Correspondent, volunteer nurse, Poet. **Organizations:** unknown. **Awards:** unknown. **Died:** Camden, N.J.

References and Credits

†Whitman W: The wound-dresser and Song of myself. In Leaves of Grass. New York, Doubleday, Page and Company, 1926, pp 176–177, 76.

Canby HS: Walt Whitman in America. Boston, Houghton Mifflin, 1943, p 227.

Whitman W: Specimen Days. New York, New American Library, 1961, p 58.

Whitman W: Specimen Days, Democratic Vistas, and Other Prose, ed L Pond. New York, Doubleday, Doran, 1935.

Walt Whitman. In Harris W, Levey L (eds): The New Columbia Encyclopedia. New York, Columbia University Press, 1975, p 2972.

Foley S, Sofer D, Jacobson J: "I am faithful. I do not give out": Walt Whitman, Civil War poet and nurse. AJN 100:48–49, 2000.

Stein AP: Walt Whitman. In Bullough V, Church OM, Stein AP (eds): American Nursing: A Biographical Dictionary, vol. 1. New York, Garland, 1988, pp 335–336.

Dolan J: History of Nursing. Philadelphia, WB Saunders, 1968.

May 29

Florence Dakin

1868–1958

"One of the most important things in life is an ability to get along with other people. Many of us find it difficult at times to work and live happily with well people and the difficulty is increased when it is necessary to be patient with someone who is irritable and cross and afraid of being hurt or who is uncomfortable and in pain most of the time. Anyone who is responsible for making a sick person comfortable, keeping her happy and amused and willing to take medicine and the food she needs, must be understanding. Sick people are often unreasonable and uncooperative. They fuss about little things and want attentions that a nurse sometimes feels are unnecessary, but sick persons are not normal persons. Therefore the nurse herself needs to be so well physically and mentally that she gives the patient strength and reassurance. She needs almost more than anything else a real sense of humor: she laughs at herself as well as with someone else." (1941)

Florence Dakin was a member of the first Board of Nurse Examiners of New Jersey. During her fifteen-year tenure nursing education in New Jersey moved from apprenticeship toward professionalism. She developed curricula for nursing schools that standardized nursing preparation throughout the state. Her model also influenced the nursing program at Teachers College of

Columbia University and those in other states and countries. She upgraded faculty, broadened course content, and modernized the nurse's work shift from twelve to eight hours. During that period nursing schools increasingly came to demand that applicants have at least a high school diploma for admission. Specialty areas, such as community health and psychiatry, were taught by nursing instructors instead of physician-lecturers. Dakin's book, *Simplified Nursing,* was designed for non-nurses to use in home care. In the section called "Getting Along with People," she helps the reader see the patient's point of view. She reminds the caretaker of the importance of rest and recreation. She pointedly cautions that caretaker fatigue may result in unspoken messages to the patient that his care is bothersome or wearisome. First published in 1925, it became available in Spanish and had seven editions.

Biography

Born: May 29, 1868, Brooklyn, N.Y. **Education:** Brooklyn Seminary; Hollins College, New York Hosp. School of Nursing (RN). **Work history:** Staff, New York Hosp.; supervisory positions, Fannie Paddock Hosp. (now Tacoma General), Tacoma, Wash.; City and County Hosp., San Francisco; Middletown Hosp., Ohio; Nursing Instructor, Patterson (N.J.) General Hosp.; N.J. Bd. of Nurse Examiners; Education Director, N.J. schools of nursing. **Organizations:** N.J. Nurses Assoc.; N.J. League for Nursing Education. **Awards:** unknown. **Buried:** Forest Hill Cemetery, Utica, N.Y.

References and Credits

†Dakin F, Thompson E. The patient's viewpoint. In Simplified Nursing, 4th ed. Philadelphia, JB Lippincott, 1941, p 3.

Fickelsson JL: Florence Dakin. In Bullough V, Church OM, Stein AP (eds): American Nursing: A Biographical Dictionary, vol. 1. New York, Garland, 1988, pp 73–74.

May 30

Doris Ruhbel Schwartz

1915–1999

"That old man taught me a great deal in his last sixty minutes of life as I sat by his bedside. Sometimes we talked, briefly and quietly. Sometimes we were just there together, not speaking yet sensing our togetherness. I learned a valuable lesson that caring about *a patient can be as important as providing care* for *the patient. Occasionally I am asked whether old people are afraid of death. That has not been my observation as a geriatric nurse. What many old people fear, it seems to me, is the thought of dying without being missed, of dying without one's absence mattering to anyone." (1990)*

Doris Schwartz kept a journal during her decades of nursing. Her career included service in the Army Nurse Corps and practice as a visiting nurse in Brooklyn. She was an early expert in transcultural nursing and wrote extensively for publication. In her later career she completed studies as a geriatric nurse practitioner and established a geriatric nurse practitioner program at Cornell, where she was a member of the faculty. She studied health care in Scotland and worked with the World Health Organization to prepare goals and priorities for geriatric service. Her approach to geriatric care conveys her commitment to individualized care and the importance of the interdisciplinary approach for community care for the elderly. Her writings reflected her commitment to humanistic, patient-centered care throughout her career.

Biography

Born: May 30, 1915, Brooklyn, N.Y. **Education:** Methodist Hosp. School of Nursing, Brooklyn, N.Y.; Univ. of Toronto; New York Univ. (BS, MS). **Work history:** Captain, Army Nurse Corps; editorial assistant, *American Journal of Nursing;* Visiting Nurse, Brooklyn; Faculty, Cornell Univ., Univ. of Pennsylvania School of Nursing. **Organizations:** charter member, American Academy of Nursing. **Awards:** Rockefeller Fellowship to Univ. of Toronto; Mary Roberts Fellowship at *American Journal of Nursing*; Fogarty Fellow, National Institutes of Health; National Science Foundation Fellowship; Pearl McIver Award, American Nurses Assoc.; Distinguished Career Award, American Public Health Assoc.; Sigma Theta Tau Founder's Award; Sigma Theta Tau Mentor Award; Lillian Wald Spirit of Nursing Award; Living Legend American Academy of Nursing, 1997. **Died:** Gwynedd, Pa.

References and Credits

†Schwartz D: Give Us to Go Blithely: My Fifty Years in Nursing. New York, Springer, 1990, preface (np).

Schorr T, Zimmerman A: Making Choices, Taking Chances: Nurse Leaders Tell Their Stories. St. Louis, CV Mosby, 1988.

Brook MJ: Doris Schwartz. In Bullough V, Sentz L (eds): American Nursing: A Biographical Dictionary, vol. 3. New York, Springer, 2000, pp 253–255.

Farr G: personal communication, 2003.

May 31

Myrtle Kitchell Aydelotte

1917–

"Nursing leadership must reorient... and restructure itself in such a way that nursing education and practice are inseparable, are symbolic, and are united in purpose. We must put aside inertia, apathy, competitiveness, personal animosities, and censorship. We must restructure a set of social relationships [that] will enable society to receive that which it has charged us to provide. If we do not do this, society will surely place the charge they have given us elsewhere. ...Nursing as an occupation is a social institution, and social institutions, many of long standing, are crumbling and changing today. ...There is a great need to accelerate the progressive movements now occurring in nursing; ...These movements are responsive to what society wants and are the directions that society will support." (1972)

Myrtle Kitchell Aydelotte, a widely honored nurse leader, stresses that nursing is a practice profession, clinical in nature. She always wanted to be a nurse and go to college. Although her family supported and encouraged her, a public health nurse visiting a family member was the person who urged her to go to the University of Minnesota. She credits her program there with giving her an excellent base for clinical nursing and for refining her thoroughness. She recognized the importance of collaboration with physicians in patient care and the value of input from the well-prepared nurse. She was the first nurse clinical instructor at St. Mary's Hospital School of Nursing in St. Paul, Minnesota, and served with the Army Nurse Corps in North Africa and Italy during World War II.

When she was the nursing director of the University of Iowa Hospital system, she elevated standards and practice when she hired nurses with college degrees for entry-level positions and nurses with master's degrees for administration and advanced practice. She was the founding dean of the School of Nursing at the University of Iowa. Her knowledgeable leadership strengthened and expanded the curriculum while making nursing independent of the College of Medicine. She promoted graduate education for nurses. Her career also included research, writing, consultation, and mentoring.

Biography

Born: May 31, 1917, Van Meter, Iowa. **Education:** Univ. of Minnesota (BS, MA, PhD). **Work history:** Head Nurse, C. T. Miller Hosp., St. Paul, Minn.; Instructor, St. Mary's Hosp. School of Nursing, St. Paul, Minn.; Nurse, Army Nurse Corps, World War II; Faculty, Univ. of Minnesota; Dean, Professor of Nursing, Iowa State Univ.; nursing research, Veterans Administration Hosp., Iowa City; Director, Nursing Service, Univ. of Iowa Hosp. and Clinics; Exec. Director, American Nurses Assoc. (ANA); American Nurses Foundation (ANF); Visiting Professor, Univ. of Illinois; Professor, Yale Univ., Univ. of Iowa College of Nursing. **Organizations:** ANA, Sigma Theta Tau; ANF. **Awards:** several from Univ. of Minnesota, Univ. of Iowa, incl. endowed research fellowship in her name at the Univ. of Iowa; elected to Institute of Medicine, National Academy of Sciences; Luther Christman Award; honorary doctorate, Univ. of Nebraska; ANF Distinguished Scholar; Distinguished Research Fellow Award, Hall of Fame, Sigma Theta Tau; Living Legend American Academy of Nursing, 1994.

References and Credits

†Newman B, Fawcett J: The Neuman Systems Model, 4th ed. Englewood Cliffs, N.J., Prentice Hall, 2002, p 4.

Schorr T, Zimmerman A: Making Choices, Taking Chances: Nurse Leaders Tell Their Stories. St. Louis, CV Mosby, 1988.

Donahue PM: Myrtle Aydelotte. In Bullough V, Sentz L (eds): American Nursing: A Biographical Dictionary, vol. 3. New York, Springer, 2000, pp 8–12.

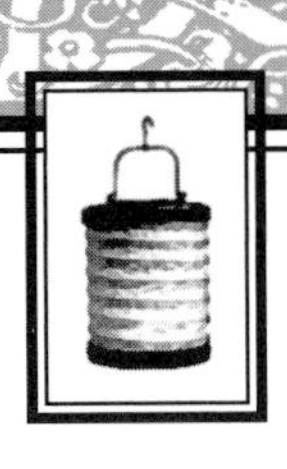

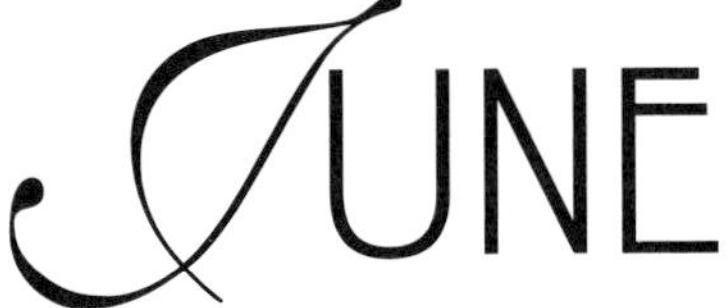

JUNE

"There are five essential points in securing the health of houses:

1. *Pure air*
2. *Pure water*
3. *Efficient drainage*
4. *Cleanliness*
5. *Light*

Without these, no house can be healthy. And it will be unhealthy just in proportion as they are deficient."

▪▪

—Florence Nightingale
Nightingale F: Notes on Nursing: What It Is, And What It Is Not. New York, D. Appleton, 1860, p 24.

June 1

Frances Reiter

1904–1977

"Practice *is the absolute primary function of our profession. ...It simply means the direct care of patients. ...In our present complex hospital situation, direct nursing care is—or should be—the one area over which nursing has complete control. ...Depending on what we do in this area, we write our own destiny and that of the future of nursing. ...The nurse-clinician, and the profession of nursing itself, must always remain closely identified with nursing practice." (1966)*

FRANCES REITER FIRST coined the term *nurse-clinician* in 1943. It defines the role as one of comprehensive involvement by a very knowledgeable nurse in providing and coordinating patient care. Inspired by the quality of clinical competence of the nurses whom she observed when she was a supervisor at Massachusetts General Hospital, she called it "curative nursing." She recognized that nurses with a broader knowledge base could collaborate with the physician and hold overall responsibility for coordinating the nursing aspects of patient care. Reiter reminds nurses that the heart of nursing continues to be the personal care of the patient, and this is enhanced by nursing knowledge. She believed that nursing faculty must be involved in practice and teaching. She also believed that when faculty members are also nurse-clinicians, they are fully prepared to demonstrate and teach the full range of nursing practice.

Biography

Born: 1904, location unknown. **Education:** Johns Hopkins Hosp. Training School for Nurses; Teachers College, Columbia Univ. (BS, MA). **Work history:** Head Nurse, Johns Hopkins; Assistant Director, Nursing Service, Montefiore Hosp., Pittsburgh, Pa.; Nursing Instructor, Johns Hopkins, Bryn Mawr; Massachusetts General Hosp.; Instructor, Professor, Teachers College, Columbia Univ.; Dean, Graduate School of Nursing, New York Medical College; Researcher, U.S. Public Health Service; member, editorial bd., *Nursing Research.*
Organizations: American Nurses Assoc. (ANA). **Awards:** Honorary Membership Award, ANA; Florence Nightingale Award, International Committee, Red Cross; Distinguished Service Award, National League for Nursing; Medal of Excellence, New York Medical College; Honorary Fellow, American Academy of Nursing; ANA Hall of Fame.
Died: Cherry, Ill.

References and Credits

†Reiter F: The nurse clinician. AJN 66:274, 1966.

Bullough V: Frances Reiter. In Bullough V, Church OM, Stein AP (eds): American Nursing: A Biographical Dictionary, vol. 1. New York, Garland, 1988, pp 268–269.

ANA Hall of Fame 10/98 American Nurses Association, Washington, D.C. http://www.nursingworld.org/hof.

Una H. Haynes

1911–

"The ultimate prevention of all forms of developmental disability is a continuing long-term goal. Until then, interdisciplinary approaches to the earliest possible detection of the nature and the scope of the disabilities, collaborative efforts toward remediation and alleviation of the dysfunctions, the promotion of health, and the prevention of illness and unwarranted secondary disabilities are effective ways to foster the potential of members of this population to achieve the highest possible degree of independence and the fullest measure of their human rights. Even if the immediate requirements to reduce expenditures tend to cloud the perspective on these salutary goals, there is little doubt that these approaches are ultimately far more cost effective than permitting the dysfunctions to cause increased handicap, which ultimately means that many individuals, who have thereby become completely dependent, may require life-long support." (1983)

UNA H. HAYNES was one of the few nurses who worked in the field of mental retardation, especially with victims of cerebral palsy. She determined that these children were unique because they had never experienced normality, as postpolio patients had. She developed and directed programs of nursing education to help nurses better administer to children with cerebral palsy, and she helped parents understand the child's limitations and improve their care-giving skills. She developed a protocol for better nursing assessment of infants and wrote the *Developmental Approach to Case Finding* in 1967. In addition, she created the accompanying "wheel of development," a tool that nurses could use to assess development and reflexes in children younger than three. She worked closely with the United Cerebral Palsy Association to generate an intensive five-day postgraduate course that taught nursing leaders the theory and clinical aspects of cerebral palsy. She also directed the development of the Nationally Organized Collaborative Project to Provide Comprehensive Services for Atypical Infants and Their Families. Staff members who attended the workshops returned to their communities throughout the United States to teach other nurses and develop "ripple" centers that eventually included sixty-five agencies and twenty-six states that helped ten thousand infants and their families. Haynes's perseverance in an area of nursing that few chose improved services for the least understood children with developmental disorders.

Biography

Born: June 2, 1911, Holyoke, Mass. **Education:** Worcester City (Mass.) Hosp. School of Nursing; Teachers College, Columbia Univ., 1934 (BSN); postgraduate courses, Teachers College. **Work history:** Public Health Nurse, Boston Community Health Assoc.; worked nights in labor and delivery; Faculty, Holyoke Hosp. School of Nursing; Director, Outpatient Services for Medically Indigent, Skinner Clinic, Holyoke, Mass.; helped local affiliate of United Cerebral Palsy Assoc. (UCPA) begin professional services committee; Consultant, UCPA Regional Program Services; Associate Director, Professional Program Services, UCPA; made film demonstrating assessment of infant during bath; member, national advisory committee to develop postgraduate nursing course in cerebral palsy and related disorders at Indiana Univ. School of Nursing, 1968. **Organizations:** Fellow, American Public Health Assoc. **Awards:** five national awards from different groups.

References and Credits

†Haynes U: Holistic Health Care for Children with Developmental Disabilities. Baltimore, University Park Press, 1983, pp 145–146.

Nehring WM: Una Haynes. In Bullough V, Sentz L (eds): American Nursing: A Biographical Dictionary, vol. 3. New York, Springer, 2000, pp 124–128.

June 3

Anna Kaplan
CA. 1888–1960

"We have introduced the eight-hour day and six-day week for our charge and staff nurses. ... This arrangement has opened ten new positions: eight for graduate nurses and two for nurses aids [sic]. It has been made possible entirely by the nursing staff themselves. ... The new schedule has been in operation since November 1 and has proved successful. We are all hoping that we may eventually return to our old salaries, but never again to the old hours on duty." *(1933)*

IN 1918 ANNA KAPLAN arrived in Palestine as part of a medical mission, the American Zionist Medical Unit for Palestine (which later became the Hadassah Medical Organization of the Zionist Organization of America, or ZOA). In Palestine she worked to establish a nursing school, following the Nightingale model. She also helped establish community health centers similar to those of the Henry Street Settlement. The nursing school curriculum and standards that she implemented were modeled after those of the National League for Nursing, and graduates took the New York state board exam for licensure. The program, which ran for three years and three months, included midwifery and public health to combat the high infant mortality rate and rampant communicable disease. She helped establish hospitals, clinics, and school and community health services to combat the many cases of malaria, tuberculosis, trachoma, dysentery, and skin diseases. Upon her return to Brooklyn she reduced the workday and the workweek for staff nurses when she worked with them to establish a work-sharing program at Beth Moses Hospital. She credited the nurses for supporting a plan to increase staff, even though it meant reduced pay because of the shorter workday.

Biography

Born: ca.1888, Bialystok, Poland. **Education:** Lebanon Hosp. Nursing School, N.Y.; coursework, Teachers College, Columbia Univ. **Work history:** Staff Nurse, Lebanon Hosp.; Head Nurse, Liberty Sanitarium; Public Health Nurse, N.Y.; ZOA medical mission, Palestine; Director, Hadassah Nursing School, Palestine; Nursing Superintendent, Rothschild Hosp., Jerusalem, and other Hadassah hosps.; Director of Nurses, Beth Moses Hosp., Brooklyn, N.Y.. **Organizations:** unknown. **Awards:** unknown. **Died:** New York City.

References and Credits

†Kaplan A: Work sharing at the Beth Moses Hospital. AJN 33:36, 1933.

Bartal N: Anna Kaplan. In Bullough V, Sentz L (eds): American Nursing: A Biographical Dictionary, vol. 3. New York, Springer, 2000, pp 155–157.

June 4

Jane Elizabeth Hitchcock

1863–1939

"On January 1, 1940, there were 23,705 public health nurses in the United States and the territories of Hawaii and Alaska. This indicates an increase of about 19% since January 1, 1937. ...However, with the additional demands for public health nursing service in connection with maternal hygiene, venereal disease control, pneumonia care, and ... [other] programs which are being developed, there are not nearly enough public health nurses to meet the needs. In many communities the already overburdened public health nurses have attempted to spread their services a little thinner in order to render some assistance in each special field. There is danger in spreading our efforts to such an extent that the work becomes less effective. If ... the ... needs of this country are to be met, twice as many public health nurses as are now on duty must be employed." (1941)

JANE HITCHCOCK WAS one of the first four nurses to work at the Henry Street Settlement. During her twenty-six years of service there, she lived at the settlement and worked as staff nurse, then supervisor. Dedicated to providing and promoting public health nursing, she recruited nurses into public health with her speeches, her writings, and her example. She developed the coursework and taught public health nursing at Lincoln Hospital School of Nursing.

She worked to have public health nursing theory and practice standardized and included in every basic nursing program. When she was a member of the New York State Board of Nurse Examiners, she prepared the public health examination questions. After the First World War she worked with the placement bureau to help nurses returning from military service find jobs. She is credited with establishing the Metropolitan Life Insurance program that provided professional nursing care as a benefit to subscribers.

Biography

Born: Aug. 1, 1863, Amherst, Mass. **Education:** Mt. Holyoke College; Cornell Univ.; New York Training School for Nurses. **Work history:** Head Nurse, Newton (Mass.) Hosp.; Public Health Nurse, Henry Street Settlement; Instructor, Lincoln Hosp. School of Nursing, N.Y.; American Red Cross, Placement Bureau; Public Health Nurse Supervisor, Ithaca, N.Y.; New York Bd. of Nurse Examiners. **Organizations:** N.Y. Hosp. Alumnae Assoc.; National Organization for Public Health Nursing. **Awards:** unknown. **Died:** Northampton, Mass.

References and Credits

†Hitchcock JE: How many public health nurses? Public Health Nursing 33:21, 23, 1941.

Sabin L: Jane Hitchcock. In Bullough V, Sentz L, Stein AP (eds): American Nursing: A Biographical Dictionary, vol. 2. New York, Garland, 1992, pp 153–154.

June 5

Ethel Swope

1859–1936

"Probably the most widely discussed question in nursing today is the eight hour day for special nurses, the benefits of which are attested to by the fact that it is in effect in approximately 150 hospitals [throughout the country] at the present time. ...Approximately 98% of the patients approve the eight hour day because... better nursing care is received due to lack of fatigue on the part of the nurse. ...Patients spoke of the comfort the patient derives from the appearance at eight hour intervals of a rested cheerful nurse. ...The people of the United States have accepted the principle of shorter periods of work in all lines of endeavor, and in consequence the membership of the American Nurses Association, with the cooperation of patients, hospitals and the medical profession are rapidly bringing about that condition which provides a more satisfactory type of bedside nursing than has ever before been realized." (1933)

ETHEL SWOPE WAS called the "Apostle of the Eight-Hour Day." Her greatest contribution to nursing may have been her determination to help hospitals see that the extremely long hours required of private duty nurses interfered with quality of care and patient safety. During her years with the California State Nurses Association (CSNA), many hospitals shortened the nurse's workday to eight hours. This achievement was credited to Swope. She later held a leadership position with the American Nurses Association (ANA) and traveled to promote the eight-hour day for nurses. She served as a Red Cross nurse and was an army nurse in France during World War I. After moving to California she established a registry of nurses, which proved to be a helpful resource to both nursing and the public.

Biography

Born: 1885, location unknown. **Education:** Connecticut Training School for Nurses, New Haven. **Work history:** Administrator, Cincinnati General Hosp.; Red Cross nurse, army nurse, World War I; Public Health Nurse, Pa., Ariz.; Superintendent, Golden State Hosp., Los Angeles; Director, Methodist Hosp., Los Angeles; Exec. Secretary, CSNA.; Assistant Director, ANA. **Organizations:** American Red Cross; American Hosp. Assoc.; National Organization for Public Health Nursing; National League for Nursing Education; Western Hosp. Assoc.; Women's Overseas League, **Awards:** unknown. **Buried:** Arlington National Cemetery.

References and Credits

†Swope E: The eight hour day makes progress. AJN 33:1147, 1152, 1933.

Stein AP: Ethel Swope. In Bullough V, Sentz L, Stein AP (eds): American Nursing: A Biographical Dictionary, vol. 2. New York, Garland, 1992, p 319.

June 6

Mary Margaret Riddle
1856–1936

"Each form of life and work demands a standard by which to estimate its usefulness and test its power, it follows as a natural sequence that there should be an established rule by which the education of nurses may be measured. . . . [State registration for nurses] will set a standard of excellence and nursing education so that the professional nurse will be the registered nurse. It will give a dignity and legal status to a profession, it will be the 'hallmark of distinction,' so to speak, or, if you please, the state's approval will set upon the nurse a stamp by which she is known to the world as 'sterling.'" (1907)

MARY MARGARET RIDDLE worked for more than a decade as a math teacher before entering nursing school. She emerged as a nursing leader whose achievements are still felt today. A strong proponent of both professional nursing organizations and state registration for nurses, she helped found the Nurses Associated Alumnae of the United States (now the American Nurses Association) as well as the group that eventually became the National League for Nursing. Her advocacy and long struggle for state registration of nurses in Massachusetts led to success in 1910, and she was issued that state's first registered nurse license. She helped launch the *American Journal of Nursing,* helped organize the Massachusetts

Red Cross, and organized army nurse units during World War I. Under her leadership the Newton (Massachusetts) Hospital Training School developed a program that was a model for others.

Biography

Born: June 6, 1856, Turbotville, Pa. **Education:** Boston City Training School for Nurses. **Work history:** numerous positions, Boston City Hosp.; Lecturer, Teachers College, Columbia Univ.; member, bd. of directors, American Journal of Nursing Co.; Editor, *Modern Hospital Magazine;* Superintendent, hospital and training school, Newton Hosp.; chair, Massachusetts Bd. of Registration in Nursing; Superintendent of Nurses, Army School of Nursing, Camp Devens. **Organizations:** Boston City Hosp. Alumnae Assoc.; Nurses Associated Alumnae of the United States; Mass. State Nurses Assoc. (MSNA); American Society of Superintendents of Training Schools for Nurses; Treasurer, Isabel H. Robb Memorial Fund, Isabel McIsaac Loan Fund for Nurses. **Awards:** honored by MSNA; Newton Hosp. initiated the Mary M. Riddle Scholar Award. **Died:** possibly Constantine, Mich.

References and Credits

†Riddle MM: Why we should have state registration for nurses. AJN 7:240, 242, 1907.

Murphy S: Mary Riddle. In Bullough V, Sentz L, Stein AP (eds): American Nursing: A Biographical Dictionary, vol. 2. New York, Garland, 1992, pp 274–276.

June 7

Virginia Cassady Clinton Kelley
1923–1994

"Life is hard; don't try to go it alone. ...I had my support group. Everybody needs people to talk with, to laugh with, to cry with. People who believe in you. People who'll keep you *believing in you." (1994)*

THE MINISTER WHO conducted Virginia Clinton Kelley's graveside service remembered her "as an American original. ...She was like a rubber ball. The harder life put her down, the higher she bounced. She didn't know what the word *quit* meant." Kelley, the daughter of a nurse, decided to become a nurse-anesthetist in high school so she could be in the "wave of the future." She developed a large successful practice in Hot Springs, Arkansas, that lasted more than three decades. She was involved locally in the national interdisciplinary dispute between doctors and nurses about who could administer an anesthetic. She believed that sexism was what defeated her and eventually caused her retirement from nursing anesthesia. Kelley was fun loving, independent, gregarious, and determined. She did not allow the severity of her breast cancer to hinder the presidential campaign and inauguration of her son Bill Clinton, as the forty-second president of the United States.

Biography

Born: June 6, 1923, Bodcaw, Ark. **Education:** Tri-State Hosp., Shreveport, La. (RN diploma); Charity Hosp., New Orleans, 1947 (nurse-anesthetist certificate). **Work history:** Private Duty Nurse; Anesthetist on Call, Josephine Hosp., St. Joseph's Hosp., Hot Springs, Ark. **Organizations:** unknown. **Awards:** unknown. **Buried:** Hope, Ark.

References and Credits

†Kelley V, Morgan J: Leading with my heart: My life, Virginia Kelley. New York, Simon and Schuster Adult Publishing Group and the Estate of Virginia Kelley, 1994, pp 136–137.

Brewer GW: Virginia Kelley. In Bullough V, Sentz L (eds): American Nursing: A Biographical Dictionary, vol. 3. New York, Springer, 2000, pp 54–57.

June 8

Dorothy Deming
1893–1972

"Patients look for something more in every nurse. ... Beyond technical skill, conscientious performance and pleasing appearance is that intangible something that makes the truly successful nurse. The quality is hard to define. ... Some call this quality 'selflessness or self-sacrifice,' some 'the true spirit of nursing,' others know it as religion. By whatever name, it is a spiritual quality that patients recognize instantly, that employers long to find in every nurse, and that can most simply and unsentimentally be called interest plus. When a nurse has this quality, it pervades all she does for patients and lights the way of those who must perform their executive and supervisory tasks far from the beds of sick people." (1952)

Dorothy Deming was a graduate student in American history when her mother died. Subsequent volunteer work with the Visiting Nurse Association (VNA) in New Haven, Connecticut, as well as the involvement of the United States in World War I, attracted her to nursing. As a student she worked with the Henry Street Visiting Nurse Association, and public health nursing became her specialty. She became a national leader with the National Organization for Public Health Nursing (NOPHN) and a national consultant on public health; she published frequently on nursing issues. She recognized the value of practical nursing for patient care and in 1944 supported different educational levels for entry into practice. A gifted and popular writer, she wrote nurse-themed fiction for adolescents that stimulated an interest in nursing as a career. Her first fictional nurse, Penny Marsh, was intelligent and committed and prompted the start of high school "Penny Marsh Clubs."

Biography

Born: June 8, 1893, New Haven, Conn. **Education:** Vassar College (bachelor's degree); graduate work, Yale Univ. Presbyterian Hosp., N.Y.C. **Work history:** Staff, VNA, New Haven, Conn., Henry Street VNA; Director, Holyoke (Mass.) VNA; Administrator, NOPHN; editorial staff, *Public Health Nursing;* Consultant, American Public Health Assoc., National Health Council. **Organizations:** NOPHN. **Awards:** unknown. **Died:** Winter Park, Fla.

References and Credits

†Deming D: Careers for Nurses. New York, McGraw-Hill, 1952, pp 17–18.

Thom LM: Dorothy Deming. In Bullough V, Church OM, Stein AP (eds): American Nursing: A Biographical Dictionary, vol. 1. New York, Garland, 1988, pp 80–82.

June 9

Daisy Dean Urch
1876–1952

"Every principal of every school of nursing in the United States could… when selecting each prospective student, put to herself these questions:

Is she the type of young woman I would like to take care of me if I were ill?
Would I choose her to teach health to my daughter?
Would I be proud to have her as a member of my profession?
Would I invite her to be a guest in my home?
Has she the mental capacity necessary to learn the sciences necessary to intelligent understanding and practice of nursing?
Is she physically and emotionally equal to the stress and strain of dealing with human beings when they are at their worst?
Is she adaptable enough to adjust herself to the fifty-seven varieties of duties a nurse must perform?" (1932)

DAISY URCH WAS raised in a large family on a farm, where she was expected to have a sense of community and to behave responsibly. She was a kindergarten teacher and a school principal before she studied nursing. An outspoken advocate for high standards of practice, she worked to attract only the best candidates to the profession. She equated improved nursing practice with a need to improve the process for selecting nursing school applicants. She recommended that desirable traits for candidates also include leadership abilities. Her goal was to enroll students who were innately capable of learning nursing and who would find fulfillment in practice. A Red Cross nurse in France during World War I, she served in both the American and British armies. At that time nurses had neither military rank nor protected rights and served at the pleasure of the commanding officer. While she was working as a temporary chief military nurse, she was demoted to staff after a dispute with the commanding officer about patient care. After the war her varied career in nursing included teaching, administration, and serving on accreditation teams as a member of the National League for Nursing Education.

Biography

Born: June 9, 1876, Clarkston, Mich. **Education:** Ferris Institute, Mich.; Illinois Training School, Chicago; Teachers College, Columbia Univ. (BS, MA). **Work history:** Private Duty Nurse; Faculty, Illinois Training School for Nurses; American Red Cross Nurse, World War I; San Francisco Hosp. School of Nursing; Inspector, California nursing schools; Director, Highland School of Nursing, Oakland, Calif.; Minnesota State Bd. of Nurse Examiners; Faculty, College of St. Teresa, Winona, Minn. **Organizations:** Calif. State League for Nursing Education; Calif. State Nurses Assoc.; Minn. League for Nursing Education; Minn. State Organization of Public Health Nursing; National League for Nursing Education. **Awards:** unknown. **Died:** Winona, Minn.

References and Credits

†Urch DD: Through better selection of students. In Birnbach N, Leweson S (eds): First Words: Selected Addresses from the National League for Nursing, 1894–1933. New York, National League for Nursing Press, 1991, p 237.

Dombrowski T: Daisy Urch. In Bullough V, Church OM, Stein AP (eds): American Nursing: A Biographical Dictionary, vol. 1. New York, Garland, 1988, pp 324–325.

June 10

Nina Diadamia Gage

1883–1946

"The progress of the nursing profession is eventually in the hands of the nurses themselves. When, as in America and Europe, they demand education, higher standards, legislation, and organize to this end, then progress is real and sure. Where they do not... the profession does not advance." (1919)

Nina Gage is credited with establishing the standards for nursing in China. She earned a degree in foreign languages before entering and completing nursing school. She then moved to China and became fluent in Chinese before she established the Hunan-Yale School of Nursing, in 1909. Despite interruptions by riots in China, a bout with typhoid fever, and the Chinese Revolution, she worked as a nurse educator, organizer, author, administrator, and supervisor. Gage successfully blended new ideas into a culture of tradition. She helped remove the bias against manual service. Her efforts replaced nursing care by coolies or family members with a model that prepared individuals to care for the sick. This new discipline needed to be defined, and her phrasing, "scholars to watch and guard," or "guard scholars," became the word for *nurse* in Chinese. She served as president of the Nurses Association of China (NAC) and the International Council of Nurses (ICN). She promoted nursing conventions in China and is credited with helping to establish a standardized curriculum for nursing schools, school accreditation, and nurse registration, all based on the American model.

Biography

Born: June 9, 1883, New York City. **Education:** Wellesley College (BA); Roosevelt Hosp. School of Nursing, N.Y.C; State Univ. New York (RN); studied Hunan dialect of Chinese, Ya-Li, Changsha, Hunan; Teachers College, Columbia Univ. **Work history:** Faculty, Superintendent, Dean, Hunan-Yale School of Nursing; Faculty, Vassar Training Camp for Nurses; Director, Nursing Service, Willard Park, N.Y.; Exec. Secretary, National League for Nursing Education (NLNE); Director, School of Nursing, Hampton Institute; Faculty, Jersey City (N.J.) Medical Center School of Nursing; Director, Nursing School of Newport (R.I.) Hosp.; Director, Nursing School of Protestant Hosp., Nashville, Tenn. **Organizations:** NAC, ICN, NLNE, American Nurses Assoc., National Organization for Public Health Nursing, American Assoc. of Univ. Women. **Awards:** unknown. **Died:** Syracuse, N.Y.

References and Credits

†Gage N: Stages of nursing in China. AJN 20:120, 1919.

Sentz L: Nina Diadamia Gage. In Bullough V, Church OM, Stein AP (eds): American Nursing: A Biographical Dictionary, vol. 1. New York, Garland, 1988, pp 128–130.

Roberts M: American Nursing: History and Interpretation. New York, Macmillan, 1954.

Jamieson E, Sewell M, Suhrie E: Trends in Nursing History. Philadelphia, WB Saunders, 1966.

June 11

Martha Jane Clement
1888–1959

The art of cooking dehydrated foods is in a class by itself. They can be made very palatable if the cooks have knowledge of the background of the food they are preparing. … We prepared fifty-two nurses as dieticians. This will be a great asset, especially in the advance areas where small hospitals have no dieticians assigned, to have a nurse trained to help in the preparation of patients' food." (1944)

Lt. Col. Martha Jane Clement, known as "Ma" Clement to the soldiers she treated, was the director of the Army Nurse Corps in the southwestern Pacific during World War II. She was assigned to various locations, including the Philippines. She later became chief nurse at Langley Field, Virginia, and was responsible for opening the Air Force Hospital. As a captain she was director of the Army Nurse Corps, Southwest Pacific Theater of Operations, in 1942, commanding four thousand nurses and running eighty-seven hospitals. She started a hospital in Australia one week after she arrived, and she and her staff nurses provided care to both American and Australian troops. She was known for her ability to maintain high morale among her nurses under the most trying conditions. Once, torrential rains washed through the tents, sweeping away the nurses' shoes. They tended 250 to 300 patients in mud up to their knees.

Gen. Douglas MacArthur cited her unit for its treatment of casualties from the Battle of Buna. She was buried in Arlington National Cemetery with full military honors.

Biography

Born: June 11, 1888, location unknown. **Education:** Southern Illinois Hosp. School of Nursing, Anna. **Work history:** Private Duty Nurse, Staff Nurse, Pacific Hosp., Missoula, Mont.; appointed to Army Nurse Corps Base Hosp., Camp MacArthur, Waco, Texas, 1918; three tours of duty, General Hosp. No. 31, Carlisle, Pa.; Base Hosp., Ft. Sam Houston, Texas; Army-Navy General Hosp., Hot Springs, Ark.; Walter Reed General Hosp., Washington, D.C.; Sternberg General Hosp., Manila; Manila Station Hosp., Ft. Mills, Philippines; Chief Nurse, Langley Field, Va. **Organizations:** unknown. **Awards:** unknown. **Buried:** Arlington National Cemetery.

References and Credits

†Clement M: Nurse dieticians trained in the Southwest Pacific. AJN 44:601, 1944.

Clement M: I'd take combat duty again. AJN 44:676, 1944.

Carson D: Martha Clement. In Bullough V, Sentz L, Stein AP (eds): American Nursing: A Biographical Dictionary, vol. 2. New York, Garland, 1992, pp 64–65.

June 12

Carolyn Conant Van Blarcom

1879–1960

"The character of the nurse's work will be influenced, in fact almost determined, by her patient's needs, mental and physical, and the earnestness with which she tries to relieve them. More than this, the nurse whose skill is warmed by a sincere desire to give of her best will, by virtue of this very desire, learn something from each patient, and will be steadily enriched and broadened by her experiences. She will have more to give, and accordingly will derive increasing satisfaction from her service to each succeeding mother and baby that she takes into her care." (1923)

Carolyn Van Blarcom was the nation's first licensed nurse-midwife. Her background in obstetrics, research in midwifery, and popular publications made a significant difference in the lives of women and babies in the United States. Her research about preventable blindness in newborns revealed that the simple intervention of silver nitrate solution was not a common practice with midwives. This led to improvements in midwives' education and practice. Although she was weakened by rheumatic fever as a child and then endured the chronic, debilitating effects of early-onset rheumatoid arthritis, she was an outstanding nursing student, instructor, researcher, organizer, and writer. Her involvement with blindness prevention and her commitment to reforming midwifery led the writer Vern Bullough to characterize Van Blarcom as "the person most responsible for bringing opthalmia neonatorum, then the leading cause of blindness, under control in the United States."

Biography

Born: June 12, 1879, Alton, Ill. **Education:** Johns Hopkins Hosp. Training School for Nurses. **Work history:** Instructor, Johns Hopkins; organized training school, St. Louis; Director, Maryland Tuberculosis Sanatorium; Director, Massachusetts Tuberculosis Sanatorium; Secretary, New York Commission for the Prevention of Blindness; researched midwifery, United States and Europe; helped establish Midwifery School, Bellevue Hosp., N.Y.C.; Secretary, Illinois Society for Prevention of Blindness; Nurse, American Red Cross, World War I. **Organizations:** unknown. **Awards:** unknown. **Died:** Arcadia, Calif.

References and Credits

†Van Blarcom CC: Obstetrical Nursing. New York, Macmillan, 1923, p 545.

Bullough V: Carolyn Conant Van Blarcom. In Bullough V, Church OM, Stein AP (eds): American Nursing: A Biographical Dictionary, vol. 1. New York, Garland, 1988, p 327.

Sicherman B, Hurd C (eds): Notable American Women: The Modern Period. Cambridge, Mass., Belknap Press, 1980.

Vernice D. Ferguson

1928–

"As we shift from the centrality of the hospital which remains notable for illness care, we soon recognize that the education of nurses must change to accommodate the increased expectations of nurses as practitioners, educators, researchers, managers and administrators as well as policy shapers. No longer must the professional nurse feel frustrated as the profession's independent function is compromised. The opportunity is now afforded to enhance collaborative and satisfying relationships between and among other health care providers and to form partnerships with those being served assuring their maximum independence and empowerment. As new partnerships are forged with the recipients of nursing services, the helping (behavioral) model so well known to nurses who practice in rehabilitation, mental health and substance abuse programs is replacing the medical model, the dominant model used in hospitals, as more appropriate." (1997)

AN OUTSTANDING ROLE model, Vernice Ferguson personifies professional achievement. Her desire to help people attracted her to the profession. Her family nurtured altruism, and she learned that support and caring toward others is a way of life. Her career was driven by her inherent belief in and her relentless pursuit of excellence, both in scholarship and practice. She taught science in public schools and taught in schools of nursing. She held leadership positions in the Department of Veterans Affairs, with the National Institutes of Health (NIH), and held the Chair in Cultural Diversity as a Senior Fellow at the University of Pennsylvania School of Nursing. Before her retirement from the VA she was its assistant chief medical director for nursing programs. When she was a guest editor for the issue of *Nursing Clinics of North America* (1990) that focused on the current nursing shortage, she wrote of the need to reformulate the role of the nurse, reposition the nurse in society, and restructure the health care environment. Highly honored, she was the second American nurse selected as an Honorary Fellow in the Royal College of Nursing of the United Kingdom.

Biography

Born: June 13, 1928, Fayetteville, N.C. **Education:** New York Univ.–Bellevue Medical Center (BS); Teachers College, Columbia Univ. (MA). **Work history:** public school science teacher; Faculty, nursing schools; DVA; National Institutes of Health; Chief Nurse, VA Medical Center, Madison, Wisc., Chicago; Author; Editor. **Organizations:** American Nurses Assoc. (ANA); International Society of Nurses in Cancer Care. **Awards:** eight honorary doctorates; two fellowships; Mary Mahoney Award, ANA; Jean McVicar Outstanding Nurse Exec. Award, National League for Nursing; Distinguished Service Awards, VA, U.S. Dept. of Health and Human Services; Lifetime Achievement in Nursing Award, Indiana Univ. School of Nursing; Living Legend, American Academy of Nursing, 1998; Fellow, Royal College of Nursing, U.K.

References and Credits

†Ferguson V (ed): Educating the 21st Century Nurse: Challenges and Opportunities. New York, National League for Nursing Press, 1997, p xxvi.

Ferguson V: personal communication, 2002.

Ferguson V (guest ed): The nursing shortage: Dynamics and solutions. Nurs Clin North Am 25:504, 1990.

June 14

Alice Fisher

1839–1888

"My dear, erase the word discouragement from your dictionary and your mind; it isn't worthy of a woman who hopes to be a nurse; never let me hear you say it again." (1904)

ALICE FISHER, WHO was born and educated in England, published two novels before graduating from the Nightingale Training School. She worked in England, where she improved hygiene conditions and nurses' training to combat typhus. Her own health problems, inflammatory rheumatism and related heart damage, did not slow her commitment to elevating the standards for nursing. Selected to reform the Philadelphia Hospital in Pennsylvania, she overcame hostilities and criticisms to reverse the horrible conditions. She was even the recipient of an explosive sent through the mail. Fortunately, the postal service intervened. The nursing program that she established attracted educated and capable women. Her determination to improve hospital conditions, combined with her superb organizational skills and personable demeanor, enabled her to improve hospital conditions, and nursing and education. These efforts resulted in a dramatic drop in the patient mortality rate.

BIOGRAPHY

Born: June 14, 1839, Queen's House, Greenwich, England. **Education:** Nightingale Training School, St. Thomas's Hosp., London, 1876. **Work history:** Assistant Superintendent, Royal Infirmary, Edinburgh; Superintendent, The Fever Hosp., Newcastle on Tyne;

Superintendent, founder of training school for nurses, Addenbroke's Hosp., Cambridge, England, May 1877; Matron, Radcliffe Infirmary, Oxford, England, April 1882; Superintendent, founder of three-year nurse training program, General Hosp., Birmingham, England, 1882; reformed Philadelphia (Blockley) Hosp., established nurse training school, November 1884. **Writings:** two novels: *Too Bright to Last* (1873), *Queen* (1875); coauthor with Rachel Williams of *Hints for Hospital Nurses* (1877). **Organizations:** unknown. **Awards:** unknown. **Died:** Philadelphia.

References and Credits

†Smith ME: The pioneer work of Alice Fisher in Philadelphia: Address to the Nurses Associated Alumnae of the United States, May 14, 1904. AJN 4:806, 1904.

Murphy S: Alice Fisher. In Bullough V, Sentz L, Stein AP (eds): American Nursing: A Biographical Dictionary, vol. 2. New York, Garland, 1992, pp 113–116.

Katherine De Witt

1867–1963

"January 19—Sunday— . . . Jennie, who for three weeks has worried me to pieces by her fussing and nervousness, repaid me for it all to-day by telling me she had never heard me say, 'I haven't time to do it.' I want to remember that; it may help me with some other patient.

January 20—Monday—A red-letter day, because I got my three patients, who have been in bed so long, up—Mrs. Appe, Jennie and Mrs. Bates. Nothing delights me as much, though I nearly broke my back in assisting them, they are so weak. . . .

February 1—Saturday—I am changed, as I expected, and to Ward E, in the public hospital. . . . I have twelve women to take care of; nearly all are in bed and pretty sick. One woman's head was covered with vermin. I cut her hair and worked over her for two hours, but even then she had to be put in a clean bed in the afternoon. It made me feel sick all day. I worked very hard. . . .

February 15—Saturday—We didn't half get through our work. We had four new cases, one on a stretcher and two in wheeled chairs. Seven of the patients have to sleep on the floor. We have over sixty." (ca. 1906)

KATHERINE DE WITT entered nursing after she first prepared and worked as a teacher. She kept a diary while she was in nursing school, and it described hospital working conditions and the demands on students. It became the basis for one of her many articles in the *American Journal of Nursing.* She did private duty nursing for mothers and babies and set the standard for care with *Private Duty Nursing,* one of her books. In that 1917 work she wrote of the value of the older nurse, saying, "There are women who have been nursing for twenty-five years or thirty who are still young in heart, active, interested, and in constant demand. Life has not palled on them, nor has their work grown stale. It is so full of interest, there is so much to learn that they begrudge the flying years, there isn't enough time for half they want to do." She was an editor at the *American Journal of Nursing* for many years, and upon her retirement several thousand nurses nationwide subscribed to the journal in recognition of her achievements.

BIOGRAPHY

Born: June 11, 1867, Troy, N.Y. **Education:** Mt. Holyoke Seminary; Illinois Training School, Chicago. **Work history:** Private Duty Nurse, Ohio, N.C., Mass.; Assistant Editor, Managing Editor, *American Journal of Nursing.* **Organizations:** Secretary, American Nurses Assoc. (ANA); President, Alumni Assoc., Illinois Training School; N.Y. State Nurses Assoc.; Secretary, Isabel Hampton Robb Scholarship Fund, Isabel McIsaac Loan Fund. **Awards:** first recipient, Honorary Recognition Award, ANA. **Buried:** Mt. Ida Cemetery, Troy, N.Y.

REFERENCES AND CREDITS

†DeWitt K: Hospital sketches. AJN 6:455, 456, 611, 1906.

Birnbach N: Katherine De Witt. In Bullough V, Church OM, Stein AP (eds): American Nursing: A Biographical Dictionary, vol. 1. New York, Garland, 1988, pp 86–88.

DeWitt K: Private duty nursing. In Reverby S (ed): The History of American Nursing. New York, Garland, 1984, p 252.

June 16

Helena Willis Render

1896–1970

"The successful psychiatric nurse understands the feelings of her patient and then through her own conscious feelings of serenity and friendliness endeavors to impart strength and confidence to him. Nor is this lost in general nursing. Everyone knows how the recently admitted patient or one expecting an operation depends on his nurse to see him through this strange and frightening experience. ...In working toward emotional composure for the patient, the nurse's initial objective is to have him feel that he is among people who are interested in him. *This is a very personal and individual approach and to pursue it we suggest three measures: friendliness, attention to trifles, and doing to the patient as you would have him do to you providing you were in his place." (1937)*

HELENA RENDER WAS a psychiatric nurse, researcher, educator, and author. She was instrumental in broadening the image of nursing, taking the profession from a focus on domestic hospital duties toward one focused on interpersonal relationships with patients. Her nursing classic, *Nurse-Patient Relationships in Psychiatry* (1947), stressed the importance of observation and recognizing the patient as a person. She wanted nurses to understand the importance of establishing a relationship with a patient and the contributions of a therapeutic relationship to improving health. In "The Understanding Heart" she writes that successful psychiatric nurses are sensitive to the patient's feelings and help convey strength and confidence by their own behavior. She broadens these qualities to general nursing and asks nurses to be a "trifle conscious." This means to take advantage of opportunities to perform small, genuine, personal acts of kindness, thoughtfulness, and caring. When the nurse focuses on the patient and tries to see things from the patient's point of view, nursing care improves. Render encouraged the study of art and literature to help nurses develop sensitivity skills in dealing with patients.

Biography

Born: June 16, 1896, St. John's, New Brunswick, Can. **Education:** Central Maine General Hosp., Lewiston; Frances Payne Bolton School of Nursing, Western Reserve Univ., Cleveland, Ohio. **Work history:** First Supervisor, Instructor, neuropsychiatric division, Cleveland City Hosp.; Chief Nurse, Iowa State Psychiatric Hosp. **Organizations:** unknown. **Awards:** unknown. **Died:** Beatrice, Neb.

References and Credits

†Render H: The understanding heart. AJN 37:1356, 1937.

Manfreda ML: Helena Render. In Bullough V, Church OM, Stein AP (eds): American Nursing: A Biographical Dictionary, vol. 1. New York, Garland, 1988, pp 269–270.

JUNE 17

Hannah Anderson Chandler Ropes

1809–1863

"The day drags heavily. I was up in the night to go my rounds; the half lit halls, the cold floors, and all over the sense of universal depression in the house made me feel as though I was all alone. I mounted to the third floor to look after some sick patients. One who I left, feeling as though he might not live through the night, I turned my steps to. ...I took a chair by him. ...This lad is the only son of his mother and she is a widow; he is unable to speak, and has been so from the time he came into the house. ...When the day dawns one of my men has gone, and before the hour of supper time comes we close the eyes of two more, one the only son of his mother!" (1862)

HANNAH ROPES BECAME a volunteer nurse during the Civil War after reading Florence Nightingale's *Notes on Nursing.* She wanted to emulate Nightingale as well as be available if her own son needed nursing care during the war. When she was appointed matron of Union Hospital in Washington, D.C., she immediately used her political resources to improve the hospital's sanitation and ventilation. Her writings demonstrated that she viewed compassion and caring as essential to patient care. She taught by example while bathing patients, brushing their hair, arranging bedding, feeding water and soup, and talking to them about their families. Louisa May Alcott, one of Rope's nurses, described her as motherly, comforting, and welcoming, making the hospital a home. An articulate social activist, Rope's writings and ideals contributed to the emerging profession.

Biography

Born: June 13, 1809, New Gloucester, Maine. **Education:** unknown. **Work history:** Civil War nurse, Author. **Organizations:** unknown. **Awards:** unknown. **Buried:** New Gloucester, Maine.

References and Credits

†Brumgardt JR (ed): Civil War Nurse: The Diary and Letters of Hannah Ropes. University of Tennessee Press, Knoxville, 1980, pp 89–90.

Stein AP: Hannah Anderson (Chandler) Ropes. In Bullough V, Sentz L, Stein AP (eds): American Nursing: A Biographical Dictionary, vol. 2. New York, Garland, 1992, pp 280–281.

Hanson K: I think you should get a job as a nurse. Nurs Hist Rev 5:71–82, 1997.

JUNE 18

Sally Lucas Jean
1878–1971

"The causes of malnutrition were known and the remedies were known. It only remained to get... the remedies to the children. ...It was realized that... the first step was to develop a method that would interest the child himself. ...We must give all children a vitalized interest in this matter of health; we must help them to form health habits so that every child in the world may grow strong and vigorous with vitality. ...We must work through the teacher if we are to build a whole world of healthy, happy, gloriously radiant children." (1924)

SALLY LUCAS JEAN is credited with popularizing the term *health education.* After service in the Spanish-American War, she worked as a school nurse in Maryland. During her career she was a leader with the World Federation of Educational Associations, the American Child Health Association, a health consultant to state and federal organizations, a prolific writer, and a renowned speaker. In 1924 she wrote that 52 percent of classroom teachers were insufficiently prepared to teach. Yet she strengthened their skills as she taught them how to integrate health teaching into the existing curricula. Her creative approaches were simple, effective, and aimed at having students take new information home. One game had students compare their monthly height and weight against the ideal and then look at how they could improve their growth by drinking milk. Other games addressed food selections, hand washing, and outdoor activity. Jean also helped develop health education programs for children in Belgium, the Panama Canal Zone, the Philippines, Japan, China, and the Virgin Islands. The Child Health Organization merged with another group to become the American Child Health Association as a result of her work on the Committee on Wartime Problems of Children. This group recognized childhood malnutrition as a serious problem. Jean valued partnerships between public health and business. She stressed the importance of school health care, and her efforts led to the formation of the school health bureau by the Metropolitan Life Insurance Company. She continued as an adviser to the bureau for forty years.

Biography

Born: June 18, 1878, Towson, Md. **Education:** Maryland State Normal School; Maryland Homopathic Hosp. Training School for Nurses (RN). **Work history:** Nurse, Spanish-American War; Private Duty Nurse, School Nurse, Baltimore; People's Institute, N.Y.C; Committee on Wartime Problems of Children; Director, Child Health Organization, then Director, American Child Health Assoc. Health Education Specialist, U.S. Bureau of Education; organized Lake Mohawk Conference, 1922; Director, health education division, American Child Health Assoc.; international consultant, health education; advisory committee member, Metropolitan Life Insurance Co. **Organizations:** American Public Health Assoc.; others unknown. **Awards:** medal from France, award from Belgium Red Cross, State Service Award from N.Y. State Assoc. for Health, Physical Education and Recreation; William Howe Award, National School Health Assoc.; honorary master's degree, Bates College.
Died: New York City.

References and Credits

†Jean SL: Health of Our School Children. Washington, D.C., U.S. Government Printing Office, 1924, pp 1, 6, 7.

Jean SL: The advance of health education. 1930. Sally L. Jean Papers, #4290, Manuscripts Department, Southern Historical Collection, Wilson Library, University of North Carolina, Chapel Hill.

Jean, SL: Health education. Western Hospital and Nurses Review, March 1926, Jean Papers.

Bullough V: Sally Lucas Jean. In Bullough V, Church OM, Stein AP (eds): American Nursing: A Biographical Dictionary, vol. 1. New York, Garland, 1988, pp 188–190.

JUNE 19

Constance Holleran

1934–

"I think interest, awareness and being informed are the key factors to developing political savvy. I grew up in a family where we had at least two and often three daily papers, and all conversation stopped for the evening news, which we then discussed. ...All I can say for developing political skills is be alert, listen carefully, be interested, learn as much as you can about both the political process and the issues, and work hard. The process and the rules are very important because you can miss just one little step and lose the whole ballgame. ...I worked extremely hard to keep nursing united on legislative issues. It took a lot of effort to communicate, educate, and coordinate all along the way, but it did pay off. As hard as it was and as understaffed as we were, we never really lost a legislative issue in ten years. We won every vote override and every budget amendment that reached the floor." (1988)

CONSTANCE HOLLERAN WAS attracted to nursing by the example of cadet nurses during World War II and the public health nurse who served her grade school. A straight talker with a good sense of humor, she says that she also learned, as a hospitalized child, what kind of nurse she did not want to be. She evolved from a shy and reluctant public speaker into an effective and politically astute advocate for nursing and public policy. Every opportunity helped her to grow. She acknowledges that she failed anatomy and physiology as a young nursing student and found that the experience helped her develop courage when she re-enrolled. Despite her early academic problems, she graduated near the top of her class. She was a consultant with the U.S. Public Health Service (USPHS), executive director of the International Council of Nurses (ICN), and helped develop the Nurses Coalition for Action in Politics (N-CAP) with the American Nurses Association (ANA) in 1974. That same year she did the legal background work that underpinned the National League for Nursing's lawsuit that forced the Nixon administration to release impounded funds in an era of budget cuts. As a result, nursing schools received almost $28 million. She thrived on the political process and was well respected on Capitol Hill as a lobbyist and excellent strategist for nursing. During her years with the ICN she initiated and obtained funding for nursing projects and carried out the planning and completion of ICN's first permanent headquarters in Geneva.

Biography

Born: June 19, 1934, Manchester, N.H. **Education:** Massachusetts General Hosp. (RN); Columbia Univ. (BS); Catholic Univ. of America (MSN). **Work history:** Consultant, USPHS; Deputy Exec. Director, ANA; Exec. Director, ICN. **Organizations:** ANA. **Awards:** University Medal, Univ. of San Francisco; Fellow, American Academy of Nursing; honorary doctorate, Villanova Univ.; alumni awards, Catholic Univ., Teachers College, Massachusetts General Hosp. School of Nursing; Living Legend, American Academy of Nursing, 1999.

References and Credits

†Schorr T, Zimmerman A: Making Choices, Taking Chances: Nurse Leaders Tell Their Stories. St. Louis, CV Mosby, 1988, p 120.

Holleran C: personal communication, December 2002.

Who's Who in American Nursing, 1996–97, 6th ed. New Providence, N.J., Reed Reference, 1995, p 289.

Irene L. Beland

1906–2000

"To justify a position among the professions, nursing must not only have some function which it can perform better than other professions, but it must be able to exercise independent judgment in the performance of these functions. Basic to sound judgment is knowledge. In fact, no group can lay claim to being truly professional until it has identified a body of knowledge which is fundamental to its practice." (1960)

After a brief stint teaching elementary school, Irene Beland finally overcame her father's opposition to nursing. During her career she had a nationally recognized positive influence on clinical nursing as a nurse educator, scholar, and scientist. She is noted for her vision, teaching, and writings. These contributions helped to organize nursing knowledge in a way that resulted in comprehensive patient care. She writes that nursing's central function is to minister to and act on behalf of an individual. Nursing's role, then, includes promoting health as well as caring for the sick. She teaches nurses to determine the patient's needs and then help meet those needs by applying a problem-solving technique. The nurse gathers information through interview, assessment, and observation. She then uses her findings to list a patient's problems and uses it to develop a plan for care. The list also provides a baseline of information for evaluating and changing the plan as necessary. Beland influenced nursing school curricula by helping the profession to see that the ability to use nursing knowledge is its foundation. She stressed that the conceptually prepared nurse is the most appropriate person to determine what care is necessary while taking the needs of the whole person into consideration.

Biography

Born: June 21, 1906, Loda, Ill. **Education:** St. Mary's Hosp. School of Nursing, Rochester, Minn.; Univ. of Minnesota (BS, MS). **Work history:** Instructor, Eitel Hosp. School of Nursing, Minnesota; Faculty, Univ. of Minnesota; Clinical Instructor, Supervisor, St. Mary's Hosp. School of Nursing; Faculty, Minneapolis Gen. Hosp., College of Nursing, Wayne St. Univ., Detroit; Author; Consultant. **Organizations:** Metropolitan Detroit Cancer Control; Detroit Nurses Assoc. **Awards:** Honorary Fellow, American Academy of Nursing. **Died:** location unknown.

References and Credits

†Beland I: Application of patient-centered curriculum in a bachelor of science program. In Abdellah F, Beland I, Martin A, Matheney R. Patient-Centered Approaches to Nursing. New York, Macmillan, 1960, p 165.

Smokvina GJ: Irene Beland. In Bullough V, Sentz L (eds): American Nursing: A Biographical Dictionary, vol. 3. New York, Springer, 2000, pp 20–22.

Beland I, Passos J: Clinical Nursing, 4th ed. New York, Macmillan, 1981.

June 21

Patricia Kathleen Scheerle

1959–

"Develop your observation and assessment skills, be an expert communicator and know your lab tests and how the results affect your patients and their care." (2001)

"Learn everything you can about the disease you're taking care of and have a knowledge of physiology that would rival that of any physician. It is your responsibility to protect your patient. If you can feel every day that your patient is lucky to have you as a nurse, then your career will be as rewarding as it could ever be. ...I've always looked for nurses who, first and foremost, love being nurses. ...The rewards as a CEO come when you find a nurse with fire in her eyes, bring her along and help her develop her potential to be the best nurse she can be." (1992)

PATRICIA K. (P.K.) SCHEERLE is a highly regarded nurse entrepreneur. She combined her own clinical experiences and observations with her enthusiasm and respect for nursing when, in 1982, she established American Nursing Services, Inc. (ANS). Her successful, nurse-owned and -operated company provides clinical staffing and home health care services, as well as nursing staff for intensive care units and clinical departments throughout much of the South. She was first attracted to nursing by the take-charge approach of the very competent nurse and the challenges and rewards of giving care. She was also sensitive to the frustration of some nurses in the clinical setting who wanted but could not gain more control over their own practice. Many of these nurses were thinking of leaving the profession. Her company provides such nurses with the opportunity to control their own schedules, assignments, and careers. In 1986 she founded The Great 100 Nurses, a Louisiana function that honors and recognizes nursing and raises thousands of dollars for nursing scholarships. Extensively involved with nursing and community organizations as a member and speaker, she has been the recipient of numerous awards and recognitions.

Biography

Born: June 21, 1959, New Orleans. **Education:** Castleton State College, Vt. (AD); exec. program, Harvard Business School. **Work history:** Pediatric Intensive Care Nurse; Administration; Founder, President, Chief Executive Officer, ANS. **Organizations:** National League for Nursing, American Nurses Assoc., Women's Health Care Exec. Network, American Organization of Nurse Execs., International Women's Forum, Sigma Theta Tau. **Awards:** Junior Achievement's Business Hall of Fame; honored by Young Women's Christian Assoc., Women Business Owners, Young Leadership Council; New Orleans Business Magazine Woman of the Year; American Business Ethics Award, New Orleans; Virginia Henderson Fellow, Sigma Theta Tau.

References and Credits

†Scheerle PK: personal communication, 2001.

†Saslow L: Making history—The R.N./CEO Revolution, Spring 1992, pp 90, 89.

New Orleans co. expands nursing frontiers. National Nurses in Business Assoc. Newsletter 4:1–8, 1988.

P.K. Scheerle, R.N.: The nurse executive behind American Nursing Services, Inc. Southwest Medical Opportunities, Feb.–March 1990, p 10.

Press packet, American Nursing Services.

Ruth Weaver Hubbard

1897–1955

"To each age comes its own peculiar problems and challenge, but to it also comes the necessary vision and strength." (1950)

RUTH W. HUBBARD was a natural leader and great communicator. She believed that general nurses could be instructed in specialized services and could promote family-oriented care in public health nursing. She was a strong advocate for nurses "to develop the understanding of the patient as an individual whose own characteristics determine needed care." Her long career used her skills as a writer, educator, resourceful fund raiser, innovator, and dedicated public health nurse. During the Great Depression she set an example at the Visiting Nurse Service (VNS) of Philadelphia by taking a greater cut in salary than any other nurse. One of Hubbard's outstanding innovations at the VNS was the intensive Home-Care Plan, which improved coordination of long-term home services to promote maximum patient recovery. She was credited with restructuring national nursing organizations during a time of crisis to develop nursing-service standards, advance various branches of nursing, and guarantee adequate salaries. She received many awards for her lifelong dedication to improving the general health of her community and the objectives and philosophy of the care providers.

Biography

Born: 1897, Brooklyn, N.Y. **Education:** Army School of Nursing, Walter Reed Hosp., Washington, D.C., 1921 (diploma); Teachers College, Columbia Univ., 1925 (BS); graduate work, Yale Univ., 1927–29, Univ. of Pennsylvania, 1935–41; used Rockefeller Foundation Fellowship to tour Eastern Europe, United Kingdom, Scandinavia to study public health nursing, general nursing, 1931. **Work history:** Staff Nurse, Brooklyn Visiting Nurse Assoc., 1922; Head Nurse, pediatric clinic, New Haven, Conn.; dispensary, 1925–27; Education Director, VNA, New Haven, Conn.; General Director, VNS, Philadelphia, 1929–55; Educator, Public Health Nursing, Yale School of Nursing; lectured on organization, administration of public health nursing, Univ. of Pennsylvania School of Nursing; Visiting Lecturer, Univ. of California, Berkeley, summer school; Univ. of Minnesota. **Organizations:** member (1930–46), Chair (1940–42), Education Committee, National Organization for Public Health Nursing (NOPHN); member, Exec. Committee, NOPHN until merger with NLN; member, Nursing Advisory Committee, Metropolitan Life Insurance Co. Nursing Service; member, Committee on Structure of National Nursing Organizations; served on Commission on Chronic Illness; member, editorial board, *American Journal of Public Health*. **Awards:** Bronze Medal for Distinguished Service to Nursing, Pa. Nurses Assoc.; Philadelphia Friendship Fete Award for outstanding service to humanity; Distinguished Daughter Award, Commonwealth of Pennsylvania; Ruth W. Hubbard Foundation established by friends and community leaders to provide scholarships. **Died:** Rush, N.Y.

References and Credits

†Hubbard RW: Public health nursing: 1900–1950. AJN 50: 608, 1950.

Dieckmann JL, Craft SN: Ruth Hubbard. In Bullough V, Sentz L, Stein AP (eds): American Nursing: A Biographical Dictionary, vol. 2. New York, Garland, 1992, pp 160–163.

Pearl McIver

1893–1976

"What are some of the principles which will influence the nursing developments of the future? ...Nursing personnel must be utilized for those functions which require nursing skill and judgment. ...The educational program must be one that will not only attract, but... retain desirable candidates. ...The learning experience must have priority over the nursing service needs of the hospital or health agency." (1952)

After one year of high school Pearl McIver completed studies at a normal school in North Dakota to prepare for teaching. She taught grade school before studying nursing at the University of Minnesota and found her niche in public health. She held the first public health nurse position in the U.S. Public Health Service (USPHS). She later helped establish and head its office of public health nursing. The Pearl McIver Award from the American Nurses Association (ANA) honors her pioneering achievements in the service, and she was the first to receive it in 1957. The survey data that she gathered during World War II about the availability of nurses proved valuable to both military and civilian leaders. She was very involved with the postwar restructuring of the major professional nursing organizations. McIver believed that nursing must be open to change. She recognized the importance of nursing research and wrote of the value of collective bargaining. She stressed that all professional nurses share the responsibilities for improving the profession and the availability of health care.

Biography

Born: June 23, 1893, Lowry, Minn. **Education:** Mayville State Normal School, N.D.; Univ. of Minnesota School of Nursing; Teachers College, Columbia Univ. (bachelor's, master's, public health nursing). **Work history:** Campus Visiting Nurse, Univ. of Minnesota; USPHS; Exec. Director, *American Journal of Nursing.* **Organizations:** ANA. **Awards:** Pearl McIver Public Health Nurse Award; Outstanding Achievement Award, Univ. of Minnesota; Lasker Award, American Public Health Assoc.; Florence Nightingale Medal, International Committee, Red Cross; Honorary Fellow, Royal Society of Health, England.
Died: Lowry, Minn.

References and Credits

†McIver P: Nursing moves forward. AJN 52:822, 823, 1952.

Harris IM: Pearl McIver. In Bullough V, Church OM, Stein AP (eds): American Nursing: A Biographical Dictionary, vol. 1. New York, Garland, 1988, pp 223–224.

June 24

Philip Edson Day
1916–1989

"A current review of nursing service disclosed the existence of many problems. One can hardly fail to be impressed with the degree of cooperation, plus the marked degree of sincerity, that characterize the approaches to nursing problems by those in nursing and related disciplines. A continued joint effort augurs well for the eventual solution of nursing's major difficulties as we mutually approach our desired goal of the best possible patient care." (1962)

PHILIP DAY WAS the first man elected president of a state nursing association. He was president of the Vermont Nurses Association from 1960 to 1962. He was director of nursing service at the Mary Fletcher Hospital in Burlington, Vermont. He served on the editorial board and wrote articles for the magazines *RN* and *Hospitals.* From 1964 until his retirement in 1971 he was president and publisher of the *American Journal of Nursing* (AJN). Day entered nursing after completing his service with the U.S. Army during World War II, when he was already married and the father of four. When he was appointed publisher of the AJN, three of the six members of his family were nurses: he, his wife, and one daughter.

Biography

Born: June 23, 1916, Ripton, Vt. **Education:** Pennsylvania Hosp. School for Men; Univ. of Pennsylvania School of Nursing, 1955 (BS); Teachers College, Columbia Univ., 1964 (MS in nursing service). **Work history:** Instructor, Pennsylvania Hosp. School for Men, 1950–55; Univ. of Pennsylvania School of Nursing; Director of Nursing Service, Mary Fletcher Hosp., Burlington, Vt., 1956–64; President, Publisher, *American Journal of Nursing,* 1964–71. **Organizations:** Treasurer, bd. member, first man elected president, Vt. Nurses Assoc., 1960–62. **Awards:** unknown. **Died:** Arnold, Calif.

References and Credits

†Day PE: Nursing service: Annual administrative reviews. Hospitals JAHA 36:124, 1962.

Bullough V: Philip Edson Day. In Bullough V, Sentz L, Stein AP (eds): American Nursing: A Biographical Dictionary, vol. 2. New York, Garland, 1992, pp 82–83.

JUNE 25

Anna Dryden Wolf

1890–1985

"Today's nurse needs, in addition to a kind heart and manual dexterity, knowledge which will permit her to carry out highly technical skills in many complicated services, and understanding of the promotion and conservation of health in its physical, mental and social aspects. ... The tendency to increase the number of nonprofessional workers must be watched very carefully. There is a danger point at which there are not enough professional persons to assure safe and appropriate services to patients and supervision to the nonprofessional staff." (1956)

ANNA WOLF WAS a catalyst for the evolution of nursing. She brought a more democratic approach to the profession in both the nursing school and staff nurse settings. Born in India of missionary parents, she completed a bachelor's degree before enrolling in and graduating from the Johns Hopkins Hospital School of Nursing and then studied with Adelaide Nutting and Annie Goodrich at Columbia University. A nurse educator and administrator, Wolf prepared U.S. nurses for service in both world wars. She taught at the Vassar Training Camp, where women with a college education prepared as professional nurses through a specialized program. Wolf held administrative positions at Johns Hopkins Hospital and was well known for her expert problem-solving skills. For example, during the nursing shortage of the war years, her strategies for managing patient care helped to defuse the excessive stress levels that nurses were experiencing. She recognized the correlation between nursing education and clinical practice and worked to improve both. After World War I she successfully applied her democratic approach in working with staff and students in the nursing program in Beijing. Her appointment as dean of the program elevated the status of the profession there.

Biography

Born: June 25, 1890, Gunthur Madras Presidency, South India. **Education:** Goucher College (BA); Johns Hopkins Hosp. School of Nursing; Teachers College, Columbia Univ. **Work history:** Faculty, Johns Hopkins Hosp. School of Nursing; Faculty, Vassar Training Camp for Nurses; Faculty, Union Medical College, Beijing; Faculty, Univ. of Chicago; Director of Nurses, New York Hospital; Director of Nurses, Johns Hopkins Hosp. School of Nursing. **Organizations:** American Red Cross; National Nursing Council for Defense and War. **Awards:** several scholarships for study; honorary doctorate from Goucher College; yearly award at Hopkins given in her honor. **Died:** St. Petersburg, Fla.

References and Credits

†Wolf A: Evolution in nursing service. Nurs Outlook 4:47, 49, 1956.

Sabrin L: Anna Wolf. In Bullough V, Church OM, Stein AP (eds): American Nursing: A Biographical Dictionary, vol. 1. New York, Garland, 1988, pp 338–339.

June 26

Frederick W. Jones

CA. 1890–1948

"We have always maintained that where the man nurse is best known there he receives the greatest recognition and the widest opportunities for constructive service. Nowhere in the nursing world does the man nurse receive the recognition nor have the opportunities that are afforded him in the United States Naval Service." (1934)

Frederick Jones was responsible for reorganizing and developing the curricula at the two outstanding U.S. nursing schools exclusively for men, the Mills School and St. Vincent. Jones was appointed director of the Mills School in New York City in 1920. Jones restructured the nursing program so men could qualify to take the New York state board examination to become registered nurses. He developed quality instruction based on innovative curricula. He was a vigorous leader as the school's superintendent of nurses, until he left in 1929 for St. Vincent's School for Nursing, also in New York City. St. Vincent's offered a three-year course that included basic science, material medica, urological nursing, psychology, massage, nutrition, professional ethics, and many additional courses related to nursing practice. Nurses who were students at the two nursing schools for men during his tenure describe him as an excellent teacher, fair, and understanding. His leadership of these institutions promoted improvements in the curricula that advanced the quality of education for men in professional nursing.

Biography

Born: ca. 1890, location unknown. **Education:** Mills School, Bellevue and Allied Hosps. Training School for Nurses, 1911. **Work history:** Assistant, Mills School; trained orderlies; Charge of Dispensary; Head Nurse, Supervising Nurse, Bellevue Hosp., N.Y.C.; Volunteer, Chanticleer Ambulance Service, World War I; Director, Mills School, Bellevue and Allied Hosps. Training School for Nurses, 1921–29; Director, St. Vincent's, 1930–38; Personnel Manager, St. Vincent's Hosp., 1946. **Organizations:** unknown. **Awards:** decorated by French government for meritorious service in ambulance corps. **Died:** location unknown.

References and Credits

†Jones FW: Vocational opportunities for men nurses. AJN 34:131–133, 1934.

Buchinger KL: Frederick Jones. In Bullough V, Sentz L, Stein AP (eds): American Nursing: A Biographical Dictionary, vol. 2. New York, Garland, 1992, pp 171–173.

June 27

Emma Goldman

1869–1940

"[Birth control is] a pressing, imperative necessity . . . [of] the larger social war; . . . a war for a seat at the table of life on the part of the people, the masses who create and who build the world and who have nothing in return. I look upon Birth Control as only one phase of that vast movement, and if I, through my agitation,—through my education, I should rather say,—can indicate a way towards the betterment of that human race, towards a finer quality, children who should have a joyous and glorious childhood, and women who shall have a healthy motherhood, if that is a crime, your Honor, I am glad and proud to be a criminal." (1916)

EMMA GOLDMAN EMIGRATED to the United States from Lithuania when she was sixteen and became a factory worker in New York City. She was involved in worker protests and socialist causes and became an outspoken anarchist. She learned practical nursing at the Blackwell's Island Prison Hospital in New York, where she was sentenced after inciting a riot by encouraging starving unemployed men to steal food. She later traveled to Vienna, completed nursing and midwife studies, returned to the States, and became an activist for women's rights. A popular prolific writer, and speaker, she helped found the journal *Mother Earth* with Alexander Berkman. She was arrested, imprisoned, and deported for opposing the draft in

World War I. She was controversial, rebellious, and dedicated to social justice; in 1922 the "*Nation* insisted that her name be on any list of the greatest living women," according to the writer Vern Bullough. After Goldman died in Canada, her body was returned to Chicago for burial in Waldheim Cemetery, "near the graves of the Haymarket 'martyrs,' those killed by the police in 1887 during the Haymarket riots," Bullough notes.

Biography

Born: June 27, 1869, Kaunas, Lithuania. **Education:** Blackwell's Island Prison, N.Y.; Allgemeines Krankenhaus, Vienna. **Work history:** Blackwell's Island Penitentiary Hosp.; Midwife, N.Y.C.; Activist, Speaker in United States, England, Canada. **Organizations:** unknown. **Awards:** unknown. **Buried:** Waldheim Cemetery, Chicago.

References and Credits

†Wexler A: Emma Goldman: An Intimate Life. New York, Pantheon, 1984, p 214.

Bullough V: Emma Goldman. In Bullough V, Church OM, Stein AP (eds): American Nursing: A Biographical Dictionary, vol. 1. New York, Garland, 1988, pp 141–143.

June 28

Clara Louise Maass

1876–1901

"I will soon send you $100.00. It will pay immediate debts and enable Sophia to come to Cuba. I can get her a position as a nurse here at $50 a month. She can take my place, Mother, for—now don't be surprised—I am soon to be married. . . . Do not worry, Mother, if you hear that I have yellow fever. Now is a good time of the year to catch it if one has to. Most of the cases are mild, and then I should be immune and not afraid of the disease any more." (1901)

"Goodby, Mother. Don't worry. God will care for me in the yellow fever hospital the same as if I were at home. I will send you nearly all I earn, so be good to yourself and the two little ones. You know I am the man of the family, but do pray for me." (1901)

JUST FOUR DAYS before her twenty-fifth birthday, Clara Maass was dead after exposing herself twice to the sting of the *Stegomyia* mosquito. This insect bite proved that mosquitoes spread yellow fever. Maass not only wanted the extra $100 offered by the army to volunteers for the experiment, she wanted to become immune to the disease so she could be more useful to those who were suffering from it. The *New York Times*'s editorial about her death in August 1901 stated:

> The ethics of the Cuban experiments would seem to depend a good deal upon the motive actuating the victims. In the case of Miss Maass, the young nurse who died on Saturday, it would seem to have been the very highest which could inspire a self-sacrificing woman to put her life in peril. She was not only willing to incur the risk of infection if thereby she might assist in establishing a scientific hypothesis of first importance in the etiology of yellow fever, but she desired to make herself immune, to the end that her usefulness in her chosen vocation might be increased and her opportunities of service to those of suffering from the disease enlarged beyond what would be possible in one liable to contract the disease. No soldier in the late war placed his life in peril for better reasons than those which prompted this faithful nurse to risk hers.

Her remains were returned to the United States, and she was buried in Fairmount Cemetery in Newark, New Jersey. The epitaph on her pink marble tombstone reads, "Greater Love Hath No Man than this ..."

Biography

Born: June 28, 1876, East Orange, N.J. **Education:** Newark (N.J.) German Hosp.; Christina Trefz Training School for Nurses, Newark, N.J., 1895. **Work history:** Private Duty Nurse, Head Nurse, 1898; volunteer contract nurse, U.S. Army, assigned to 7th U.S. Army Corps at Jacksonville, Fla.; Savannah, Ga.; and Santiago, Cuba; honorably discharge, 1899; signed second contract and was sent to Philippines for communicable disease nursing; assigned to Cuba, 1900. **Organizations:** unknown. **Awards:** Newark (N.J.) German Hosp. renamed Clara Maass Memorial Hosp., 1952 (now in Belleville, N.J.); Cuban postage stamp in her honor, 1951; U.S. commemorative stamp, 1976; American Nurses Assoc. Hall of Fame. **Buried:** Fairmount Cemetery, Newark, N.J.

References and Credits

†Cunningham JT: Clara Maass: A Nurse, A Hospital, A Spirit. Cedar Grove, N.J., Rae Publishing, 1968, pp 44, 46, 76.

Fickelssen JL: Clara Mass. In Bullough V, Church OM, Stein AP (eds): American Nursing: A Biographical Dictionary, vol. 1. New York, Garland, 1988, pp 216–217.

ANA Hall of Fame 10/98 American Nurses Association, Washington, D.C. http://www.nursingworld.org/hof.

June 29

Rozella May Schlotfeldt

1914–

"There is little question that nurses themselves must create a new and improved future appropriate for the challenges that lie ahead for their profession. ... There is a relatively small group of nurses who are involved in making important changes in the profession. They are those who are dedicated to inquiry and scholarship; to designing and offering new approaches to preparing nurse practitioners, administrators, educators and investigators; and to planning and evaluating innovative means for delivering high quality nursing care. Some nurses are also involved in working to improve the nation's outmoded, inefficient, and costly health care system. ...It is difficult to know how many additional nurses espouse neither of the commitments set forth above, but rather, can be accurately described as unconcerned and uninvolved; perhaps they are even oblivious to their need to anticipate the changes that will inevitably be forced upon them as a consequence of changes that are occurring in the rapidly changing information and service-oriented society." (1982)

Rozella Schlotfeldt always wanted to be a nurse. Although her mother had almost completed nursing studies before becoming ill with typhoid fever, marriage made her ineligible for further study. Then, widowed young, she did private duty nursing to support her family. Rozella Schlotfeldt credits the positive influence of her mother and her maternal grandmother, and the advantages of her midwestern childhood, for her strong work ethic, ambition, and love of learning. Her nursing practice included staff nursing in maternity care, with the Veterans Administration, and as a member of the Army Nurse Corps in France and Austria. She recalls the first use of antibiotics and the caution associated with early post-operative ambulation. Her wartime experiences helped her to see how nursing can work with the human spirit. Her nursing experiences in teaching and leadership evolved into her work as a nursing scholar, researcher, and writer. Schlotfeldt is recognized as a major influence on the development of professional nursing. She says that her contributions to the future of nursing "have been guided by the firm conviction that nursing is an essential human service that must become a uniformly beneficial, consequential, and respected profession whose practitioners have mastered vast amounts of professional knowledge that they wisely, skillfully, humanely, and ethically apply." She is a highly accomplished, recognized authority and leader in nursing education. She helped establish the School of Nursing at the University of Colorado. While at Case Western Reserve University, she developed the Collaborative Model, which linked nursing students with community agency affiliations in a way that recognized the interdependence between school and agency and upheld a standard of excellence. She was also instrumental in designing the professional doctoral degree for nursing (ND) there. A highly respected and much sought-after consultant on nursing, she was also a visiting professor of nursing at major universities and a prolific writer about critical issues in nursing and nursing research.

Biography

Born: June 29, 1914, DeWitt, Iowa. **Education:** State Univ. of Iowa (BS); Univ. of Chicago (MS, PhD). **Work history:** Staff Nurse, Univ. of Iowa Hosp. and Veterans Administration Hosp., Des Moines; Instructor, Univ. of Iowa; Faculty/administration, Univ. of Colorado School of Nursing, Wayne State College, Case Western Reserve Univ.;

Biography continued on page 768

June 30

Amy Elizabeth Pope

1869–1949

"The more important obligations that a nurse owes her patients are: that she faithfully carry out the doctor's orders, give the patients conscientious care, treat them and their friends with courtesy, and that she keep inviolable any secrets of patients or their family or friends that come to her knowledge. When people are ill or in trouble they are apt to talk of things which in their calmer moments they would not mention, and it is exceedingly dishonorable to repeat anything learned under such conditions. ...If nurses would follow more closely the principles of the pledge... which they... take at graduation, they would be less likely to commit... indiscretions." (1934)

A Red Cross nurse during the Spanish-American War, Amy Elizabeth Pope served in the Philippines, Puerto Rico, and Cuba. Her greatest contributions, however, were in nursing education. She was a nursing instructor and one of nursing's earliest and most influential textbook writers. Her extensive range of publications for student nurses started in 1904 with *Home Care of the Sick.* This was followed by more than twenty books whose topics included anatomy and physiology, physics, chemistry, nursing procedures, dietetics, and pharmacology. She also wrote a medical dictionary. The popular text *Art and Principles of Nursing: Pope's Manual of*

Nursing Procedure pulled together the students' knowledge of anatomy, physiology, chemistry, and principles of physics and hygiene in a text designed to teach by explanation and demonstration. She wrote *Practical Nursing: A Textbook for Nurses* at the request of nursing school superintendents who were setting up new schools of nursing. Written with Anna Maxwell, it had five editions and was later translated into Spanish.

Biography

Born: June 30, 1869, Quebec, Can. **Education:** Presbyterian Hosp. School of Nursing, N.Y.C.; postgraduate courses, St. Bartholomew's Hosp., London; Gardner Gymnasium, N.Y.C; Pratt Institute; Teachers College, Columbia Univ. **Work history:** Nurse, Presbyterian Hosp., N.Y.C.; Red Cross nurse, Spanish-American War; Instructor, Presbyterian Hosp. Training School for Nurses, N.Y.C.; Staff Nurse, Isthmian Canal Commission; organized nurse training school, San Juan, Puerto Rico; Instructor, St. Luke's Hosp. Training School, San Francisco; Private Duty Travel Nurse. **Organizations:** unknown. **Awards:** unknown. **Buried:** Cypress Lawn Cemetery, San Francisco.

References and Credits

†Pope A, Young V: The Art and Principles of Nursing. New York, Putnam, 1934, p 8.

Cooper SS: Amy Pope. In Bullough V, Church OM, Stein AP (eds): American Nursing: A Biographical Dictionary, vol. 1. New York, Garland, 1988, pp 263–265.

Pope A: Pope's Manual of Nursing Procedure. New York, GP Putnam's Sons, 1919.

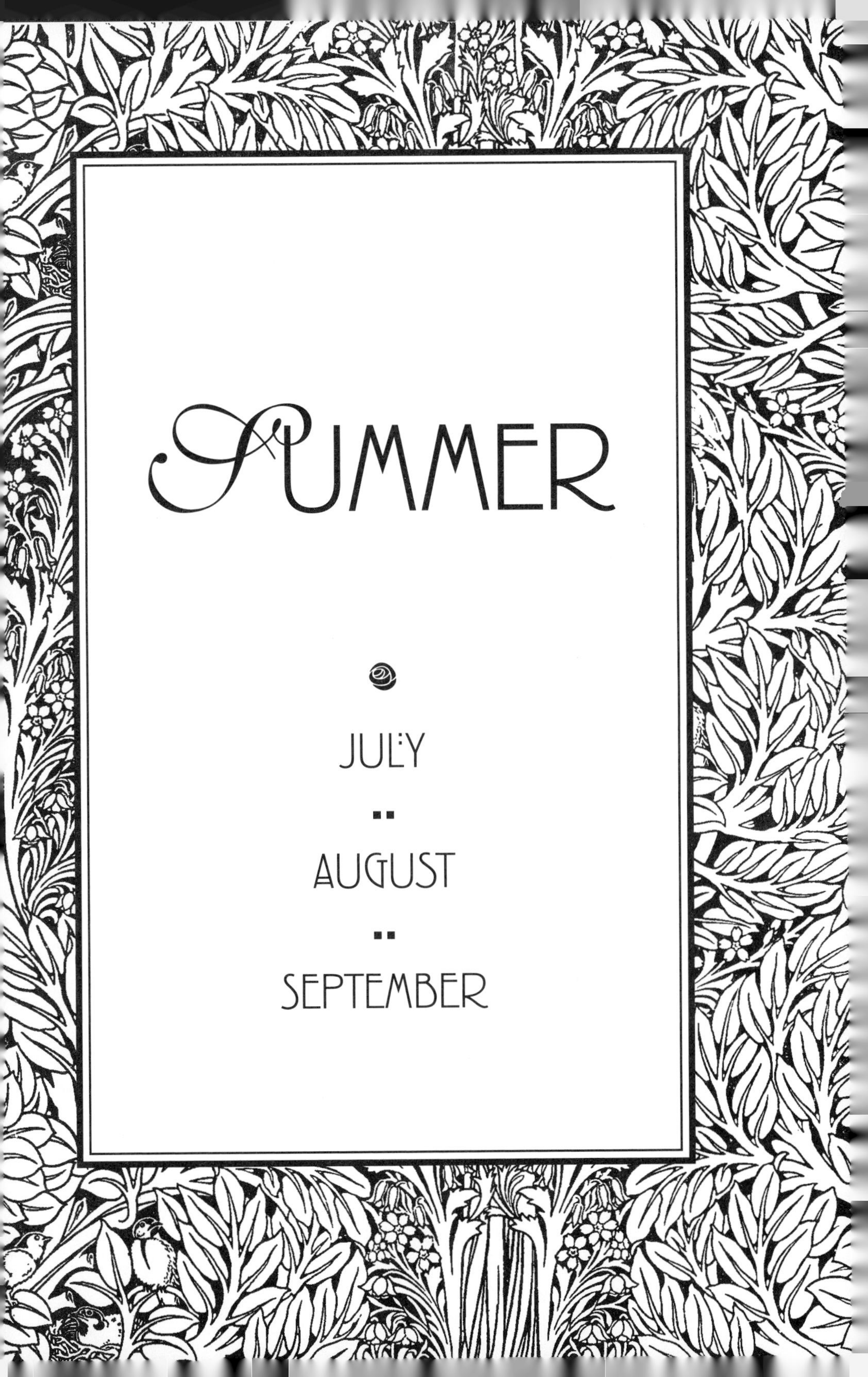
SUMMER
JULY
AUGUST
SEPTEMBER

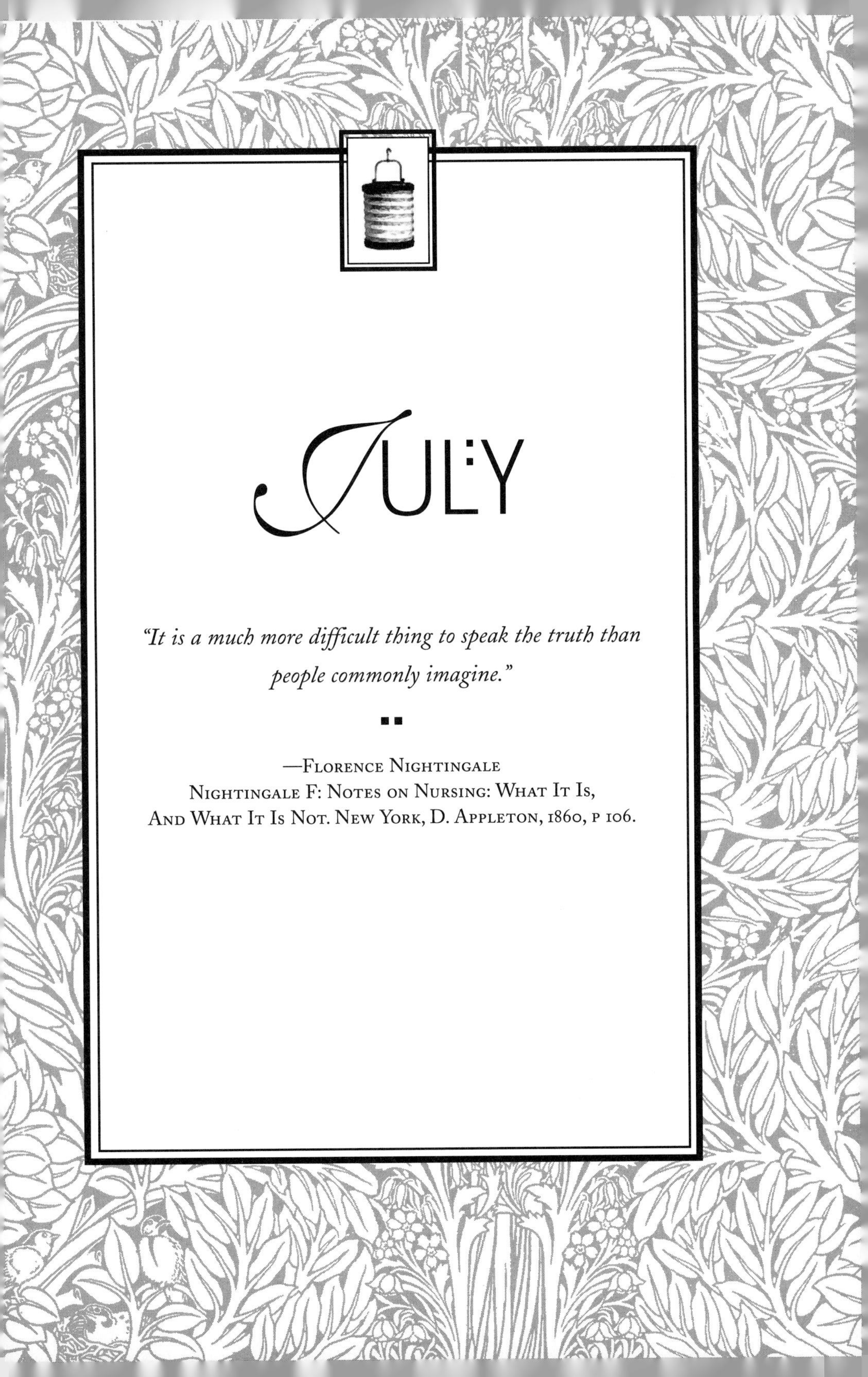

JULY

"It is a much more difficult thing to speak the truth than people commonly imagine."

—Florence Nightingale
Nightingale F: Notes on Nursing: What It Is, And What It Is Not. New York, D. Appleton, 1860, p 106.

July 1

Mildred Emily Newton
1901–1972

"Nurses—trained from the first day in the classroom to respect thoroughness and precision—are well qualified to participate in research. ...Research is the key to a profession's progress and a measure of its stature. For years, nurses stood aside or played a secondary role while others did research concerning their profession. Today, nurses seeking out new truths about themselves and nursing are finding that research offers an exciting, demanding and desperately needed contribution to nursing art and science." (1962)

Mildred Newton was a nurse-educator, researcher, and Nightingale scholar who reminded all nurses that they have a role in nursing research. She explained that nurses were often resources for researchers in other disciplines, and she encouraged nurses to recognize their ability to do research about nursing concerns. She was known for recognizing and encouraging colleagues and others she knew. One of the earliest nurse historians, she had a special interest in studying the life of Florence Nightingale and the lives of early American nurses. Her doctoral dissertation at Stanford University was titled "Florence Nightingale's Philosophy of Life and Education." Newton coauthored textbooks on surgical nursing and nursing practice and published many articles about nursing. She was actively involved with the National League for Nursing (NLN), especially the accreditation of college programs, for almost two decades. One of her university surveys in the early 1950s focused on whether the University of Florida had sufficient facilities to start a nursing program. She was later involved in surveys of existing nursing programs at the university level. Newton received many awards in recognition of her leadership abilities and accomplishments. Her four-volume stamp collection traces the history of nursing and medicine; she donated it to Ohio State University.

Biography

Born: July 1, 1901, Cedar Falls, Iowa. **Education:** Colorado State Teachers College; Univ. of California; Evanston (Ill.) Hosp. School of Nursing; Northwestern Univ. (BS); Univ. of Southern California (MA); Stanford Univ. (EdD). **Work history:** Faculty, Administrator, Pasadena (Calif.) Hosp. and Junior College, Univ. of California, Ohio State Univ.; Consultant to U.S. Army, U.S. Defense Dept., Kellogg Foundation; Chair, grant committee, U.S. Public Health Service; member, editorial bd., *Nursing Research.* **Organizations:** American Nurses Assoc.; American Red Cross Nursing Service; NLN; American Council on Education. **Awards:** Sigma Theta Tau, Alpha Tau Delta, Pi Lambda Theta honor societies; award from Pi Lambda Theta, Ohio Chapter; Adelaide Nutting Award, NLN; numerous awards from Ohio State Univ., which named a building at the nursing school for her. **Died:** San Francisco.

References and Credits

†Newton M: As nursing research comes of age. AJN 62:46, 1962.

Donahue PM: Mildred Newton. In Bullough V, Church OM, Stein AP (eds): American Nursing: A Biographical Dictionary, vol. 1. New York, Garland, 1988, pp 240–242.

July 2

Mary Jane Morrow Ward

1921–

"It is rewarding, in the sense of having shared the results of your work and efforts with colleagues, of having contributed in some small way to the nursing profession, and of having learned much about yourself in the process." (2000)

MARY JANE WARD entered nursing after she was a grandmother. Her husband and only child both died in accidents within four years of each other. "I realized that in order to help myself, I had to get my focus on others," she says. She entered a two-year nursing program and then found nursing research. For twenty years her career as a principal investigator and a research evaluator enabled her to consult for national agencies and university schools of nursing that were beginning research projects. She wrote more than forty books and articles, lectured internationally, and taught research strategies to nursing administrators and faculty. She was the primary author of three reference books. She served as codirector, then director of the Western Interstate Commission for Higher Education (WICHE) project, in Boulder, Colorado, in 1976. A two-volume work is entitled *Instruments for Measuring Nursing Practice and Other Health Care Variables.* She served as professor and associate dean at several university and college schools of nursing. She consulted and presented research data at professional and academic meetings throughout the United States, Canada, and abroad. During her retirement she has audited courses and done volunteer work for a television health fair and Habitat for Humanity. She lives in Boulder and continues to review manuscripts for a book publisher.

Biography

Born: July 2, 1921, Salina, Okla. **Education:** Univ. of Arkansas, Texas State College for Women (premedical studies); Univ. of Virginia (BS in education); Graduate School of Nursing, New York Medical College; predoctoral Nurse Research Fellowship, U.S. Public Health Service (USPHS); Univ. of Colorado, 1975 (PhD). **Work history:** Teacher, Charlottesville, Va.; Clinical Staff Nurse; Charge nurse; Instructor, medical-surgical nursing; Professor, Associate Dean for research, Univ. of Colorado School of Nursing, Univ. of Tennessee, Memphis College of Nursing; Professor, Exec. Associate Dean, Nell Hodgson Woodruff School of Nursing, Emory Univ.; Professor, Associate Dean, Academic Programs, College of Nursing, Univ. of Oklahoma, Oklahoma City, until retirement in 1994. **Organizations:** National Nursing Advisory Council; American Indian Health Services USPHS; Department of Human Services. **Awards:** Elizabeth Buford Phillips Scholarship for academic excellence, leadership potential, Univ. of Virginia; Margaret Mahoney Adams Award for excellence in nursing care of children, N.Y. Medical College.

References and Credits

†Robinson TM: Mary Jane Ward. In Bullough V, Sentz L (eds): American Nursing: A Biographical Dictionary, vol. 3. New York, Springer, 2000, pp 282–284.

July 3

Lystra Eggert Gretter
1858–1951

The Florence Nightingale Pledge
"I solemnly pledge myself before God and in the presence of this assembly, to pass my life in purity and to practice my profession faithfully. I will abstain from whatever is deleterious and mischievous, and will not take or knowingly administer any harmful drug. I will do all in my power to maintain and elevate the standard of my profession, and will hold in confidence all personal matters committed to my keeping and all family affairs coming to my knowledge in the practice of my calling. With loyalty will I endeavor to aid the physician in his work, and devote myself to the welfare of those committed to my care." (1893)

LYSTRA GRETTER WAS a widow with a small child when she first studied nursing. Her progressive ideas and leadership abilities were evident early in her career. She upgraded a hospital nursing school program in Detroit by reducing the workday from twelve to eight hours, arranging for ward supervision, extending the length of the program, and improving the academic and clinical courses. She organized a nursing group when women's clubs were rare and assembled handwritten lecture notes before textbooks were available. A coalition builder, she held a variety of leadership positions in public health nursing. She was the catalyst for the creation of the

Nightingale Pledge, and it is credited to her. It was first used by nursing students on April 25, 1893.

Biography

Born: 1858, Bayfield, Ontario, Can. **Education:** Buffalo (N.Y.) General Hosp. Training School for Nurses. **Work history:** Principal, Farrand Training School for Nurses, Harper Hosp., Detroit; Superintendent, Detroit Visiting Nurse Assoc.; helped establish chair of Public Health Nursing, Univ. of Michigan. **Organizations:** Society of Superintendents of Training Schools for Nurses; Mich. State Nurses Assoc.; Mich. Red Cross; Mich. League for Nursing Education; Detroit Council on Community Nursing; National Organization for Public Health Nursing. **Awards:** honorary master's degree, Wayne Univ., Detroit. **Died:** Grosse Pointe, Mich.

References and Credits

†http://www.nursingworld.org/pressrel/nnw/nnwpled.htm.

Smith VH: Lystra Gretter. In Bullough V, Church OM, Stein AP (eds): American Nursing: A Biographical Dictionary, vol. 1. New York, Garland, 1988, pp 156–158.

JULY 4

Harriet (Araminta) Ross Tubman

1820–1913

"God's time is always near. ...He gave me my strength, and he set the North star in the heavens; he meant I should be free." (ca. 1861)

"I looked at my hands, to see if I was the same person now I was free. There was such a glory over everything, the sun came like gold through the trees, and over the fields, and I felt like I was in heaven....I had crossed the line of which I had been dreaming. I was free; but there was no one to welcome me to the land of freedom." (1869)

HARRIET TUBMAN, CALLED one of the bravest women in the world and compared to Joan of Arc, was known as the Moses of her people. Born a slave in Maryland, Tubman escaped to Philadelphia when she was twenty-nine; she traveled alone and was guided only by the North Star. A woman of great spirituality, she made nineteen return trips to the South and shepherded three hundred slaves, including her parents, to freedom in Canada via the Underground Railroad. A small, resourceful woman with the strength of a man, she carried a rifle for protection and used music to communicate with runaway slaves. Her familiar turban covered the scar from a head injury that she suffered when a slaveowner accidentally hit her with a heavy weight during his dispute with another slave. The injury left her with narcolepsy and pain for the rest of her life. At the request of Gov. John A. Andrew of Massachusetts, she worked for the Union Army as a scout, spy, and camp and hospital nurse, skillfully treating serious illnesses with roots and herbs. She nursed in Virginia, the Carolinas, and Florida during the war. After the war this great humanitarian opened her home in Auburn, New York, to the sick and needy, but she never received the government pension that she earned and deserved. However, she was given a military funeral.

Biography

Born: ca. 1820, Bucktown, Md. **Education:** no formal education. **Work history:** slave; Abolitionist; Union Army liaison and nurse; caretaker for the aged and indigent; Suffragette; speaker on women's rights. **Organizations:** National Federation of Afro-American Women. **Awards:** People of Auburn, N.Y., established the Harriet Tubman Home for Aged and Indigent Colored People (now the Harriet Tubman Home, on the National Register of Historic Places); honored by the Woman's State Assoc. of New York and the New England Woman Suffrage Assoc.; the Liberty ship *Harriet Tubman* was christened by Eleanor Roosevelt during World War II; commemorative stamp, U.S. Postal Service; March 10, 1990, designated "Harriet Tubman Day" by U.S. Congress. **Died:** Auburn, N.Y.

References and Credits

†Blassingame JW (ed): Slave Testimony. Baton Rouge, Louisiana State University Press, 1977, p 464.

†Loewenberg B, Bogin R: Black Women in Nineteenth-Century American Life. State College, Pennsylvania State University Press, 1976, p 220.

Bradford S: Harriet Tubman: The Moses of Her People (1869). Reprint, Secaucus, N.J., Citadel Press, 1961.

Stein AP: Harriet (Araminta) Tubman. In Bullough V, Church OM, Stein AP (eds): American Nursing: A Biographical Dictionary, vol. 1. New York, Garland, 1988, pp 321–322.

Carnegie ME: The Path We Tread: Blacks in Nursing, 1854–1984. Philadelphia, JB Lippincott, 1986.

Guy-Sheftall B: Words of Fire: An Anthology of African-American Feminist Thought. New York, New Press, 1995.

Toppin E: A Biographical History of Blacks in America since 1528. New York, David McKay, 1971.

Davidson N: Harriet Tubman "Moses." In Smith JC (ed): Notable Black American Women, vol. 1. Detroit, Gale, 1992, pp 1152–1155.

The Life of Harriet Tubman, available on-line at http://www.nyhistory.com/harriettubman/life.html, 2003.

July 5

Marjorie E. Sanderson
1911–1996

"A clearly defined concept of nursing and a conviction concerning its unique service to society requires that each nursing practitioner should be able to enunciate a definition of nursing which is meaningful to him and which he can interpret to others. The practitioner should also hold a firm conviction that the service he renders is unique and is needed by society.... Quality evolves as the professional practitioner experiences a freedom of spirit, resulting in eagerness to share in change or even to initiate change for improvement of care." (1964)

MARJORIE SANDERSON HAD a versatile career as an outstanding nurse educator and influenced nursing programs in seven states for more than fifty years. Her achievements included the establishment of academic nursing programs for practical nurses as well as professional nursing programs that culminated in undergraduate and graduate degrees. In 1964 she proposed five elements of quality nursing care: "a clearly defined concept of nursing and a conviction concerning its unique service to society, a differentiation of technical and professional skills, an increased emphasis on the science of nursing practice, an acceptance of specialization in the clinical nursing services, and a program for continuity of nursing care." According to Sanderson, a basic function of the director of nursing is to define nursing as a professional service. She also was a nurse-researcher, with interests ranging from community health needs to nurses' attitudes. When she was involved with patient care at a large hospital, she successfully applied her own ideas about staffing patterns in the clinical setting. She was a charter member of the American Academy of Nursing (AAN).

Biography

Born: July 5, 1911, Cedarville, Ohio. **Education:** Grant Hosp. School of Nursing, Columbus, Ohio; Ohio State Univ. (BSNE); Teachers College, Columbia Univ. (MNE, PhD); postgraduate study, Univ. of Southern California; Reformed Theological Seminary, Jackson, Miss. **Work history:** Nursing Educator, Director, School of Nursing, Bethany Hosp., Kansas City, Mo.; Henry Ford Hosp., Detroit; member, Kansas State Bd. for Nursing; Director, Miami Valley (Ohio) Hosp. School of Nursing; Nursing Administrator, Univ. Hosp., Baltimore; Faculty, Associate Dean, School of Nursing, Univ. of Maryland; Director, Walter Reed Army Institute of Nursing; Faculty, Administrator for nursing programs, Medical College of Georgia; Univ. of South Carolina; York College, Pa.; Mercer College, Ohio; Pennsylvania State Univ., East Stroudsburg (Pa.) State Univ. **Organizations:** American Nurses Assoc.; Sigma Theta Tau; American Assoc. for Higher Education. **Awards:** Isabelle Hampton Robb Fellow, Teachers College, Columbia Univ.; Distinguished Professor Award, Univ. of South Carolina; charter member, AAN; nursing writing award estab. in her memory, East Stroudsburg (Pa.) Univ. **Died:** location unknown.

References and Credits

†Sanderson M: Quality patient care. In Blueprint for Action in Hospital Nursing. New York, National League for Nursing, 1964, p 53.

Hertz JK: Marjorie Sanderson. In Bullough V, Sentz L, Stein AP (eds): American Nursing: A Biographical Dictionary, vol. 2. New York, Garland, 1992, pp 285–287.

Champagne C: personal communication, 2003.

July 6

Alice Magaw Kessel

1860–1928

"There is a great deal yet to be learned about anesthetics and their administration. To the anesthetist there is little, in a financial way, to be hoped for. Is it strange that there are so few who will be faithful to the work long enough to gain sufficient experience in that which all surgeons know to be a most important factor in the operating-room? There is little that is attractive or encouraging unless one cultivates a fondness for the work, and is determined to become as proficient as possible in an art both difficult and important." (1904)

In 1893 the Doctors Mayo, Charles and William W., chose Alice Magaw to give anesthesia to their surgical patients. They gave her a training period. They believed that the great care and soothing, undivided attention that a nurse like Magaw brought to her work demonstrated her superiority in giving anesthetics. Thus this first clinical nurse specialty developed because surgeons were seeking a solution to the high morbidity and mortality from anesthesia. By 1906 Magaw had administered anesthesia to fourteen thousand patients without any deaths attributed to anesthesia. The Mayos praised her as "the Mother of Anesthesia, a peerless anesthetist." Magaw refined and developed anesthetic techniques such as open-drop ether administration. She wrote about her findings in medical journals, emphasizing the importance that she attached to individual care, and she reported on the efficacy of nitrous oxide as a supplement to ether anesthesia. Before her marriage to Dr. George Kessel in 1908, she trained other nurses to give anesthetics. She retired from nursing after her marriage.

Biography

Born: 1860, Rochester, Minn. **Education:** Woman's Hosp., Chicago; instruction by William W. Mayo in administering anesthesia, St. Mary's Hosp., Rochester, Minn. **Work history:** worked for Drs. William and Charles Mayo, St. Mary's Hospital, Rochester, Minn. **Organizations:** unknown. **Awards:** Alice Magaw Award, American Assoc. of Nurse Anesthetists. **Died:** location unknown.

References and Credits

†Transactions of the Minnesota State Medical Association: 99, 1904.

Magaw A: Observations drawn from an experience of eleven thousand anesthesias. Transactions of the Minnesota State Medical Association: 91–102, 1904.

Thatcher VS (ed): History of Anesthesia with Emphasis on the Nurse Specialist. Philadelphia, JB Lippincott, 1953.

Obst TE: Alice Magaw Kessel. In Bullough V, Church OM, Stein AP (eds): American Nursing: A Biographical Dictionary, vol. 1. New York, Garland, 1988, pp 200–201.

American Association of Nurse Anesthetists on-line, available at http://www.aana.com.

July 7

Stella Goostray

1886–1969

"Nursing has gotten where it is today because of indomitable courage, foresight, and self-sacrifice of countless women, some of whose names we do not even know. It will be so again. The first thing that lies ahead then is the adoption of an adequate system of nursing education which will advance nursing to new levels of effectiveness. ...The second major adjustment which is necessary is to secure an adequate system of providing basic economic security for all groups of nurses. ...Those of us who have been concerned with nursing education have been so afraid that the spiritual values in nursing would not receive due emphasis that we have kept saying over and over again that man cannot live by bread alone. We have not always added what is equally true that man cannot live without bread." (1935)

Stella Goostray began her nursing studies during World War I at Children's Hospital in Boston, and her interest in the health care of children was evident throughout her career. When she later returned to the hospital, as director of the nursing service, some of what she did to improve the quality of care included modernizing nursing procedures and increasing the number of qualified nursing staff. Pediatric nursing education benefited from her involvement with President Herbert Hoover's White House

Conference on Child Health and Protection. When she began teaching nursing, she first worked with Isabel Stewart at Teachers College, Columbia University, and later with S. Lillian Clayton in Philadelphia. Goostray earned her reputation for high standards and was an example of dedication and excellence. She improved nursing education through her efforts to strengthen curriculum. She maintained high expectations of those who taught nursing and was involved with ongoing program evaluations, accreditation reviews, and extensive writing for publication. She wrote books on drugs and solutions, chemistry, math, and nursing history, as well as many professional articles. Her work to help establish the Nursing Council for National Defense focused on improving military nursing and inclusion of black nurses.

Biography

Born: July 8, 1886, Boston. **Education:** Boston Children's Hosp. School of Nursing (RN); Teachers College, Columbia Univ. (BS); Boston Univ. (MEd). **Work history:** Nursing Instructor, St. Mary's Children's Hosp., N.Y.C.; Teachers College–Presbyterian Hosp. School of Nursing; Philadelphia General Hosp. School of Nursing; Director, Nursing Service, Boston Children's Hosp.; Faculty, Boston Univ. School of Nursing. **Organizations:** member, bd. of directors, President, American Journal of Nursing Co.; Secretary, National League for Nursing Education; adviser, Joint Nursing Commission on Education Policies; Consultant, Commission on Grading of Nursing Schools; President, National Nursing Council for War Service; Consultant, National League for Nursing; nurse historian–consultant, Boston Univ. School of Nursing. **Awards:** honorary doctorate, Boston Univ.; several awards in Mass. for outstanding contributions to nursing; Adelaide Nutting Award, National League for Nursing; McManus Medal, Teachers College; American Nurses Assoc. Hall of Fame. **Buried:** Mt. Auburn Cemetery, Boston.

References and Credits

†Goostray S: What lies ahead for the nursing profession? AJN 35:768–769, 1935.

Wells MR: Stella Goostray. In Bullough V, Church OM, Stein AP (eds): American Nursing: A Biographical Dictionary, vol. 1. New York, Garland, 1988, pp 149–152.

ANA Hall of Fame 10/98 American Nurses Association, Washington, D.C. http://www.nursingworld.org/hof.

Alyce Faye Wattleton
1943–

"My training and experience as a nurse and nurse-midwife were invaluable in teaching me, as Margaret Sanger's profession taught her, that a woman's health and her right to control her reproduction are inextricably linked to her ability to achieve equality. My determination has been driven by the repugnant idea of the government in a free society intruding into the most private aspects of a woman's life and body. ...Nothing is more essential to your personal liberty than protecting your body from the intrusions of government edicts. ...Be especially mindful that women's reproductive rights will continue to be at the heart of the struggle for women's equality. Within your rights to control your fertility is vested enormous power, the power to control entry of life into the world. Some believe such power should not be entrusted to you, for they fear the destruction of the old order of women living in subservience to sexual and reproductive control. ...The irony of this struggle is that if the women of our country, of our world, united to end inequality, it would be eradicated. The potential is within us, within you. In solidarity, women need not fear the price of claiming what is ours—our right to full equality and opportunity." (1996)

FAYE WATTLETON, WHO as a young child thought of being a missionary nurse in Africa, credits the influence of her mother, a devout and popular fundamentalist preacher, for instilling in her compassion, integrity, and determination. Faye Wattleton learned the importance of social justice and service to others from the example of family, and all these qualities blended in her professional practice. Her public health nursing experiences in Ohio and her midwifery internship at Harlem Hospital exposed her to the tragedies of illegal abortion and unwanted children. In her memoir, *Life on the Line,* she wrote that, during her year at Harlem Hospital, "approximately 6500 women entered... suffering from the complications of incomplete abortions." After her work as director of Planned Parenthood in Dayton, Ohio, she was approached to lead the Planned Parent Federation of America (PPFA). She was its youngest president and the first woman to hold the position since Margaret Sanger founded the organization. Wattleton's leadership saw the organization grow in scope and financial support. For fourteen years she was a consistent and articulate advocate for birth control, sex education, and the right to have an abortion. She also was a popular radio and television guest, who used the media to reach the general public for support in the struggle for women's rights. She spoke out against punitive policies and legislation that were barriers to a woman's freedom of choice, enduring verbal and physical hostility but never shying away from addressing a woman's right to reproductive freedom. Wattleton has been featured in and honored by numerous national magazines. *Glamour* said of her, in 1990, "Even pro-life activists concede she is everything you don't want in an opponent—articulate, strikingly telegenic, bright, and most importantly, messianic on this subject. In short, she has star quality." *Money* magazine selected her as one of five outstanding Americans, and *Esquire* named her as one of the twenty-five most influential people in the United States.

Biography continued on page 768

July 9

Frances Charlotte Thielbar

1908–1962

"The ultimate purpose of any program of nursing education is the development of an individual who is capable of giving the best possible care to the patient and who, in her practice, demonstrates the principles of prevention.... We wish students to carry their knowledge of mental hygiene and mental nursing into the whole nursing field, and apply the principle of caring for the whole individual in the general hospital and in the public health field. We also wish our psychiatric training to develop better adjusted nurses who do not repress their conflicts but who solve them on a conscious plane." (1934)

Frances Thielbar promoted nursing research, particularly that regarding nursing coursework and nursing care. Her psychiatric nursing background influenced the inclusion of high-quality instruction in psychiatric nursing early in the program for undergraduate students. She believed this would help students learn more about themselves, as well as provide a good foundation in mental health that they could apply in all areas of practice. She opposed student affiliations with state mental hospitals because those hospitals lacked the quality and the commitment necessary to meet the educational objectives. She stressed the importance of qualified, individual instruction as well as supervision during the student's psychiatric rotation. Thielbar was instrumental in obtaining federal funding that allowed qualified clinical instructors to accompany students to their clinical experiences. Students were taught to be patient centered and holistic in the care they provided, and Theilbar called on graduate nurses to be good role models, particularly in their attitudes and behaviors toward patients. She was a pioneer for higher education in nursing and developed one of the earliest graduate programs for nurses when she established the master's program at the University of Pennsylvania.

Biography

Born: July 10, 1908, River Forest, Ill. **Education:** Wellesley College (AB); Yale School of Nursing (BSN); Univ. of Chicago (MSN, PhD). **Work history:** Butler Hosp., R.I.; Univ. of Chicago; Univ. of Pennsylvania; Director, American Journal of Nursing Publishing Co.; founder, editorial bd. member, *Nursing Research.* **Organizations:** American Assoc. of Univ. Women; R.I. League for Nursing; member, R.I. Bd. of Nursing; Assoc. of Collegiate Schools of Nursing; National League for Nursing. **Awards:** unknown. **Died:** Wynnewood, Pa.

References and Credits

†Thielbar F: Ward teaching in a mental hospital. AJN 34:710, 1934.

Manfreda ML: Frances Thielbar. In Bullough V, Church OM, Stein AP (eds): American Nursing: A Biographical Dictionary, vol. 1. New York, Garland, 1988, pp 305–307.

July 10

Minnie Goodnow

1875–1952

"History tends to make us humble. It many times shows us that the work which we think original is only a repetition of that which has been done before. It shows us how our predecessors struggled with problems almost exactly like those which we meet. It makes us see that the conditions under which they worked were markedly similar to those of today; that their methods were not wholly unlike ours; and that their results resembled ours, being no less conspicuous than those which we today laud as remarkable. ...History discourages by its habit of repeating itself, evincing how tenacious the race is of outworn ideas and methods. It encourages by revealing the progress which has been made, and the part which earnestness and persistence have played in the advance." (1916)

Minnie Goodnow left her college studies of Greek to study architecture in her father's office, but family financial problems detoured her to nursing. She combined her professional expertise and her interest in architecture to give valuable nursing suggestions for hospital design. She also designed practical equipment to be used by nurses. She worked as an ambulance nurse during World War I and studied occupational therapy so that she would be prepared to work with veterans upon their return home. A versatile author, she published texts on nursing, chemistry, physics, and pediatrics.

She wrote *Outlines of Nursing History* in 1916; its eleventh edition was printed in 1963. This well-illustrated work, which is fascinating to read, was adopted as a teaching text by many training schools. It was a valuable resource for teachers, as her editions included chapter summaries, comprehensive examination questions, and a teaching outline for fifteen lessons in nursing history. In addition, she included listings of important dates in nursing and an updated summary of nursing organizations and worldwide nursing publications. She met with nurses everywhere during a two-year trip around the world.

Biography

Born: July 10, 1875, Albion, N.Y. **Education:** Univ. of Denver; Las Vegas Hot Springs Sanitarium School of Nursing, N. Mex.; General Memorial Hosp., N.Y.; New York Infant Asylum; George Washington Univ.; Univ. of Pennsylvania. **Work history:** Private Duty Nurse; Superintendent of Nursing, Denver Women's Hosp.; Milwaukee County (Wisc.) Hosp.; Park Avenue Hosp., Denver; Bornson Hosp., Mich.; Staff, hospital architects, Boston; Harvard ambulance unit, France, World War I; Army Hosp., Wheeling, W.Va.; Institute for Crippled Men, N.Y.C.; Superintendent of Nursing, Children's Hosp., Washington, D.C.; Director of Nurses, General Hosp., Philadelphia; Superintendent of Nurses, Newport (R.I.) Hosp.; Superintendent of Nurses, Somerville (Mass.) Hosp.; Superintendent of Nursing Schools, Mass.; Superintendent of Nurses, Pratt Diagnostic Hosp., Boston. **Organizations:** unknown. **Awards:** unknown. **Died:** Boston.

References and Credits

†Goodnow M: Foreword to Outlines of Nursing History. Philadelphia, WB Saunders, 1916, pp 3–4.

Bullough V: Minnie Goodnow. In Bullough V, Church OM, Stein AP (eds): American Nursing: A Biographical Dictionary, vol. 1. New York, Garland, 1988, pp 143–144.

Clara Leach Adams-Ender

1939–

"If a person does not normally and naturally care, she or he should not consider nursing as a profession. One of my basic passions and the foundation of nursing is that we care about ourselves and other people. ...You have to care about yourself first before you ever know how to care for another person. ...I mean you have got to be sure that you learn to take care of yourself well. One of the things nurses have talked about for years and years is 'burnout.' ...I do not believe in burnout....You have not taken care of yourself well if you have gotten burned out....You've got to figure out how you can nurture yourself in order to keep up with the pace of nursing." (2001)

CLARA LEACH ADAMS-ENDER was born into a large sharecropper family where poverty, hard work, and determination taught her responsibility at an early age. *Working Woman* magazine recognized her as one of 350 women who changed the world. Although she was first attracted to law because it offered challenge, she studied nursing instead because that is what her father wanted her to do. She soon found challenges in nursing as well. Her professional satisfaction was enhanced by her ability to overcome obstacles related to gender, race, and tradition. She sees countless opportunities in the military, where nursing's mission is clear and strengthened by its ability to control its own practice. Enthusiastic about nursing, opportunities, and life, Adams-Ender stresses her philosophy that self-care is essential if nurses are to provide quality nursing care. She was promoted to brigadier general during her thirty-four-year career with the army, and when she retired, she had been chief nurse of the Army Nurse Corps and the first nurse to serve as commanding general of an army base. Her recently published memoir, *My Rise to the Stars: How a Sharecropper's Daughter Became an Army General*, traces her professional journey from her early days in the fields of North Carolina to brigadier general.

Biography

Born: July 11, 1939, Willow Springs, N.C. **Education:** North Carolina Agricultural and Technical State Univ. (BSN); Univ. of Minnesota (MS); U.S. Army Command Staff and General College (master's of military art and science); U.S. Army War College. **Work history:** numerous positions in the Army Nurse Corps., incl. Faculty, Ft. Sam Houston, Texas; Walter Reed Army Institute of Nursing (WRAIN); Adjunct Faculty, Georgetown Univ., Oakland (Mich.) Univ. School of Nursing; Chief Nurse, Germany, Recruiting Command, Walter Reed Army Center; Chief Nurse Exec., Army Nurse Corps; Deputy Commanding General, Military District of Washington, D.C.; Deputy Commanding General, Military District of Washington, D.C.; Commanding General, Ft. Belvoir, Va.; member, editorial bd., *Journal of Professional Nursing*. **Organizations:** American Nurses Assoc.; Credit Union Exec. Society; The Rocks, Inc.; Delta Sigma Theta Sorority; American Organization of Nurse Execs. **Awards:** recognition, *Working Woman* magazine; Expert Field Military Badge; Fellow, American Academy of Nursing; Lifetime membership, NAACP; Roy Wilkins Award for Meritorious Service in Civil Rights and Public Service; Legion of Merit; Meritorious Service Medal with Three Oak Leaf Clusters; Distinguished Service Medal with Oak Leaf Cluster; ten honorary doctoral degrees.

References and Credits

†Adams-Ender C: Rise to the stars! In Reflections on Nursing Leadership, fourth quarter: 15, 2001, Honor Society of Nursing, Sigma Theta Tau International.

Hawkins WL: African American Biographies. Jefferson, N.C., McFarland, 1992, pp 4–5.

Davis AT: Clara Leach Adams-Ender. In Smith JC (ed): Notable Black American Women. Detroit, Gale, 1992, pp 1–2.

Adams-Ender C: personal communication, 2002.

Lucille Notter

1907–1993

"Nurses are assuming increasingly demanding professional responsibilities in the health care system and can be expected to assume more ...responsibility for their own contribution to the improvement of health care. ...Every nurse has a part to play in research, whether it be participation in research itself or as a use of the products of research. ...The research nurse and the practitioner have a common goal—to provide the best nursing care possible. ...The findings of research must be applied in practice if they are to effect improvement in patient care. This goal can be achieved only if practicing nurses are aware of research projects being carried out and can read and evaluate the findings in terms of their implications for nursing." (1983)

LUCILLE NOTTER WAS attracted to nursing when she observed nurses while she was working as a hospital records clerk and because she had a friend who had recently finished nursing school. Notter was a catalyst for and an outstanding leader in nursing research. Her influence was strengthened by her own example, her encouragement of others, and her belief that the goal of nursing research is to improve clinical practice. Her 1974 book, *Essentials of Nursing Research,* had several editions. As first full-time editor of the highly regarded journal *Nursing Research,* she stimulated study in such areas as nursing education, nursing practice, and nursing history. She directed annual programs for the American Nurses Association that allowed nurse-researchers to network and share findings. She was also involved in the open curriculum project of the National League for Nursing (NLN), which offered academic opportunities to registered nurses who wanted to earn a baccalaureate degree.

Biography

Born: July 13, 1907, Frankfort, Ky. **Education:** St. Mary and Elizabeth Hosp. School of Nursing Louisville, Ky. (BSNE, MA, EdD); Teachers College, Columbia Univ. **Work history:** Head Nurse, Superintendent, Instructor, Michael Reese Hosp., Chicago; various positions, Visiting Nurse Service of New York; Assistant Exec. Director, Visiting Nurse Assoc. of Brooklyn; Faculty, Hunter College; Faculty, writers workshop, Boston Univ. School of Nursing; Author; Researcher; Editor, *Nursing Research, International Nurse Index, Cardiovascular Nursing.* Director, special programs, American Nurses Assoc. (ANA). NLN. **Organizations:** ANA, NLN. **Awards:** ANA Hall of Fame. **Died:** location unknown.

References and Credits

†Notter L: Essentials of Nursing Research, 3d ed. New York, Springer, 1983, pp xi, xiii.

Safire G: Contemporary American Leaders in Nursing. New York, McGraw-Hill, 1977.

Buchinger KL: Lucille Notter. In Bullough V, Sentz L, Stein AP (eds): American Nursing: A Biographical Dictionary, vol. 2. New York, Garland, 1992, pp 246–248.

ANA Hall of Fame 10/98 American Nurses Association, Washington, D.C. http://www.nursingworld.org/hof.

July 13

Madeleine M. Leininger

1925–

"As the founder of transcultural nursing, it looks promising to see transcultural nursing become a full reality in the 21st Century. Quality of health care will become the focus in many countries. Managed care practices will be passe largely because of the limited emphasis on quality care and consumers will be active in what they want and need according to their cultural values. Consumers will take charge *of what they want and expect of health providers. Providing effective, meaningful, and culturally based care for diverse and similar care needs will be expected. Transcultural nurse experts will be in demand and different nursing practices will become evident. Uniculturalism will of necessity be replaced with multicultural care philosophy, goals, and practices in education and service. ...The new generation of nurses will be in a good position to advance transcultural nursing knowledge as ... a discipline that has revolutionized and transformed nursing education and practice." (1997)*

Madeleine Leininger is a nursing pioneer, researcher, theorist, creative leader, and futurist. An internationally renowned speaker, consultant, author, and certified transcultural nurse specialist, she initiated and directed the first graduate child psychiatric nursing program in the country and was the first professional graduate nurse to pursue a doctoral degree in anthropology. Leininger's keen observations of nurses and patients made her aware of the need to significantly broaden and deepen nursing's understanding of the relationship between culture and care and the need to integrate this knowledge into nursing education, practice, and research. Her subsequent theory of culture care, diversity and universality, based on care as the essence of nursing, recognizes that nursing practice must be holistic, integrating broad, humanistic, and scientific knowledge that is culturally appropriate in order to provide care that is appropriate, therapeutic, and safe. She conceptualized and established the discipline of transcultural nursing, which blended selected knowledge from anthropology and nursing care. Leininger's ideas are now being used worldwide. Her book, *Nursing and Anthropology: Two Worlds to Blend* (1970) was the first on the subject. She founded the Transcultural Nursing Society (1974) and the National Care Research Conferences (1978). Leininger hopes that all nurses will be prepared in transcultural nursing and able to practice effectively with diverse cultures by 2015.

Biography

Born: July 13, 1925, Sutton, Neb. **Education:** St. Anthony's Hosp. School of Nursing, Denver; Benedictine College, Atchison, Kans. (BS); Creighton Univ.; Catholic Univ. of America (MS); Univ. of Washington (PhD). **Work history:** Staff Nurse, Instructor, Head Nurse, Director of psychiatric unit, St. Joseph's Hosp., Omaha, Neb.; Faculty, School of Nursing, Univ. of Cincinnati; Professor of nursing and anthropology, Univ. of Colorado; Dean, Professor of nursing, Univ. of Washington; Dean, Professor, Univ. of Utah; Distinguished Professor, Troy State Univ., Ala.; Professor, Director, Transcultural Nursing Program, Wayne State Univ., Detroit; Researcher; Author; Speaker; Consultant; Scholar; Founder, *Journal of Transcultural Nursing;* originator of certification in transcultural nursing. **Organizations:** President, American Assoc. of Colleges of Nursing (AACN); Founder, Transcultural Nursing Society; founded National Research Caring Conference (later, International Assoc. of Human Caring); initiated Commission on Nursing and Anthropology; member, American Anthropological Assoc.; American Nurses Assoc. **Awards:** Distinguished Order of the Royal College of Nursing, Australia; Distinguished Nurse Scholar, Troy State Univ., Ala.; Professor Emeritus, Wayne State Univ., Detroit; Fellow, American Academy of Nursing (AAN); Living Legend, AAN, 1998; emeritus member, AACN; honorary doctorates, Univ. of Indianapolis; Scholastic Benedictine College; Univ. of Kuopio, Finland; nominated for Nobel Peace Prize, 2001.

References and Credits continued on page 769

July 14

Mildred Garrett Primer

1905–2003

"I don't remember a time when I didn't want to be a nurse." (Date unknown)

"We would like to see each school child taking increasing responsibility for his own health. Remembering that example as well as precept has much to do with what he learns. We try to surround him with people who are themselves healthy in mind, body, and spirit." (1950)

MILDRED GARRETT PRIMER DEVELOPED her career in public health nursing in Texas, where she rose to the position of director of the Division of Public Health Nursing at the state Department of Health in Austin. She began her public health nursing career in 1930 with supplies she bought from Walgreen's Drug Store, a black bag, and her home-styled gray uniform. She started to work at the state level as a nurse adviser in 1936 and remained until her retirement in 1972. She was also active in public health nursing organizations and held many high offices. She implemented in-service education for public health nurses, and she was influential in providing nursing services to migrant farm workers in Texas in 1962. Garrett played a pivotal role in ending discrimination in wages and educational scholarships for black nurses.

Biography

Born: July 13, 1905, near Hempstead, Texas. **Education:** Northwest Texas Hosp. School of Nursing, Amarillo; John Sealy Hosp., Galveston; Montezuma Baptist College, N. Mex., 1928; Vanderbilt Univ., 1931, 1936 (course in public health nursing, BSN). **Work history:** Nurse's Aide, Baptist Hosp., Clovis, N. Mex.; Private Duty Nurse, 1928; College Nurse, summer 1929; Public Health Nurse, Potter County and children's clinic, Texas Dept. of Health, 1930; obtained Works Progress Administration project for state health dept., 1931; State Advisory Nurse, state health dept., Austin, 1936; Director, nurse education, Texas Dept. of Public Health, 1938. **Organizations:** President, Texas Graduate Nurses Assoc.; Vice President, Texas Organization of Public Health Nursing; First Vice Chair, Public Health Nurses Section, American Nurses Assoc.; Chair, Council of State Directors of Public Health Nursing. **Awards:** unknown. **Died:** Texas.

References and Credits

†Crowder ELM: Mildred Garrett Primer. In Bullough V, Sentz L, Stein AP (eds): American Nursing: A Biographical Dictionary, vol. 2. New York, Garland, 1992, pp 127–130.

†Garrett M: Nursing contributions to health programs for school children. Texas Public Health Association Newsletter 1:225, 1950, p 225.

JULY 15

Maria Francesca Cabrini

1850–1917

"This [establishing a hospital] is the work that needs to be done."
(1892)

"Difficulties! Difficulties! What are difficulties? Childish trifles magnified by our imagination, which is not yet accustomed to focus itself upon, or to plunge itself into, Almighty God."
(Date unknown)

"The earth is so very small because we must limit ourselves to only one point of it. I want to embrace the whole world and contact it everywhere. ...My mission is the world."
(Date unknown)

MOTHER FRANCES CABRINI was affectionately called "the Immigrant Saint" and was described by the writer Mary Sullivan as the "Italian Immigrant of the Century." When she was a young woman, her health interfered with her aspirations to do missionary work in China. Although she was turned down by a religious order, she was determined to serve, made general vows, and started the Missionary Sisters of the Sacred Heart of Jesus. Pope Leo XIII asked these sisters to travel to the United States to work with Italian immigrants in New York City, where the nuns established schools, orphanages, and the much-needed Columbus Hospital. The charitable work of Cabrini and her congregation effectively addressed the basic social and health care needs of poor Italian immigrants. She later helped establish hospitals in Chicago and Seattle. She was a legend in her own time and the first canonized U.S. citizen; her congregation spread worldwide.

Biography

Born: July 15, 1850, near Lodi, Italy. **Education:** teacher's license, Italy. **Work history:** Teacher; Founder, Missionary Sisters of the Sacred Heart; missionary work, United States. **Organizations:** unknown. **Awards:** Canonization, 1946; National Women's Hall of Fame, 1996. **Buried:** New York City.

References and Credits

†Shumway F: The Social Contributions of Mother Cabrini in the United States with Emphasis on the Immigrant [thesis]. Washington, D.C., Catholic University of America, 1950.

†James E (ed): Notable American Women, 1607–1850. Cambridge, Mass., Belknap Press, 1971, p 275.

†Martignoni A: My Mission Is the World. New York, Vatican Religious Book Co., 1949.

Clifford AE: Mother Cabrini. In Bullough V, Sentz L, Stein AP (eds): American Nursing: A Biographical Dictionary, vol. 2. New York, Garland, 1992, pp 53–54.

Saint Frances Xavier Cabrini. In Harris W, Levey J (eds): The New Columbia Encyclopedia. New York, Columbia University Press, 1975, p 414.

Sullivan Mary: Mother Cabrini: Italian Immigrant of the Century. New York, Center for Migration Studies, 1992.

National Women's Hall of Fame, available on-line at http://www.greatwomen.org/profile.

July 16

Isabel McIsaac

1858–1914

"The increasing knowledge of the importance of the prevention of disease makes the study of hygiene and sanitation one of the most valuable factors in the education of nurses, who may by their understanding of the conditions which preserve health or cause disease, render as effective assistance in the prevention as in the cure of the manifold ills which afflict mankind. In the nursing care given every patient, no matter how trivial his ailment, as much or more time is devoted to protecting him from further or other ills, than is given to the care intended for his cure." (1922)

ISABEL McISAAC, ONE of the first students supervised by Isabel Hampton, went on to work with Hampton as well as other illustrious nursing leaders such as Edith Draper and Lavinia Dock. When McIsaac was the assistant superintendent of nursing at Presbyterian Hospital in Chicago, she made changes that improved and helped standardize the training program for nurses. First, she extended the program to three years, then introduced clinical demonstrations and added grading of practical work and conduct as well as theory. She expanded coursework to cover administration and ethics while establishing continuing education programs for graduate nurses. She helped form nursing organizations at the state, national, and international levels. She wrote and successfully lobbied for the nurse registration act in Illinois and then helped convince Congress to establish the Army Nurse Corps. She served as president of the American Journal of Nursing Company, and in retirement she wrote and published three texts for nurses as well as a text for the Red Cross on home nursing. She then left retirement to travel extensively for nursing organizations, give nursing recruitment talks, head the Army Nurse Corps and the American Red Cross nursing division, and take part in the 1913 suffrage parade in Washington, D.C.

Biography

Born: 1858, Waterloo, Iowa. **Education:** Illinois Training School for Nurses, Chicago. **Work history:** Assistant Superintendent for Nursing, Superintendent of Nurses, Presbyterian Hosp., Chicago; helped form national, international nursing organizations; Lobbyist; Columnist, *American Journal of Nursing;* President, American Journal of Nursing Co.; head of Army Nurse Corps.; Vice Chair, American Red Cross Nursing Committee. **Organizations:** charter member, Alumnae Assoc. of Ill. Training School for Nurses; American Society of Superintendents of Training Schools for Nurses; Nurses Associated Alumnae of United States and Canada; International Council of Nurses; American Federation of Nurses. **Awards:** Isabel McIsaac Fund for Nurses, established by Robb Memorial Fund Committee; honorary member, Matron's Council, International Congress for Nurses at the Pan-American Exposition, 1901. **Buried:** Waterloo, Iowa.

References and Credits

†McIsaac I: Hygiene for Nurses. New York, Macmillan, 1922, p 1.

Milauskas J: Isabel McIsaac. In Bullough V, Church OM, Stein AP (eds): American Nursing: A Biographical Dictionary, vol. 1. New York, Garland, 1988, pp 220–223.

July 17

Marie Manthey

1935–

"This book is dedicated to Florence Marie Fisher, a nurse who cared for me when I was hospitalized at the age of five with scarlet fever, in St. Joseph's Hospital, Chicago. Although I never saw her again, her personalized and humane care of me became a model I have followed throughout my professional career. This dedication is also made to all those nurses who recognize the profound influence this special kind of nursing practice will have on the lives of their patients and who, by practicing it themselves, perpetuate the proud tradition and invaluable legacy of all the nurses like Ms. Fisher—ultimately the highest tribute of all." (1980)

Marie Manthey cherishes a lifelong memory of a compassionate nurse who cared for Manthey when she was five. As her own career progressed, she worked with others, in the 1960s, to develop the concept of primary nursing as an alternative to team nursing. She built on literature that defined the therapeutic relationship between nurse and patient as the essence of nursing. She became an effective public speaker about nursing. She saw primary nursing as the realm of the hospital staff nurse, the essential person to ensure that high-quality and individualized patient care is provided. She believes it requires decentralized decision making by staff nurses, who recognize their ability to be self-directed and patient centered. She helps nurses recognize their own knowledge and authority in directing and providing nursing care. Although she left bedside nursing years ago, Manthey continues to identify with its learning experiences, including its challenges, joys, and stresses. She introduced primary nursing when she was at Yale–New Haven Hospital and later pioneered a consulting service, now international, to assist the implementation of primary nursing. She wrote the acclaimed *The Practice of Primary Nursing* in 1980. Manthey consults with nurses internationally, from Indonesia to Iceland, Canada, Europe, and the former Soviet Union, about ways to adapt primary nursing to their systems.

Biography

Born: July 17, 1935, Chicago. **Education:** St. Elizabeth's Hosp. School of Nursing, Chicago (RN); Univ. of Minnesota (BNA, MNA). **Work history:** President, Creative Health Care Management (CHCM), Minneapolis; Consultant; Educator; Author; Vice President, Yale–New Haven Hosp.; Assistant Administrator, Director of Nursing, United Hosps. of St. Paul, Minn.; Associate Director of Nursing, Univ. of Minnesota Hosp.; Faculty, Yale School of Nursing, Univ. of Minnesota School of Nursing. **Organizations:** Minn. League for Nursing; Council of Minn. Nursing Organizations; Minn. Nurses Assoc. **Awards:** Honorary Fellow, Royal College of Nursing, U.K.; Fellow, American Academy of Nursing; Lifetime Mentoring Award, CHCM; Marguerite R. Kinney Award for Distinguished Career, 2001, American Assoc. of Critical Care Nurses (AACCN); Pioneering Spirit Award, AACCN; first honorary doctorate given by Univ. of Minnesota School of Nursing.

References and Credits

†Manthey M: The Practice of Primary Nursing. Boston, Blackwell Scientific, 1980.

Schorr T, Zimmerman A: Making Choices, Taking Chances: Nurse Leaders Tell Their Stories. St. Louis, CV Mosby, 1988.

Manthey M: personal communication, 2002.

Creative HealthCare Management on-line, available at http://www.chcm.com/experts/contact.shtml.

Manthey M: resume.

Dorothy M. Smith

1913–1997

"The words 'taking care of patients' or 'giving nursing care to patients' are meaningless in themselves. We need to think more specifically of (1) What are the patients' nursing problems, both predictive and actual? (2) How and where should they be defined and recorded? (3) What are the ways of dealing with these problems? (4) How can we insure that they are dealt with properly? (5) How can we validate the rightness of both the assessment and the measures used?...We can guarantee to each patient that his nursing problems will be evaluated, managed, and followed up as indicated. Certainly we need more nursing personnel, better motivated and better prepared. But this is not enough. We need a system or a method of nursing practice, *such as the five-step one just described—and we must begin to recognize, respect, and reward the intellectual and scientific component in nursing." (1964)*

DOROTHY SMITH WAS a nurse-educator and administrator who helped students develop patient-centered nursing practice. She recommended a process for identifying, addressing, and documenting responses on a problem list. She believed that it was essential to combine education with practice and ultimately gained practice privileges for faculty so that students could learn by example.

While serving as the founding dean of the University of Florida College of Nursing, she also was chief of nursing practice at the Shands Teaching Hospital, where her ongoing clinical practice was a model for both faculty and students. Her philosophy stressed that patient care was the central point for teaching and research. She is credited with a shift in emphasis in graduate nursing programs to clinical practice and, in research to patient outcomes.

Biography

Born: 1913, Bangor, Maine. **Education:** Quincy (Mass.) City Hosp. School of Nursing (RN); Teachers College, Columbia Univ. (BS). **Work history:** Staff Nurse, Instructor, Education Director, Quincy (Mass.) Hosp.; Assistant Director of Nursing Education, Duke Univ.; Consultant, National League for Nursing; Assistant Director of Nursing, Hartford (Conn.) Hosp.; Dean, School of Nursing, Univ. of Florida, Gainesville. **Organizations:** Fla. Nursing Assoc.; American Nurses Assoc. (ANA) **Awards:** honorary doctorate, Univ. of Rochester; honorary member, Fellow, American Academy of Nursing (AAN); Living Legend, American Academy of Nursing, 1996; ANA Hall of Fame. **Buried:** Weld, Maine.

References and Credits

†Smith D: Myth and method in nursing practice. AJN 64:72, 1964.

Safier G: Contemporary American Leaders in Nursing: An Oral History. New York, McGraw-Hill, 1977.

Brook M: Dorothy Smith. In Bullough V, Sentz L (eds): American Nursing: A Biographical Dictionary, vol. 3. New York, Springer, 2000, pp 262–263.

ANA Hall of Fame 10/98 American Nurses Association, Washington, D.C. http://www.nursingworld.org/hof.

"Mother" Mary Ann Ball Bickerdyke

1817–1901

"I did the work of one, and tried to do it well." (Date unknown)

"I'll go to Cairo [Illinois, where Union soldiers were dying of dysentery], and I'll clean things up down there. You don't need to worry about that, either. Them generals and all ain't going to stop me. This is the Lord's work you're calling me to do. And when I'm doing the Lord's work, they ain't nobody big enough to stop me." (1861)

ILLINOIS ERECTED A statue in a park in Galesburg in 1906 in honor of "Mary Ann Bickerdyke, a Sanitary Commission worker in the West who ministered to the needs of the wounded in no less than nineteen battles." The inscription on the statue reflects the enormity of her accomplishments:

> "'Mother Bickerdyke (1861—Army Nurse—1865) She Outranks Me." Quoted from General Sherman.

Born on a farm, Bickerdyke listened and observed farming techniques and the use of herbal remedies from her grandparents and uncles in their everyday work. She later proclaimed herself a "botanic physician." There are no records of her having a formal education.

She started her career before nursing schools were established. At that time women, like Charles Dickens's character Sairey Gamp, were recruited from prisons, almshouses, and asylums to tend the wounded and sick. Her friends Ulysses S. Grant and William Tecumseh Sherman helped cut red tape so she could nurse sick and dying soldiers. She followed Sherman's army during the Civil War, first cleaning the filthy treatment centers, then ministering to the wounded, comforting the dying, and rehabilitating the veterans by counseling, fund raising, and returning many soldiers to work on the farm. She continued to work until last soldier was discharged.

Biography

Born: July 19, 1817, Knox County, Ohio. **Education:** self-taught botanic physician and nurse. **Work history:** volunteered to take medical supplies to southern Illinois to help in Civil War effort. **Organizations:** unknown. **Awards:** Citizens of Kansas commissioned her portrait for the state capitol; pension awarded by U.S. Congress, 1886. **Buried:** Linwood Cemetery, Galesburg, Ill.

References and Credits

†Holland MAG: Our Army Nurses. Boston, B. Wilkins, 1895, p 517.

†Baker NB: Cyclone in Calico: The Story of Mary Ann Bickerdyke. Boston, Little, Brown, 1952, p 11.

Feller CM, Moore CJ (eds): Highlights in the History of the Army Nurse Corps. Washington, D.C., U.S. Army Center of Military History, 1995, p 83.

Church OM: Mary Ann Ball Bickerdyke. In Bullough V, Church OM, Stein AP (eds): American Nursing: A Biographical Dictionary, vol. 1. New York, Garland, 1988, pp 26–28.

Undine Sams

1919–1999

"The adoption of the E & GW [economic and general welfare] program by the ANA [American Nurses Association] House of Delegates in 1946 has got to be the most significant event. It was the beginning of nurses really having a say in their working conditions. ... With numbers, there is strength and power!" (1990)

Undine Sams held continuous membership in the Florida Nurses Association (FNA) and the ANA for fifty-eight years. She translated to action her dedication to strengthening and advancing the nursing profession. Her leadership of the FNA in the 1940s opened the doors to membership for black nurses. She recognized the value of each professional, despite existing segregation laws. Tenacious and articulate, she was especially committed to issues surrounding economic and general welfare at the state and national levels. The writer Patricia Messmer has attributed the start of FNA's strong and enduring economic and general welfare program to Sams's leadership and skill. In 1951 her efforts helped enact Florida's first mandatory nurse practice act. She spearheaded the establishment of a charitable foundation by the FNA and was a major donor. Committed to nursing issues, she was a regular participant in the ANA's annual House of Delegates and, shortly before her death, asked her doctor's permission to attend the upcoming meeting. Undine died where she had nursed five decades before, at Mt. Sinai Medical Center in Miami Beach.

Biography

Born: July 21, 1919. Wachula, Fla. **Education:** Jackson Memorial Hosp. School of Nursing (RN); Barry College (now Univ. of Florida) (BSN). **Work history:** Private Duty Nurse, ER Nurse, Industrial Nurse, School Nurse, volunteer Red Cross nurse. **Organizations:** FNA, ANA, Sigma Theta Tau. **Awards:** Army-Navy Excellence Award, World War II; one of the "Faces of the Century," in T. Schorr and M. Kennedy's *100 Years of American Nursing;* Special Recognition Awards, ANA, FNA; Florida Nurse of the Year, economic and general welfare award in her name, FNA; ANA Hall of Fame; honorary doctorate, Florida International Univ. **Died:** Miami Beach, Fla.

References and Credits

†Messmer P et al.: Nursing loses staunch advocate. American Nurse:4, 1999, available on-line at http://www.nursingworld.org/tan/julaug99/news.htm.

ANA Hall of Fame 10/98 American Nurses Association, Washington, D.C. http://www.nursingworld.org/hof/sams.htm.

Schorr T, Kennedy M: 100 Years of American Nursing: Celebrating a Century of Caring. Philadelphia, JB Lippincott, 1999.

July 21

Clare Dennison

1891–1954

"Staff nurses in our hospitals (must) receive remuneration in proportion to the work they do and the responsibility they carry… (nursing must be) a career in which women can live normally and make provision for old age." (1942)

Clare Dennison spent most of her nursing career at the Strong Memorial Hospital in New York as the superintendent of nurses and director of the School of Nursing of the University of Rochester. Her approach to nursing addressed two needs: hospital management of nursing, and clinical specialists to teach students. She improved the quality of nursing education while reducing the students' workload. At the same time she gained parity for the nursing faculty with other professors at the university. She made clear distinctions between nursing services and nursing care and made certain that nursing care was the nurses' primary responsibility. She worked to ensure that nurses would be paid well for this professional work. She received many professional nursing awards, and scholarships for outstanding students were established in her name. Upon retirement she continued with her varied interests in the League of Women Voters, gardening, and children's theater.

Biography

Born: July 21, 1891, Grand Pre, Nova Scotia, Can. **Education:** Massachusetts General Hosp. School of Nursing, 1918; Teachers College, Columbia Univ., 1931 (BS). **Work history:** Clinical Instructor in medicine, Assistant Superintendent of Nursing, Head Nurse, Massachusetts General Hosp., Boston; Superintendent of Nurses, Director, School of Nursing, Strong Memorial Hosp., Rochester, N.Y., 1951. **Organizations:** unknown. **Awards:** Strong Memorial Hospital sponsored student in her memory; University of Rochester Dept. of Nursing estab. memorial lectureship in her name. **Died:** Rochester, N.Y.

References and Credits

†Cohen KF: Claire Dennison. In Bullough V, Sentz L, Stein AP (eds): American Nursing: A Biographical Dictionary, vol. 2. New York, Garland, 1992, pp 86–89.

July 22

Rosemary Ellis

1919–1986

"There are very few nurses who have become philosophers. It is essential that this pool be enlarged. Continuing inquiry is needed to examine and explicate other meanings, to further methodology for nursing knowledge, and to identify and explicate nursing values and ethics. The domain of human experience in illness must be explored further to provide knowledge vital for nursing practice. Practice requires a synthesis of the various ways of knowing. This synthesis must be manifest in the ways of being, in doing for and with another person. . . . Finally; it is easy to differentiate science, history, and philosophy in the abstract. Ultimately, in the human experience of knowing, they must become a whole. By and large, philosophy has been neglected by nurses, or it has been considered only superficially. The neglect and superficiality are a detriment to nursing and nursing-knowledge development. The potential of philosophic inquiry for nursing is largely unrealized." (1983)

Rosemary Ellis was a career nurse-researcher-scientist, educator, and author. Called "one of nursing's most penetrating thinkers and treasured scholars," by the authors Joyce Fitzpatrick and Ida Martinson, Ellis was one of the most outstanding teachers of the twentieth century. A pioneer in the development of nursing theory, she defined ways to obtain nursing knowledge through research and encouraged nurse-scholars to make this their specific focus. Her research on the sensory disturbances of surgical patients relative to noise in intensive care units gave her international recognition as a scholar. This study also helped nursing gain recognition as a science. Challenged by a stroke that left her with hemiplegia, she wrote about the experience and then, with the use of a leg brace, continued to travel and teach for more than a decade.

Biography

Born: July 22, 1864, Berkeley, Calif. **Education:** Univ. of California, Berkeley (AB in economics); Univ. of California, San Francisco (BSN); Univ. of Chicago (MA in nursing education, PhD in human development). **Work history:** First Lt., U.S. Army Nurse Corps; Professor, Frances Payne Bolton School of Nursing, Case Western Reserve Univ., Cleveland, Ohio. **Organizations:** member, scientific advisory bd., National Stroke Assoc.; American Nurses Assoc., National League for Nursing, U.S. Public Health Assoc. **Awards:** Fellow, American Academy of Nursing; Sigma Theta Tau; Alpha Xi Delta; Distinguished Nursing Science Award, American Nurses Foundation; Rosemary Ellis Scholarship for Ph.D Education in Nursing, Frances Payne Bolton School of Nursing, Case Western Reserve Univ., Cleveland, Ohio. **Buried:** Arlington National Cemetery.

References and Credits

†Fitzpatrick J, Martinson I (eds): Selected Writing of Rosemary Ellis: In Search of the Meaning of Nursing Science. New York, Springer, 1996, p 70, back cover.

Hawkins JW: Rosemary Ellis. In Kaufman M (ed): Dictionary of American Nursing Biography. New York, Greenwood, pp 113–117.

Brook M: Rosemary Ellis. In Bullough V, Sentz L, Stein AP (eds): American Nursing: A Biographical Dictionary, vol. 2. New York, Garland, 1992, pp 97–98.

Stella S. Mathews

1868–1949

"Nurses must always be on the lookout for contagion, report it and try to impress the parents with the importance of isolation. With the many language difficulties this seems at times impossible. We feel that our most fertile field for teaching the need of isolation lies in the prenatal clinics and the child health conferences. ...Like all public health nurses we realize that the better the teaching in the health conferences the less our problems will become in other activities." (1930)

BECAUSE HER MOTHER did not want her to study nursing, Stella Mathews first worked as a clerk for the Minnesota legislature. She then prepared as a teacher and taught school. This career was interrupted when she needed to care for her sick mother. After her mother's death she studied nursing in Wisconsin. She later spearheaded the establishment of what became the Wisconsin Nurses Association. The knowledge that she gained about the political process while working as a clerk helped the group to gain passage of the Nurse Practice Act in Wisconsin in 1911. The surgeon John Yates encouraged Mathews to learn about anesthesia, and she worked for him in Milwaukee after taking additional related coursework at Johns Hopkins University. After deciding that anesthesia was not for her, she moved to San Francisco and studied hospital management with

Amy Pope at St. Luke's Hospital. During World War I she was a chief nurse and served in France. She was highly honored for her work with the Red Cross to organize nursing schools and health programs for children in Greece. She later joined her sister in Hawaii, where she did public health nursing and helped establish the Territorial Nurses Association (TNA).

Biography

Born: July 23, 1868, Albion, Ill. **Education:** Knowlton (later Columbia) Hosp. Training School Milwaukee, Wisc. (RN). **Work history:** Head Nurse, Allegheny (Pa.) Hosp.; Superintendent, Milwaukee Children's Hosp.; Chief Nurse, Milwaukee Hosp. unit in Europe, World War I; Red Cross nurse, Poland, Greece; Superintendent, Hilo Hosp., Hawaii; Public Health Nurse, Hawaii. **Organizations:** Wisc. Nurses Assoc., Milwaukee County Nurses Assoc., American Red Cross, TNA. **Awards:** Victory Medal of the United States; Silver Medal, Polish Red Cross; Gold Cross of Merit, Poland; Chevalier of the Royal Order of George the First of Greece; Florence Nightingale Medal, International Committee, Red Cross. **Died:** Berkeley, Calif.

References and Credits

†Mathews S, MacOwan A: Public health nursing in Honolulu. Public Health Nurse 22:523–524, 1930.

Cooper SS: Stella Mathews. In Bullough V, Church OM, Stein AP (eds): American Nursing: A Biographical Dictionary, vol. 1. New York, Garland, 1988, pp 229–231.

July 24

Vern L. Bullough

1928–

"Nursing is a profession without borders, offering all kinds of opportunities." (2002)

"[Nursing] has become quite a different profession from the one Nightingale first visualized, but the caring element remains its foundation. …Men will undoubtedly help change nursing, but they will be joining with the women to do so. Nursing is radically different at the beginning of the 21st century than it was at the beginning of the 20th century, and men have finally arrived at a position where they can help shape its future. Nevertheless the only prediction possible to make is that nursing will continue to change, preserving the best of the past but growing with the future." (2001)

Vern Bullough was a late entrant into nursing and was attracted by its image of service to other human beings. He felt he had something to offer, namely, his expertise as a researcher who knew much about the obstacles that nursing had to overcome. He was upset that in the early years the resurgent feminist movement downplayed nursing, and he felt that its story should be told. He spent a good part of his career teaching history and social science. He has also published books and monographs in medieval history and in the history of medicine, science, and nursing. He and his first wife, Bonnie, researched and wrote extensively about nurses and their contributions to nursing. He is especially known for his three-volume *American Nursing: A Biographical Dictionary.* He founded the Center for Sex Research and established the Bonnie and Vern Bullough Collection on Sex and Gender at the library of California State University, Northridge; it is one of the largest such collections in the world. Bullough has published in several different fields, but he has increasingly concentrated on the area of sex and gender. Bullough is a caring nurse and scholar who has played a major role in nursing by analyzing and reporting on its trends.

Biography

Born: July 24, 1928, Salt Lake City, Utah. **Education:** Univ. of Utah (BA); Univ. of Chicago (MA); Univ. of Chicago (PhD); California State Univ., Long Beach (BSN). **Work history:** Faculty, Youngstown (Ohio) Univ., California State Univ.; taught history, social science; Instructor, history of medicine, California College of Medicine; Instructor, School of Public Health, Univ. of California, Los Angeles; Adjunct Professor of Nursing, Dean, Distinguished Professor, State Univ. of New York, Buffalo; Professor, Univ. of Southern California. Outstanding Professor Emeritus, California State Univ., Northridge. **Writings:** *Nursing: A Historical Bibliography; The Frontiers of Sex Research; An Annotated Bibliography of Homosexuality; Florence Nightingale and Her Era: A Collection of New Scholarship.* **Organizations:** member, exec. bd., American Assoc. for History of Nursing (AAHN); editor, AAHN newsletter, 1980–90; member, American Academy of Nursing. **Awards:** Nurse of the Year, *Nurse Week,* 2001; Ray Cox Award, California Nurses Assoc., 2002.

References and Credits

†Bullough VL: personal correspondence, June 2002.

†Bullough, Vern L. Finally we have arrived: Men in nursing. In Dochterman JM, Grace HK: Current Issues in Nursing, 6th ed. St. Louis, CV Mosby, pp 509–510.

About the editors. In Bullough V, Sentz L (eds): American Nursing: A Biographical Dictionary, vol. 3. New York, Springer, 2000, p vi.

July 25

M. Helena McMillan

1869–1970

"Fewer hours for the nurse ... means ... a consciousness of just treatment of the student; a possibility, on the part of the nurse, to profit as she should by her training, ... and in the end better results for the hospital and better results for the school. ... This improvement will have to be made if the schools expect to hold the respect of the public and to continue to attract women of ability. ... The time has come when ancient regulations (such as twelve-hour duty) will no longer be tolerated and we will be compelled to abolish such and substitute modern organization." (1907)

Helena McMillan was a concerned and effective nurse-educator, organizer, activist, and reformer. Her advocacy for the health and welfare of student nurses helped change the focus from training to education. She substituted an eight-hour day for the traditional twelve-hour day, which then was followed by evening classes. She was a leader in professional organizations, and she lobbied repeatedly until Illinois passed the nurse practice act. Her determination to make nursing education a university-level field of study led to programs in Chicago and Cleveland. She is credited with starting the nursing program at the University of Chicago. The school of nursing that she established at Lakeside Hospital in Cleveland became the Frances Payne Bolton School of Nursing at Case Western Reserve University.

Biography

Born: 1869, Montreal. **Education:** McGill Univ., Montreal (BA); Illinois Training School, Chicago; postgraduate course, public health nursing, Henry Street Settlement, N.Y.C. **Work history:** Kingston General Hosp., Ontario, Can.; Superintendent of Nurses, Lakeside Hosp., Cleveland; Superintendent, Presbyterian Hosp., Chicago. **Organizations:** Cleveland Graduate Nurses Assoc.; Ill. Nurses Assoc.; National League for Nursing Education; adviser for coursework, Teachers College, Columbia Univ. **Awards:** Saunders Medal, American Nurses Assoc. **Died:** Boulder, Colo.

References and Credits

†McMillan MH: The physical effect of the three years' course. AJN 7:770, 1907.

Cooper SS: Helena McMillan. In Bullough V, Church OM, Stein AP (eds): American Nursing: A Biographical Dictionary, vol. 1. New York, Garland, 1988, pp 224–226.

July 26

Helen Nahm

1901–1992

"After years of national experience, I have come to the conclusion that in order to solve problems, one has to do it on the local scene. Nursing leaders must get involved at home and challenge younger nurses to do the same. Younger nurses must get involved to bring about important changes in our community and our society." (1977)

"Professional nursing is independent and interdependent practice, in addition to its collaborative functions." (Date unknown)

HER PROFESSIONAL PEERS remember Helen Nahm as one of the most influential American nurse-educators of the midtwentieth century. Her leadership style was characterized by one of her colleagues as one of "pride in achievement as opposed to vanity of ambition." She was sensitive to others yet was someone who could make decisions with which other people might disagree. Her innovations at the University of California, San Francisco, brought an undergraduate program leading to a bachelor of science degree in nursing, an expanded clinical specialty program leading to a master of science in nursing, and a doctoral program in nursing. At that time the San Francisco campus had one of the few advanced nursing programs in the country and the only one in the West. Nahm also is credited with doubling the nursing faculty and student enrollment. In San Francisco she facilitated the growth of the social and behavioral sciences in the nursing department, which led to the first basic science department within a school of nursing. Under her leadership San Francisco's nursing school rose to the very top ranks of American university schools of nursing. While working with the National League for Nursing (NLN), she pioneered efforts to accredit nursing programs. She was a prolific writer and published more than fifty articles in scholarly journals. According to Nahm, "the primary function of graduate programs is to prepare nurses for leadership positions in nursing education and nursing service and for research."

Biography

Born: 1901, Augusta, Mo. **Education:** Univ. of Missouri School of Nursing, (diploma, 1924; BA in zoology, 1926); Univ. of Minnesota, 1946 (MS, PhD). **Work history:** Univ. Hosp., Columbia, Mo.; Instructor, Scott and White Hosp., Temple, Texas, 1927; Surgical and Maternity Nurse, Washington Univ. Hosps., St. Louis, 1930; Instructor, Missouri School of Nursing; Director, Hamline Univ. School of Nursing, St. Paul, Minn.; Director, Division of Nursing Education, Duke Univ.; Dean, School of Nursing, Univ. of California, San Francisco, 1958–60. **Organizations:** Director, National Nursing Accrediting Service, 1950; Director, Dept. of Baccalaureate and Higher Degree Programs, NLN, 1952; Director, Division of Nursing Education, NLN, 1953. **Awards:** Adelaide Nutting Award, NLN, 1967; four honorary doctoral degrees; Distinguished Service Award, Univ. of Minnesota Alumni Assoc., 1977; Honorary Fellow, American Academy of Nursing, 1978; Helen Nahm Research Award, Univ. of California School of Nursing, San Francisco. **Died:** Missouri.

References and Credits

†Safier G: Contemporary American Leaders in Nursing: An Oral History. New York, McGraw-Hill, 1977, p 273.

†Tribute to Dean Helen Nahm, University of California, San Francisco, on-line, available at http://www.sunsite.berkeley.edu.

Dean Helen Nahm, In Memoriam, on-line, available at http://www.library.ucsf.edu.

Struckam P, Styles MM: Helen Nahm. In Bullough V, Sentz L, Stein AP (eds): American Nursing: A Biographical Dictionary, vol. 2. New York, Garland, 1992, pp 239–241.

July 27

Linda Ann Judson Richards
1841–1930

"The nurse is a human being, and the patient is a human being. All your skill will not make you a nurse, if you do not have the right feeling in your heart for your patient. It is lonely to be sick. The nurse can help the sick person in his loneliness by being there to help, not just with the head and the hands, but with the heart." (Date unknown)

LINDA RICHARDS WAS a young teenager when her mother died. She then lived with the family of a local physician, and he allowed her to help with patient care. She later worked as an "assistant nurse" at Boston City Hospital. Although she had no formal nursing preparation, the hospital offered her the position of head nurse after only three months. However, she realized that the position required specific education, so she entered the first class of the nursing school of the New England Hospital for Women and Children. One of the first five graduates of the yearlong program, she is known as "America's first trained nurse," although other schools were in operation. She demonstrated the value of professionally prepared nurses to initially resistant hospital staff. She is credited with introducing patient records and nurses' uniforms. She consulted with Florence Nightingale, studied the Nightingale system, and introduced it at Boston City Hospital, after which it was widely imitated.

She later served as a missionary to Japan and started nursing education programs there. Richards established several nurse training schools, significantly upgraded nursing care in mental hospitals, and helped establish the hospital economics course at Columbia. She was the first stockholder of the American Journal of Nursing Company.

Biography

Born: July 27, 1841, near Potsdam, N.Y. **Education:** New England Hosp. for Women and Children, Boston; studied the Nightingale system in England. **Work history:** Superintendent, Bellevue Training School, N.Y.C.; Superintendent, Boston Training School; helped develop Training School at Boston City Hosp.; missionary work, Japan; established nursing program, Doshisha Hosp., Kyoto, Japan; helped establish hosp. economics program, Columbia Univ.; headed Visiting Nurse Society, Philadelphia; established training school, Philadelphia Methodist Episcopal Hosp.; reorganized nursing schools at Northeast Hosp. for Women and Children, Brooklyn Homeopathic Hosp., and Hartford (Conn.) Hosp.; Superintendent, Training School, Univ. of Pennsylvania Hosp., Philadelphia; improved nursing in mental hospitals, Taunton and Worcester, Mass., Kalamazoo, Mich. **Organizations:** American Society of Superintendents of Training Schools for Nurses. **Awards:** Linda Richards Award, National League for Nursing; member, American Nurses Assoc. Hall of Fame. **Buried:** Forest Hills Cemetery, Boston.

References and Credits

†Baker R: Linda Richards: America's First Trained Nurse. New York, Julian Messner, 1960, p 184.

Bullough V: Linda Ann Judson Richards. In Bullough V, Church OM, Stein AP (eds): American Nursing: A Biographical Dictionary, vol. 1. New York, Garland, 1988, pp 270–272.

ANA Hall of Fame 10/98 American Nurses Association, Washington, D.C. http://www.nursingworld.org/hof.

July 28

Gladys Sellew

1887–1977

"The standard by which to judge good direction ... from poor direction of nursing service on the ward is: Does the patient receive the maximum benefit from the available nursing service? We must never forget that many intangible factors are comprised in the term 'benefit received'—kindness, an atmosphere of peace and quiet, etc. ... The term 'available' must also be interpreted in a spirit of fairness to the ... nurse who carries the work. ... Let the most experienced members in ... nursing ... show what good direction of nursing care under the existing circumstances means. If we cannot achieve the very perfection of nursing, if we cannot give each patient as good nursing care as we desire, let us teach in class what is the ideal and also what we intend to put in practice on the wards. ... We hope for continual improvement, a continual advance toward a continually receding ideal." (1929)

Gladys Sellew was influenced by the work of Jane Adams, and Sellew worked as a volunteer in social services before she answered the 1917 call for nurses by the director of the School of Nursing of the University of Cincinnati. The need for nurses during World War I had created a shortage. Although she was drawn to pediatrics, during her career she also worked as a staff nurse, educator, and author. She wrote many articles and coauthored several books about nursing, some that reflected her interest in sociology and nursing. The influential text that Sellew wrote about ward administration was the first to address time studies and nursing by looking at the number of hours of nursing care required by patients. Her doctoral dissertation about black families in Washington, D.C., is thought to be the first by a nurse to digress from a focus on nursing education. A kind and privately generous person, Sellew quietly demonstrated trust and belief in other people. For example, she provided personal loans to families in need, and all were repaid. She also provided rooms in her home to needy students, without incident.

Biography

Born: July 29, 1887, Cincinnati, Ohio. **Education:** Univ. of Cincinnati (AB, BSN, AM); Catholic Univ. of America (PhD). **Work history:** Pediatric Nurse, Cincinnati General Hosp.; Superintendent, Nursing Service, Babies and Children's Hosp., Cleveland. Ohio; Director of Pediatrics, Cook County Hosp., Chicago; Faculty, Univ. of Cincinnati, Western Reserve, Illinois Training School for Nurses, Catholic Univ., Rosary College, Univ. of Maryland. **Organizations:** American Nurses Assoc. **Awards:** Senior Citizens Award, Oberlin (Ohio) Health Commission; Distinguished Service Award, Oberlin College; Man of the Year Award, *(Oberlin) News Tribune;* recognition by President Richard Nixon. **Died:** Oberlin, Ohio.

References and Credits

†Sellew G: Correlation of theory and practice in relation to ward administration. AJN 29:859–860, 1929.

Sentz L: Gladys Sellew. In Bullough V, Sentz L, Stein AP (eds): American Nursing: A Biographical Dictionary, vol. 2. New York, Garland, 1992, pp 298–300.

Logan L: Eminent teachers: Gladys Sellew, A.B., B.S., A.M., R.N. AJN 29:565–566, 1929.

Renilda E. Hilkemeyer

1915–

"By empowering the nurses we empower the patients." (2000)

"The case studies point out that regardless of how expert we might be in the field of cancer nursing, whenever cancer touches us, the same individual and family reactions and emotions occur as they do in lay individuals. At times like these, we may need to be made aware of the need for help and accept it." (1996)

Renilda Hilkemeyer is renowned internationally as a leader in the specialty of cancer nursing. She helped to write the protocols and policies that provide education for nurses to improve patient care and administer chemotherapy. She was one of the original twenty oncology nurses who founded the Oncology Nursing Society in 1973–1975. It now has more than twenty thousand members. Her courage and determination played a central function in shaping the role of the oncology nurse today. From 1955 to 1977 she was the director of the Department of Nursing and professor of oncology nursing at the University of Texas System Center, M.D. Anderson Hospital and Tumor Institute, in Houston. While there she founded an on-site child care center for Anderson employees, one of the first such sites in the nation. Hilkemeyer served on many local and national committees on nursing and cancer.

She chaired the American Cancer Society (ACS) subcommittee to establish scholarships for graduate work in cancer nursing, as well as the committee to develop the proposal for clinical professorships in oncology nursing. These professorships and scholarships subsequently produced leaders in oncology nursing throughout the country. She was a productive writer and presenter, with more than fifty papers about cancer nursing for national and international journals and audiences.

Biography

Born: July 29, 1915, Martinsburg, Mo. **Education:** St. Louis Univ. School of Nursing and St. Mary's Hosp., St. Louis, 1936 (diploma); George Peabody College for Teachers, Nashville, Tenn., 1947 (BSNE). **Work history:** OR Nurse, Staff Nurse, St. Mary's Hosp., Jefferson City, Mo.; District Public Health Nurse, Mo. Division of Health; Assistant Director, School of Nursing General Hosp. No. 1, Kansas City, Mo.; Consultant, nursing education, Bureau of Cancer Control, Mo. Division of Health; Director, Dept. of Nursing, Professor, Oncology Nursing, Univ. of Texas System Cancer Center, M.D. Anderson Hosp. and Tumor Institute, Houston. **Organizations:** Assistant Exec. Secretary, Mo. State Nurses Assoc. **Awards:** first nurse to receive Distinguished Service Award, American Cancer Society (ACS), 1981, as "an internationally recognized pioneer whose sensitivity and extraordinary effort helped to create the specialty of cancer nursing"; Nursing Leadership Award, ACS, 1989 (first recipient); Distinguished Merit Award, International Society of Nursing in Cancer Care; Renilda Hilkemeyer Child Care Center, which she founded in 1969, named in her honor.

References and Credits

†Hilkemeyer RE: Nurses: Oncology nursing. AJN 100:76, 2000.

†Hilkemeyer R: Foreword to McCorkle R, Grant M, Frank-Stromborg M, Baird SB: Cancer Nursing: A Comprehensive Textbook, 2d ed. Philadelphia, WB Saunders, 1996.

Dudas S: Renilda Hilkemeyer. In Bullough V, Sentz L (eds): American Nursing: A Biographical Dictionary, vol. 3. New York, Springer, 2000, pp 137–140.

July 30

Linda H. Aiken

1943–

"The magnet hospital concept has endured for more than two decades as the single most successful organizational reform to attract and retain highly qualified professional nurses in hospital practice. Magnet hospitals are living evidence that creating professional nurse practice environments is the solution to the flight of nurses from hospital practice. ...Magnet designation to institutions that meet magnet standards of excellence is far more than a reward to an institution and its nurses. It provides valuable information to consumers that enables them to select good hospitals. Magnet status also serves as a guide to nurses in selection of employment, and nursing schools should educate their students about the advantages of magnet hospitals to ensure that nurses themselves support these exemplary institutions." (2002)

As a young girl, Linda Aiken read the Cherry Ames nursing series, the Frank Slaughter medical novels, and was influenced by her mother, a professional who believed that women need careers for economic independence. Linda Aiken was mentored by the nursing leader Dorothy Smith. An early clinical nurse specialist, Aiken is interested in clinical care, research, and advanced coursework. Her studies in medical sociology led to her increased involvement in health policy and nursing research. She stresses the value of risk taking, networking, research, and writing and urges nurses to work with professional groups that reach beyond nursing. Her extensive and continuing professional involvement reinforces her highly regarded expertise on national health care policy and nursing practice. As vice president of the Robert Wood Johnson Foundation, she initiated its decision to fund research that shows care by nurse practitioners improves patient outcomes and is cost effective. She influenced the decision to allow Medicare to give direct reimbursement to nurse practitioners. In 1990 she proposed a restructuring of hospital nursing that recognized different levels of nurse preparation and proposed new roles, such as that of attending nurse. Her current research on patient outcomes and magnet hospitals reinforces the positive relationship between an adequate and empowered professional nursing staff and quality patient care.

Biography

Born: July 29, 1943, Roanoke, Va. **Education:** Univ. of Florida, Gainesville (BSN, MSN); Univ. of Texas, Austin (PhD); Univ. of Wisconsin, Madison (postdoctoral work). **Work history:** Staff Nurse; Clinical Nurse Specialist; Administrator, Robert Wood Johnson Foundation; Professor of Nursing, Professor of Sociology, Univ. of Pennsylvania; Director, Center for Health Outcomes and Policy Research, Univ. of Pennsylvania; Consultant to President Bill Clinton's Health Care Reform Task Force; Research Associate, Population Studies Center, Univ. of Pennsylvania; Senior Fellow, Leonard Davis Institute for Health Economics, Pennsylvania. **Organizations:** numerous committees, Institute of Medicine, National Academy of Sciences (NAS); past president, American Academy of Nursing; committees, National Academy of Social Insurance (NASI); Physician Payment Review Commission; Council on Health Care Economics and Policy; National Advisory Council for Health Care Policy, Research, and Evaluation; Pa. State Nurses Assoc.; American Nurses Assoc. (ANA). **Awards:** Barbara Thomas Curtis Award, ANA; Baxter Episteme Laureate, Sigma Theta Tau International; Distinguished Pathfinder Research Award, Friends of National Institute of Nursing Research (NINR); one of eleven nurses nationally to receive continuous funding from NINR; Media Award, American Academy of Nursing (AAN); member, American Academy of Arts and Sciences; election to Institute of Medicine, NAS; Fellow, AAN; Distinguished Fellow, Assoc. for Health Services Research; NASI; Honorary Fellow, Royal College of Nursing, U.K.; honorary doctorates, Emory Univ., Georgetown Univ., Univ. of Wisconsin.

References and Credits

†Aiken L: Superior outcomes for magnet hospitals: The evidence base. In McClure M, Hinshaw A: Magnet Hospitals Revisited: Attraction and Retention of Professional Nurses. Washington, D.C., American Nurses Publishing, American Nurses Association, 2002, p 77.

References and Credits continued on page 769

JULY 31

Isabel Adams Hampton Robb

1860–1910

"In your professional life you have learned that we may dress and nurse a wound ever so carefully, but that all of your work represents time and energy expended in vain, that a breakdown of the wound is inevitable did not the surgeon first clean and scrape away all the diseased tissues, reaching deep down into the fresh healthy part until no germ or disease was left to impair the growth of new, healthy flesh. And so it is with our work in caring for humanity in other ways—we are but staying a worse condition perhaps, but not removing the cause if we rest satisfied with mere treatment and do not direct our best energies towards prevention." (1907)

ISABEL ROBB HAS been called "the architect of American nursing" by the writer Nancy Noel. Robb initiated major changes in nursing education and organization. While in Chicago, she introduced the first grading policy for nursing studies and practices in the country. She also increased affiliations for students and eliminated private duty nursing by students, which benefited hospitals and took away from valuable study time. She also helped to develop the school of nursing at the highly regarded Johns Hopkins Hospital. Her classic text, *Nursing: Its Principles and Practice,* was published in 1894. She helped establish the American Society of Superintendents of

Training Schools for Nurses (later the National League for Nursing), the Nurses Associated Alumnae of the United States and Canada (later the American Nurses Association), and the *American Journal of Nursing*. Although she stopped working as a nurse after marriage and motherhood, she continued to be involved with nursing issues as a volunteer. She proposed a three-year program for nursing education, a reform that was eventually adopted. She helped develop the course in hospital economics that led to the Department of Nursing at Columbia University, and, in the interest of educational standards, she helped form the International Council of Nurses (ICN). Robb died at fifty when she was struck by a streetcar en route to see her son.

Biography

Born: July 1860, Welland, Ontario, Can. **Education:** St. Catherines Collegiate Institute, Ontario (teaching certificate); Bellevue Hosp. Training School for Nurses, N.Y.C. **Work history:** Nurse, St. Paul's House, Rome, Italy; Superintendent, Illinois Training School for Nurses, Cook County Hosp., Chicago; helped develop, then administer School of Nursing, Johns Hopkins Hosp.; Instructor, Lakeside Hosp. Training School for Nurses, Cleveland, Ohio. **Organizations:** founder, ICN; bd. member, Lakeside Hosp., Cleveland; Cleveland Visiting Nurse Assoc.; American Red Cross; numerous other groups. **Awards:** Isabel Hampton Robb Scholarship Fund; American Nurses Assoc. Hall of Fame. **Buried:** Burlington, N.J.

References and Credits

†Robb IH: Educational Standards for Nurses: With Other Addresses on Nursing Subjects. Cleveland, Ohio, EC Koekert, 1907, p 218.

Noel NL: Isabel Robb. In Bullough V, Church OM, Stein AP (eds): American Nursing: A Biographical Dictionary, vol. 1. New York, Garland, 1988, pp 274–276.

ANA Hall of Fame 10/98 American Nurses Association, Washington, D.C. http://www.nursingworld.org/hof.

Noel N: Isabel Hampton Robb: Architect of American Nursing [thesis]. New York, Teachers College, Columbia University, 1978.

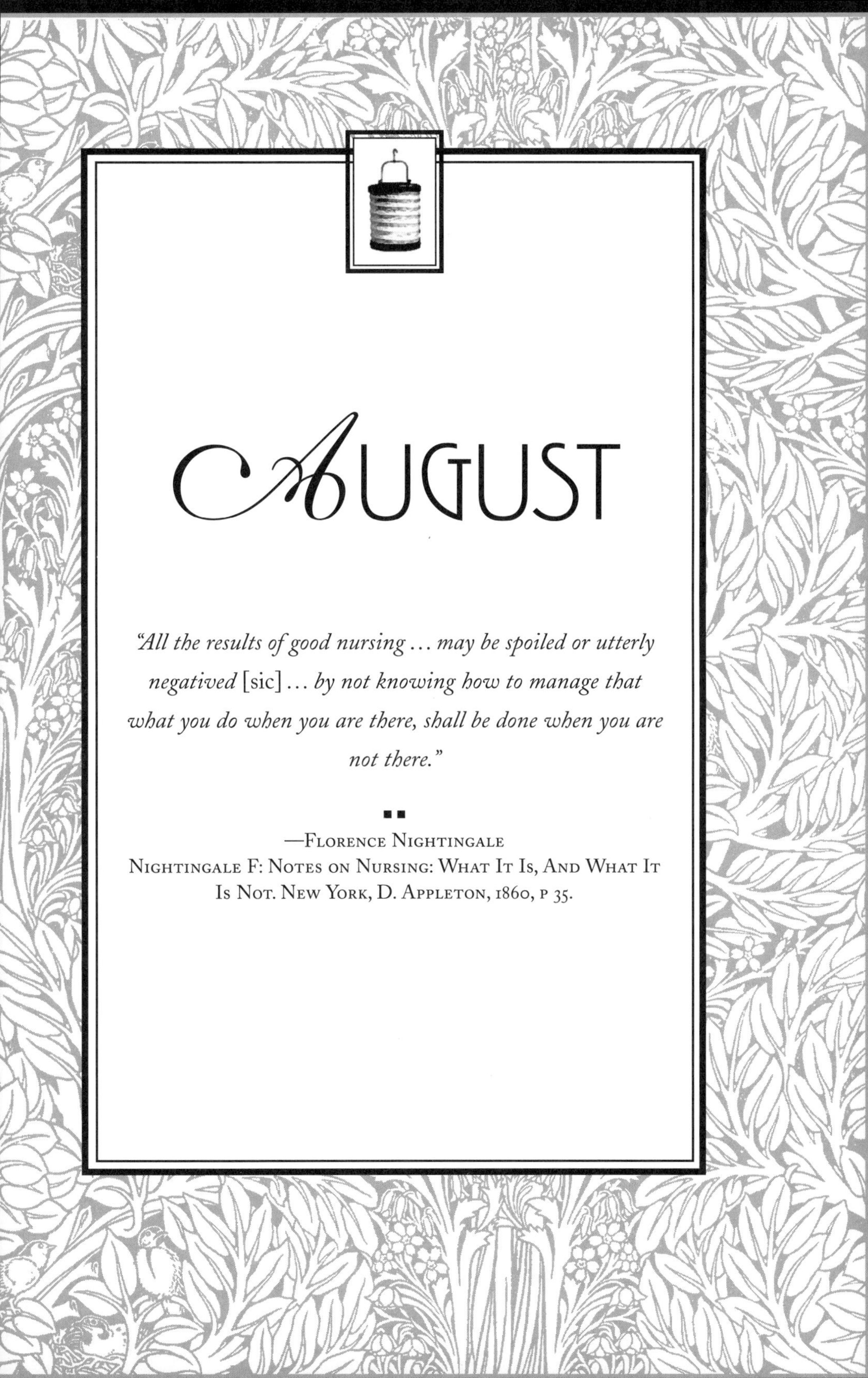

AUGUST

"All the results of good nursing ... may be spoiled or utterly negatived [sic] *... by not knowing how to manage that what you do when you are there, shall be done when you are not there."*

—Florence Nightingale

Nightingale F: Notes on Nursing: What It Is, And What It Is Not. New York, D. Appleton, 1860, p 35.

August 1

Dolores Krieger

1921–

"Healing, which is the foremost function of Therapeutic Touch, could be called a humanization of energy in the interest of helping or healing others or oneself. The first thing you do when learning Therapeutic Touch, and frequently the major factor for learning it, is to heal yourself, which is proper and perhaps even necessary. ...How the process proceeds depends on your ability to discriminate among the subtle cues of the healee's energy-field dynamics. ...In general, healing might be described as the conscious, full engagement of your energies in the interest of helping another. With Therapeutic Touch, this interest arises from a sense of compassion and a recognition that there is an underlying order in the universe." (1993)

INSPIRED BY SISTER KENNY, the Australian physical therapist who brought an innovative polio treatment to the United States, Dolores Krieger decided to become a nurse and work her way through college to study physical therapy. But after six months she wanted to study only nursing. Health professionals now know her as the nursing pioneer whose research and development gave the world therapeutic touch. What began as postdoctoral research in 1972, with colleague Dora Kunz, is now acknowledged as a widely used alternative healing approach. When Krieger taught

"Frontiers of Nursing" at New York University, in the mid-1970s, she recalled during a 1994 lecture, "it was the first time in recorded history that healing had been taught within a fully accredited university curriculum." Since then she has taught the technique, which she describes as a contemporary interpretation of ancient healing practices, to more than forty thousand health professionals. Based on science, it has been taught in more than eighty colleges and universities in this country, and in seventy-three foreign countries. Therapeutic touch allows a skilled healer to focus on the illness by working to correct the imbalance in the patient's energy field. Krieger reminds health professionals that old perceptions change based on knowledge and experience and that they need to be open to new ideas and findings that expand the human potential for healing.

Biography

Born: Aug. 1, 1921, Paterson, N.J. **Education:** Westchester (N.Y.) School of Nursing (RN); New York Univ. (BS, MA, PhD). **Work history:** Clinical Nurse, Faculty, New York Univ. Division of Nursing; Writer; Lecturer; Researcher; developed therapeutic touch. **Organizations:** founder, N.Y. Student Nurses Assoc.; Founder, honorary member, Nurse Healers–Professional Associates International. **Awards:** New York Univ. Distinguished Alumnus Award; Harry S. Truman Lecturer, Avila College; Martha E. Rogers Award, National League for Nursing; Alyce and Elmer Green Award for Excellence, International Society for the Study of Subtle Energies and Energy Medicine; New York Univ. Scholarship in Nursing Award; Professor Emerita, New York Univ.

References and Credits

†Krieger D: Accepting Your Power to Heal. Rochester, Vt., Bear, 1993, pp 16–18.

Krieger D: Therapeutic touch: An optional and radical perception. Distinguished Guest Lecture for Alternative and Complementary Medicine Elective. New York, College of Physicians and Surgeons, Columbia Univ., March 9, 1994, p 4.

Krieger D: personal communication, 2002.

AUGUST 2

Nell Viola Beeby

1896–1957

"The nurse recognizes ... that her patient will not learn unless he is interested. ... Her unintentional as well as her intentional teaching must be considered. She has been eminently successful if she has shown by her own attitudes and activities how to manage and conserve one's mental and physical health with what one has, how to get along with the family, how to give one's work a little more than is required." (1936)

NELL VIOLA BEEBY specialized in obstetrics after graduating from nursing school. Her practical and caring nature while working with mothers and babies made her popular with the families. The daughter of missionary parents, she wanted to do missionary nursing. When there were no openings, she applied to the Yale-in-China program and taught in China until the Chinese Civil War in 1927. Upon her return to the United States she was hired by the *American Journal of Nursing.* While working as an editor there she accepted an short assignment to serve as a foreign correspondent in Europe in 1945. When she returned to the *Journal,* she promoted a focus on new developments in nursing as well as educational and international issues. To publicize and promote nursing research she proposed the formation of the American Journal of Nursing Company and saw *Nursing Research* and *Nursing Outlook* begin under her leadership. Research funding for nursing issues was made possible with the Roberts Fellowship and the establishment of the Sophia Palmer Library. The National League for Nursing (NLN) honored Beeby "for her adaptation of nursing practice to universal need."

Biography

Born: Aug. 1, 1896, Secunderabad, India. **Education:** St. Luke's Hosp., Chicago; Teachers College, Columbia Univ. (BS). **Work history:** Private Duty Nurse, OB Nurse, Supervisor, St. Luke's Hosp., Chicago; Instructor, Supervisor, Yale-in-China Nursing School; Editor, Foreign Correspondent, Editor in Chief, *American Journal of Nursing;* Exec. Editor, American Journal of Nursing Co. **Organizations:** Ill. State Nurses Assoc.; American Nurses Assoc.; International Council of Nurses. **Awards:** Adelaide Nutting Award, NLN. **Died:** Jackson Heights, N.Y.

References and Credits

†Beeby NV: The private duty nurse as teacher. AJN 36:780, 1936.

Cleveland S: Nell Beeby. In Bullough V, Church OM, Stein AP (eds): American Nursing: A Biographical Dictionary, vol. 1. New York, Garland, 1988, pp 24–26.

Hazel Avis Goff

1892–1973

"Be ready to give our best and then, wherever we go, all persons will have the highest regard for what we represent in nursing. ...There is but one legitimate reason for undertaking pioneer nursing work in another land—that is deep interest in the people and the confidence that your knowledge of nursing care can be used to help those people help themselves—*in improving their nursing methods ...Plant the seeds of your idea with a key person. Water it from time to time with smiles and jokes and compliments and, one day, you will be presented with a lovely blossom which she thinks is hers. Do you care? Emphatically no; you are seeking results not commendation for bright ideas. ...Keep on sowing similar seeds, and at the end of a year when you count your blossoms or compile your report, you will be surprised at the harvest." (1943)*

Hazel Goff did international nursing with the Red Cross, the Rockefeller Foundation, and the League of Nations. After service as an army nurse in France during World War I, she was sent by the Red Cross to start a nursing program in Bulgaria. She recruited American nurses to establish or help develop nursing schools in war-torn countries and taught those nurses to be effective leaders. She taught the nurses how important it was to learn about and respect the existing culture, and she explained why it was necessary to integrate into the community and to involve community leaders in decision making. She was also a nurse consultant to many European countries when she was field director for the Rockefeller Foundation. She was sponsored by the International Council of Nurses to be the first nurse in the health division of the League of Nations. After the league asked her to survey public health needs in ten countries, her subsequent specific recommendations led to changes in public health coursework.

Biography

Born: Aug. 1892, Leeds, Quebec, Can. **Education:** Normal School, Framingham, Mass.; Massachusetts General Hosp. Training School for Nurses, Boston; Teachers College, Columbia Univ. (BS). **Work history:** Red Cross army nurse; Superintendent of Nurses, Blodgett Memorial Hosp., Grand Rapids, Mich.; helped establish, then directed Red Cross nursing school in Bulgaria; European Field Director, Rockefeller Foundation; League of Nations health section; organized rural public health, Balkans; organized nursing school, Istanbul; Director of Nursing, St. Luke's Hosp., Cleveland, Ohio; Lecturer, Columbia Univ.; reorganized technical nursing school, Lisbon, Portugal; Staff, National League for Nursing Education; Director of Nursing, Allegheny (Pa.) General Hosp.; Director of Nursing, Madison (Wisc.) General Hosp.; Lecturer, Univ. of Pennsylvania School of Nursing. **Organizations:** Sigma Theta Tau; Chi Eta Phi. **Awards:** special recognition by queen of Bulgaria for work in public health nursing; Honorary Recognition Award, Pennsylvania Nurses Assoc. **Buried:** Riverside Cemetery, Grafton, Mass.

References and Credits

†Goff H: Preparing for postwar work abroad. AJN 43:169–171, 1943.

Cooper SS: Hazel Goff. In Bullough V, Church OM, Stein AP (eds): American Nursing: A Biographical Dictionary, vol. 1. New York, Garland, 1988, pp 139–141.

August 4

Lucy Lincoln Drown

1848–1934

"When you have done everything that you can do for a dangerously ill patient, remember to say a little prayer for him." (Date unknown)

"I still seem to be one of the links between the distant past and the present. …My mind has gone back many times to that coterie of women, profound earnest women, who met together so many years ago to consider the problems that are so familiar to you. They came so fast that we hardly knew which one to choose first. The proper admission qualifications for the candidates for the training schools, the length of the course, the curriculum of study, the better character of the nurses, the better preparation of the teachers—all these and many more had to be met as best we could. And as I look back on all the pictures on memory's walls there come before me some of the faces that I wish could assemble here tonight …Miss Hampton … Miss Darche … Miss Kimber … Miss Dock … Miss McIsaac … Miss Palmer. … I would like to go on and name those dear names and have you see some of them as I and others see them. Years have gone … progress thus has become manifest … [and] as years go on we begin to look to you for leaders to a higher sphere." (1923)

LUCY LINCOLN DROWN taught public school for twelve years before she entered nursing school in Boston. Her strong administrative abilities were evident while she was a student, and after she finished the program, she worked as an assistant to Linda Richards, the then-superintendent of nurses and director of the Nurse Training Program at Boston City Hospital. Drown succeeded Richards when Richards left. During the next twenty-five years Drown did much to improve nursing and nursing education through her commitment to the profession. She was compassionate and thoughtful in contacts with students and patients. The alumnae group that she helped establish later merged with the alumnae group of Massachusetts General Hospital and became the Massachusetts State Nurses Association to support nursing registration. She wrote a column on nursing issues for the *American Journal of Nursing* and started a journal club at the school, where students would read and discuss professional publications. Drown was involved with nursing at the local, national, and international levels, always focused on improving standards for nursing.

Biography

Born: Aug. 4, 1848, Providence, R.I. **Education:** normal school, Salem, Mass. (course in teaching); Boston City Hosp. **Work history:** Assistant, Superintendent of Nurses, Head of Nurse Training Program, Boston City Hosp. **Organizations:** Alumni Assoc., Boston City Hosp. Training School for Nurses; International Congress of Nurses; Suffolk County (Mass.) Nurses Assoc.; Mass. State Nurses Assoc.; charter member, American Society of Superintendents of Training Schools for Nurses. **Awards:** residence at Boston City Hosp. named in her honor. **Buried:** near Concord, N.H.

References and Credits

†Gladwin, Mary. Ethics: Talks to Nurses. Philadelphia, WB Saunders, 1930, p 95.

†Drown LL: An address. AJN 23:923, 1923.

McNeely AG, Palmer IS: Lucy Drown. In Bullough V, Church OM, Stein AP (eds): American Nursing: A Biographical Dictionary, vol. 1. New York, Garland, 1988, pp 101–103.

August 5

John Devereaux Thompson

1917–1992

"The new nurse has heightened responsibilities in addition to her redefined role and critical interrelationships with the individual patient. There is a strong bond between these newer professional roles, on the one hand, and broader nurse involvement in the total health care delivery system, on the other. For unless nurses can effectively bring about changes in the way health care is evaluated and delivered in this country, their new roles may never emerge from the inadequacies, illogical constraints, and irrational decision options which now characterize both the system itself and the nurses role in it." (1980)

A PHYSICIAN UNCLE ENCOURAGED John Thompson to attend nursing school because it was a practical way to get an education during the depression. When Thompson finished nursing school, he worked for a short time as a hospital staff nurse, then joined the navy. He served as a pharmacist's mate aboard ship during World War II and later studied hospital administration at Yale University. This allowed him to combine his growing interest in the value of statistics and nursing history, specifically, Nightingale and her use of statistics to improve hospital management. He worked for several years as an assistant to the director of Montefiore Hospital in New York before he returned to Yale as a faculty member in hospital administration. The recipient of numerous grants, he collaborated on research that studied and influenced hospital services, economics, and nurse staffing by applying statistical data to hospital costs and operations. He taught hospital administration for decades and held a joint appointment to the School of Nursing. The writer Edward J. Halloran has described him as patient centered, "a unique and special teacher who helped humanize hospital administration." He saw the "new nurse" evolve from the nurse practitioner movement, primary nurse responsibilities, and the expanded expectations of technical expertise. He is noted as the originator of the concept of the diagnostic-related groups (DRGs), which changed the method of hospital payments for patients to a rate determined by physicians and became the standard for reimbursement for Medicare.

Biography

Born: Aug. 6, 1917, Franklin, Pa. **Education:** Ohio State Univ.; Mills Training School for Men Nurses, Bellevue Hosp., N.Y.C.; City College of New York (bachelor's degree in business); Yale Univ. (hosp. administration). **Work history:** Staff Nurse; Pharmacist's Mate, U.S. Navy, World War II; Assistant to the Director, Montefiore Hosp., Bronx, N.Y.; Assistant Director, Professor, Director of hosp. administration program, Yale Univ.; joint appointment to Yale School of Nursing. Writings: *Leuven Lectures* (Belgium) on reimbursement. **Organizations:** member, bd. of directors, New Haven Visiting Nurse Assoc.; Adviser, Trustee, Conn. Hospice. **Awards:** Baxter Prize for contributions to Health Service Research (shared with Robert Fetter). **Died:** New Haven, Conn.

References and Credits

†Thompson JD: The passionate humanist: From Nightingale to the new nurse. *Nurs Outlook* 28:291, 1980.

Halloran EJ: John Thompson. In Bullough V, Sentz L (eds): American Nursing: A Biographical Dictionary, vol. 3. New York, Springer, 2000, p 271.

August 6

Susie (Baker) King Taylor
1848–1912

"It seems strange how our aversion to seeing suffering is overcome in war,—how we are able to see the most sickening sights, such as men with their limbs blown off and mangled by the deadly shells, without a shudder; and instead of turning away, how we hurry to assist in alleviating their pain, bind up their wounds, and press the cool water to their parched lips, with feelings only of sympathy and pity. ... There are many people who do not know what some of the colored women did during the war. There were hundreds of them who assisted the Union soldiers by hiding them and helping them to escape. Many were punished for taking food to the prison stockades for the prisoners. ... These things should be kept in history before the people. There has never been a greater war in the United States than the one of 1861, where so many lives were lost—not men alone, but noble women as well. I gave my services willingly for four years and three months without receiving a dollar. I was glad, however, to be allowed to go with the regiment, to care for the sick and afflicted comrades." (1902)

SUSIE (BAKER) KING TAYLOR was born a slave off the coast of Georgia. As a young child she moved to her grandmother's home in Savannah, where she was secretly and illegally taught to read and write. The writer Karen Buchinger reports that, in 1862, Taylor fled with an uncle and others to St. Catherine's Island, which was controlled by the Union Army. She married a black volunteer for the Union Army when she was fourteen and traveled with his regiment for four years. She worked first as a laundress, but her literacy, compassionate nursing skills, and ability to use medicinal plants made her a more valuable asset in the care of the sick and wounded. She also worked with Clara Barton in South Carolina and the Sea Islands. Despite Taylor's documented service as a volunteer nurse, she was never able to collect benefits because she had not signed contract papers, a technicality. When she was living in Boston after being widowed and remarrying, she did much to help war veterans claim their entitlements. Her *Reminiscences of My Life in Camp* ...preserves her observations about the war, her involvement, and its effect on the human spirit. The cruelty to blacks in the South after the war made her wonder whether the war had been waged in vain, and her own postwar travels there to care for her terminally ill son exposed her to continued discrimination and prejudice.

Biography

Born: Aug. 6, 1848, Isle of Wight, Va. **Education:** home schooled. **Work history:** volunteer nurse, Civil War; opened schools for black children, adults, Savannah, Ga.; domestic helper for northern families; organized Boston branch of the Woman's Relief Corps. **Organizations:** Woman's Relief Corps. **Awards:** unknown. **Died:** Boston.

References and Credits

†Taylor SBK: Reminiscences of My Life in Camp with the 33rd U.S. Colored Troops, Late 1st South Carolina Volunteers: A Black Woman's Civil War Memoirs. New York, Markus Wiener, 1988, pp 88, 52, 142.

Buchinger K: Susie (Baker) King Taylor. In Bullough V, Sentz L, Stein AP (eds): American Nursing: A Biographical Dictionary, vol. 2. New York, Garland, 1992, pp 319–321.

August 7

Anne Lucippa Austin

1891–1986

"Direct contact with the actual words of those who took part in the events ... has the power to evoke a strong sense of reality, as well as to make a deep and lasting impression not always created by a secondhand account. Those who were eyewitnesses or participants have much to teach us, if we listen to them judiciously. We read them to gain not only a feeling of the times but also the facts recorded at the time, albeit with human bias but without the intrusion of the interpretation of others which may throw shadows on them or detract from their charm. ... The extent to which it is possible for the reader to enter into the spirit of the times of which the narrator writes will somewhat determine his degree of understanding of the present." (1957)

ANNE LUCIPPA AUSTIN instilled in her students the importance of precise, meticulous documentation. This was also an essential and important quality of her own historical nursing research. She wrote several books and articles on nursing history and received the Columbia University Nursing Education Alumni Award in recognition of her *History of Nursing Source Book.* She collaborated with Isabel Stewart to write *A History of Nursing from Ancient to Modern Times,* and Austin contributed the biography of Stewart for *Notable American Women.* Austin was drawn to firsthand accounts of history makers. She served as an army nurse during World War I, a Red Cross instructor, and taught nursing at the university level. Her unpublished papers see nursing's need to define itself clearly to the public. She also addressed the need for male nurses, writing: "The place for men nurses: Two questions: Is there a future for men from the standpoint of their own personal careers and lives? Is there a major place for men from the standpoint of the patient? Now in 1977, I answer 'yes' to both questions."

Biography

Born: Aug. 7, 1891, Ischua, N.Y. **Education:** Buffalo (N.Y.) Homeopathic Hosp. Training School (diploma). **Work history:** private practice, Buffalo, N.Y.; Army Nurse Corps; Red Cross nurse; Lockport (N.Y.) City Hosp.; Instructor, Buffalo Homeopathic Hosp. School of Nursing; Administrator, Farrand Training School of Nurses, Harper Hosp., Detroit; Faculty, Frances Payne Bolton School of Nursing, Western Reserve Univ., Cleveland, Ohio; Teachers College, Columbia Univ.; Univ. of California, Los Angeles; Univ. of Pennsylvania School of Nursing. **Organizations:** National League for Nursing. **Awards:** honorary member, Alumni Assoc. of Frances Payne Bolton and Fillmore Hosp. Schools of Nursing; Alumni Award, Teachers College, Columbia Univ. **Buried:** Cold Springs Cemetery, Lockport, N.Y.

References and Credits

†Austin AL: History of Nursing Source Book. New York, GP Putnam's, 1957, pp 7–8.

Brunner LS: Anne Austin. In Bullough V, Church OM, Stein AP (eds): American Nursing: A Biographical Dictionary, vol. 1. New York, Garland, 1988, pp 13–14.

AUGUST 8

Elizabeth Kerr Porter

1894–1989

"It is impossible to carry well our share of the responsibility for adequate service in hospitals and homes, for joint action with allied professional and lay groups, for research projects, for International Exchange–Visitor Programs, and for membership in World Health Organization teams, unless we understand conditions responsible for man's present ills and his impaired health. Parallel with this first challenge, especially in this Florence Nightingale Centennial Year, is the call to study anew the history of nursing that we may accept added responsibilities imposed by a legacy such as ours in nursing education, nursing experience, and nursing opportunity, and that, without making a break with the past, we may emerge from past professional performance to a broader and more efficient service." (1954)

ELIZABETH PORTER WAS committed to organizing and protecting the economic security of nurses. She spoke out in defense of nurses' rights to organize for that purpose. Her leadership, educational, and administrative skills made her contributions to nursing legendary. She served two terms as president of the American Nurses Association (ANA). During her tenure she played an essential role in consolidating the six existing national nursing organizations into two major associations. She also strengthened the ANA's economic security program; improved employment conditions for nurses; increased nursing representation on national boards and commissions; eliminated racial restrictions for membership in the ANA; and formed the National Student Nurses Council. She served on many boards and in high offices of other nursing associations. She reminded nurses in 1952 that "the American Nurses Association can be only as strong as individuals are strong for collective action, and that strength must be fostered in district and state groups."

Biography

Born: 1894, Pittsburgh, Pa. **Education:** Western Pennsylvania Hosp. School of Nursing, 1930; Teachers College, Columbia Univ., 1935 (BS); Univ. of Pennsylvania, 1936 (MS); Univ. of Pennsylvania School of Nursing, 1946 (EdD). **Work history:** coordinator, advanced clinical nursing program, Professor, Univ. of Pennsylvania Hosp. School of Nursing; Faculty, Professor, Director, graduate program in nursing, Dean, Francis Payne Bolton School of Nursing, Case Western Reserve Univ., Cleveland, Ohio. **Organizations:** President, ANA, 1950–54; President, Ohio Nurses Assoc., 1958–60; Vice President, American Nurses Foundation; member, bd. of directors, National Health Council. **Awards:** Pa. Ambassadorial Award, 1954; Florence Nightingale Medal, International Committee, Red Cross; honorary doctorate, Univ. of Pennsylvania; ANA Hall of Fame. **Died:** location unknown.

References and Credits

†Porter E: Calling American Nurses to Action, speech to Thirty-Ninth Convention of ANA, April 26–30, 1954, Chicago. In Flanagan L: One Strong Voice: The Story of the American Nurses Association. Kansas City, Mo., Lowell Press, 1976, pp 510–526.

American Nurses Association on-line, available at http://www.ana.org/hof/portek.htm.

ANA Hall of Fame 10/98 American Nurses Association, Washington, D.C. http://www.nursingworld.org/hof.

August 9

Frances Slanger

1913–1944

"It is 0200 and I have been lying awake for about one hour, listening to the steady, even breathing of the other three nurses in the tent. Thinking about some of the things we had discussed during the day. The rain is beating down on the tent with a torrential force. The wind is on a mad rampage. The fire is burning low and just a few live coals are on the bottom. With the slow feeding of wood, and finally coal, a roaring fire is started. I couldn't help thinking how similar to a human being a fire is; if it is allowed to run down too low and if there is a spark of life left in it, it can be nursed back. So can a human being. It is slow, it is gradual, it is done all the time in these Field Hospitals and other hospitals in the ETO [European Theater Operations]. ...We have learned a lot about our American boy and the stuff he is made of. The wounded do not cry. ...It is we who are proud of you, a great distinction to see you open your eyes and with that swell of American grin, say "Hiya, Babe."" (1944)

SECOND LT. FRANCES SLANGER was an army nurse who stood less than five feet tall, had a terrific sense of humor, and nearly drowned as she waded ashore in Normandy with the 45th Field Hospital's second platoon three days after D-Day. She was outspoken and a hard worker. Shortly after she wrote the letter quoted,

German artillery attacked the field hospital near Elsenborn, Belgium, about twenty miles from the German border, and hit Slanger's tent with fragments. She was mortally wounded on October 21, 1944, the first American nurse to die in action in Europe. Dr. John Bonzer, who was with Slanger when she died, said she was as brave in the face of death as she was in life. She is buried in a military cemetery in France between the fighting men whom she had so admired and tried to save. Many soldiers wrote to *Stars and Stripes* after reading her moving remarks. As the columnist Bob Welch recounted more than fifty years later, one soldier wrote, "You were here merely because you felt you were needed. ...If the world had a few more people like you in it, there wouldn't be any wars."

Biography

Born: Aug. 9, 1913, Poland. **Education:** Boston City Hosp., 1937. **Work history:** U.S. Army Nurse Corps. **Organizations:** unknown. **Awards:** Lt. Frances Slanger Memorial Post, chapter of Jewish War Veterans of the USA formed in Boston by Jewish women veterans of World War II. **Died:** Elsenborn, Belgium.

References and Credits

†Slanger F: An army nurse writes an editorial. AJN 45:1, 1945.

Welch B: Frances Slanger. (Eugene, Ore.) Register-Guard, Dec. 19, 2000.

August 10

Mildred L. Montag

1908–

"The purpose of the project was to prepare the bedside nurse, for it was felt that the need for this kind of nurse was great. The graduates expressed pleasure in giving direct care to patients and concern when they were not permitted to do so because auxiliary personnel were so assigned. Nursing service must answer the question of who shall give direct nursing care to patients. If all nursing care is to be given by auxiliary nursing personnel, are they not in effect nurses? Is there not a place at the bedside for the highly skilled technician and for the professional nurse as well? It is not enough to place the blame for the present situation on the so-called shortage of nurses. It requires a re-evaluation of what constitutes nursing care, and by whom it should be given. ...There is a need for the registered nurse at the bedside. ...The nurse must be permitted to do nursing and to do it well if she is to receive satisfaction from the job of nursing and to wish to continue doing it." (1959)

MILDRED MONTAG IS a nurse educator, researcher, and author who supports levels of entry for practice. Her doctoral dissertation explored the possibility of preparing bedside duty nurses through a technical nursing education program at the community college level. She then served as director of the research project that put her proposal into practice. She worked with Louise McManus, who obtained funding to carry out the study, which was based on Montag's thesis. This landmark effort established the associate degree program in nursing. The study showed that a two-year program, with carefully planned coursework and clinical affiliations, could produce competent direct care nurses whose state board examination scores and performance were equal to and often better than those of diploma graduates. Montag saw a need for technical nurse preparation at community colleges and envisioned a complimentary health care approach that would use skills of both the professional practitioner and nurse technician. Influenced by the findings and ideas of McManus, Montag developed and taught the first course on leadership and team nursing and saw the team approach defined by patients' needs.

Biography

Born: Aug. 10, 1908, Struble, Iowa. **Education:** Hamline Univ., St. Paul, Minn. (BA); Univ. of Minnesota (BS in nursing); Teachers College, Columbia Univ. (master's, doctorate). **Work history:** Faculty, Univ. of Minnesota School of Nursing, St. Luke's School of Nursing, N.Y.C.; Director, School of Nursing, Adelphi College; Professor of Nursing, Teachers College, Columbia Univ.; Professor Emeritus, Teachers College, Columbia Univ.; Author. **Organizations:** unknown. **Awards:** first recipient, Linda Richards Award, National League for Nursing, for pioneering work in nursing; honorary doctoral degrees from Bridgeport (Conn.) Univ., Adelphi Univ., State University of New York, Eastern Kentucky Univ.; Distinguished Alumni Awards, Univ. of Minnesota, Hamline Univ., Teachers College, Columbia Univ.; Honorary Fellow, College of Nursing, New South Wales, Australia.

References and Credits

†Montag M: Community College Education for Nursing: An Experiment in Technical Education for Nursing. New York, McGraw-Hill, 1959, pp 359–360.

Safier G: Contemporary American Leaders in Nursing: An Oral History. New York, McGraw-Hill, 1977.

Kalisch P, Kalisch B: The Advance of American Nursing. Philadelphia, JB Lippincott, 1995.

Buchinger KL: Mildred L. Montag. In Bullough V, Sentz L, Stein AP (eds): American Nursing: A Biographical Dictionary, vol. 2. New York, Garland, 1992, pp 228–230.

Montag M: personal communication, 2003.

August 11

Margene Olive Faddis

1900–1983

"What do I believe about nursing? After 45 years one has many beliefs and after retirement one has more time to ... look at one side and then turn them over and look at the other. Life is made up of contrasts. Perhaps you can see progress more clearly. You may be a little more patient about the present and a little more hopeful about the future. We will expect much more from the present generation of nurses, chiefly because they have had more education in critical areas. The problems are many and serious, but we have increasing numbers of nurses who are prepared to help solve them and who are eager to be about it because they have little patience with the status quo. Most important of all is a growing emphasis on the basic function of nursing without which we can never be a true profession. Many of our most urgent and frustrating problems have arisen, at least in part, because we have often wandered too far from that focus." (1965)

ILLNESS CLAIMED BOTH her brothers, one as an adult and one as an adolescent, and this may have drawn Margene Faddis to nursing. During her career as an educator she emphasized clinical competence and believed that the educational standards in baccalaureate programs for nursing were the basis for professional recognition. As a faculty member at the Frances Payne Bolton School of Nursing at Case Western Reserve University, her visionary leadership influenced curriculum and practice. While teaching, she also cared for her ill and aging parents at home. This may have heightened her commitment to integrating geriatric nursing coursework into the nursing program. An accomplished woman with wide-ranging interests, she published nursing texts as well as histories of the Frances Payne Bolton School of Nursing. She was compassionate, dedicated, scholarly, and exceptional.

Biography

Born: Aug. 15, 1900, Mt. Vernon, Ohio. **Education:** Lakeside Hosp. School of Nursing, Cleveland; Western Reserve Univ. (BS, MA). **Work history:** Lakeside Hosp., Cleveland; Pasadena Calif. General Hosp.; Faculty, Frances Payne Bolton School of Nursing, Cleveland; member, editorial bd., *American Journal of Nursing*. **Organizations:** American Nurses Assoc. (ANA); American Assoc. of Univ. Professors; American Gerontological Society. **Awards:** Professor Emeritus, Case Western Reserve Univ.; Distinguished Alumnus Award, Frances Payne Bolton School of Nursing; honorary doctorate, Case Western Reserve Univ.; ANA award for contributions to the profession. **Died:** Cleveland, Ohio.

References and Credits

†Faddis M: This I believe ... Nurs Outlook 13:26, 28, 1965.

Cooper SS: Margene Faddis. In Bullough V, Sentz L, Stein AP (eds): American Nursing: A Biographical Dictionary, vol. 2. New York, Garland, 1992, pp 105–108.

August 12

Mary Roberts Rinehart

1876–1958

"This story has been honest, as honest as I have been able to make it. It is the truth, but it is not all of the truth. … I have no desire to hurt the living, and I have respected the dead. How accurate I have been I do not know. …Our very memories deceive us. For the unpleasant we set up the defensive machinery of forgetfulness, and not all of us can bear all of the truth, even about ourselves. I am not through. I am still going on. This look backward has been indeed but to refresh the eye, for its prime function of looking forward. I am still strong, very active. …And I still work very hard. I have left this manuscript … to see friends … to go about, to live and learn. …We have many friends, my husband and I, and often it seems to me that all of life comes down to that, to human relationships, and that nothing else really matters." (1931)

As a high school student, Mary Roberts Rinehart had some personal experience in nursing her very sick mother. But her initial goal was to be a doctor. She enrolled in nursing school because she was too young to be admitted to medical school, and she was one of the five hundred qualified nurses in the country when she graduated in 1896. She married a surgeon soon after school and began writing as a young mother in order to help with family finances. Called nursing's most prolific author of fiction, this popular writer produced more than sixty books during her lifetime. During World War I she was a war correspondent for the *Saturday Evening Post* and later a Red Cross nurse in Paris. While other reporters were banned from the front, Rinehart capitalized on her nursing background to gain entry to Belgian military hospitals and war-torn areas. Her work, *Kings, Queens and Pawns* (1915), includes her observations of the brutality of war. Some of her fictional characters were nurses, such as Miss Pinkerton in *Adventures of a Nurse Detective,* a device she used to demonstrate nurse-patient relations. After her personal experience with breast cancer and surgery in 1936, she wrote *I Had Cancer* to increase awareness among women. With John Farrar two of her sons started the Farrar and Rinehart Publishing Company (which later became Rinehart Publishing).

Biography

Born: Aug. 12, 1876, Allegheny, Pa. **Education:** Pittsburgh Training School for Nurses; postgraduate surgical course. **Work history:** War Correspondent, World War I; Red Cross nurse, World War I; Journalist; Author. **Organizations:** unknown. **Awards:** Mystery Writers of America Special Award; medal from Queen Elizabeth of Belgium; honorary membership, Blackfoot Indian Tribe; honorary doctorate, George Washington Univ. **Buried:** Arlington National Cemetery.

References and Credits

†Rinehart M: My Story. New York, Farrar and Rinehart, 1931, pp 429–431.

Stein AP: Mary Rinehart. In Bullough V, Church OM, Stein AP (eds): American Nursing: A Biographical Dictionary, vol. 1. New York, Garland, 1988, pp 273–274.

Cohn J: Improbable Fiction: The Life of Mary Roberts Rinehart. Pittsburgh, Pa., University of Pittsburgh Press, 1980.

Claribel Augusta Wheeler

1881–1965

"To be a nurse is to belong to a profession which has the highest ideals of service, and one in which the lives of its followers are dedicated to the service of humanity. ...Her opportunities for personal service are very great, she comes into intimate contact with human lives at a time when they are most dependent, and in a subtle way creeps into their hearts so that she has a marvelous opportunity not only for giving sympathy and comfort, but for teaching her message of health. ...Never before in the history of nursing have there been such rare opportunities for service as are now offered in this work." (1921)

Claribel Wheeler was a nursing leader who established two major nursing programs, one at Mt. Sinai Hospital in Cleveland, Ohio, in 1916, and another at Washington University in St. Louis in 1923. She chose nursing because she saw its potential for personal fulfillment as well as its value to society. She wrote persuasively of the opportunities in nursing, especially the expanding roles for public health nurses, in "factories, stores, schools, boards of health, social work, and in rural districts." She saw the importance of education in public health for nurses at both the basic and graduate levels and worked to make such coursework available. Wheeler was emphatic about the qualifications necessary for those considering the profession, cautioned against correspondence schools, and stressed the importance of attending an accredited school. She was in the forefront of the accreditation movement for nursing schools and a skilled, effective volunteer in professional organizations. When she wrote "The Profession of Nursing" in 1921, she proudly claimed that the country had 100,000 nurses and 50,000 students.

Biography

Born: Aug. 13, 1881, Prospect, N.Y. **Education:** Vassar Bros. Hosp. School of Nursing, N.Y.; Sloane Maternity Hosp., N.Y.C.; Teachers College, Columbia Univ. **Work history:** Administrator, Vassar Bros. Hosp.; United Hosp., Port Chester, N.Y.; Mt. Sinai Hosp. School of Nursing, Cleveland, Ohio; Washington Univ. School of Nursing, St. Louis; Exec. Secretary, National League for Nursing Education. **Organizations:** Cleveland League for Nursing Education; Ohio State Nurses Assoc.; Mo. League for Nursing Education; American Nurses Assoc. **Awards:** unknown. **Died:** Richmond, Va.

References and Credits

†Wheeler C: The profession of nursing. Public Health Nurse 13:201, 204, 1921.

Sentz L: Claribel Augusta Wheeler. In Bullough V, Sentz L, Stein AP (eds): American Nursing: A Biographical Dictionary, vol. 2. New York, Garland, 1992, pp 349–350.

Lyle Morrison Creelman

1908–

"What of the future? It is to a very large extent in our own hands. We will make many errors but as long as we know our goal and keep it ever in mind our future is bright and secure." (1943)

LYLE MORRISON CREELMAN was Canada's first nurse to serve with the World Health Organization (WHO). An editorial in the *International Council of Nurses Journal* stated, "In these fourteen years with WHO, she has probably achieved more for nursing throughout the world than any other nurse of her time." Her first role on the international scene began in 1944 when she became the chief nurse in the British zone of occupied Germany. She organized nursing services to help millions of people of many nationalities who had been displaced from their homes during the war. Later she served in Canada as field director of an extensive study of Canadian public services, and she coauthored a greatly acclaimed report on this project. The study outlined the direction for public health nursing in Canada and was used for many years as a reference for public health professionals there. Her outstanding administrative skills, grounded in the public health principles of self-sufficiency in health care, allowed her to recruit, prepare, and collaborate with nurses from many nations to commence international projects that could later be carried on alone by the individual countries. Her vision guaranteed that countries would achieve self-sufficiency in health care through primary nursing care. She was the WHO consultant to the International Council of Nurses (ICN) and official observer for many nongovernment organizations. She chaired the membership committee of the ICN. WHO commissioned her to study maternal and child health service in Southeast Asia. She was the recipient of many awards for her contributions to nursing.

Biography

Born: Aug. 14, 1908, Upper Stewiacke, Nova Scotia, Can. **Education:** Vancouver Normal School (teaching certificate); Univ. of British Columbia, 1936 (BSN); Teachers College, Columbia Univ., 1939 (master's). **Work history:** taught elementary school for three yrs.; Public Health Nurse, Cranbrook, British Columbia; Metropolitan Health Committee, British Columbia; Public Health Nurse, Director of Nursing, 1940s; Chief Nurse, U.N. Relief and Rehabilitation Administration, Germany, 1944; Public Health Nurse, Vancouver; Nursing Consultant, maternal and child health, Nursing Unit of WHO, 1950; Chief Nursing Officer, WHO, 1954. **Organizations:** Canadian Nurses Assoc. (CNA); WHO consultant to ICN; chair, membership committee, ICN; Canadian Public Health Assoc. **Awards:** numerous Canadian awards, incl. Jeanne Mance Award, highest honor of CNA; Medal of Service of the Order of Canada, government of Canada; Queen's Golden Jubilee Medal in recognition of her nursing work, 2002.

References and Credits

†Creelman L: What of the future? *Canadian Nurse* 39:35–37, 1943.

†Zilm G: Lyle Creelman. In Bullough V, Sentz L (eds): American Nursing: A Biographical Dictionary, vol. 3. New York, Springer, 2000, pp 61–63.

August 15

Lillian Bessie Carter

1898–1983

"I am seventy years old today, and I think of where I am, and what I'm doing and why. When Earl died, my life lost its meaning and direction. For the first time, I lost my will to live. Since that time, I've tried to make my life have some significance. I felt useful when I was at Auburn, serving as housemother for my bad sweet K.A.'s [Kappa Alphas]. And I'm glad I worked at the Nursing Home, but God forbid that I ever have to live in one! I didn't dream that in this remote corner of the world, so far away from the people and material things that I had always considered so necessary, I would discover what Life is really all about. Sharing yourself with others, and accepting their love for you, is the most precious gift of all. If I had one wish for my children, it would be that each of you would dare to do the things and reach for goals in your own lives that have meaning for you as individuals, doing as much as you can for everybody, but not worrying if you don't please everyone." (1968)

LILLIAN BESSIE CARTER was an independent person even as a youngster. She became a nurse against her family's wishes. She married a farmer, James Earl Carter, and had four children. She was a civil rights activist and a peace activist in the 1920s and 1930s, again against her family's wishes. Her husband was elected to the Georgia legislature and died while in office, leaving "Miss Lillian" alone in the 1950s, when her children were all grown. She pulled herself together and became a housemother for the Kappa Alpha fraternity at Auburn University in Alabama for many years. Later, she returned to Plains, Georgia, and managed a nursing home. In her own words, her most enduring and rewarding life experience came when she was sixty-seven. She applied for and was accepted into the Peace Corps and went to India for two years. She wrote a book detailing the adverse conditions and her achievements in that role. She felt her time in India was far more meaningful and fulfilling than any time she spent as a goodwill ambassador for her son, President Jimmy Carter.

Biography

Born: Aug. 15, 1898, Richland, Ga. **Education:** attended Wise Hosp. for Nursing; Grady Memorial, Atlanta. **Work history:** nursed black population of Plains and Archery, Ga.; Volunteer, Peace Corps, family-planning clinic, Godrej Industries near Bombay; raised money to support efforts in India; worked for civil rights, women's causes, and senior citizens programs. **Organizations:** unknown. **Awards:** first woman to receive Covenant of Peace Award, Synagogue Council of America; Ceres Medal, U.N. Food and Agriculture Organization. **Buried:** Plains, Ga.

References and Credits

†Carter, Lillian. Away from Home: Letters to My Family. New York, Simon and Schuster, Lillian Carter, and Gloria Carter Spann, 1977, p 153.

Curson D: Lillian Carter. In Bullough V, Sentz L, Stein AP (eds): American Nursing: A Biographical Dictionary, vol. 2. New York, Garland, 1992, pp 54–56.

August 16

Susan C. Francis

1873–1962

"You will be interested to know that the analysis of turnover among general staff nurses included in this study shows that hospitals which have adopted the eight-hour day and have increased salaries over those common during the depression have less turnover among the nursing staff. Yet there are other factors which seem to influence the staff turnover almost as much. And these factors relate to the type of care which the nurse is allowed to give to her patients. When her patient load is too heavy so that good nursing care is impossible, the staff turnover is relatively high even though hours and salaries are satisfactory." (1938)

SUSAN C. FRANCIS was a hospital administrator and a natural organizer for the American Nurses Association (ANA). During her presidency of the ANA (1934–1938) she worked to attain unity and vigor for the nursing profession. She endeavored to make the state and national rules of the ANA consistent so that nurses moving to a different state could easily retain their association membership. Her objective was to educate each nurse about the strength that comes from individuals with common goals working together to improve conditions in the community and the profession. She emphasized the necessity of each nurse's efforts to strengthen the profession and protect the community. She served as secretary of the board of directors of the *American Journal of Nursing* and on the Committee on the Grading of Nursing Schools. A colleague praised her loyalty, tolerance, objectivity, sense of justice, and steadfastness of purpose.

Biography

Born: Aug. 16, 1873, Bridgeport, Pa. **Education:** Training School of Reading Hosp., 1894. **Work history:** Private Duty Nurse; Superintendent of Nurses, City Hosp., Washington, D.C. (now Gallinger Memorial); Superintendent, Touro Infirmary, New Orleans; Superintendent of Nurses, Jewish Hosp., Philadelphia; Director, Pennsylvania-Delaware division, American Red Cross, World War I; Superintendent, Children's Hosp., Philadelphia, and Director, nursing school, Philadelphia. **Organizations:** first secretary, Philadelphia League for Nursing Education; President, Pa. State Nurses Assoc.; Chair, headquarters committee, ANA; Secretary, President, ANA. **Awards:** unknown. **Buried:** St. Paul's Cemetery, Amityville, Pa.

References and Credits

†Francis, SC: President's address to Thirty-First Convention, 1938. In Flanagan L (ed): One Strong Voice: The Story of the American Nurses Association. Kansas City, Mo., Lowell Press, 1976, pp 477–478.

Dombrowski T: Susan Francis. In Bullough V, Church OM, Stein AP (eds): American Nursing: A Biographical Dictionary, vol. 1. New York, Garland, 1988, pp 119–120.

AUGUST 17

Marian Alford

1904–1989

"I see the urgent need for nurses to work with all others so nothing pertaining to nursing will go on without our participation."
(Date unknown)

THE TWENTIETH-CENTURY image of American nursing is largely the result of the commitment and involvement of Marian Alford. She used quality nursing care as the standard for negotiations with hospital administrators. Her diplomatic skill enabled her to improve nursing conditions and salaries. She was the director of the California Nurses Association (CNA) from 1956 to 1966. During her tenure hospital-based professional performance committees (PPCs) were established so nurses could discuss practice conditions, salaries, employment conditions, and quality of patient care. She celebrated the emergence of "a new generation of nurses" who "see themselves as a profession" and "refuse to compromise their ideals" to accept "a pattern in which the motives of industry are smothering the basic human ideal of giving quality nursing care." She supported the thousands of nurses who resigned in San Francisco Bay area because of "the gradual deterioration over the past 25 years in the quality of patient care."

BIOGRAPHY

Born: Aug. 17, 1904, Humboldt County, Calif. **Education:** Univ. of California School of Nursing, 1936 (BS); Teachers College, Columbia Univ., 1948 (MA). **Work history:** Private

OB Nurse; General Duty Nurse, OB; Night Supervisor, Univ. of California and Stanford Hosp., Palo Alto; Assistant Director of Nursing, Stanford Hosp.; Director of Nursing, Peralta Hosp., Oakland, Calif. **Organizations:** Alameda County Nurses Assoc.; President, bd. member, CNA. **Awards:** unknown. **Died:** Oakland, Calif.

References and Credits

†Stanley J: Marian Alford. In Bullough V, Sentz L, Stein AP (eds): American Nursing: A Biographical Dictionary, vol. 2. New York, Garland, 1992, pp 4–6.

August 18

Phoebe Yates Levy Pember

1823–1913

"In the midst of suffering and death, hoping with those almost beyond hope in this world; praying by the bedside of the lonely and heart stricken; closing the eyes of boys hardly old enough to realize man's sorrows, much less suffer by man's fierce hate, a woman must *soar beyond the conventional modesty considered correct under different circumstances." (ca. 1863)*

Phoebe Pember was widowed shortly after her marriage. Seeking a challenge, she courageously accepted an offer from the wife of the Confederacy's secretary of war to serve as matron of the largest hospital. The Chimborazo Hospital in Richmond, Virginia, took care of more than seventy-six thousand patients during the war. The matron's duties were diverse and demanding. She supervised all the workers, ensured that doctors' orders were carried out, and was responsible for sanitation and food service. Most hospital care in the South was provided by men, who saw no need to be supervised by a woman. Undaunted, Pember made sure that they provided high-quality care as she demonstrated compassion and dedication to the patient, particularly to those who were dying. According to the writer Hannah Williamson, historians say that Pember's diary, *A Southern Woman's Story,* is one of the best accounts of life in a Confederate hospital. Among the entries is her delightful account of making chicken soup for her patients. Pember also guarded the whiskey barrel so that the whiskey would be available for medicinal use. She was memorialized in the twentieth century on a U.S. postage stamp as part of a Civil War series.

Biography

Born: Aug. 18, 1823, Charleston, S.C. **Education:** unknown. **Work history:** Matron, Chimborazo Confederate Hosp., Richmond, Va. **Organizations:** unknown. **Awards:** depicted on U.S. postage stamp. **Died:** Pittsburgh, Pa.

References and Credits

†Pember P: A Southern Woman's Story. New York, Carlton, 1879, p 192.

Williamson H: Phoebe Pember. In Bullough V, Sentz L, Stein AP (eds): American Nursing: A Biographical Dictionary, vol. 2. New York, Garland, 1992, pp 261–262.

Pearl Parvin Coulter

1902–2002

"The 'past' from which nursing education needed to free itself lay not in its concern with meeting the nursing needs of society, but rather in the time and . . . place at which that concern should be manifested. The welfare of the patient is the primary focus of both nursing service and nursing education—and the success of the two are irrevocably entwined. Nursing education is not an end in itself—its only reason for being is to produce a nurse who can fill the role of a competent practitioner. Nursing service should . . . look to the graduating classes of schools of nursing to fill its need for professional workers, rather than expect that need to be met by nursing students." (1961)

Pearl Parvin Coulter exemplified professional excellence in public health nursing through practice, her work with professional organizations, teaching, and publications. While at the University of Colorado she influenced the course of public health nursing education when she designed a new approach to fieldwork. She implemented a learning strategy that ensured that a full-time faculty member was available to work with the students during their practicum. The baccalaureate nursing program that she started at the University of Arizona gained national prominence, especially for its focus on adequate practicum in its community health nursing and its focus on the family. Her landmark 1954 book, *The Nurse in the Public Health Program,* outlined her ideas about community health and provided a framework for changes in education and practice that was adopted by many schools of nursing across the country.

Biography

Born: Aug. 19, 1902, Almyra, Ark. **Education:** Univ. of Denver (AB, MS); Univ. of Colorado (nursing diploma); George Peabody College for Teachers, Nashville, Tenn. (certificate in public health nursing). **Work history:** public school teacher; Staff Nurse, Colorado Visiting Nurse Assoc.; Faculty, George Peabody College for Teachers, Nashville, Tenn.; Director, public health nursing, Nashville (Tenn.) Health Dept.; Faculty, Univ. of Colorado, Univ. of Arizona; member, bd. of directors, American Journal of Nursing Co.; committee work, U.S. Public Health Service, Arizona State Bd. of Nursing. **Organizations:** Colo. Nurses Assoc., Ariz. Nurses Assoc.; American Nurses Assoc. (ANA); Council of Higher Education for Nursing; Western Interstate Commission for Higher Education; National League for Nursing. **Awards:** Honorary Membership Award, Pearl McIver Public Health Nursing Award, ANA; honorary doctorates, Univ. of Colorado, Univ. of Arizona; Dean Emeritus, Univ. of Arizona. **Died:** Sun City, Ariz.

References and Credits

†Coulter P: The Winds of Change: A Progress Report of Regional Cooperation in Collegiate Nursing Education in the West, 1956–1961. Boulder, Colo., Western Interstate Commission for Higher Education, 1963.

Anglin LT: Pearl Coulter. In Bullough V, Sentz L, Stein AP (eds): American Nursing: A Biographical Dictionary, vol. 2. New York, Garland, 1992, pp 67–69.

University of Arizona on-line, available at http://www.ahsc.arizona.edu/opa/news/feb02/pearl.htm.

August 29

Jane Van de Vrede

1889–1972

"The knowledge of the training school was not broad enough. There the patient was considered only for the period of acute illness in home or hospital, disassociated from his past and his family: in a new environment with only the nurse in charge. All this is changed in the public health field. The nurse keeps constantly in mind the family environment, the previous conditions and social causes which bear upon the illnesses. ...To this phase of health work the nurse, and in the immediate future the nurse only, can make the greatest contribution." (1921)

As a young adult, Jane Van de Vrede had surgery, with complications, in a hospital setting characterized by poor sanitation and inadequate care. This prompted her to leave teaching and study nursing. Her influence on nursing in the South dramatically improved nursing care by upgrading nursing educational standards, granting licensure by examination, and requiring mandatory registration. She understood the importance of public health nursing and successfully involved the Red Cross to make related coursework available for nurses in schools in the South. When she was working with the Georgia State Board of Examiners of Nurses, she urged nursing schools to adopt such standards as entrance requirements, qualified faculty, clinical assignments, nurse-patient ratios, and adequate supervision.

During her tenure four out of five hospital nursing schools in the state were closed because they were substandard. She was an advocate for health insurance and retirement benefits for nurses and is noted for promoting interracial cooperation among nurses during the early twentieth century.

Biography

Born: Aug. 12, 1880, Wausau, Wisc. **Education:** County Teacher Training School, Wausau, Wisc.; Milwaukee (Wisc.) General Hosp. School of Nursing. **Work history:** lab work in bacteriology, Milwaukee General Hosp. and Savannah, Ga.; Nursing Instructor, Savannah, Ga.; Director of Nursing Service, American Red Cross, Southern Division; Ga. State Bd. of Examiners of Nurses; Dept. of Public Health Nursing, Work Projects Administration. **Organizations:** American Red Cross; Ga. Nurses Assoc. (GNA); American Nurses Assoc.; Atlanta Business and Professional Women's Assoc.; Ga. Hosp. Assoc.; Ga. State Assoc. of Graduate Nurses; Ga. State League for Nursing (GSLN); Ga. Chapter, National League for Nursing. **Awards:** memorial resolution, board room named in her honor, GNA; Jane Van de Vrede Award, GSLN. **Died:** Smyrna, Ga.

References and Credits

†Zalumas JC: Jane Van de Vrede. In Bullough V, Sentz L, Stein AP (eds): American Nursing: A Biographical Dictionary, vol. 2. New York, Garland, 1992, pp 333–336.

August 21

Dorothy Johnson

1919–1999

"Nursing care, which is provided to individuals or groups under stress of a health-illness nature, has as its primary purpose to relieve tension and discomfort to the end of restoring or maintaining internal and interpersonal equilibrium. Internal and interpersonal equilibrium—which I hold to be the specific goal of professional nursing—does not imply a state of health or well-being. It is rather a state in which opposing forces—biological, psychological, or social—are balanced momentarily. ...A state of equilibrium ... makes possible more effective utilization of available energy, facilitating recovery from illness or promoting health." (1959)

A CREATIVE THINKER and a pioneer nurse-theorist, Dorothy Johnson defined nursing as both a science with its own body of knowledge and an essential service with a "common core." She also emphasized that "ministering to the basic human needs of individuals is the essence, the very heart, of professional nursing." She developed the concepts of nursing diagnosis and the identification of nursing problems and differentiated them as separate from medicine and unique to nursing practice. She stressed that nursing practice builds on its own foundation of scientific knowledge. When she was a student at Vanderbilt University, she was inspired and influenced by Lulu Hassenplug, who continued to serve as her mentor. Through courses, writings, and presentations Johnson in turn inspired many other nurses to become researchers and theorists.

Biography

Born: Aug. 21, 1919, Savannah, Ga. **Education:** junior college, Savannah, Ga.; Vanderbilt Univ. (BSN); Harvard Univ. (MPH). **Work history:** Faculty, Vanderbilt Univ.; Staff Nurse, Chatham-Savannah (Ga.) Health Council; Faculty, Univ. of California, Los Angeles; helped establish nursing programs in India. **Organizations:** unknown. **Awards:** Lulu Hassenplug Award, Calif. State Nurses Assoc. **Died:** location unknown.

References and Credits

†Johnson D: The nature of a science of nursing. Nurs Outlook 7:292, 1959.

Ross-Kerr J, Brink PJ: Dorothy Johnson. In Bullough V, Sentz L (eds): American Nursing: A Biographical Dictionary, vol. 3. New York, Springer, 2000, pp 149–152.

Johnson D: A philosophy of nursing. Nurs Outlook 7:198–200, 1959.

Mathild Helen Krueger Lamping

1869–1948

"On our arrival at Gievgili there were about twelve hundred patients, mostly surgical, sheltered in the tobacco factory; two days later we received 560 more wounded, many of them being Austrian prisoners of war. In this unsanitary locality, the building crowded to its utmost capacity, with vermin and filth on every hand and no prospects of obtaining vitally needed equipment for the promotion of better sanitary conditions, we went to work, not optimistic nor sanguine of results, but with a determination to do our best. ...Badly infected wounds were the rule, not the exception. Each day we realized more and more how pitifully inadequate our force was for the proper care of the wounded soldiers, and each day conditions grew worse and more disheartening. Our only encouragement was the marvelous fortitude, heroic courage and gratitude of our patients, who rarely even so much as groaned under the suffering of painful dressings." (1915)

THROUGHOUT HER NURSING career Mathild Lamping worked to make things better. When she headed the nursing school at Harper Hospital in Detroit, she upgraded admissions criteria and added student nurse affiliations in visiting nursing.

Her greatest challenge, however, came when she joined a delegation to Serbia for the Red Cross before the United States entered World War I. The twelve nurses and six doctors worked in a cold and overcrowded converted tobacco factory; sanitation was deplorable, prevention of the spread of disease was impossible, and supplies and food were scarce. She developed typhus and was returned home. She later helped gain passage of the nurse practice act in Michigan and defined specific health problems in a Wisconsin county during a demonstration project in 1915. She worked again with the Red Cross during World War I.

Biography

Born: Aug. 21, 1869, Wolf River Twp., Winnebago Co., Wisc. **Education:** Illinois Training School, Chicago (RN); Teachers College, Columbia Univ. **Work history:** Farrand Training School for Nurses/Harper Hosp., Detroit; American Red Cross nurse abroad; County Nurse, Dunn Co., Wisc.; Superintendent, La Crosse (Wisc.) Lutheran Hosp.; President, Wisconsin Bd. of Nurse Examiners; Public Health Nurse, Texas. **Organizations:** American Nurses Assoc.; member, bd. of directors, Ill. Training School for Nurses; Infant Welfare Assoc., Oak Park; Art Institute of Chicago. **Awards:** Cross of Mercy and diploma from king of Yugoslavia. **Died:** Neenah, Wisc.

References and Credits

†Krueger M: Personal experiences in Serbia. AJN 15:1014–1015, 1915.

Cooper SS: Mathild Lamping. In Bullough V, Church OM, Stein AP (eds): American Nursing: A Biographical Dictionary, vol. 1. New York, Garland, 1988, pp 205–206.

August 23

Joanne C. Gladden

1943–

"It is clear to me that the quality of the interpersonal relationship with homeless persons is the most significant element in determining the nurse's effectiveness. ...It is important that the nurse be able to convey, early in the relationship, an attitude of presence, respect, and caring. ...A single act of kindness such as obtaining a pair of properly fitting shoes for a resident with aching feet can be a simple but powerful way of communicating understanding and care. A sense of personal worth and connectedness can be fostered ... through active listening, expressions of empathy and encouragement, and an accepting, positive regard. 'Mattering' to at least another person is a potentially significant seed for personal growth." (1991)

A NURSE PRACTITIONER and educator, Joanne Gladden was drawn to the profession by the healing nature of nursing. Greatly influenced by her father's suffering with cancer and her mother's deep respect for nurses, she was also influenced by a deeply caring nurse who guided Gladden's recovery from a serious illness when she was seven. Widely published and highly honored, Gladden has had a broad-based and versatile career that includes clinical nursing, community health, occupational health, independent practice, consulting, speaking, and teaching. She is knowledgeable about homelessness in rural America and helped establish a homeless shelter in North Dakota. She was one of several providers of health care and health counseling at a rural shelter-based nurse-run clinic, later named in her honor. Her work as a gerontology nurse practitioner includes presentations and publications about the health care transitions of older adults and the implications for nursing. She writes that at such times nursing's mission is essential. As facilitative, caring, and sensitive health care providers, nurses have the knowledge and skill for a meaningful presence with patient and family. She concludes that "person-to-person connections can never be overstated as critical pathways for health and healing."

Biography

Born: Aug. 23, 1943, Cleveland, Ohio. **Education:** St. John's College, Ohio (BSN); Univ. of Minnesota (MS); Univ. of Colorado Health Sciences Center (PHD). **Work history:** Clinical Nurse, St. Vincent Hosp., Ohio; Community Health Nurse, Occupational Health Nurse, Visiting Nurse Assoc. Ohio; Nurse Practitioner, Montana, Alaska, North Dakota. Faculty. Western Interstate Commission for Higher Education, Alaska, North Dakota, Maryland; Consultant; Lecturer; Author. **Organizations:** American Nurses Assoc. (ANA); Maryland Nurses Assoc.; National Gerontological Nursing Assoc.; Sigma Theta Tau; Gerontological Society of America; Health Resources Committee, Salem Lutheran Church; N.D. Coalition for Homeless Persons and Families. **Awards:** recognition awards from N. Dakota, JC Penny; Outstanding Faculty Award, Univ. of Alaska; Regents Faculty Award, Univ. of Maryland, Univ. of North Dakota; *Who's Who in American Nursing;* Outstanding Young Women of America; ANA Search for Excellence Award; N.D. Nurse Researcher of the Year; several research awards; N.D. medical clinic named in her honor.

References and Credits

†Bushy A. (ed): Rural Nursing, vol. 1. Newbury Park, Calif., Sage, 1991, p 388.

Gladden J: Critical connections to older adult decision-making during health care transitions. Geriatric Nursing 21:7, 2000.

Gladden J: resume.

Gladden J: personal correspondence, 2002.

AUGUST 24

Joanna Mabel Johnson
1891–1971

"Our first nursing experience in the cherry orchards of Wisconsin was ... the experiment of seeing what a rather intensive nursing service would do to reduce losses. ...Probably 20,000 itinerant cherry pickers come to this area each year for the short intensive season of picking. ...This temporary population, which brought many of its ills with it and contracted its share after arrival, presented a problem of sufficient importance. ...Inspection of drinking water ... was continued throughout the season. We established ... a health station and averaged about fifty service calls a day. ...We were particularly interested in the complications resulting from a farming community suddenly turning industrial for ... one month out of twelve. ...Those operators to whom service was rendered came out of the season in a much more cooperative attitude toward the health service of the nurses than they entered it." (1931)

JOANNA JOHNSON WAS studying to be a teacher when she developed pneumonia; this experience attracted her to nursing. She was the first occupational health nurse to be hired by an insurance company when what is now Wausau Insurance Companies hired her in 1928. She worked for companies that held policies, and she defined the role of the nurse in areas of worker safety, disease and accident prevention, and rehabilitation. She was the first to define standards and guidelines for industrial nurses and wrote and lectured frequently about this. Her work expanded the role of the nurse and influenced the development of university coursework in the specialty of industrial nursing. In 1978 the first professional chair in occupational health was named in her honor when it was established at the Milwaukee School of Nursing of the University of Wisconsin.

Biography

Born: Aug. 16, 1891, Shawano County, Wisc. **Education:** Oshkosh State Normal School (now Univ. of Wisconsin, Oshkosh); St. Mary's Hosp. School of Nursing, Rochester, Minn. (RN). **Work history:** various nurse positions, Columbia Hosp., Milwaukee, Wisc., Pasadena, Calif.; Industrial Nurse, Northwestern Malleable Iron Co., Milwaukee, Wisc.; Public Health Nurse, Milwaukee, Wisc.; Industrial Nurse, Employers Mutual Insurance Co. (now Wausau), Wausau, Wisc.; helped establish National Safety Council; consultant on industrial health to Case Western Univ., Wayne State Univ., Marquette Univ.; Teachers College, Columbia Univ., Univ. of Illinois, Univ. of Pennsylvania; Exec. Director, Green Bay Visiting Nurse Assoc. (VNA). **Organizations:** American Nurses Assoc.; Industrial Health Council of American Medical Assoc.; National Society for Prevention of Blindness; National Safety Council; Chicago and Milwaukee Industrial Nurses Clubs. **Awards:** issue of *Nursing World* dedicated to her; award from Los Angeles County Heart Assoc.; professional chair in her name at Milwaukee School of Nursing. **Died:** Pasadena, Calif.

References and Credits

†Johnson J: Nursing problems when farming becomes an industry. Public Health Nurse 23:81, 1931.

Cooper SS: Joanna Johnson. In Bullough V, Church OM, Stein AP (eds): American Nursing: A Biographical Dictionary, vol. 1. New York, Garland, 1988, pp 194–196.

AUGUST 25

Edith Patton Lewis
1914–

"We in nursing know, or think we know, what it is we do for people. Anywhere along the health-illness continuum, our concern is less with the immediate problem and more with the person with the problem and the forces—past, present, and future—that impinge upon it. Ours can be a lifetime contribution to this person's total health care, not a short-term one. ...If the nurse is identified and used as a person with a different orientation than the physician—one who provides a different kind of health care service—then we have the potential for a new pattern of health manpower deployment and some overdue restructuring of our health care delivery system." (1972)

EDITH PATTON LEWIS edited journals owned by the American Journal of Nursing Company from 1945 to 1980. She served as managing editor of *Nursing Research* from 1952 to 1957; editor of the *American Journal of Nursing* from 1963 to 1970; contributing editor of the *American Journal of Nursing* from 1957 to 1959; and editor of *Nursing Outlook* from 1970 to 1980. She also served as a valuable nurse recruiter for the U.S. Cadet Nurse Corps during World War II. In her books she upheld nursing as an important field because it is so varied. Her own career as a journalist exemplified her point. Her articles supporting nurses who were violating the no-strike pledge of the American Nurses Association contributed to the improvement of salaries and benefits and helped change the opinion among nurses about the ethics of collective bargaining activities. She wrote analytically about the three competing systems of education: diploma, the associate of arts curriculum, and the baccalaureate course. While she was editor of *Nursing Outlook,* the official organ for the National League for Nursing, her editorials focused on the changing roles for nurses as clinical nurse specialists and nurse practitioners. She gave personal attention to writers and would-be writers and was proud that she never sent a writer a form letter. In her speeches and editorials she advised authors to use plain, straightforward writing—she deplored nurses' tendency to write what she called "pretentious prose." She was a freelance writer in the intervals between full-time employment and after her retirement in 1980. She conducted writing workshops and wrote reports on professional conferences, conventions, and histories of the *American Journal of Nursing.* She lives in Connecticut.

Biography

Born: Aug. 27, 1914, Philadelphia. **Education:** Smith College (BS in psychology); Worcester (Mass.) State Hospital (yearlong internship in psychology); Frances Payne Bolton School of Nursing, Western Reserve Univ., Cleveland, Ohio, 1939 (MS). **Work history:** Psychiatric Staff Nurse, New York Hosp., Westchester Co.; Head Nurse, Supervisor, Instructor, Massachusetts General Hosp., Boston, 1940–42; Director of Nursing Education, Norwich (Conn.) State Hosp., 1942–45; recruited students for U.S. Cadet Nurse Corps; editor, *American Journal of Nursing;* Managing Editor, *Nursing Research;* Editor, *Nursing Outlook.* **Writings:** wrote two books, *Opportunities in Nursing* (1952) and *Nurse: Careers within a Career in Professional Nursing* (1962); with Mary H. Browning compiled *The Dying Patient: A Nursing Perspective* (1972). **Organizations:** unknown. **Awards:** Distinguished Alumna Award, Francis Payne Bolton School of Nursing, 1975; honorary recognition, Conn. Nurses Assoc., for Distinguished Service to the Profession, 1978, and for Outstanding Contribution to Nursing Education, 1982; Fellow, American Academy of Nursing, 1977.

References and Credits

†Lewis EP: A nurse is a nurse—Or is she? editorial. Nurs Outlook 20:21, 1972.

Bullough B: Edith Lewis. In Bullough V, Sentz L, Stein AP (eds): American Nursing: A Biographical Dictionary, vol. 2. New York, Garland, 1992, pp 194–196.

Mary Lou de Leon Siantz

1948–

"Parents have an important role in mediating the effects of poverty and stress on the lives of their children. ...It is crucial to identify isolated mothers and fathers who are most at risk, as well as to provide them with culturally sensitive social and emotional support. This action will ... also indirectly prevent or alleviate potential behavioral and social problems their children may experience. ...Immigration is ... about children and their families. Research, intervention, and social policy must ... consider a life-span perspective that focuses on the well-being, developmental potential, and successful integration of immigrant parents and children into American society while respecting their cultures, histories, beliefs, and migration experiences." (1997)

MARY LOU DE LEON SIANTZ, a Mexican American nurse, scholar, and leader, was attracted to nursing by the example of others. She recalls childhood conversations about health care with the family doctor who made home visits to treat her asthma. Later, working as a candy striper, she enjoyed hearing about nursing from students and registered nurses. Her research, writings, and professional example make a difference in the lives and health care of children and families often overlooked by society, particularly minorities and migrant farmworkers. Her research areas include mental retardation, the stigma of mental illness for children of color, developmental outcomes in the migrant Head Start child, and depression in Mexican migrant mothers. She sees her involvement in professional organizations as a way to give back to the profession. Additionally, she is shaping the future of nursing by recruiting students from ethnic minority backgrounds, a rich resource that she says has traditionally been overlooked. An advocate for a foreign-language requirement in nursing school, she encourages nurses to learn Spanish, because it will build trust and help eliminate discrimination when Latinos seek health care. She encourages nurses to learn more about the health concerns of underserved populations, especially the migrant farmworker families.

Biography

Born: Aug. 26, 1948, Los Angeles. **Education:** Mt. St. Mary's College, Los Angeles (BSN); Univ. of California, Los Angeles (MN); Univ. of Maryland, College Park (PhD).
Work history: Staff Nurse, Children's Hosp., Los Angeles; Nurse Therapist, Neuropsychiatric Institute, Mental Retardation Unit, Univ. of California, Los Angeles; Director of Training in Nursing, Univ. Affiliated Program, Univ. of South California; Faculty, School of Nursing, Univ. of California, Los Angeles; Faculty, Univ. of Michigan School of Nursing; Program Assoc., Univ. of Michigan Institute for Study of Mental Retardation and Related Disabilities; Director, Division of Nursing, Georgetown Univ. Affiliated Program for Child Development; National Mental Health Coordinator, Migrant Head Start Program; Nursing Faculty, Georgetown Univ., Indiana Univ., Univ. of Washington. **Organizations:** Sigma Theta Tau; Society for Research in Child Development; Sigma Xi; National Assoc. of Hispanic Nurses; Assoc. of Child and Psychiatric Nurses; member, Committee on Health of Immigrant Children and Families and Committee on Workforce Diversity in Health Professions; member, National Advisory Council on Nursing Research; Secretary's Advisory Committee on Infant Mortality; member, Technical Advisory Evaluation Panel, Secretary's Advisory Committee on Infant Mortality; member, Committee on Work Environment for Nurses and Patient Safety. **Awards:** Kennedy Fellowship in Bioethics, Kennedy Institute, Georgetown Univ.; Ildaura Murillo Rhode Award for Educational Excellence; Fellow, American Academy of Nursing; Harris Distinguished Lecturer, San Diego State Univ.; Nowik International Fellowship; election to Institute of Medicine, National Academy of Sciences.

References and Credits

†Siantz de Leon ML: Factors that impact the developmental outcomes of immigrant children. In Booth A, Lansdale N (eds): Immigration and the Family. Mahwah, N.J., Erlbaum Associates, 1997, p 159.

Siantz de Leon ML: personal correspondence, December 2002.

Steefel L: Third-world life in a first-world country. Spectrum 2:26–27, 2001.

Siantz de Leon ML: resume.

August 27

Mother Teresa

1910–1997

"We ourselves feel that what we are doing is just a drop in the ocean. But if that drop was not in the ocean, I think the ocean would be less because of that missing drop. I do not agree with the big way of doing things." (Date unknown)

"The biggest disease today is not leprosy or tuberculosis, but rather the feeling of being unwanted, uncared for and deserted by everybody." (1971)

"There is something else to remember—that this kind of love begins at home. We cannot give to the outside what we don't have on the inside. This is very important. If I can't see God's love in my brother and sister then how can I see that love in somebody else? How can I give it to somebody else? Everybody has got some good. Some hide it, some neglect it, but it is there." (Date unknown)

Born Gonxha (Agnes) Bojaxhiu, Mother Teresa practiced her daily devotion to her Catholic faith as her mother did. Her father, Nikola Bojaxhiu, was poisoned, and her mother, Drana Bojaxhiu, fed her family and many of the local Yugoslav poor by operating an embroidery and textile business. Mother Teresa was touched by missionaries' stories of the suffering in India. She learned from her mother and understood the one-on-one ministry with a single patient, and she taught this to others. She was a master organizer and could use the media to her advantage, which enabled her to reach those who could finance her efforts around the world. She was steadfast in her commitment to ease the suffering of any individual. She received the Nobel Peace Prize in 1979.

Biography

Born: Aug. 26, 1910, Skopje, Yugoslavia. **Education:** entered order of Sisters of Loreto, who founded mission in India, and went to Motherhouse, Rathfarnham, Ireland; took final vows as Sister Mary Teresa, 1937. **Work history:** led young Christian, Hindu, and Muslim members of Sodality of Mary in ministering to poor, sick, and dying in the street; established more than 600 missions, 180 receiving centers, in 130 countries staffed by 275 brothers, 4,000 nuns, and 120,000 volunteers. **Organizations:** unknown. **Awards:** Nobel Peace Prize, 1979. **Died:** Calcutta.

References and Credits

†Teresa, Mother: A Gift for God. In Knowles E (ed.): The Oxford Dictionary of Quotations. Oxford, England, New York, Oxford University Press, 1999, p 768. Used with permission of the Missionaries of Charity, Calcutta, India.

†Teresa, Mother: The Observer. In Knowles E (ed.): The Oxford Dictionary of Quotations. Oxford, England, New York, Oxford University Press, 1999, p 768. Used with permission of the Missionaries of Charity, Calcutta, India.

†Mother Teresa: A Simple Path. Comp L Vardey. New York, Ballantine, 1995, back jacket. Used with permission of the Missionaries of Charity, Calcutta, India.

Mother Teresa. In Snodgrass M: Historical Encyclopedia of Nursing. Santa, Barbara, Calif., ABC-CLIO, 1999, pp 247–251. Used with permission of the Missionaries of Charity, Calcutta, India.

Mother Elizabeth Ann Bayley Seton

1774–1821

"Human passions and weakness to be sure are never extinct—but they cannot triumph in the heart which is possessed by [piety], this friend of love and Peace—she is very lovely. ... Make acquaintance with her—she will not be angry that you have neglected her so long." (1809)

Elizabeth Bayley Seton, a descendent of one of New York's first families, was raised in the city when it was a financial and political center with a population of thirty thousand. Her father was a prominent physician and medical inspector for arriving immigrants. Elizabeth Bayley married into a family of fortune, but her husband's poor business sense, compounded by the effects of war in Europe as well as his poor health, led to financial ruin. When doctors advised that the Setons go to Italy to help his worsening tuberculosis, they left their four younger children with relatives and took their eight-year-old daughter along. William Magee Seton died in Italy in 1803, and Elizabeth Seton's exposure to Catholicism there led to further religious study and eventual conversion. The resultant rejection by family and friends caused her to move to Maryland, where Bishop John Carroll invited her to establish a school for girls.

In this more tolerant setting, with her small following, she then started the first new community of apostolic religious women founded in the United States. In addition to teaching, the sisters also began to provide bedside nursing care. This met a need of people in rural Maryland who had communicable diseases and no resources for care. The sisters later provided nursing care to both Union and Confederate soldiers during the Civil War. The American Sisters of Charity, based on the traditions of St. Vincent de Paul and Louise de Marillac, began to provide leaders in nursing education early in the nineteenth century and are now involved in hundreds of facilities in North America and around the world.

Biography

Born: Aug. 28, 1774, New York City. **Education:** unknown. **Work history:** Established school for girls, Baltimore; Established religious order, Sisters of Charity; initiated nursing care, rural Maryland. **Organizations:** unknown. **Awards:** canonized by the Roman Catholic Church, 1975. **Died:** Emmitsburg, Md.

References and Credits

†Bechtle R, Metz J (eds): Elizabeth Bailey Seton: Collected Writings, vol. 2. Hyde Park, N.Y., New City Press, 2002, p 86.

Sabin L: Mother Elizabeth Seton. In Bullough V, Church OM, Stein AP (eds): American Nursing: A Biographical Dictionary, vol. 1. New York, Garland, 1988, pp 288–290.

Kelly E: Numerous Choirs: A Chronicle of Elizabeth Bayley Seton and Her Spiritous Daughters, vol. 2: Expansion, Division, and War, 1821–1865. St. Meinrad, Ind., Abbey Press, 1996.

Myers R: American Women of Faith. Huntington, Ind., Sunday Visitor Publication Division, 1989.

August 29

Sister John Gabriel
1875–1951

"A [teaching] method is good, just in the degree that it challenges the student's intellect and forces her to work at her maximum capacity. ...The unit of thought and practice, however, should always be directed to the patient whose welfare is the pivot around which all the activity of the student nurse and the institution as a whole circulates." (1928)

Sister John Gabriel was a young member of the Sisters of Charity of Providence and a practicing pharmacist at Columbus Hospital in Great Falls, Montana, when she had an opportunity to comfort a hospitalized patient. Realizing that nursing would allow her to do more to help sick people, she enrolled in the nursing school and dedicated her life to her new profession. Soon after her graduation, in the early 1900s, she provided nursing care in frontier towns of the Pacific Northwest to native Americans, miners, lumberjacks, and railroad workers. She continued to study and teach nursing while consistently working to improve the preparation, supervision, and curriculum of the religious sisters who taught in nursing programs. She was an effective speaker and writer who published several books and articles about nursing education.

Biography

Born: Aug. 30, 1875, Manville, R.I. **Education:** Sisters of Charity of Providence, Montreal; Columbus Hosp. School of Nursing, Great Falls, Mont.; St. Vincent. Hosp. School of Nursing, Portland, Ore.; Univ. of Washington, Seattle (BA). **Work history:** pharmacy, Columbus Hosp., Great Falls, Mont.; General Nurse, Pacific Northwest; Teacher, Pacific Northwest; Instructor, Loyola Univ., Chicago; Holy Name College, Oakland, Calif.; Holy Cross Hosp., Salt Lake City, Utah; Creighton Univ., Omaha, Neb. **Organizations:** American Nurses Assoc.; member, editorial bd., *American Journal of Nursing;* Washington Nurses Assoc. **Awards:** honorary member, Eugene Field Society; Fellow, American College of Hosp. Administrators. **Buried:** Seattle.

References and Credits

†Gabriel J: The relative value of various types of teaching in schools of nursing. AJN 28:273, 276, 1928.

Dombrowski T: Sister John Gabriel. In Bullough V, Church OM, Stein AP (eds): American Nursing: A Biographical Dictionary, vol. 1. New York, Garland, 1988, pp 126–128.

August 30

(Mary) Maureen Cushing
1937–

"I think nursing is set apart from other disciplines because nurses as a group consistently perform tasks in an above average manner and they are honest in accounting for the care they render. It took me a long time to realize that to be happy in practicing law I had to surround myself with attorneys who placed the same value on high standards as I did. In nursing I loved the responsibility, the challenge of making decisions, and the people. ...There were values in nursing which I wanted to transfer to my law practice. These included attention to detail, honesty, compassion, and, particularly, the need to work with people who would not level off professionally." (1988)

"Nursing knows no parallel. It is solitary and communal at the same time." (2002)

Maureen Cushing recalls being first attracted to nursing when she was five. To her it was "romantic, mysterious, and dramatic," as she was covertly led up a wooden stairway to a screened porch to visit a sibling enduring a long hospitalization. After two decades of bedside nursing Cushing became a practicing attorney and acknowledges that she never really left nursing behind. As life events trigger recall of certain patients, she is reminded of the devotion of family, memories of the struggles, fears, and courage of patients and the many forms of loss and suffering experienced by both. She looks back on the special camaraderie of hospital nursing. She recognizes the qualities of good nursing that enhance her legal practice and knows that the drama of law pales next to the daily challenges and achievements that nurses experience. Her nursing background and her high regard for what nurses do is integrated into her law practice. Saying that she gave more thought to the essence of nursing after leaving it than she ever did when she was active in the profession, she credits family and nursing for the values that influence her work as a trial lawyer and her dedication to service. The author of legal issues chapters in nursing textbooks, she also wrote *Nursing Jurisprudence* (1988) and "The Legal Side," a column for the *American Journal of Nursing* (1981–1989).

Biography

Born: Aug. 30, 1937, North Andover, Mass. **Education:** Lawrence General Hosp. School of Nursing (RN); Boston College School of Nursing (BSN); New England School of Law, Boston (JD). **Work history:** all nursing in medical-surgical acute care, various Boston hospitals; Nursing Instructor, Northeast Baptist Hosp.; legal lectures for nurses in United States and Germany; Civil Trial Lawyer; Author. **Organizations:** American Trial Lawyers Assoc.; Mass. Trial Lawyers Assoc.; Northeast Chapter, American Assoc. of Nurse Attorneys; Mass. Bar Assoc. **Awards:** Boston College Alumni Assoc. Award for Excellence in Public Service as a Nurse-Attorney; Recognition Award, American Society of Law and Medicine.

References and Credits

†Schorr T, Zimmerman A: Making Choices, Taking Chances: Nurse Leaders Tell Their Stories. St. Louis, CV Mosby, 1988, p 58.

†Cushing M: personal communications, 2002.

August 31

Annie Turner Wittenmyer

1827–1900

"Nearly every soldier in that hospital was prostrated by fever or severe wounds. ... Typhoid fever and acute dysentery was the verdict in regard to my brother. There was little hope. ... An old, experienced surgeon said, 'If he can have good care and nursing his recovery is possible, not probable.' ... [he was] removed into a little inner room, and my fight with death began in earnest. Oh! Those dreadful days and nights of watching; no joys on earth can obliterate their memory. The restless tossing of the fever-stricken ones in the adjoining room, the groans of the wounded, the drip, drip, drip of the leaking vessels hung above the worst wounded ones to drop water on the bandages and keep them cool and moist, put every nerve on the rack, and pulsated through heart and brain until it seemed as though I should go wild. It was an inside view of the hospitals that made me hate war as I had never known how to hate it before. ... The pitiful cry of helpless ones calling, 'Nurse, nurse! water, water!' ... still rings in my ears." (1895)

Annie Turner Wittenmyer was a financially independent young widow who devoted her life to charitable causes. As a volunteer worker during the Civil War, she helped gather and distribute supplies, provided nursing care, and worked to improve nutrition in the military field hospitals. She recognized that, like sanitation and medicine, diet was important to recovery. Dying soldiers appealed to her to help their families, and several orphanages for war victims were funded in Iowa because of her efforts. After the war she was involved in church-related charities and then was elected several times as president of the National Woman's Christian Temperance Union. She opposed women's suffrage but worked for pensions to be awarded to Civil War nurses. She also helped to establish homes for Civil War nurses, widows, and mothers of veterans through the National Woman's Relief Corps. Some of her papers are stored at the Library of Congress.

Biography

Born: Aug. 26, 1827, Sandy Springs, Ohio. **Education:** schools in Kentucky, Ohio. **Work history:** Civil War volunteer; Matron, Iowa Soldiers' Orphans' Home; editor, founder, *Christian Woman;* President, Woman's Christian Temperance Union; Chaplain, Woman's Relief Corps; Director, National Woman's Relief Corps Homes, Ohio, Pa. **Organizations:** Founder, Ladies and Pastors Christian Union; Non-Partisan Woman's Christian Temperance Union. **Awards:** special pension from Congress in recognition of Civil War related efforts. **Died:** Sanatoga, Pa.

References and Credits

†Wittenmyer A: A rich reward for services: Saving the life of a brother. In Under the Guns: A Woman's Reminiscences of the Civil War. Boston, EB Stillings, 1895, pp 73–74.

Greenblatt E: Annie Wittenmyer. In Bullough V, Sentz L, Stein AP (eds): American Nursing: A Biographical Dictionary, vol. 2. New York, Garland, 1992, pp 360–362.

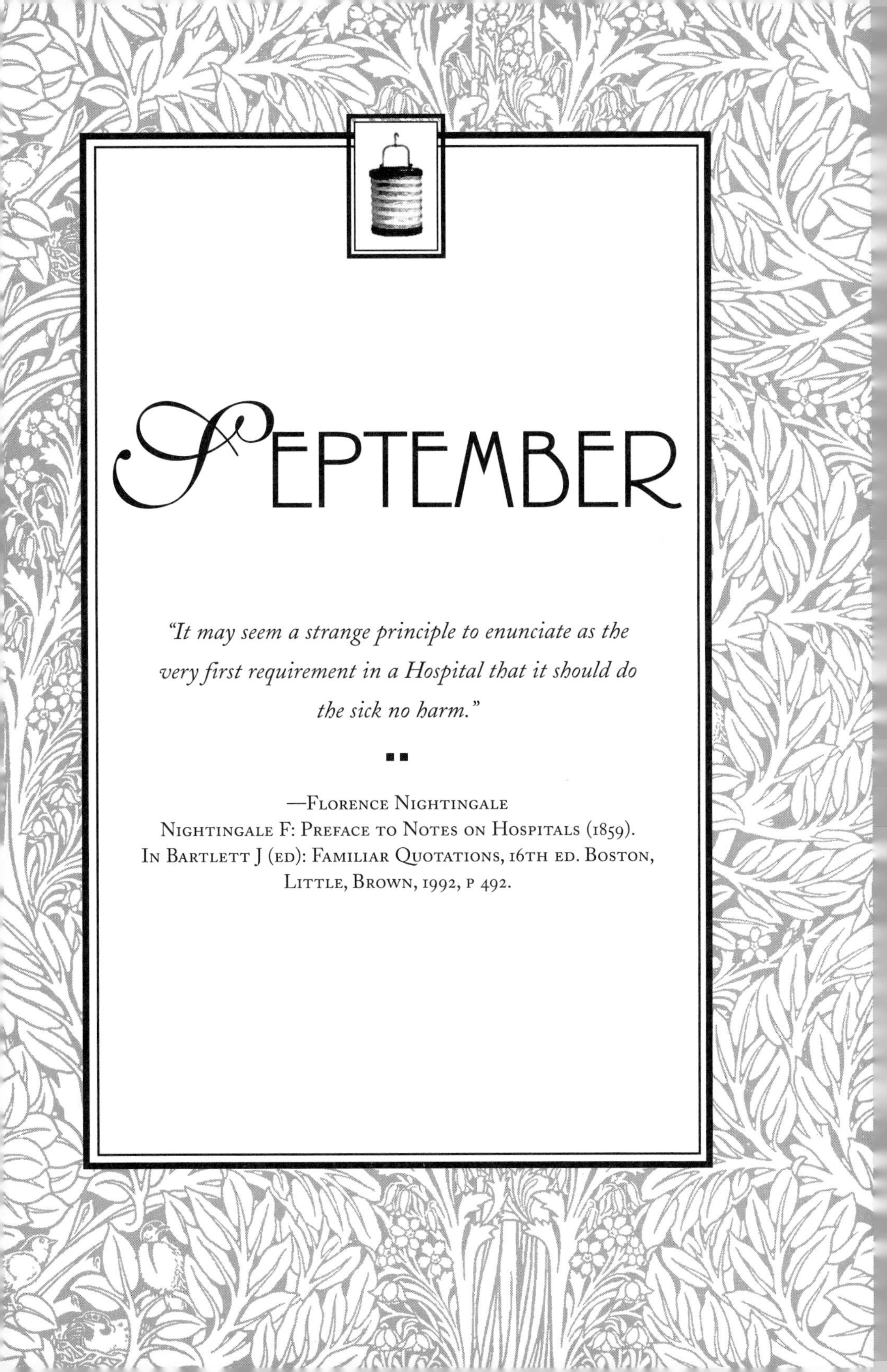

September

"It may seem a strange principle to enunciate as the very first requirement in a Hospital that it should do the sick no harm."

▪▪

—Florence Nightingale
Nightingale F: Preface to Notes on Hospitals (1859). In Bartlett J (ed): Familiar Quotations, 16th ed. Boston, Little, Brown, 1992, p 492.

September 1

Hildegard E. Peplau

1909–1999

"Nursing is a significant, therapeutic, interpersonal process. It functions co-operatively with other human processes that make health possible for individuals in communities. In specific situations in which a professional health team offers health services, nurses participate in the organization of conditions that facilitate natural ongoing tendencies in human organisms. Nursing is an educative instrument, a maturing force, that aims to promote forward movement of personality in the direction of creative, constructive, productive personal, and community living." (1952)

HILDEGARD PEPLAU WAS the first nursing leader to identify the significance of the patient-nurse relationship. In the late 1950s she created an awareness in patients that they should participate in their own care. She spoke with precision and exigency, urging the profession to assume full responsibility for its expansion. She is known as the "mother of psychiatric nursing." She is the only nurse to serve the American Nurses Association as executive director and later as president. She received the highest award in nursing, the Christiane Reimann Prize, at the Quadrennial Congress of the International Council of Nurses (ICN). Her renowned book, *Interpersonal Relations in Nursing,* was completed in 1948 and published four years later. The publication was delayed because the publisher believed that publishing a book by a nurse with no physician coauthor would be provocative. Peplau's book is credited with transforming nursing from a group of skilled workers into a mature, complete profession. Her theory and practice were directly responsible for the development of the specific clinical field of psychiatric nursing. Many agree that Hildegard Peplau's life and work created the greatest changes in nursing practice since Florence Nightingale. Peplau said that she wanted to be remembered "as a responsible citizen and a nurse and leave the rest to history."

Biography

Born: Sept. 1, 1909, Reading, Pa. **Education:** Pottstown (Pa.) Hosp. School of Nursing, 1931 (diploma); Bennington College, full scholarship, 1936–43 (BA in interpersonal psychology); Teachers College, Columbia Univ., 1945, 1947 (MA, PhD). **Work history:** School Nurse, Bennington College, Vt.; worked with Eric Fromm, Freda Fromm-Reichman, and Harry Stack Sullivan; First Lt., U.S. Army Nurse Corps, 1943–45; assigned to U.S. School of Military Neuropsychiatry, England, during World War II; New York State Psychiatric Institute; wrote *Interpersonal Relations in Nursing;* Educational Director, postgraduate program in psychiatric nursing, Highland Hosp., Ashville, N.C.; Instructor, Director, advanced program in psychiatric nursing, Instructor in nursing education, Teachers College, N.Y.; Private Duty Psychiatric Nurse, N.Y.C.; Instructor, Chair, Director, psychiatric nursing, Professor Emerita, Rutgers State Univ. of New Jersey, College of Nursing; maintained a part-time psychotherapy practice; developed workshops in clinical psychiatric nursing; Consultant to surgeons general of air forces of U.S., Turkey, and Labrador; lectured in Canada, Africa, and South America; Visiting Professor in nursing, Univ. of Leuven, Belgium, two yrs.; Interim Exec. Director, American Nurses Assoc. (ANA); Nursing Consultant, National Institute of Mental Health; major contributor to "Nursing: A Social Policy Statement," paper published by ANA, 1980. **Organizations:** member, first expert advisory committee to World Health Organization, 1948; member, bd. of directors, ICN; President, ANA; Director, N.J. State Nurses Assoc.; Third Vice President, ICN; **Awards:** Living Legend, American Academy of Nursing, 1996; numerous honorary doctorates; Hildegard E. Peplau Award, 1990, ANA bd. of directors and Council of Psychiatric Mental Health Nursing, ANA Hall of Fame. **Died:** Sherman Oaks, Calif.

References and Credits

†Peplau HE: Interpersonal Relation in Nursing: A Conceptual Frame of Reference for Psychodynamic Nursing. New York, GP Putnam's Sons, 1952, p 16.

Visone EMB, Church OM: Hildegard Peplau. In Bullough V, Sentz L, Stein AP (eds): American Nursing: A Biographical Dictionary, vol. 2. New York, Garland, 1992, pp 262–264.

Sills G, Peplau LA, Reppert B: The Hall of Fame Inductees: Hildegard Peplau obituary, available on-line at http://www.ana.org/hof/peplauh2.htm.

ANA Hall of Fame 10/98 American Nurses Association, Washington, D.C. http://www.nursingworld.org/hof.

Peplau A: personal communication, 2003.

September 2

Anne Larson Zimmerman

1914–2003

"We're going to have to be willing to make choices, and, once a choice is made, ... defend it even though it may not be unanimous. We nurses seem to have great difficulty in making choices and then living with them. We make a choice, and then we go back and reexamine it and reexamine it. ... We seem to think that all decisions must be unanimous ... rather than accepting ... a seven-to-six decision, ... biting the bullet ... and moving on. ... I think that if we could get ourselves in a position where we're strong enough to defend the majority decision and have respect for a minority opinion, we would be much better off." (1978)

As a young girl, Anne Zimmerman was drawn to nursing by the example of those who cared for her sick mother, her own experiences when she was hospitalized with a fractured femur, and the Great Depression. She became a leading national advocate for the economic and general program of the American Nurses Association (ANA). She credits an instructor, Margaret Bottinelli (Troxel), for teaching her social justice and instilling in her the realization that "a just wage need not be at the expense of the patient." When Zimmerman applied for work as a young staff nurse, she was newly divorced and had a small child. She found hospitals were hesitant to hire her because she had a dependent; she also found that her earnings as a single parent were inadequate. This led to her involvement with professional nursing organizations and specifically to leadership roles in pushing for economic security for nurses. She promoted active political involvement at all levels and encouraged nurses to get experience by running for office or managing campaigns in their own nursing organizations. Nurses could then build on their successes to become more politically sophisticated and influential in the legislative arena, especially when working to improve health care. Above all, she calls membership in the ANA the hallmark of professional nursing. When she was president of the ANA, she said, "I think nurses are beginning to realize that just because we are lovable people does not mean that people will treat us in a lovable way. ...We are going to have to make our voices heard more strongly if we expect to exert influence on national health policy." Her respected and knowledgeable voice on collective bargaining as a responsibility of professional nursing and her commitment to work-related issues had national and international influence. In addition, in 1988 she and Thelma Schorr published a collection of candid personal histories of some contemporary nurses who influenced the profession, *Making Choices, Taking Chances: Nurse Leaders Tell Their Stories.*

Biography

Born: Sept. 1, 1914, Marysville, Mont. **Education:** St. John's Hosp., Helena, Mont. **Work history:** Staff Nurse, St. John's Hosp.; Associate Administrator, Calif. Nurses Assoc. (CNA); Director, ANA Economic and General Welfare Program; Administrator, Illinois Nurses Assoc. (INA); President. ANA; Faculty, Loyola Univ., Chicago; American Journal of Nursing Co.; Commission on Graduates of Foreign Nursing Schools; International Lecturer; Consultant. **Organizations:** Mont. State Nurses Assoc., CNA, INA, ANA, International Council of Nurses. **Awards:** honorary member, Sigma Theta Tau International; Fellow, American Academy of Nursing (AAN); Living Legend, AAN, 1997; Sage Award, Power of Nursing Conference, Univ. of Illinois College of Nursing; Honorary Membership Award, INA, 1964; Shirley Titus Award for contributions to the Economic and General Welfare Program, ANA, 1980; Catholic Nurse of the Year, Archdiocesan Council of Catholic Nurses of Chicago, 1989; Anne Zimmerman Research Endowment Fund, American Nurses Foundation; honorary doctorates, Montana State Univ., Loyola Univ., Chicago. **Died:** Chicago.

References and Credits continued on page 770

Emilie Willms

1888–1969

"I am a great believer in that each individual is on this earth for a purpose. Mine was to serve many and not be confined to a few. I follow my destiny." (ca. 1955)

EMILIE WILLMS WAS a nursing pioneer. She answered an advertisement in the *American Journal of Nursing* for nurses needed in Greece and served from 1928 until her retirement in 1955. She upgraded hospital standards, established schools of nursing, and promoted programs for public health and rehabilitation. She worked under adverse conditions to provide health care to wounded Greek military as they courageously fought oppression. She was committed to the country and its people, who lovingly called her "the second Florence Nightingale."

BIOGRAPHY

Born: Sept. 1, 1888, Bremen, Germany. **Education:** Homeopathic Hosp., Newark, N.J.; New York School of Social Work. **Work history:** welfare worker, Silver Lake, N.J.; New Jersey Tuberculosis League; Dover (N.J.) General Hosp.; Superintendent, American Women's Hosp. School of Nursing, Kokkinia, Greece; Municipal Hosp., Athens; Children's Hosp., Athens; 7th Military Hosp., Athens; Jersey City (N.J.) Medical Center; member of medical team of Near Eastern Foundation: assisted in Sinai Desert, Cyclades Islands; Rehabilitation Center for Civilian Disabled. **Organizations:** Hellenic National Graduate Nurses Assoc. **Awards:** Knight of the Order of Phoenix, Greece; British Red Cross Medallion; Greek War Services Medal; acknowledgment by East Orange (N.J.) General Hosp. (as her alma mater is now known). **Died:** East Orange, N.J.

References and Credits

†Beer ES: The Greek Odyssey of an American Nurse. Mystic, Conn., Lawrence Verry, 1972, pp 96, vi.

Sentz L: Emilie Willms. In Bullough V, Church OM, Stein AP (eds): American Nursing: A Biographical Dictionary, vol. 1. New York, Garland, 1988, pp 337–338.

September 4

Mary Grant Seacole

1805–1881

"I would pass the night restlessly, awaiting with anxiety the morning, and yet dreading the news it held in store for me. I used to think it was like having a large family of children ill with fever, and dreading to hear which one had passed away in the night. And as often as the bad news came, I thought it my duty to ride up to the hut of the sufferer and do my woman's work. But I felt it deeply. How could it be otherwise? There was one poor boy in the Artillery … whom I nursed through a long and weary sickness … and whom I grew to love like a fond, old-fashioned mother. I thought if ever angels watched over any life, they would shelter his; but one day, a short time after he had left his sick bed, he was struck down. … It was a long time before I could banish from my mind the thought of him as I saw him last … the blue eyes closed in the sleep of death." (1857)

Mary Seacole learned Creole herbal folk medicine from her mother in Jamaica and later applied it successfully to treat cases of yellow fever, cholera, and wounds in Panama and the Caribbean. She had a reputation as a healer, which prompted the military to call on her to treat a yellow fever outbreak in a Jamaican camp. After the death of her husband she traveled to England, where Florence Nightingale was organizing nurses for the Crimean

War effort. Convinced that she could be helpful, Seacole volunteered but was rejected. Undaunted, she traveled to Balaklava and established a "British Hotel" where the wounded could recover with good food in comfortable surroundings. Seacole, who considered herself a "doctress," worked on the battlefield, caring for injured soldiers from both sides of the conflict. Her accomplishments were overshadowed by those of Florence Nightingale. Scholars suspect that Seacole may have been rejected for nursing service because she was a woman of color, neither British nor upper class, and her medical knowledge raised fears that she would practice independently rather than assume the expected subservient role of following doctors' orders.

Biography

Born: 1805, Kingston, Jamaica. **Education:** learned folk medicine from her mother. **Work history:** "Doctress" in Jamaica, Panama, Caribbean, Turkey; Author. **Organizations:** unknown. **Awards:** Mary Seacole Assoc., founded 1980, "to raise public's awareness of this great black woman." **Died:** England.

References and Credits

†Edwards P, Dabydeen D: Black writers in Britain, 1760–1890. Edinburgh, Scotland, Edinburgh University Press, 1991, p 174.

Griffon DP: "A Somewhat Duskier Skin": Mary Seacole in the Crimea. Nurs Hist Rev 6:115–127, 1998.

Internurse.com, available on-line at http://www.internurse.com/history/seacole/MarySeacole.htm.

Marion W. Sheahan

1892–1994

"I think that nurses should recognize the imminence of an entire change in the organization for health care. Nurses have to be prepared to take their part in the change that's coming, organizationwise and socially. There are too few of our group who really have a concept of where we are going and how we are moving. ... There are personalities that lend themselves to being willing to take responsibility, and that's the essence of leadership—not only deciding what to do and having commitments to certain objectives. ...I think all leadership is the willingness to be committed and take responsibility for the mistakes you make as well as the successes you have. ...Important, too, is the ability to interpret your concepts and goals to the end [that] nursing leadership is accepted on a coequal basis with other components in agency and community affairs." (1977)

Marion Sheahan's commitment to social reform was influenced by her contacts with Margaret Sanger and Annie Goodrich. Sheahan's work with the Henry Street Settlement sparked a nursing career that influenced national public health and policy. She was instrumental in including nursing service under the Temporary Relief Act during the depression, and the resulting nursing preparation and service programs that she developed in

New York became national models. She recognized that the advent of social security provided opportunities for government scholarships to prepare nurses in public health. She was an actively involved member of the National League for Nursing, as well as numerous national committees that addressed nursing issues. One result of her work with the National Nursing Council for War Service led to equal treatment of black nurses in the military. The highlight of her national involvement was serving as the only nurse on President Truman's health commission, which prepared the comprehensive report, *Health Care of the Nation,* in 1952.

Biography

Born: Sept. 5, 1892, New York City. **Education:** St. Peter's Hosp. School of Nursing, Albany, N.Y.; additional coursework, Syracuse Univ., Columbia Univ. **Work history:** Public Health Staff Nurse, Henry Street Settlement, Albany (N.Y.) City Health Dept., Niagara County (N.Y.) Health Dept., New York State Health Dept.; Administrator, New York State Health Dept.; member, National Council for War Service, National Nurses Planning Committee, President's Commission to Study Health Needs of the Nation, Surgeon General's Consulting Group on Nursing, National Social Welfare Assembly, New York Hosp. Review and Planning Council. **Organizations:** N.Y. State Nurses Assoc., National Organization for Public Health Nursing, American Public Health Assoc. (APHA). **Awards:** Lasker Award, Sedgwick Award, APHA; honorary doctorates, Adelphi Univ., Case Western Reserve Univ.; Florence Nightingale Medal, International Committee, Red Cross; Distinguished Service Award, National League for Nursing; McIver Award, American Nurses Assoc.; Honorary Fellow, American Academy of Nursing. **Died:** Albany, N.Y.

References and Credits

†Safier G: Contemporary American Leaders in Nursing. New York, McGraw-Hill, 1977, p 366.

Pavri JM: Marion Sheahan. In Bullough V, Sentz L (eds): American Nursing: A Biographical Dictionary, vol. 3. New York, Springer, 2000, pp 257–260.

September 6

Mary Starke Harper
1919 –

"Statistics reveal that the elderly are a rapidly growing population in the United States and also indicate that this population is at risk, both physically and mentally. Yet this group all too often 'falls through the safety net' of health services. Because the interrelationship between physical and mental illness becomes more prominent in old age, many of the elderly's behavioral disorders go unrecognized and untreated. Many suffer physical and mental discomfort because of lack of knowledge and resources. It is important to keep in mind that the overall goal in working with the elderly is to enhance the quality of life, help to develop and/or maintain independent functioning, and to empower the elderly and prevent iatrogenic dependency. ... This is a population that can benefit greatly by the nursing model of care. ... There is an extreme shortage of geropsychiatric nurses, a need that must be addressed if the medical and nursing communities are to help this population in the coming years." (1991)

Mary Starke Harper, a highly regarded patient advocate, researcher, scholar and consultant, has a broad clinical, academic, and professional background and a lifetime of versatile and ongoing achievement. She worked for the federal government for sixty years, and her present focus is on psychogeriatrics and primary health care for the rural elderly. A creative and inquisitive child, she was raised in a family that highly valued discipline and study. Harper studied business administration at her father's request, but after his death she changed her major to nursing. As a student nurse doing fieldwork in public health, she participated in the now infamous Tuskegee syphilis study. That experiment defined control and treatment groups by assigning numbers to patients. The nurses then administered medications according to number but were not given specific information about diagnosis or treatment. In a recent lecture at Yale University, Harper referred to that experience as cautionary, reminding nurses to remain vigilant in their duties to protect patients against risk in research projects. She was the cofounder of the National Black Nurses Association. Since the early 1980s she has been involved in the development of health policy, minimum data sets, nursing home care, home health care, and assisted living care. Harper conceived, then implemented, the National Fellowship Programs, which provided opportunities for eight thousand minority students to earn doctoral degrees in psychology, nursing sociology, and social work and provided residencies in psychiatry. Her concern about barriers to health care for many minorities resulted in the first National Minority Health Research and Development Centers, the first to be managed by minority scholar-researchers. She held faculty positions at several university schools of nursing and continues to apply her expertise on mental health and aging.

Biography

Born: Sept. 6, 1919, Ft. Mitchell, Ala. **Education:** nursing, Tuskegee Institute; Univ. of Minnesota (BS, MS); St. Louis Univ. (PhD). **Work history:** Faculty, Schools of Nursing, Univ. of Minnesota, University of California, Los Angeles, St. Joseph College, New York, Virginia Polytechnic Institute and State Univ.; Veterans Administration Hosps., Mich., Calif., N.Y., Ohio, Ala.; U.S. Dept. of Health and Human Services; National Institute of Mental Health; Director, Office of Policy Development and Research, White House; Researcher; Author; Editor. Consultant. **Organizations:** Secretary, American Assoc. of International Aging; National Council of Home Health; Hillcrest Children's Center, Washington, D.C. **Awards:** chair endowed in her name and research conference in her name, Tuskegee Institute;

Biography continued on page 770

SEPTEMBER 7

Clara S. Weeks Shaw

1856–1940

"The importance of the art of nursing can scarcely be overestimated; in many cases the recovery of the patient will depend more upon the care he receives than upon medical skill. ...A natural aptitude for nursing is a valuable basis for instruction, but will not take the place of it, nor will good intentions ever compensate for a lack of executive ability. Unimpaired health and power of endurance, intelligence and common sense are primary essentials for a nurse. She should be a person of even, cheerful temperament, not easily irritated or confused—for to lose temper or presence of mind in the sick-room is fatal to usefulness. She must have acute perceptions, habits of correct observation and accurate statement, and some manual dexterity. She needs to be quiet, neat and systematic, and capable of eternal vigilance." (1897)

CLARA WEEKS SHAW was educated and worked as a schoolteacher before entering nursing school. While working as a nurse administrator in the nursing school that she established in Patterson, New Jersey, she recognized and met the need for a nursing textbook written by a nurse. Only two textbooks for nurses existed before the publication of hers, and both were written primarily by physicians. When her *Textbook of Nursing* was published in 1885, it was the first by an American nurse. Her introductory remarks addressed the concerns of some doctors who felt threatened when educated nurses would initiate treatment and trespass into the doctor's realm. She reminded them that educated nurses understand their duties and limits. She suggested that the doctors should worry more about the untrained helpers who picked up bits and pieces of information and acted upon it.

Biography

Born: 1856, location unknown. **Education:** Rhode Island State Normal School; New York Hosp. Training School. **Work history:** organizer, Superintendent, Patterson (N.J.) General Hosp. School of Nursing. **Organizations:** unknown. **Awards:** unknown. **Died:** Mountainview, N.Y.

References and Credits

†Shaw CW: A Textbook of Nursing. New York, D. Appleton, 1897, pp 13–14.

Bullough V: Clara S. Weeks Shaw. In Bullough V, Church OM, Stein AP (eds): American Nursing: A Biographical Dictionary, vol. 1. New York, Garland, 1988, p 290.

SEPTEMBER 8

Karren Kowalski

1943–

"Mastery of knowledge and skills begins with ordinariness. ...There are many roads from ordinariness to mastery, and the road I chose is but one of them. However, I believe each of these roads requires a passion, a commitment—a willingness to do whatever it takes to reach desired goals. Early nursing leaders such as Dorothea Dix, Linda Richards, and Mary Breckenridge loved what they did. Their work was a passion, a mission. ...I love creating women's health care the way women want it. Hand in hand with the passion comes the knowledge that the 'essence' of life is not the mission. ...Regardless of the nobility of that mission, the ends never justify the means. What keeps life in perspective for me is knowing that the essence of living is the process or the journey—it is the lives I have touched, the people I have helped along the way, and knowing that I have made a difference." (1988)

KARREN KOWALSKI SERVED as a nurse in Vietnam before returning to Colorado, where her determination and persistence reformed women's health care. As she worked in obstetrics, she discovered that her mission was to change the hospital environment, especially for indigent women, to one that was more caring and supportive. She designed a patient-centered program that provided continuity of care by nurses for maternity patients and worked for legislation to allow for the practice of nurse-midwives. She recognized the importance of parents' seeing their baby in cases of infant death, and her efforts changed hospital policy. Her doctoral dissertation examined bereavement, and she started a support group for bereaved parents. She recognizes the importance of mentors and credits those who encouraged her to achieve all that she could. Kowalski cherishes the time that she spent working as the assistant vice president and administrator of the Women's and Children's Hospital at Rush-Presbyterian–St. Luke's Medical Center in Chicago. She commuted weekly from Denver for five years so that she could work there in Luther Christman's unification model, where one leader was responsible for both service and education. She is a courageous, creative thinker who now runs her own consulting firm. She recognizes that the work environment is the major factor in the nursing shortage, and she defines a supportive environment that values the nurse as one that would attract and retain the best nurses. Her numerous civic, academic, and professional awards pay tribute to her achievements.

Biography

Born: Sept. 10, 1943, Alameda, Calif. **Education:** Indiana Univ. (BSN); Univ. of Colorado (MSN, PhD). **Work history:** Army Nurse Corps., Vietnam; Head Nurse, labor and delivery, Univ. Hosp., Denver; Administrator, Women's and Children's Hosp., Rush-Presbyterian–St. Luke's Medical Center, Chicago; Chair, Dept. of Maternal-Child Nursing, College of Nursing, Rush-Presbyterian–St. Luke's Medical Center, Chicago; Faculty, Indiana Univ., Univ. of Colorado; Author; Speaker; Consultant. **Organizations:** American Nurses Assoc. (ANA); Colorado Nurses Assoc.; Sigma Theta Tau International; Nurses Assoc. of the American College of OB-GYN; Assoc. of Women's Health, Obstetric, and Neonatal Nursing (AWHONN); American Sociological Assoc. **Awards:** Fellow, American Academy of Nursing; Certificate of Merit, U.S. Army; Distinguished Alumnae Award, Univ. of Colorado School of Nursing; March of Dimes award for contributions in perinatal care; ANA Award for Outstanding Leadership; American Journal of Nursing Book of the Year Awards; Career Achievement Awards, Colorado Nurses Assoc.; Mary Beth O'Holleran Mentorship Award and Distinguished Service Award, Rush-Presbyterian–St. Luke's Medical Center; Distinguished Professional Service Award (highest national honor), AWHONN; Univ. of Colorado School of Nursing Alumni of the Century.

References and Credits

†Schorr T, Zimmerman A: Making Choices, Taking Chances: Nurse Leaders Tell Their Stories. St. Louis, CV Mosby, 1988, p 161.

References and Credits continued on page 770

September 9

Rena E. Boyle

1914 –

"Both nurse and non-nurse interviewers found it difficult to judge the student's estimate of the patient's condition, and it was a bit of a shock to find that the patient whom the student described as 'pleasant, happy, and loving to talk' was truly characterized by all of the comments—but, in addition, was hard of hearing and quite senile! None of the interviewers have indicated their own profession to the patients, and nurses and non-nurses alike have found it most illuminating to look at hospital situations through the eyes of patients and students." (1958)

RENA BOYLE ALWAYS wanted to be a teacher. Her interest in teaching, coupled with her innovations, was a spark for nursing education internationally, nationally, and regionally. She was a dean of nursing education and a consultant to the International Cooperative Administration in Haiti, Guatemala, and the University of Panama. While she was dean at the University of Nebraska, the school of nursing became an autonomous college and student enrollment increased significantly. She streamlined the curriculum to accommodate working nurses so they could matriculate with associate and baccalaureate degrees in off-campus programs. She wrote many articles on nursing education, nursing research, and teacher preparation. She served as director of the Department of

Baccalaureate and Higher Degree Programs at the National League for Nursing, and from the NLN she received the organization's highest award, the Adelaide Nutting Award.

Biography

Born: Sept. 9, 1914, Chicago. **Education:** Methodist Hosp. School of Nursing, Peoria, Ill., 1938 (diploma); Univ. of Minnesota, 1941, 1946, 1953 (BS, MS, PhD). **Work history:** Instructor, Associate Professor, Univ. of Minnesota; Chief of Nursing, Research and Consultant Branch, Division of Nursing, U.S. Public Health Service, 1956; Director, Department of Baccalaureate and Higher Degree Programs, NLN; Dean, Univ. of Nebraska. **Organizations:** unknown. **Awards:** Outstanding Achievement Awards, Univ. of Minnesota, Neb. Nurses Assoc., NLN; Professor Emerita; Distinguished Service to Nursing Award, Univ. of Nebraska College of Nursing; honorary doctorate, Univ. of Nebraska.

References and Credits

†Boyle R: How well do we know the patients we know best? AJN 58:1542, 1958.

Sentz L: Rena E. Boyle. In Bullough V, Sentz L, Stein AP (eds): American Nursing: A Biographical Dictionary, vol. 2. New York, Garland, 1992, pp 33–34.

September 10

Fay Louise Bower

1929–

"Taking the lead is being influential... skillful... [and] capable of initiating change. ...Seeing the big picture is an important aspect of leadership because it allows the leader to place the present situation and the decisions that need to be made into a larger context. ...It is looking at how the present situation is connected to or affected by other situations. It is the ability to see beyond the obvious, beyond the current activity, beyond the present. ...Paying attention, networking, and connecting what is known with what is learned form a model that has worked for me when I needed to get the full perspective. It has helped me make wise decisions... and it opened doors for me as a professional. I doubt that any leader at any level is able to provide leadership without the full picture, regardless of the issue." (2000)

FAY BOWER WAS born at a time when professional options for women seemed limited to teaching and nursing, and she recalls always wanting to be a nurse. Her decision enhanced nursing with a career of achievement and influence that spans a half century. She experienced every aspect of nursing. She has been a clinical nurse, educator, researcher, consultant, and speaker, as well as an author, editor, and administrator. Her first book, *The Process of Planning Nursing Care,* introduced the nursing process and nursing practice models. She defined nursing's unique role in comprehensive client care as dependent on the nurse's decision-making skills. This includes the ability to consider alternative approaches, as nurses assess patient needs and determine interventions. Her membership in professional and civic organizations is characterized by active involvement. A widely published and highly honored professional, she has served as president of the second-largest organization in nursing, Sigma Theta Tau International (STTI), and as consultant to numerous schools of nursing in the United States and Canada. She says that her most rewarding experiences have been her opportunities to mentor other nurses, researchers, clinicians, and leaders.

Biography

Born: Sept. 10, 1929, San Francisco. **Education:** St. Mary's Hosp. School of Nursing (RN); San Jose State College (BSN); Univ. of California, San Francisco (MSN, DNSc). **Work history:** Neonatal Intensive Care Nurse, Stanford Hosp.; Faculty, Nursing Administrator, nursing schools, San Jose State College; Univ. of San Francisco; Holy Names College, Oakland, Calif.; Univ. of California, San Francisco; Faculty, nursing schools, Univ. of Mississippi; Harding College, Ark.; Univ. of American, Beirut; President, Clarkson College, Neb.; Author; Editor; Speaker. **Organizations:** STTI, National League for Nursing, Assoc. of Episcopal Colleges, Neb. Nurses Assoc., Neb. Assoc. of Independent Colleges, American Assoc. of Colleges of Nursing, Calif. League for Nursing, Calif. Nurses Assoc., Assoc. of OB/GYN Nurses, Western Gerontological Assoc., American Assoc. of Univ. Professors; Jesuit Deans of Nursing; Calif. Teachers Assoc.; numerous community service organizations. **Awards:** several scholarships established in her name; numerous recognitions by *Who's Who* publications; Fellow, American Academy of Nursing; Phi Kappa Phi; Sigma Theta Tau; Phi Beta Gamma; Outstanding Professor Award, San Jose State College.

References and Credits

†Bower FL: Nurses Taking the Lead: Personal Qualities of Effective Leadership. Philadelphia, WB Saunders, 2000, pp 13, 67, 87.

Bower F: The Process of Planning Nursing Care: Nursing Practice Models, 3d ed. St. Louis, CV Mosby, 1982.

Bower F: resume.

Bower F: personal correspondence, 2002.

Fay Louise Bower. In Who's Who in American Nursing, 1996–97, 6th ed. New Providence, N.J., Reed Reference, 1995.

SEPTEMBER 11

Betty Reynolds Neuman

1924–

"In the Neuman Systems Model, health promotion is subsumed within the area of primary prevention and becomes one of the specific goals with it for nursing action. …Intervention goals would include education and appropriate supportive actions toward achieving optimal client wellness. …Primary prevention as intervention with inherent health promotion is an expanding, futuristic, proactive concept with which the nursing field must become increasingly concerned. It has unlimited potential for major role development that could shape the future image of nursing as world health care reform continues to evolve in the twenty-first century." (2002)

As a young child, Betty Neuman saw her father hospitalized many times for treatment of Bright's Disease until his death at thirty-six. Limited family finances precluded thoughts of college. During World War II she took a job in a defense plant, where she worked until she learned of the wartime nursing shortage and the Cadet Nurse Corps. In 1947 she completed the Corps's accelerated nursing program. She then moved to California, where she held several clinical nursing positions. As a graduate student, then faculty member, at the University of California, Los Angeles (UCLA), she focused her interests on mental health and community health.

She became a renowned theorist, speaker, consultant, and author while maintaining a practice as a licensed marriage and family counselor. In 1967 while at UCLA she developed the first post-master's community mental health program for nursing, and she chaired the program there for more than six years. She is noted worldwide for her holistic systems model, now called the Neuman Systems Model, which she developed in 1970. Her "whole person approach to patient problems" views people and their environment as dynamic interactive systems, where wellness changes on a continuum influenced by the energy exchange between people and their environment. She also views nursing as a system, one of internal and external environmental forces that affect the health of clients, whether individual, group, or community. Within nursing's own system Neuman calls for education and practice to be more closely connected. The interdisciplinary Neuman Systems Model is especially popular in Holland and England; in Holland it directs interdisciplinary psychiatric care and also is prominent in nursing education.

Biography

Born: Sept. 11, 1924, Lowell, Ohio. **Education:** People's Hosp. (now General Hosp.) School of Nursing, Akron, Ohio; City College and East Los Angeles Junior College; UCLA (bachelor's, master's); Pacific Western Univ., Los Angeles (PhD); National Fellow, American Assoc. of Marriage and Family Therapy. **Work history:** hosp. nursing, school nursing, occupational health nursing, private duty, program development, and administration, researcher, teacher, theorist, author, consultant, lecturer; State Mental Health Consultant, W. Va. **Organizations:** unknown. **Awards:** honorary doctorate, Neumann College, Pa.; Grand Valley State Univ., Mich.; Honorary Fellow, American Academy of Nursing.

References and Credits

†Neuman B, Fawcett J (eds): The Neuman Systems Model, 4th ed. Englewood Cliffs, N.J., Prentice Hall, 2002, p 29.

Brook M: Betty Neuman. In Bullough V, Sentz L (eds): American Nursing: A Biographical Dictionary, vol. 3. New York, Springer, 2000, pp 218–221.

Maude E. Callen

1900–1990

"My desire is to live as long as I can so that I can help. And 'let me live in a house by the side of the road and be a friend to man' the rest of my days, helping all I can." (Date unknown)

ONCE DESCRIBED BY *USA Today* as a "publicity shy Mother Teresa for backwoods America," Maude Callen first traveled to South Carolina's Low Country as a missionary nurse in 1923, and her life of service continued well into her eighties. The area had no phones, electricity, or a hospital when she arrived. She was an African American graduate nurse-midwife, teacher, and public health professional. For forty-eight years she was often the only person available to give maternal and child care in this isolated area of the segregated South. In 1951 she was one of only nine qualified midwives in South Carolina, where she assisted in the delivery of at least one thousand babies as she covered a four-hundred-square-mile area with ten thousand people. She provided midwife training institutes for lay midwives, many of whom were illiterate, to reduce the high maternal and infant death rates. Her supportive, nonthreatening style improved the quality of care by replacing traditional practices with formal, understandable instruction. She taught "granny" midwives maternal and infant care, hygiene, nutrition, communicable disease prevention, and the necessity of immunizations and established literacy classes for them as well. She founded and ran a health clinic with money donated after a 1951 *Life* magazine story focused on her dedication and nursing activities. Eugene Smith, the renowned photojournalist who did the story, called it his "most rewarding experience" and described her as the greatest person that he had ever been privileged to know. Her partnerships with white public health professionals in the pre-civil rights years significantly improved health care for women and children in South Carolina.

Biography

Born: 1900, Quincy, Fla. **Education:** Florida A&M College; Georgia Infirmary, Savannah; Homer G. Phillips Hosp., St. Louis (tuberculosis care); Tuskegee Institute (midwifery). **Work history:** Missionary Nurse, Protestant Episcopal Church, Berkeley County, Ala.; Founder, Teacher, Midwife Training Institute, S.C.; Founder, Volunteer, Senior Citizen Nutrition Site, Pineville, S.C. **Organizations:** unknown. **Awards:** Outstanding Older South Carolinian, 1981; named "A Top Achiever" by *USA Today,* 1984; Alexis de Tocqueville Award, United Way of America; Jefferson Award, American Institute for Public Service; honorary doctorates, Clemson Univ., Medical Univ. of South Carolina; featured on CBS's *On the Road with Charles Kuralt;* J. Marion Sims Award, S.C. Public Health Assoc., 1973; S.C. Hall of Fame. **Died:** Pineville, S.C.

References and Credits

†University of South Carolina College of Nursing Callen Scholarship Brochure, 2003.

O'Driscoll P: Maude Callen is one very busy woman. USA Today. 1984.

Magner L: Doctors, Nurses, and Medical Practitioners. Westport, Conn., Greenwood, 1997.

Smith E: Nurse midwife. Life, Dec. 3, 1951.

Nurse and midwife Maude Callen dies. (Charleston, S.C.) Evening Post, Jan. 24, 1990, p 7A.

Singletary R: Maude Callen's legacy lives. Currently 4:1–2, 1993.

Pooser C: MUSC honors nurse-midwife-teacher Callen. (Charleston, S.C.) News and Courier/Evening Post, May 20, 1989, p 9A.

Maude Callen receives public health award. J Nurse-Midwifery, undated clipping, p 30.

Bear B: personal communication, 2003.

Johnson S: personal communication, 2002.

September 13

Dita Hopkins Kinney

1854–1921

"Those who have had a large experience in life have learned to look with suspicion upon methods which promise great results and which call for small expenditure, be it of money, effort, or time. Everything in this world must be paid for. So much for so much is the inexorable law, and he who expects something for nothing invites disappointment and chagrin, the intensity of those being in exact proportion to the value of the thing he hoped to secure." (1905)

Dita Kinney was a widow with a young child when she entered nursing. During her career she countered the ubiquitous advertisements for questionable and fraudulent nursing schools with speeches and writings that supported educational standards and nursing registration. She then worked as a contract nurse for the army and cared for soldiers with communicable diseases after the Spanish-American War. Meanwhile, an ongoing government investigation was concerned with the high number of wartime mortalities. Major contributing factors were mismanagement by the War Department and conservative-led efforts that prevented the recruitment of qualified nurses. The subsequent reorganization established the Army Nurse Corps, with Kinney as its first superintendent. However, she found herself in a position with little authority. Her observations and recommendations to improve conditions for nurses were ignored. Her successor, Jane Delano, implemented several changes that were first proposed by Kinney.

Biography

Born: Sept. 13, 1854, New York City. **Education:** Mills Seminary (now College), Oakland, Calif.; Massachusetts General Hosp. Training School for Nurses (RN); studied hosp. administration, Massachusetts General Hosp. **Work history:** Nursing Instructor, Lecturer, New England; Administrator, Long Island Almshouse; City and County Hosp., St. Paul, Minn.; French Hosp., San Francisco; General Hosp., Presidio, San Francisco; Army Hosp., N. Mex.; Office of Surgeon General, Washington, D.C.; Superintendent, Addison Gilbert Hosp., Gloucester, Mass. **Organizations:** unknown. **Awards:** unknown. **Buried:** Trinity Cemetery, N.Y.C.

References and Credits

†Kinney D: Some questionable nursing schools and what they are doing. AJN 5:225, 1905.

Danis EM, McCarthy RT: Dita Kinney. In Bullough V, Church OM, Stein AP (eds): American Nursing: A Biographical Dictionary, vol. 1. New York, Garland, 1988, pp 201–204.

Margaret Higgins Sanger

1879–1966

"More than ever in history, women need to realize that nothing can ever come to us from another. Everything we attain we must owe to ourselves. Our own heart must feel it. For we are not passive machines. We are not to be lectured, guided, and molded this way or that. We are alive and intelligent, we women, no less than men, and we must awaken to the essential realization that we are living beings, endowed with will, choice, comprehension, and that every step of life must be our own initiative." (1920s)

MANY WOULD SAY that Margaret Louise Higgins Sanger should be the "Person of the Century" for she truly influenced the people of the entire world. Sanger was deeply affected by the early death of her Irish Catholic mother, who had given birth to eleven children. This is believed to have inspired her daughter's lifelong quest for education and family planning for the poor populations of women in the world. In October 1916 Margaret Sanger was jailed for thirty days in New York City for violating the Comstock Law, which forbade dissemination of birth control literature. She overcame the death of her only daughter, five-year-old Peggy, and continued to lobby for birth control legislation that allowed physicians to legally prescribe contraceptives. She founded Planned Parenthood, organized the Birth Control International Information Center, and is credited with helping to find funding for research to develop the first effective anovulant contraceptive, or birth control pill.

Biography

Born: Sept. 14, 1879, Corning, N.Y. **Education:** Claverack College, Hudson River Institute, 1896; White Plains Hosp., 1900; postgraduate training, Manhattan Eye and Ear Hosp. **Work history:** Public Health Nurse, New York's Lower East Side; opened first U.S. birth control clinic, Brooklyn, 1916; Editor, *Woman Rebel (*1914); *Birth Control Review (*1910–40), *Human Fertility (*1940–48). **Writings:** autobiography, 1938. **Organizations:** Founder, President, American Birth Control League; organized first World Population Conference, Geneva, 1927; first president, International Planned Parenthood Federation. **Awards:** American Nurses Assoc. Hall of Fame. **Died:** Tucson, Ariz.

References and Credits

†Sanger M: Margaret Sanger promotes birth control as an "ethical necessity for humanity." In Torricelli R, Carroll A (eds): In Our Own Words: Extraordinary Speeches of the American Century. New York, Kodansha International, 1999, p 69.

Bullough V: Margaret Sanger. In Bullough V, Church OM, Stein AP (eds): American Nursing: A Biographical Dictionary, vol. 1. New York, Garland, 1988, pp 279–282.

Chesler E: Woman of Valor: Margaret Sanger and the Birth Control Movement in America. New York, Simon and Schuster, 1992.

New York University on-line, biographical sketch of Margaret Sanger, June 8, 2000, available at http://www.NewYorkUniversity/educationalproject/sanger/ms-bio.htm, pp1–4.

ANA Hall of Fame 10/98 American Nurses Association, Washington, D.C. http://www.ana.org/hof/sangmh.htm.

SEPTEMBER 15

Laura Rebekah Logan

1879–1974

"The value of the response which the graduate nurse makes depends very largely upon the understanding which is given her as a student of the part she plays in the social welfare of her time. ... The education of the nurse must have incorporated into it all that will fit her to live as a good citizen and to do her part in promoting a high quality of human life. ... *The goal of nursing education, our ethical ideal, is to insure the best service which with knowledge and skill in our field we may render throughout the whole cross-section of social need." (1925)*

"More and more nursing educators and nurses must remember that above all methods of teaching and above all acquirements schools of nursing can give it is the individual woman who counts and that the nursing profession will increase or lose its public power in proportion to the collective expressions of the people's faith in each nurse who touches them." (1923)

ALTHOUGH LAURA REBEKAH LOGAN initially studied nursing as a way to earn money to go to medical school, she decided to remain in nursing and became an outstanding leader in nursing education. A true visionary, she was the second nursing professor in the country and established the first five-year U.S. nursing program at the University of Cincinnati. Students there took classes in liberal arts and nursing, earning a baccalaureate degree as well as a diploma in nursing. Logan was noted for initiating advanced and innovative coursework and inspiring others to excel as nurse leaders. She was active in professional organizations, particularly the National League for Nursing Education (NLNE), and served as an editor at the *American Journal of Nursing.*

Biography

Born: Sept. 15, 1879, Amherst Point, Novia Scotia, Can. **Education:** Acadia Univ. (BA); Mt. Sinai Hosp. School of Nursing, N.Y.C. (RN); Teachers College, Columbia Univ. (BS). **Work history:** various positions in nursing education at Mt. Sinai Hosp., N.Y.C.; Hope Hosp. School of Nursing, Ft. Wayne, Ind.; Cincinnati General Hosp.; Univ. of Cincinnati; Illinois Training School, Chicago; Flower Fifth Ave. Hosp., N.Y.C.; Boston City Hosp.; St. Louis City Hosp.; Stanford Univ.; Univ. of Chicago; Marquette Univ.; Nursing Education Editor, *American Journal of Nursing.* **Organizations:** various leadership positions, NLNE; Red Cross Nursing Service Committee; National Commission for Grading of Nursing Schools; National Organization for Public Health Nursing; American Nurses Assoc.; adviser, U.S. Veterans Bureau; Council of National Defense; Ohio State Nurses Assoc. **Awards:** honorary degrees, Acadia Univ., Univ. of Cincinnati; Residence Hall named Logan Hall, Univ. of Cincinnati. **Died:** Sackville, Nova Scotia, Can.

References and Credits

†Logan L: The goal of nursing education. AJN 25:544, 1925.

†Logan LR: Retrospect and prospect AJN 23:922, 1923.

Fickelssen JL: Laura Logan. In Bullough V, Church OM, Stein AP (eds): American Nursing: A Biographical Dictionary, vol. 1. New York, Garland, 1988, pp 214–217.

Ella Phillips Crandall

1871–1938

"Let me point out still one other public service which I believe public health nursing is destined to render in constantly increasing measure (and now, I refer primarily, but not solely, to those who give bedside care). The system of hourly nursing, already well established in a few cities, forecasts a larger and more satisfactory and more economical service to the sick public than has yet been provided. ...It is bound to grow rapidly, though not as an enterprise separate from visiting nursing, but as an integral part of it. ...Both the nurses and the public see the practicability and dignity... of a service which sells the nurse's skill rather than her time." (1921)

ELLA PHILLIPS CRANDALL was a nursing leader in both clinical and public health nursing. When she started the school of nursing at Miami Valley Hospital in Ohio, she worked closely with S. Lillian Clayton to modernize the hospital and the nursing program. When Crandell joined the Visiting Nurse Service (VNS) in New York City, she recognized the sense of isolation felt by nurses in the field and how it was affected by the wide range of their training and performance. She then took a faculty position at Teachers College for two years to develop related coursework. She was a friend and adviser to nurses and health agencies that worked to standardize preparation and practice for public health nursing. Her work with Lillian Wald at Henry Street and Mary Adelaide Nutting at Columbia led Crandell to spearhead the development of a professional organization, the National Organization for Public Health Nursing (NOPHN), and a professional journal for public health nurses.

Biography

Born: Sept. 16, 1871, Wellsville, N.Y. **Education:** Philadelphia General Hosp. School of Nursing (RN); New York School of Philanthropy. **Work history:** Superintendent, Nursing Instructor, Miami Valley Hosp., Dayton, Ohio; Superintendent, VNS, N.Y.C; Faculty, Teachers College, Columbia Univ.; Organizer, Administrator, NOPHN; Administrator, Council of National Defense; Exec. Director, Payne Fund (to promote education of youth for peace). **Organizations:** NOPHN; American Nurses Assoc., American Red Cross, Committee to Study Community Organization for Self Support for Health Work for Women and Young Children; Bureau of Educational Nursing of the Assoc. for Improving the Condition of the Poor; American Child Health Assoc. **Awards:** unknown. **Died:** New York City.

References and Credits

†Crandell, EP: An historical sketch of public health nursing. AJN 22:644, 1922.

Mernitz KS: Ella Crandell. In Bullough V, Church OM, Stein AP (eds): American Nursing: A Biographical Dictionary, vol. 1. New York, Garland, 1988, pp 68–70.

James E (ed): Notable American Women, 1607–1959, vol. 1. Cambridge, Mass., Belknap Press, 1971.

September 17

Mary Kelly Mullane

1909–1999

"If nursing could get itself together and provide the public with a well-defined redefinition of the role of nursing in modern society—what it ought to be—we couldn't fail, given our large numbers. ...I hope the next generation of professional nurses will demonstrate their expertise and dedicate their money and energies to speaking with one voice about future goals of American's health care. If they can, the public and nursing itself will be better for it. ...We need to recognize that we are kept at the forefront of public confidence only when we serve the public's needs in their terms, not ours." (1977)

A WIDELY PUBLISHED and highly honored nursing visionary, Mary Kelly Mullane was called the statesman of nursing during her career. She influenced nursing education during a career of high achievement. She was committed to high standards and believed that nursing required higher education. She helped establish the nursing program at Mercy College in Detroit, worked for inclusion of the nursing program at Wayne State University in the university system, and promoted the development of the doctoral program in nursing at the University of Illinois in Chicago. While at Wayne State, she and Kathryn Faville gained equal clinical opportunities for black nurses, and Mullane is credited with helping integrate black nurses into the American Nurses Association (ANA). While at the University of Iowa she transferred the authority for curriculum and clinical experience from the hospital to the university. She saw the nursing program at the University of Illinois in Chicago become a nationally prominent leader in doctoral education. She participated in a seminar on nursing administration that led to the development of fourteen graduate-level nursing programs in nursing administration.

Biography

Born: Sept. 25, 1909, New York, N.Y. **Education:** Holy Name Hosp., New York (RN); Teachers College, Columbia Univ. (BS, MA); Univ. of Chicago (PhD); postdoctoral studies, Dept. of Systems Engineering, Univ. of Illinois. **Work history:** Private Duty Nurse, OR Supervisor, Holy Name Hosp., New York; Instructor, St. Joseph Hosp., Patterson, N.J., and St. Francis Hosp., Jersey City, N.J.; founder, Mercy College School of Nursing, Detroit; Faculty, Administrator, Wayne State Univ.; Dean, Univ. of Iowa School of Nursing; Dean, School of Nursing, Univ. of Illinois, Chicago; Exec. Director, American Assoc. of Colleges of Nursing. **Organizations:** National Council of Catholic Nurses; Mich. and Ill. State Nurses Assocs.; Michigan and Illinois League for Nursing; National League for Nursing (NLN); Assoc. of Collegiate Schools of Nursing; **Awards:** Detroit Nurse of the Year; Mich. State Pharmaceutical Award; scholarship in her name, Providence Hosp., Detroit; member, Pi Lambda Theta, Sigma Theta Tau, Phi Kappa Phi; honorary member, Institute of Medicine, Chicago, Chicago Pediatric Society; ongoing annual symposium in her name, Alpha Lambda Chapter, Sigma Theta Tau, Univ. of Illinois, Chicago; Distinguished Honorary Award, ANA; honorary doctorates, Southern Illinois Univ., Univ. of Illinois, Loyola Univ.; Adelaide Nutting Award, NLN; Founders Award, Sigma Theta Tau; McManus Award, Columbia Univ.; Univ. of Illinois Distinguished Alumnae Award; member, American Academy of Nursing. Living Legend, American Academy of Nursing, 1997. **Died:** Naples, Fla.

References and Credits

†Safier G: Contemporary American Leaders in Nursing: An Oral History. New York, McGraw-Hill, 1977, pp 252–253.

Dudas S: Mary Mullane. In Bullough V, Sentz L (eds): American Nursing: A Biographical Dictionary, vol. 3. New York, Springer, 2000, pp 233–237.

Martha Montague Russell

1867–1961

"During the last twenty years a new recognition of social obligation has grown up in the community, and it is now generally conceded that ... it is essential ... to consider the problems of accident, illness, disability and unemployment not as individual, but as social problems. The first legislation in this country regarding accident insurance was enacted about seven years ago, and now thirty-four states have workman's compensation laws. ... The next step in social insurance which is receiving the attention of those interested in equalizing the burdens of society, is that of health insurance. ... The democratic character of an effective health insurance is most pronounced in a government system." (1917)

"Compulsory health insurance is the next step to be taken." (1917)

Martha Russell served in France as a Red Cross nurse during World War I. She worked almost to the point of exhaustion to see that nursing services were provided to approximately three million soldiers. She made sure that nurses working in the base hospitals had warm clothing for winter, and she encouraged American nurses abroad to join the Red Cross effort. She chaired the committee on health insurance of the National League for Nursing, and its report supported government involvement in compulsory health insurance. She cited health insurance programs and benefits in other countries, especially the positive effect on lifespan. She used a report from Metropolitan Life Insurance about the health of families in Rochester, New York, to show the differences in accessibility to quality care based on income. She said caregivers recognized that one of the greatest benefits of health coverage for everyone would be "the promise of prevention" and that coverage for nursing care was essential.

Biography

Born: Sept. 18, 1867, Pittsfield, Mass. **Education:** Mt. Holyoke College; New York Hosp. School of Nursing. **Work history:** Administrator, Providence (R.I.) Lying-In Hosp.; Director of Nurses, West Pennsylvania Hosp., Pittsburgh; Superintendent of Nurses, Sloan Hosp.; Administrator, Red Cross Nursing Service; other stateside nursing positions, incl. Superintendent of School of Nursing, Univ. of Colorado. **Organizations:** American Red Cross; National League for Nursing Education. **Awards:** Florence Nightingale Medal, International Committee, Red Cross. **Died:** Front Royal, Va.

References and Credits

†Russell MM: What social insurance will mean to nurses. AJN 17:388–389, 1917.

†Russell MM: Report of the Committee on Health Insurance: AJN 17:864, 1917.

Sentz L: Martha Montague Russell. In Bullough V, Sentz L, Stein AP (eds): American Nursing: A Biographical Dictionary, vol. 2. New York, Garland, 1992, pp 281–282.

September 19

R. Faye McCain

1917–1982

"Patient assessment is the responsibility of the professional nurse. ...A patient, today, is expected to do for himself whatever he is capable of doing; in other words, he is expected to participate in his therapeutic regimen. But in order to help him be a participant, the nurse must know his functional abilities as well as his disabilities. When she plans nursing care and writes nursing orders, the nurse will capitalize on the patient's abilities but, at the same time, she will endeavor to assist him to live with his disabilities, whether they are temporary or permanent." (1965)

Faye McCain was a pioneer in medical-surgical nursing and in her role as a clinical nurse specialist. Her work proved fundamental to defining both nursing diagnoses and the role of clinical nurse specialist. She was an advocate for graduate study for nurses and developed a "nursing symptom" framework to direct nursing interventions. She taught students to define the patient's symptoms; study the related physiology to understand the cause; then plan appropriate care by researching and applying related nursing knowledge. She stressed that it was essential for professional nurses to develop assessment skills based on science and knowledge. In 1965 she outlined how nursing assessment of functional abilities directed subsequent nursing care in her now classic article, "Nursing by

Assessment—Not Intuition." She contrasted nursing, which she described as "primarily intuitive," with other professions that were more "precise." She acknowledged the assessment recommendations of other nurse-researchers but said they were not being applied. She called on nursing to use its knowledge and learned skills of interview, observation, inspection, review of known data, and professional judgment to plan ongoing patient care.

Biography

Born: Sept. 16, 1917, Texas. **Education:** Parkland Hosp., Dallas (RN); San Francisco College for Women (BSNE); Teachers College, Columbia Univ. (MA). **Work history:** Staff Nurse, Head Nurse, Flight Nurse, Army Nurse Corps.; Head Nurse, Supervisor, San Francisco Veterans Administration Hosp.; Teacher, San Francisco College for Women; Supervisor, medical-surgical nursing, Univ. Hosp., Ann Arbor, Mich.; Chair, medical-surgical nursing, Univ. of Michigan School of Nursing, Ann Arbor; Clinical Nurse Specialist; Acting Director of Graduate Study in Nursing, Univ. of Michigan, Ann Arbor. **Organizations:** National League for Nursing, Sigma Theta Tau, Phi Kappa Phi. **Awards:** student symposium to honor her work and graduate scholarship in her name, Univ. of Michigan, Ann Arbor. **Died:** Washington, D.C.

References and Credits

†McCain RF: "Nursing by assessment—Not intuition. AJN 65:83, 82, 1965.

Strodtman LK: Faye McCain. In Bullough V, Sentz L (eds): American Nursing: A Biographical Dictionary, vol. 3. New York, Springer, 2000, pp 199–201.

SEPTEMBER 29

Eleanor J. Sullivan

1938–

"We affect the future by what we do or fail to do today. . . . The future is a wide-open vista, a blank canvas on which to transform our vision into reality. There is no inextricable mystery here—we simply pose the questions: what is best for our clients, our patients? What is best for our profession? What can I do to make a difference? What works? What doesn't work? In a perfect world, how would nursing and health care be configured? Generations of nurses and their patients are relying on our imagination, intellect, and daring. By examining the issues, seizing the opportunities, and accepting the challenges, nursing is poised to create a vision for the future into the years to come. The future of nursing depends on it. And on you." (1999)

WHEN ELEANOR SULLIVAN'S husband was injured in an accident, she stayed at the hospital until his death several weeks later. She watched and listened to the nurses. She saw what they did and how they cared for him and for her. She decided then that she wanted to become a nurse. With five small children, and the youngest just six weeks old, she started nursing school. Although many people tried to discourage her, she persisted. The profession has been enhanced by her scholarship, leadership, research, and publications. She, in turn, gratefully acknowledges that nursing has provided immeasurable satisfaction through the many opportunities she has had to pursue her goals and contribute to nursing. Her book, *Creating Nursing's Future: Issues, Opportunities and Challenges,* provides the expertise, direction, and vision for nursing to take the lead in determining its own future rather than following a path defined by others. She has served as president of Sigma Theta Tau International (1997–99) and is the editor of the highly ranked *Journal of Professional Nursing,* the official journal of the American Association of Colleges of Nursing. A highly regarded researcher and author on substance abuse, nursing education, and health care policy, she more recently has turned to fiction, writing mysteries with a nurse protagonist.

Biography

Born: Sept. 20, 1938, Indianapolis, Ind. **Education:** St. Louis Community College (ADN); St. Louis Univ. (BSN); Southern Illinois Univ. (MSN); St. Louis Univ. (PhD); Fellowship in Academic Administration and Health Policy, Assoc. of Academic Health Centers. **Work history:** Associate Dean, Faculty, School of Nursing, Univ. of Minnesota; Faculty, Univ. of Missouri, St. Louis; Dean, Faculty, School of Nursing, and Faculty, School of Medicine, Univ. of Kansas; Editor; Author. **Organizations:** Sigma Theta Tau; American Assoc. of Colleges of Nursing. **Awards:** Fellow, American Academy of Nursing; research awards; American Journal of Nursing Book Awards; honorary alumnus, Univ. of Kansas; Alumnus of Year, St. Louis Univ.; L. Christman Award, Assembly of Men in Nursing.

References and Credits

†Sullivan E: Creating Nursing's Future. St. Louis, CV Mosby, 1999, p xiv.

Sullivan E: personal communication, 2001, 2002.

Futuristic issues in nursing, 2001, press release on course. American Association of Colleges of Nursing, available on-line at http://www.classes.kumc.edu/son/nrsg962/content/Sullivan.htm.

Sullivan E: resume.

September 21

Lydia Eloise Hall

1906–1969

"We, at Loeb Center, believe the public deserves and can profit from professional nursing care. Here, patients and families are acutely aware that they are receiving such care. ... When the patient has passed the first stage of illness he is able, with his family and the nurse, to face and solve the problems involved in achieving maximum health. We encourage the patient to become engaged in a learning process which helps his body heal and his personality grow. We place emphasis on what the problem is and how to overcome it. ... In turn, the patient and family learn how to face problems and ways of solving them. ... He and his family re-enter the world of active living better prepared to cope with it than before the period of illness." (1963)

Lydia Hall's professional career included public health, research, consulting, and teaching, all of which influenced her innovative approach to rehabilitation nursing. She had the opportunity to help establish and then direct the Loeb Center for Nursing and Rehabilitation at New York's Montefiore Hospital when it opened in 1963. She applied the findings of Carl Rogers and Harry Stack Sullivan to her model for professional nursing care. The first priority was to identify the patients' needs; then the professional nurse would provide the personalized, one-on-one care that focused on identifying and meeting those needs. The professional nurse was the essential ingredient in the therapeutic relationship so that the patient could improve and benefit from the art as well as the skill of nursing. Hall often spoke about and published accounts of her experiences and ideas for nursing practice.

Biography

Born: Sept. 21, 1906, New York, N.Y. **Education:** Gettysburg (Pa.) College, York (Pa.) Hosp. School of Nursing (RN); Teachers College, Columbia Univ. (BS in public health nursing, MA, ABD). **Work history:** various nurse positions in New York and Pennsylvania; Metropolitan Life Insurance Co.; research, New York Heart Assoc.; Staff Nurse, then administrator, Visiting Nurse Service, New York; Faculty, Fordham Hosp. School of Nursing; Faculty, Teachers College; Research, U.S. Public Health Service; Faculty, North Carolina School of Nursing, Marquette Univ. School of Nursing; established, then directed Loeb Center, Montefiore Medical Center. **Organizations:** American Nurses Assoc. (ANA), National League for Nursing, National Organization for Public Health Nursing; N.Y. State Nurses Assoc.; Kappa Delta Pi; numerous voluntary committees in New York. **Awards:** Teachers College Alumni Award for Distinguished Achievement in Nursing Practice; Doctors Hosp., Freeport, N.Y. renamed Lydia E. Hall Hosp.; ANA Hall of Fame. **Died:** Queens, N.Y.

References and Credits

†Hall LE: A center for nursing. Nurs Outlook 11:806, 1963.

Birnbach N: Lydia Hall. In Bullough V, Church OM, Stein AP (eds): American Nursing: A Biographical Dictionary, vol. 1. New York, Garland, 1988, pp 161–163.

ANA Hall of Fame 10/98 American Nurses Association, Washington, D.C. http://www.nursingworld.org/hof.

September 22

Mary A. Brewster

1822–1878

"Thursday, June 25 [1846]... I have today commenced the office of ship's nurse. The lame sick and bruised all come to me. Doctoring done free of all expense."

"Sunday Sept. 20th, 1846 ...[Her actual birthday] Finds me well on a pleasant but foreign shore. Far from my own native land. This day completes my 23rd year. In looking upon the past which has so quickly fled I can see much misspent time and many hours unprofitably passed—and wasted—many good resolves which were made and broken. How often have I felt that I would try and be more useful and live better—and yet have lived the same. Shall I ever see another birthday Lord thou alone knowest. *May this be my desire, to commence anew from this time by living a life which will bear reviewing, which will save me much sad reflection. May this be my aim, to live up to the profession I have made, striving to do all the good I can in whatever circumstances I may be placed or wherever I may be."*

"Monday July 6 [1846]... The last part of the day I have spent in making doses for the sick, in dressing some hands and feet, 5 sick and I am sent to for all the medicine. I am willing to do what can be done for any one particularly if sick for in whaling season a whaleship is a hard place for comfort for well ones and much more sick men."

MARY BREWSTER WAS a nurse, wife, and author. She kept a journal from 1845 to 1851, while she was sailing on the American whaling vessel *Tiger* with her husband, the ship's captain, William E. Brewster. According to the author Joan Druett, this journal was the earliest publicly held diary kept by an American whaling wife. Mary Brewster held the distinction of being the first white woman to travel to the Arctic. She was born in and retired to Stonington, Connecticut, where her home stands today as a historical treasure.

Biography

Born: Sept. 20, 1822, Stonington, Conn. Little is known about education, work, or other aspects of her life. **Died:** Stonington, Conn.

References and Credits

†Druett J (ed): She Was a Sister Sailor: The Whaling Journals of Mary Brewster. Mystic, Conn., Mystic Seaport Museum, 1992, pp 98, 128, 102.

September 23

Amelia Howe Grant

1887–1967

"Our modern corollary [to Florence Nightingale's definition of 'health nurses'] is that the nurse must know and understand her patient's ways of living, his attitudes concerning health, his work, his recreation, his desires, and his needs, whether they be physical, mental, social or economic, in order to give her best service. The early visiting nurses took care of the sick, using all of the knowledge, experience, and technical skill of the day. . . . They learned much about the causes of sickness, the reasons why people did not have adequate medical care, the relationship of poverty and poor living conditions to health, the influence of social maladjustment, and the effect of sickness in the home upon other members of the family." (1942)

Amelia Grant was a true leader in the field of public health nursing education. She made major contributions to the basic concepts and philosophy of public health nursing for both its practice and education through her example as the head of the New York City Health Department and as a faculty member at Teachers College of Columbia University and the Yale School of Nursing. She developed theories and philosophies that identified the outpatient department as a link between the hospital and the family. She wrote about the importance of social hygiene and connected it to the prevention and cause of disease. She characterized the role of the nurse as educator in the home and school, and she advocated the adoption of these basic public health principles. Grant was a well-organized administrator, and she used these skills to unify the seven hundred nurses in the New York City Health Department and to create and implement an in-service educational program.

Biography

Born: Sept. 23, 1887, Utica, N.Y. **Education:** Afton (N.Y.) High School; Faxton Hosp. School of Nursing, Utica, N.Y.; one-year course in public health nursing, Simmons College, Boston; Teachers College, Columbia Univ. (BS, MS). **Work history:** Private Duty Nurse; Public Health Nurse, Supervising Nurse, Henry Street Visiting Nurse Assoc.; Assistant Instructor, Teachers College, Columbia Univ.; Assistant Professor, nursing education, Yale Univ. School of Nursing; Administrator, Assistant Director, Bellevue Yorkville Health Demonstration Project, funded by the Millbank Memorial Foundation for Research in Community Health, N.Y.C.; Director, New York City Bureau of Nursing, Dept. of Health. **Writings:** wrote for *Public Health Nursing*. **Organizations:** President, National Organization for Public Health Nursing; Chair, National League for Nursing Education; Chair, Joint Committee, American Social Hygiene Assoc.; member, many community organizations. **Awards:** numerous professional honors. **Died:** Amsterdam, N.Y.

References and Credits

†Grant AH: Nursing: A Community Health Service. Philadelphia, WB Saunders, 1942, pp 14–15.

Calley LM: Amelia Grant. In Bullough V, Sentz L, Stein AP (eds): American Nursing: A Biographical Dictionary, vol. 2. New York, Garland, 1992, pp 135–137.

September 24

Sister Elizabeth Kenny

1886–1952

"Though it is no longer fashionable to be thought an idealist, I cannot quite free myself of the conviction that a Power greater than ourselves must shape human destiny to its final purpose. ...I have striven to set down the brief record of a life that has little claim to distinction beyond the fact that within its narrow limits a battle has been fought against forces entrenched in precedent and armoured with tradition. A measure of victory has been won, and honors have been bestowed. ...But honors fade or are forgotten, and monuments crumble into dust. It is the battle itself that matters—and the battle must go on. One human life alone cannot encompass the full extent of the struggle. ...To the men and women of the future, therefore, I give freely what I have done. May they ..., equipped with all that modern science can provide, dedicate the labor of their hands and the devotion of their hearts to the end that healing may be brought to the suffering children of every land, of every creed, and of every race. Only thus can we prove ourselves worthy of the heritage of freedom that has been bequeathed to us." (1943)

Sister Elizabeth Kenny is credited with the medical community's acceptance of physical therapy as a valued practice. She first studied muscle function when she was fourteen so that she could help a young sibling with physical weakness. He improved after she worked with him, and a physician friend encouraged her to pursue additional studies. When she was a young rural visiting nurse in Australia, traveling on horseback to remote areas, she first successfully used hot wet compresses to relieve the muscle contractures of a small child. Sister Kenny—all Australian nurses who achieved the rank of naval officer were known as *Sister*—reasoned that infantile paralysis (polio) was characterized by muscle weakness and spasms that led to contractures and that massage and exercise would strengthen muscles, prevent contractures, and lead to improvement. She recommended warm soaks and exercise when the accepted medical treatment was immobilization of affected muscles. When the Mayo Clinic accepted her methods of palliative care, it ended more than twenty years of rejection and ridicule by the medical community. She is said to never have accepted income of any kind from her care of patients but supported herself with income from her books and royalties from the two devices ("an improved stretcher and a devise for stabilizing wounded bodies for transport") that she developed and patented during World War I.

Biography

Born: Sept. 20, 1886, Warialda, New South Wales, Australia. **Education:** St. Ursula's College, Australia. **Work history:** Visiting Nurse, South Wales; Transport Nurse, World War I; operated clinics in Australia and England for treatment of infantile paralysis, before and after the war; Author; Lecturer, Univ. of Minnesota; opened Kenny Institute, Minn.; started Sister Kenny Foundation, opened clinics across United States. **Writings:** biography, which became the eponymous film *Sister Kenny.* **Organizations:** unknown. **Awards:** Gold Key from Congress of Physical Therapists; honorary doctorates from Univ. of Rochester, New York Univ. **Died:** Toowoomba, Queensland, Australia.

References and Credits

†Kenny E, Ostenso M: And They Shall Walk. New York, Dodd, Mead, 1943, vii, 272.

Stein AP, Bullough V: Sister Elizabeth Kenny. In Bullough V, Church OM, Stein AP (eds): American Nursing: A Biographical Dictionary, vol. 1. New York, Garland, 1988, pp 198–200.

September 25

Sue Sophia Dauser

1888–1972

"Womanly compassion has been expressed through the ages by individuals and by religious devotees in the care of the sick and unfortunate. But modern professional nursing was born in War. Ever since Florence Nightingale led her courageous little band to the Crimea, nurses have been going to war, sharing the work and sacrifices of the fighting men." (1946)

Sue Sophia Dauser was appointed superintendent of the Navy Nurse Corps on January 30, 1939, and remained in that position until her retirement in November 1945. She was the first woman to receive the rank of captain. Her great accomplishment was to see that navy nurses received commissions, equal pay, and privileges for their rank. While superintendent she expanded the Navy Nurse Corps from six hundred nurses in the period before World War II to more than eleven thousand commissioned officers in 1945. All these nurses had volunteered to serve. She worked closely with the American Red Cross, Allied armed services, and the army head of services to improve nursing care on the battlefield and to supply nursing personnel on all fronts. She established postgraduate training programs for navy nurses and made certain that the navy participated in the Cadet Nurse Training Program. The first black woman nurse, Phyllis Daley, was sworn in to the Navy Nurse Corps as an ensign in March 1945 while Dauser was superintendent. Dauser was a veteran of both world wars. After her retirement, she became one of the founders and a resident of the retirement home Mt. Angel Towers in southern California. She was known for her ready smile, her eagerness to assist others, and her interest in everything. She rarely spoke of herself.

Biography

Born: Sept. 20, 1888, Anaheim, Calif. **Education:** Fullerton High School, 1907; attended Stanford Univ., 1907–9; California Hosp. School of Nursing, Los Angeles, 1917 (RN). **Work history:** Surgical Supervisor, California Hosp. School of Nursing, Los Angeles; joined Naval Reserve, April 1917; prepared for military nursing, San Diego Naval Hosp.; Chief Nurse, Naval Reserve, Base Hosp. #3, Los Angeles; regular navy, July 10, 1918; Chief Nurse, HMS *Mandingo,* 1918; converted existing facility to U.S. Navy Base Hosp. #3, Edinburgh, Scotland; Chief Nurse, Naval Hosps., Brooklyn, N.Y., San Diego, Calif.; Night Nurse for President Warren G. Harding on Alaskan cruise on *Henderson* and was attending him when he died in 1923; provided nursing care, directed activities of Red Cross volunteer nurses, Naval Reserve and regular navy staff nurses, and naval corpsmen on ships, 22 yrs.; Superintendent, Navy Nurse Corps, 1939–45. **Organizations:** unknown. **Awards:** first navy nurse to receive Distinguished Service Medal. **Died:** Anaheim, Calif.

References and Credits

†Dauser S: Preface to Navy Nurse by P Cooper. New York, McGraw-Hill, 1946, p ix.

Cohen KF: Sue Dauser. In Bullough V, Sentz L, Stein AP (eds): American Nursing: A Biographical Dictionary, vol. 2. New York, Garland, 1992, pp 77–79.

Mount Angel Newsletter 24: 1972.

September 26

Cora E. Simpson

CA. 1880–CA. 1960

"A few years ago, a few of us came to China. There was no association, no textbooks, no schools of nursing, and no word for 'nurse' in the Chinese language. We were told that China did not want us, did not need nurses. . . . But a few slipped by . . . and began the education of nurses. Let me raise the curtain for you again in 1922. The Nurses Association of China has a roll of over five hundred members, over sixty schools of nursing are registered, with a standard, uniform curriculum. It holds its own national examinations and issues its own diplomas to successful candidates. It offers two postgraduate courses, so when the complete course is taken the student holds three school and three national diplomas. It holds a national convention. . . . The journal . . . is published in English and Chinese. . . . The Association . . . was admitted to membership in the International Council of Nurses. This work has grown beyond the fondest dreams of the founders." (1923)

Cora Simpson began her service as a missionary nurse in Foochow, China, in 1907, before the Chinese had a word or a role for such a professional person. She was sent by the Women's Board of the Methodist Episcopal Mission of the United States, and she is considered the chief founder of the Nurses Association of China (NAC). Through the efforts of the NAC nursing schools were established, with the first graduates in 1915. Simpson recognized needs to be met by nurses' service and initiated school and community health care, care for lepers, and baby and child services. Through her efforts the medical community saw the value of nursing care and increased support for her programs. She was instrumental in having the NAC recognized by the International Council of Nurses (ICN). She remained actively involved despite the political upheaval in China. Upon her return to the States she continued to be supportive by giving speeches about her years in China, the NAC, and what nursing had accomplished.

Biography

Born: 1880, location unknown. **Education:** Methodist Hosp. School of Nursing, Neb.; additional coursework in theology, Bible, social services, Chinese, pharmacy, public health nursing. **Work history:** Missionary Nurse, China; established nursing schools, China; established NAC. **Organizations:** NAC, ICN. **Awards:** General Secretary Emeritus, NAC; Alumni Service Medal (posthumous), Neb. Methodist Hosp. **Died:** location unknown.

References and Credits

†Simpson C: A wireless from China for you! AJN 23:504, 1923.

Stein AP: Cora E. Simpson. In Bullough V, Sentz L, Stein AP (eds): American Nursing: A Biographical Dictionary, vol. 2. New York, Garland, 1992, pp 302–304.

September 27

Jessie C. Sleet (Scales)

CA. 1875–1950

"I have never hesitated to visit anyone when I have felt that a word of advice or a friendly warning was all they needed. I have visited forty-one sick families and made one hundred and fifty-six calls in connection with these families, caring for nine cases of consumption, four cases of peritonitis, two cases of chicken pox, two cases of cancer, one case of diphtheria, two cases of heart disease, two cases of tumor, one case of gastric catarrh, two cases of pneumonia, four cases of rheumatism, two cases of scalp wound. I have given baths, applied poultices, dressed wounds, washed and dressed new-born babes, cared for mothers. ...I have instructed them how to care for the sick one. ...I have made daily visits if... required..., caring for them until they were able to care for themselves." (1901)

JESSIE SLEET BROKE the color barrier when she persevered in the face of racial discrimination and became the first graduate black nurse hired, in 1900, as a district public health nurse in New York City. She was given a trial period of employment with what later became the New York Tuberculosis Association. The agency was concerned about the high incidence of tuberculosis in the black community, and Sleet focused on home visits to encourage medical care. In addition, she made frequent visits to churches, physicians, and organizations about the needs of the community and her work. This resulted in approval and strong support. She was competent and effective and received a permanent job with the organization. She worked there for ten years, and before she left she prepared the nurse who would fill her position, thus ensuring both the quality of nursing service and the continued option of public health nursing for black graduate nurses.

Biography

Born: ca. 1875, Stratford, Ontario, Can. **Education:** nursing school, Provident Hosp., Chicago; additional coursework, Freedman's Hosp., Washington, D.C. **Work history:** Private Duty Nurse, Lakewood, N.J.; Public Health Nurse, New York Tuberculosis Assoc. **Organizations:** unknown. **Awards:** unknown. **Died:** location unknown.

References and Credits

†Sleet J: A successful experiment. AJN 1s:729, 1901.

Buchinger K: Jessie Sleet (Scales). In Bullough V, Sentz L, Stein AP (eds): American Nursing: A Biographical Dictionary, vol. 2. New York, Garland, 1992, pp 305–307.

September 28

Alma Elizabeth Gault

1891–1981

"Is it economically sound to promote comprehensive nursing which encompasses a constellation of services to the patient and family, including case findings, promotion of health and rehabilitation as well as care of the sick? Research ... might reveal savings to the community and to the hospital. ...Nurses must help with or do this research if it is to be done properly. The pediatric nurse who understands the child and his mother, who comforts, sustains and helps them to meet the problems of pain, separation and even death has a discipline of mind and skill in interpersonal relationships that is second to no other professional worker. With these abilities the nurse can make valuable contributions to research." (1954)

ALMA ELIZABETH GAULT influenced nursing in Tennessee through her involvement with Meharry Medical College and later Vanderbilt University. When she took the position of dean at Nashville's Meharry Medical College School of Nursing in the mid-1940s, she was a white nurse in a segregated southern school for black students. Her leadership resulted in an accredited diploma school, followed by a highly ranked baccalaureate program with inclusion in the American Association of Collegiate Schools of Nursing. In addition, the Rockefeller Foundation provided opportunities for foreign nursing students to study there and for Meharry students to study in Canada. Long before the civil rights movement, Gault was actively involved in integration issues and efforts for racial and professional justice in such areas as public transportation, public eating areas, and hospital cafeterias. Her diplomacy and skill helped defuse community problems in Nashville after the slaying of Martin Luther King Jr.

Biography

Born: Sept. 28, 1891, Fernwood, Ohio. **Education:** College of Wooster, Ohio (bachelor's degree in philosophy); Vassar Training Camp for Nurses; Philadelphia General Hosp. School of Nursing; graduate study, Univ. of Chicago. **Work history:** Head Nurse, Philadelphia General Hosp.; Nurse, tuberculosis clinic, Ohio State Health Dept.; Nurse, pediatric clinic, Johns Hopkins Hosp.; Faculty, Illinois Training School and Cook County School of Nursing, Chicago; Director, Union Memorial Hosp. School of Nursing, Baltimore; Director of Nursing Service, Memorial Hosp., Springfield, Ill.; Dean, Meharry Medical College School of Nursing, Nashville, Tenn.; Faculty, Vanderbilt Univ. School of Nursing, Nashville, Tenn.; Tennessee Bd. of Nursing. **Organizations:** American Nurses Assoc. (ANA); Sigma Theta Tau; Delta Kappa Gamma; National League for Nursing (NLN); Council on Aging; American Assoc. of Univ. Women; Senior Citizens, Inc. **Awards:** Certificate of Merit, American Cancer Society; Distinguished Alumnae Award, Wooster College; Distinguished Service Award, NLN; honorary recognition, Hall of Fame, ANA; Alma Gault Day, Nashville, Tenn. **Died:** Columbus, Ohio.

References and Credits

†Gault A: Nursing's professional reach. Nurs Outlook 2:377, 1954.

Baldwin PE: Alma Gault. In Bullough V, Church OM, Stein AP (eds): American Nursing: A Biographical Dictionary, vol. 1. New York, Garland, 1988, pp 132–133.

ANA Hall of Fame 10/98 American Nurses Association, Washington, D.C. http://www.nursingworld.org/ hof.

September 29

Margo McCaffery
1938–

"My own experience with migraines not only made me more aware of the pain of others but brought into sharp focus the fact that the existence and character of pain cannot be proved. ... It was clear to me that most patients had some difficulty with discomfort or pain—brief to prolonged, mild to severe—and that nurses spent more time with patients who were in pain than did any other member of the health team. ... I had become irrevocably committed to nursing's role in the care of patients with pain. I believed that nursing could make a unique contribution there. ... If nurses were to identify their unique and significant contributions to patient care—then helping the patient with pain would play a major part. ... We can at least minimize the physical pain and suffering. ... Compared to the myriad problems faced by a patient, it is one problem we can do something about." (1988)

After her father suffered an accident that resulted in brain damage, Margo McCaffery became so angry with a neurosurgeon to want to become one. Then, because she wanted a shorter course of study, she decided to study practical nursing instead. Meanwhile, her mother had submitted a university application for her, and Margo McCaffery learned that she had been accepted and offered a scholarship. She entered a nursing program without knowing much about it, saying she thought she would become a "junior doctor." She soon learned the true nature of nursing. She worked as a staff nurse and later taught nursing. Personal experience with migraine headaches and her work with burn patients sparked her interest in pain control, which became the focus of her graduate study. Because little had been written on the subject, she developed her own investigative methods, and in 1968 she published what has become one of the most frequently cited definitions of pain: Pain is whatever the person experiencing it says it is, and it exists whenever the patient says it does. Her interest in and findings about pain extend to teaching, writing, research, consulting, and widespread lecturing. She is an internationally recognized specialist in the nursing care of patients with pain, an award-winning author on pain management, and a current member of the World Health Organization's Expert Committee on Cancer Pain Relief and Active Supportive Care.

Biography

Born: Sept. 29, 1938, Corsicana, Texas. **Education:** Baylor Univ. (BS); Vanderbilt Univ. (MS). **Work history:** Staff Nurse, Corsicana, Texas; Faculty, Texas Woman's Univ., Vanderbilt Univ., Univ. of California, Los Angeles; Nurse-Clinician, pain management, Inglewood, Calif.; Researcher; Author; Lecturer; Workshop Leader on pain management; national and international consultant on pain management, Calif. **Organizations:** American Nurses Assoc.; American Pain Society (APS); American Society of Pain Management Nursing (ASPMN); founding member, International Assoc. for the Study of Pain; Sigma Theta Tau; Alpha Chi. **Awards:** Fellow, American Academy of Nursing; American Nurses Foundation Scholar; Univ. of Southern California Comprehensive Cancer Center Award; several Book of the Year Awards, *American Journal of Nursing;* Linda Richards Award, National League for Nursing; Nurse Exemplar Award, ASPMN; Elizabeth Narcessian Award, APS.

References and Credits

†Schorr T, Zimmerman A: Making Choices, Taking Chances: Nurse Leaders Tell Their Stories. St. Louis, CV Mosby, 1988, pp 269–271.

McCaffery M: personal correspondence, November 2002.

Franz J, Vandervort-Jones P (eds): Who's Who in American Nursing, 1986–87, 2d ed. Owings Mills, Md., Society of Nursing Professionals, 1987, p 410.

September 30

Barbara Fassbinder

1953–1994

"My biggest fear was how the community would react to me and my kids and my husband." (1994)

"I will have to pay with my life for caring for the sick and dying. ... Our best and only weapons are good techniques and strict use of barrier precautions. ... Depriving large, well-educated segments of society of their civil rights and their constitutional rights to privacy, to say nothing of assigning criminal penalties to persons that are already terminally ill, is simply cruel. ... Those actions will not prevent one single infection. They will only perpetuate fear and misunderstanding." (1991)

Barbara Fassbinder was one of the first health care providers to be infected with the AIDS virus. In 1986, in an emergency room setting, she was asked to remove an arterial line in the forearm of a dying young man. She applied pressure to the site with a gauze pad for ten minutes. Later, when she was washing her hands, she noticed that she had small cuts on her fingers from gardening. The patient died and his autopsy showed he had AIDS. She did not learn of her own infection, however, until she tried to donate blood in 1987. She and her family kept the diagnosis secret at first. She later toured the country, telling her story to warn other health care workers and to comfort AIDS patients. In 1991 she testified before a joint session of Congress against mandatory testing of health care providers. Dr. Michael Osterholm, an AIDS expert who befriended the Fassbinder family, said she "helped bridge the gap between the worlds of the health care provider and the AIDS patient in need of competent and compassionate care like no one else could." Fassbinder was a member of the Iowa Nurses Association (INA). She also served on the National Health Care Reform Task Force convened by Hillary Rodham Clinton. Fassbinder received national recognition in 1992 from the U.S. surgeon general and the Department of Health and Human Services (HHS) for her efforts in AIDS education. In 1992, at the American Nurses Association (ANA) convention, she was given special recognition for her courage. Upon Fassbinder's death in 1994, the ANA stated, "We commend Barbara for her personal courage and her sense of professional responsibility in taking her story public. She was an outspoken advocate of education, the use of universal precautions and the need to protect the rights of health care workers. Upon her death, we must rededicate our efforts to challenge the greatest enemy in the battle against AIDS—ignorance."

Biography

Born: Sept. 29, 1953, Cedar Rapids, Iowa. **Education:** Univ. of Iowa College of Nursing. **Work history:** ER Nurse, Memorial Hosp., Prairie du Chien, Wisc. **Organizations:** INA. **Awards:** national recognition, HHS, U.S. surgeon general for AIDS education efforts; Iowa Nurses Foundation Memorial Fund for Barbara Fassbinder–AIDS Education and Research, INA; subject of filmography, *The Barbara Fassbinder Story*, Univ. of Iowa College of Medicine, Iowa City. **Buried:** Monona City Cemetery, Monona, Iowa.

References and Credits

†Hilchey T: Barbara Fassbinder, 40, nurse with AIDS traced to her job. New York Times, Sept. 22, 1994, p D23.

†Congress kills AIDS penalties, Orders states to oversee testing. AJN 91:81, 1991.

McElwaine S: HIV positive courage and compassion in a small town. Family Circle, Jan. 7, 1992, pp 94–97.

Cooper SS: Barbara Fassbinder. In Bullough V, Sentz L (eds): American Nursing: A Biographical Dictionary, vol. 3. New York, Springer, 2000, pp 87–88.

Profession mourns loss of Barbara Fassbinder. American Nurse 26:3, 1994.

Fassbinder D: personal communication, 2003.

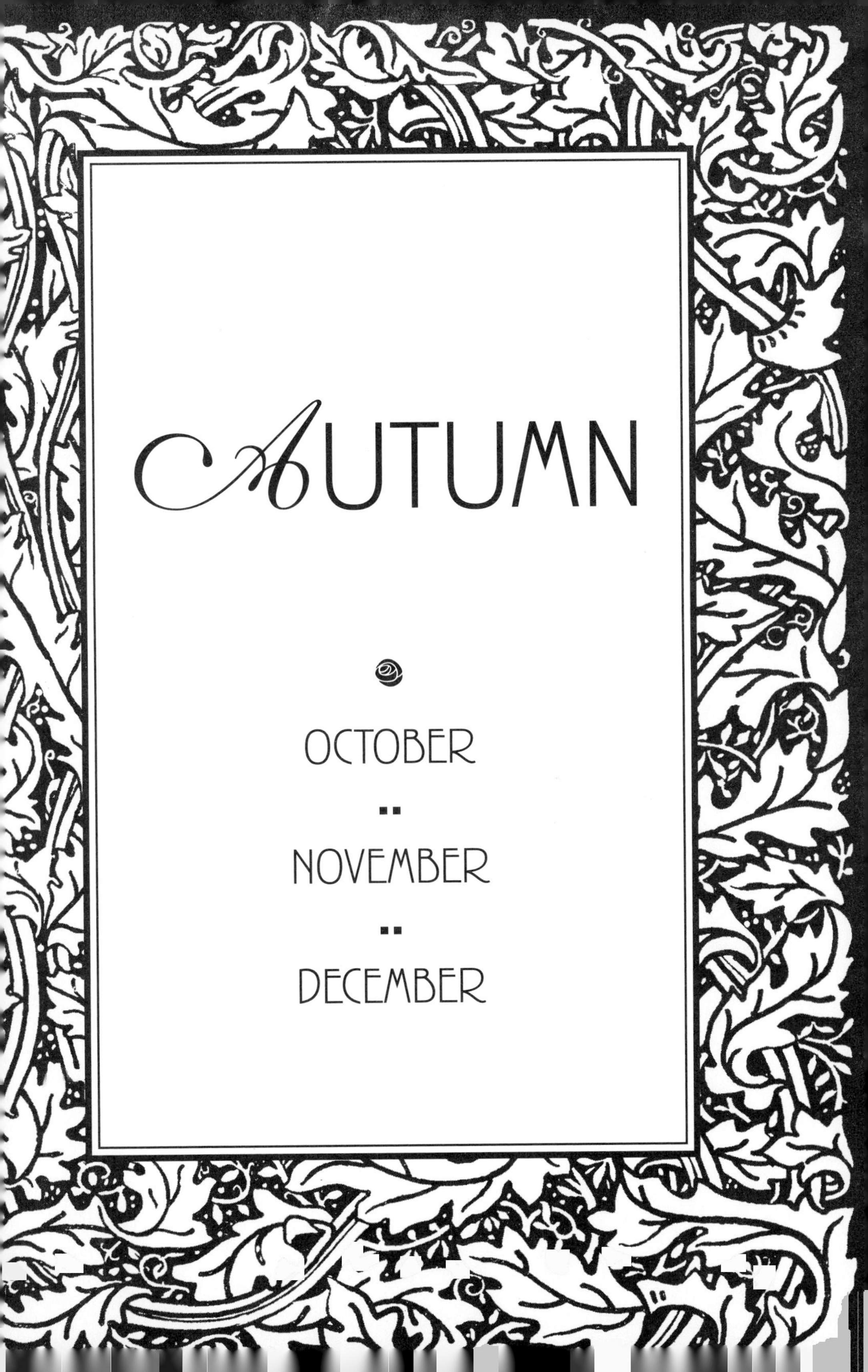

AUTUMN

OCTOBER

NOVEMBER

DECEMBER

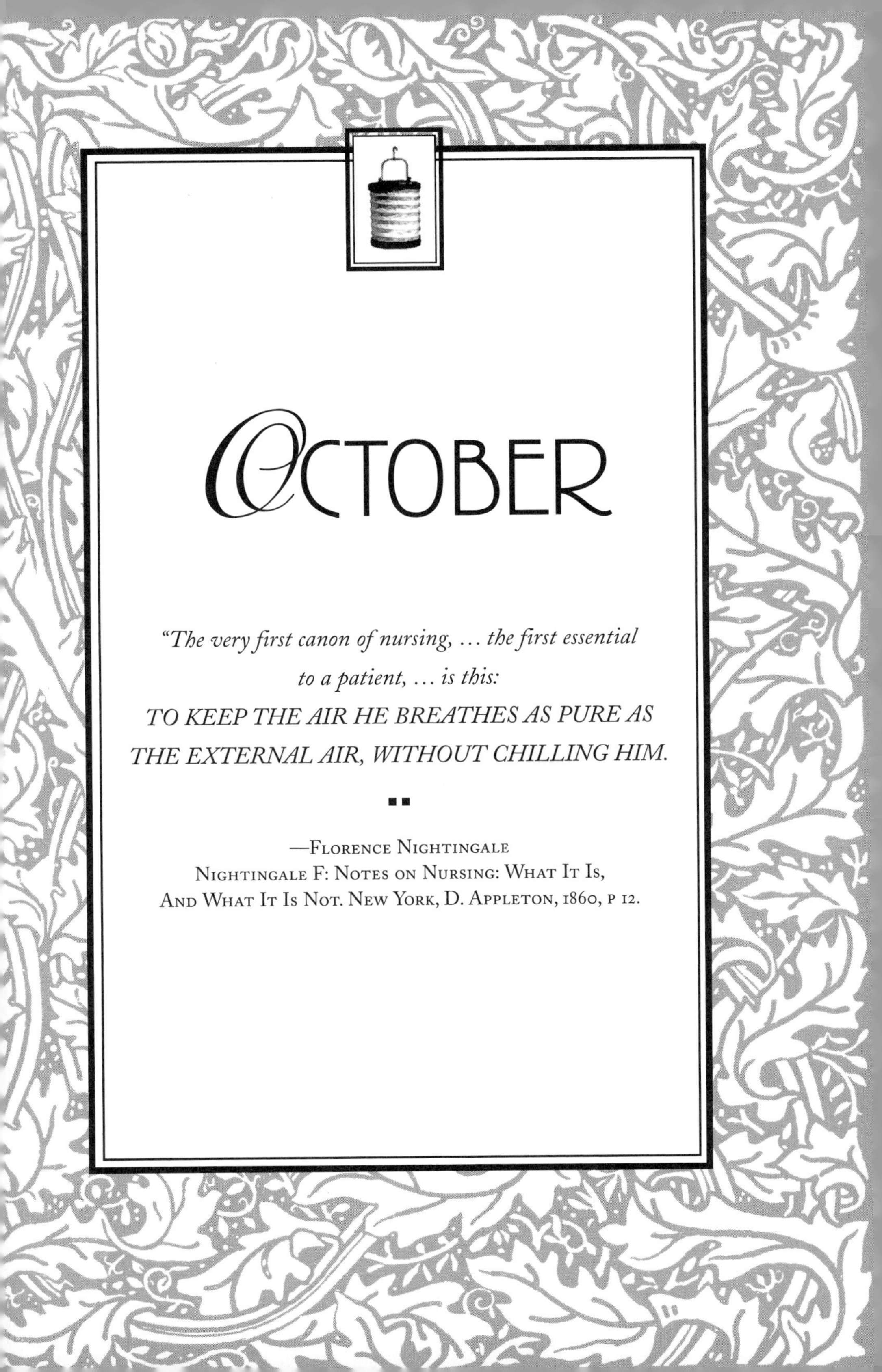

October

"The very first canon of nursing, … the first essential to a patient, … is this: TO KEEP THE AIR HE BREATHES AS PURE AS THE EXTERNAL AIR, WITHOUT CHILLING HIM.

—Florence Nightingale
Nightingale F: Notes on Nursing: What It Is, And What It Is Not. New York, D. Appleton, 1860, p 12.

October 1

Clara Dutton Noyes

1869–1936

"If we are a profession, then surely there is an absolute necessity for advanced study. If we wish to see this profession placed on a strong basis, then we must be strong as a body in the fundamental principles underlying our work. If we attempt to take a position in the front ranks of the progressive movements of the age and, what is more important, stay there, we must as individuals be thoroughly prepared, and this can only be done by courses of study which have been organized on a permanent educational basis." (1905)

CLARA NOYES ASSISTED, then succeeded, Jane Delano as a leader in Red Cross nursing. As the Red Cross director of nursing service, Noyes assessed the health needs of recovering European countries after World War I, then assigned Red Cross nurses to help develop programs accordingly. For example, she designated Red Cross funds to build a nursing school in Bordeaux, France. During the depression years in the United States, she designed and upgraded Red Cross nursing programs to meet the health needs of the people. She was firm in her belief that nurses needed to take ongoing coursework to stay clinically current and that they needed to be involved in their professional organization. She encouraged postgraduate study. She contrasted the active interest of older physicians in continuing their education with the indifference that she saw among some older nurse graduates. This, in turn, led to difficulty placing these nurses for employment. Noyes managed to remain active in leadership positions in professional organizations while heavily involved with her Red Cross nursing duties.

Biography

Born: Oct. 3, 1869, Port Deposit, Md. **Education:** Johns Hopkins Hosp. School of Nursing. **Work history:** Johns Hopkins Hosp.; New England Hosp. for Women and Children, Boston; Director of Nurses, St. Luke's Hosp., Mass., Bellevue Hosp., N.Y.C.; Director, American Red Cross, active in European and U.S. programs. **Organizations:** leadership positions in National League for Nursing Education; International Council of Nurses; American Nurses Assoc. (ANA); active in alumni assoc. of Johns Hopkins Hosp. School of Nursing. **Awards:** Florence Nightingale Medal, International Committee, Red Cross; several Red Cross medals; French medals of honor; Walter Burns Saunders Medal, ANA; ANA Hall of Fame. **Buried:** Old Lyme, Conn.

References and Credits

†Noyes C: Post-graduate study for nurses. AJN 5:614, 1905.

Sabin LE: Clara Noyes. In Bullough V, Church OM, Stein AP (eds): American Nursing: A Biographical Dictionary, vol. 1. New York, Garland, 1988, pp 242–243.

ANA Hall of Fame 10/98 American Nurses Association, Washington, D.C. http://www.nursingworld.org/hof.

OCTOBER 2

Jean Barrett

1903–1993

"Perhaps we have been slow to act. Now we have come to the place where something must *be done to conserve time in order that we may care adequately for our patients in spite of the growing shortage of nurses. It has become a matter of doing less or of devising simpler ways of giving the same care. ...First we can eliminate from our nursing procedures those aspects which are nonessential to the patient's welfare and comfort. ...Every moment of nursing time must be used to the greatest benefit of patients." (1943)*

When Jean Barrett was twelve, she visited her grandmother, who had a fractured femur, and this influenced the girl's decision to become a nurse. Barrett's career included private duty nursing, teaching, administration, and international nursing. She established the nursing program at Syracuse University, enhanced nursing education in Taiwan through her work with the United Nations, and worked with nurses in the Middle East. Her major interests, as reflected in her writings, included ward management, the head nurse and her relationship with patient care, and new practice roles. For example, one aspect of Barrett's study of the nurse specialist practitioner showed that surgeons working with these nurses found their patient care to be of significantly high quality and welcomed the nurses' observations and communication on rounds.

Biography

Born: Oct. 4, 1903, San Francisco. **Education:** Upper Iowa Univ. (BA); Iowa Methodist School of Nursing; Teachers College, Columbia Univ. (MA). **Work history:** Private Duty Nurse; Nursing Instructor, schools of nursing in Washington; Iowa; Decatur-Macon County (Ill.) Hosp.; New Haven (Conn.) Hosp.; Faculty, Yale Univ. School of Nursing; Chair, Nursing Education, Syracuse Univ.; Nursing Professor, Dean, Yale Univ. School of Nursing; Consultant, World Health Organization; member, U.N. National Citizens Committee. **Organizations:** unknown. **Awards:** Woman of Achievement in Health Award, *Syracuse Post Standard.* **Died:** Eugene, Ore.

References and Credits

†Barrett J: Simplifying nursing procedures. AJN 43:713, 716, 1943.

Cooper SS: Jean Barrett. In Bullough V, Sentz L (eds): American Nursing: A Biographical Dictionary, vol. 3. New York, Springer, 2000, pp 16–17.

Barrett J: The nurse specialist practitioner: A study. Nurs Outlook 20:524–527, 1972.

Lulu Wolf Hassenplug

1903–1995

"Do we fully appreciate our own worth as nurses and the importance of our work as a major component of the health care system? Or, as members of a female dominated profession, have we been socialized to be so passive and nonassertive that we are content to have health agency administrators, physicians, business managers and legislators define and control what we do? ... In numbers we are the largest of the health professions. Think what power we could generate in the legislature if all of us, one million and a quarter strong, approached Congress as a unified group demanding changes in the delivery of health care and reimbursement practices." (1977)

Lulu Wolf Hassenplug had a lifelong love of the theater and first wanted to be an actress. Her father opposed this, as well as her subsequent decision to study nursing, saying that she was too talented for nursing. When she worked at Vanderbilt University in 1938, the school already required two years of college for admission and granted a bachelor's degree in nursing upon completion of its three-year nursing program. Hassenplug wanted nursing students to integrate with the rest of the student body. She gained respect for nurses there as students, rathar than as a captive workforce for the university hospital. A visionary, reformer, and prolific author, she revolutionized nursing education while wielding her influence as a leader in professional organizations. She supported a broader education in the humanities as a foundation for nursing practice and recognized that preparation for public health nursing should be a basic part of baccalaureate programs. She is credited with establishing the first nursing program at the University of California at Los Angeles (UCLA). When she was appointed dean there, she literally took the program from a basement setting and transformed it into a first-class nursing school that offered undergraduate and graduate degrees. Hassenplug supported levels for entry into practice. She saw the nurse practitioner movement as a necessary way to provide appropriate health care and to keep nursing focused on care.

Biography

Born: Oct. 3, 1903, Milton, Pa. **Education:** Army School of Nursing; Teachers College, Columbia Univ. (BS); Fellow, Florence Nightingale International Foundation, London; Rockefeller Fellow, Johns Hopkins Univ. (MPH). **Work history:** Education Director, Jewish Hosp., Philadelphia; Faculty, Medical College of Virginia, Vanderbilt Univ.; Faculty, Dean, UCLA; Consultant to numerous universities and government committees. **Organizations:** founder, Western Council for Higher Education of Nurses; National League for Nursing (NLN); American Nurses Assoc. (ANA); Calif. Nurses Assoc. (CNA). **Awards:** fellowships from Rockefeller Foundation, Nightingale Foundation; honorary doctorates, Univ. of New Mexico, Bucknell Univ.; Isabel Hampton Robb Scholarship; Rockefeller Travel Grants; *Los Angeles Times* Woman of the Year (education); Vanderbilt Univ. video series; Arizona State Univ. Achievement Award Medallion; Adelaide Nutting Award, NLN; Jessie M. Scott Award, ANA; Distinguished Service Award, nursing scholarship in her name, UCLA; award in her honor, CNA. **Died:** location unknown.

References and Credits

†Hassenplug L: Nursing can move from here to there. Nurs Outlook 25:434, 1977.

Safier G: Contemporary American Leaders in Nursing: An Oral History. New York, McGraw-Hill, 1977.

Sentz L: Lulu K. Wolf Hassenplug. In Bullough V, Sentz L, Stein AP (eds): American Nursing: A Biographical Dictionary, vol. 2. New York, Garland, 1992, pp 144–146.

October 4

Margaret Stafford

1922–

"I believe, without equivocation, that health care systems cannot survive without us, and we must represent ourselves in the practice arena. ... By joining together and supporting each other, nurses can achieve for patients and for themselves what no individual nurse can achieve alone. I ... believe to this day that collective action of and for nurses and their patients is one of the most professional activities in which I have been involved. ... I view the collective bargaining process as a means of making things better and not an end unto itself. I feel strongly that it is a rightful and ethical means to accomplish a rightful and ethical goal, a goal that is two-fold—the provision of high-quality care for the patient and the achievement and maintenance of the professional integrity of the nurse. One is contingent upon the other." (1988)

MARGARET STAFFORD IS a distinguished clinical nurse specialist, researcher, author, teacher, and advocate for professional nursing and quality care. Her ongoing involvement with critical issues in nursing began in the mid-1960s. She was concerned about hospital conditions for both patient care and clinical practice, and she saw a solution in nursing's need to organize. Inspired by the keynote speaker at an American Nurses Association (ANA) convention in 1966, she became active in collective bargaining with the

Illinois Nurses Association that same year. This resulted in dramatic changes at Cook County Hospital in Chicago. The improved working conditions included better staffing ratios, competitive salaries, and a policy of no admissions if staffing levels were deemed inadequate. As a result, patient care was better and so was nurse recruitment and retention. Stafford views collective bargaining as the key to quality patient care by professional nurses. She was one of the nation's first clinical nurse specialists in cardiology, and her practice set the standard for these nurses with masters degrees. While at the Hines Veterans Administration Hospital in Illinois, she started a nurse-run pacemaker clinic. She taught, published, mentored others, and consulted about her practice. In recognition, an unprecedented annual lecture program in her name was established and funded at Hines from 1990 to 1999. She continues to remind hospital administrators that advocacy is essential to quality care and that quality care must be addressed by improvements in nurse staffing.

Biography

Born: Oct. 4, 1922, Chicago. **Education:** Cook County Hosp. School of Nursing, Chicago; Loyola Univ. School of Nursing (BSN, MSN). **Work history:** Clinical Nurse Specialist, Cook County Hosp., Hines VA Hosp.; appointed to numerous government and professional nursing and health planning groups; Faculty, nursing schools, Univ. of Illinois, Northern Illinois Univ., Loyola Univ., all in Chicago; Consultant; Mentor; Author; Researcher. **Organizations:** ANA; INA; Chicago Nurses Assoc.; American Heart Assoc.; Sigma Theta Tau; Nurses Coalition for Action in Politics; Southern Poverty Law Center; Critical Care Assoc.; American Nurses Foundation. **Awards:** Fellow, American Academy of Nursing; Illinois award for service in comprehensive state health planning; honorary membership award, INA; Founder's Day Award, Loyola Univ., 1975, 2002; Clinical Nurse Specialist of the Year Awards, ANA, INA; Economic Security and General Welfare Citation of Achievement Award, ANA; Hines VA Hosp. award for exemplary achievement; award from Chicago Heart Assoc.

References and Credits

†Schorr T, Zimmerman A: Making Choices, Taking Chances: Nurse Leaders Tell Their Stories. St. Louis, CV Mosby, 1988, pp 333, 336.

Stafford M: To err is human: Building a safer health system. CHART for Nurses (publication of the Illinois Nurses Association) 97:1, 6–9, 2000.

Stafford M: resume.

Stafford M: personal communication, August 2002.

Irene Mortenson Burnside

1923–

"The overall goal for group work is to make the later years the very best that they can be instead of the very worst, as they now are for some elderly, especially the frail aged. ...Regardless of what we write or expound, the true teachers are the aged group members." (1994)

A CHILDHOOD ROLE MODEL attracted Irene Burnside to nursing. She is credited with the development of gerontological nursing as a specialty. A noted nursing leader, her sensitive involvement and clear direction moved the nursing profession forward. She is an internationally renowned speaker, consultant, and author about the care of the aged, particularly the psychosocial aspects of aging. She researched and wrote about the value of reminiscence therapy in group work. Her group work with the elderly began when she was working on her certification in adult psychiatric nursing, and from her pioneering interest nursing's role expanded into the psychosocial care of older persons. She writes that nurses are ideally suited to do group work with adults who may be impaired. Among nurses' many qualities is that they are oriented to wellness and prevention, she notes. She found that nurses' abilities to handle difficult situations and to work with a variety of personalities are especially valuable in working with the older population. She defined the nurse's role in her writings about group process and technique. Burnside is a prolific writer whose award-winning books and other publications have enhanced both professional practice and the quality of life for older adults. In 1982 she was the first nurse to present grand rounds, when she did so at the St. Paul–Ramsey Medical Center in Minnesota. Her oral history is preserved in the archives of Baylor University Waco, Texas.

Biography

Born: Oct. 4, 1923, Grove City, Minn. **Education:** Ancker Hosp. School of Nursing, St. Paul, Minn.; Denver Univ. (BFA); Univ. of California, San Francisco (MSN); certificate in adult psychiatric nursing, Univ. of California, San Francisco; Andrus Gerontology Center, Univ. of Southern California; Univ. of Texas, Austin (PhD). **Work history:** Army Nurse Corps, Japan; various staff nursing positions; Charge Nurse, Gladman Psychiatric Hosp., Oakland, Calif.; Faculty, Univ. of California, San Francisco; Coordinator, Andrus Gerontology Center; Faculty, San Jose State Univ.; Consultant; Lecturer; Author; Visiting Professor, numerous nursing schools. **Organizations:** Honor Society; American Geriatrics in Higher Education; American Nurses Assoc. (ANA); Gerontology Society of America (GSA); International Assoc. of Gerontology; Sigma Theta Tau International (STTI). **Awards:** Fellow, GSA; Fellow, American Academy of Nursing; other awards from U.S. Nurse Cadet Corps, STTI; ANA; National League for Nursing; Andrus Gerontology Center; book awards; numerous listings in *Who's Who* publications.

References and Credits

†Burnside I, Schmidt M (eds): Working with Older Adults, 3d ed. Boston, Jones and Bartlett, 1994, p 314.

Garand LJ: Irene Burnside. In Bullough V, Sentz L (eds): American Nursing: A Biographical Dictionary, vol. 3. New York, Springer, 2000, pp 39–42.

Burnside I: Nursing and the Aged, 3d ed. New York, McGraw-Hill, 1988, p v.

October 6

Ernest Grant

1958–

"I have the best job in the world. I know I make a difference every day." (2002)

"My dream is to work myself out of a job. ...I look forward to the day that my skills as a nurse will no longer be needed because no one is being burned anymore!" (1999)

HIS COLLEAGUES DESCRIBE Ernest Grant as a man with a mission and a heart of gold. He is known as "Mr. Burn" throughout North Carolina. His communication skills get his message across. His passion is prevention, and he proves it every day by teaching burn prevention to senior citizens and children. He also teaches firefighters, teachers, and health care workers the latest in proper care at the scene of an injury, as well as emergent, acute, and rehabilitative care. He convinced the North Carolina legislature to restrict the sale of fireworks to people sixteen and older and to mandate that hot water heaters be preset to 120 degrees Fahrenheit and labeled with information about preventing scalds. He developed and disseminated the "Learn Not to Burn" program throughout North Carolina and other areas of the Southeast. He helped devise and implement the "Remembering When" program for senior citizens about preventing falls and fires. He also developed the long-term

National Burn Awareness Campaign that spotlights different topics each year, such as prevention of camping and recreational burns, scald injuries, and gasoline injuries. Grant estimates that he educates more than eight thousand citizens about burn prevention each year. During the fall of 2001 he volunteered for ten days at the burn center at New York–Presbyterian University Hospital of Columbia and Cornell to care for victims of the World Trade Center attack on September 11. *Nursing Spectrum* named Grant its 2002 Nurse of the Year.

Biography

Born: Oct. 6, 1958, Asheville, N.C. **Education:** Buncombe Technical Institute, Asheville, N.C., 1977 (LPN); North Carolina Central Univ., Durham, 1985 (BSN); Univ. of North Carolina, Greensboro, 1993 (MSN). **Work history:** Staff Nurse, Medical-Surgical Intensive Care Unit, orthopedics, Memorial Mission Hosp., Asheville, N.C.; Clinical Nursing Instructor, Skills Lab Coordinator, North Carolina Central Univ. Dept. of Nursing, Durham; Staff Nurse, Outreach Nurse-Clinician, North Carolina Jaycee Burn Center, Univ. of North Carolina Hosps., Chapel Hill; **Organizations:** Secretary, President, Vice President, Nominating Committee Chair, American Assembly for Men in Nursing, N.C. Chapter; American Assoc. of Univ. Professors; American Burn Assoc.; International Burn Society–Congress on Burn Injuries; National Fire Protection Assoc.; founder, Nursing Honor Society, N.C. Central Univ. Dept. of Nursing; Chair, Commission on Member Services, N.C. Nurses Assoc.; N.C. State Fire Education Committee; Univ. of N.C., Greensboro, School of Nursing Advisory Bd.; Sigma Theta Tau International; National Honor Society, Alpha Chapter, Univ. of N.C., Chapel Hill. **Awards:** *Nursing Spectrum Magazine* Nurse of the Year, 2002; Honorary Nurse Practice Award, American Nurses Assoc., July 2002; 1998 Governor's Award of Excellence.

References and Credits

†Mitiguy JS: Ernest Grant, Nurse of the Year: A man with a message and a mission. Nursing Spectrum 3:8–9, 2002.

†Grant E: Burn nursing. Advance for Nurses 1:1999.

Grant E: resume.

Grant E: personal communication, 2002.

October 7

St. Francis of Assisi

1182–1226

"Lord make me an instrument of Thy peace. Where there is hatred, let me sow love; where there is injury; pardon; where there is doubt, faith; where there is despair, hope; where there is darkness, light, and where there is sadness, joy. O, divine Master, grant that I may not so much seek to be consoled, as to console; to be understood as to understand; to be loved, as to love, for it is in giving that we receive, it is in pardoning that we are pardoned, and it is in dying that we are born to eternal life." (Date unknown)

The Peace Prayer is attributed to St. Francis of Assisi, who steadfastly practiced a dedication to reform and a concern for the common good for all people. He renounced wealth and lived with and nursed lepers, the sick, and poor. He dignified his freedom from possessions and practiced an extraordinary communication with all creatures that he encountered. He never became a priest, yet he was founder of the Franciscan Order, a writer, and a poet. Francis Bernardone, known as the Little Poor Man, died when he was forty-five and was canonized at the Church of St. George's by Pope Gregory IX, two years later, on July 16, 1228. St. Francis sought and taught peace, yet he never judged or admonished. The historian Gilbert K. Chesterton describes Francis's nature and character in his book *St. Francis of Assisi:*

> What distinguishes this very genuine democrat from any mere demagogue is that he never either deceived or was deceived by the illusion of mass-suggestion. ...To him a man was always a man and did not disappear in a dense crowd any more than in a desert. He honored all men; that is, he not only loved but respected them all. What gave him his extraordinary personal power was this; that from the Pope to the beggar, from the sultan of Syria in his pavilion to the ragged robbers crawling out of the wood, there was never a man who looked into those brown burning eyes without being certain that Francis Bernardone was really interested in *him;* in his own inner life from the cradle to the grave; that he himself was being valued and taken seriously, and not merely added to the spoils of some social policy or the names in some clerical document.

Biography

Born: 1182, Assisi, Italy. **Education:** unknown. **Work history:** restored ruined churches; fed, washed, clothed, housed lepers, poor, and sick; audience with Pope Innocent III; wrote what is now known as Rule of Saint Francis and Canticle of the Sun. **Organizations:** unknown. **Awards:** unknown. **Died:** Porziuncola, Italy.

References and Credits

†Peace prayer of St. Francis of Assisi, available on-line at http://www.americancatholic.org/features/francis/peaceprayer.asp.

†Chesterton GK: St. Francis of Assisi. New York, George H. Doran Co., 1924, pp 141–142.

Spoto D: Reluctant Saint: The Life of Francis of Assisi. New York, Viking Compass, 2002.

Green J: God's Fool: The Life and Times of Francis of Assisi. Trans. Heinegg P. San Francisco, Harper and Row, San Francisco, 1985.

St. Francis of Assisi. Catholic Encyclopedia on-line, available at http://www.newadvent.org/cathen/06221a.htm.

Benen FM, Herman P: Introduction and notes. The Writings of St. Francis of Assisi. Chicago, Franciscan Herald Press, 1964.

October 8

Josephine Beatrice Bowman

1881–1971

"Is there anything unpleasant in the work of the Navy Nurses? Most certainly, but it would be hard to tell just what one would call unpleasant. As the work deals with human beings with their frailties, it is easy to see that unpleasant things do arise. What one nurse finds hard, another gets her greatest pleasure from and no one need be unhappy if she has the altruistic spirit necessary to get the most out of life. The pleasure one gets is usually in proportion to the amount of service one renders." (1925)

JOSEPHINE BOWMAN WAS born into a medical, military, and seafaring family in Des Moines, Iowa. She was educated at the Medico-Chirurgical Hospital Training School for Nurses in Philadelphia. After her graduation in 1904 she worked with the American Red Cross Service in disaster relief. She was one of twenty nurses to join the new Navy Nurse Corps, and she rose to the rank of chief nurse and served on the SS *Red Cross.* When the United States entered World War I, she returned from duty in Asia to organize and supervise the U.S. Naval Hospital in Great Lakes. She realized that her nurses would benefit from the postgraduate nursing courses she offered, and she earned a reputation for outstanding administrative and nursing skills. She was appointed superintendent of the Navy Nurse Corps and in her truly efficient style organized regional supervisors who understood local needs. She retired in 1935.

Biography

Born: Dec. 19, 1881, Des Moines, Iowa. **Education:** Medico-Chirurgical Hosp. Training School for Nurses, Philadelphia, 1904. **Work history:** Nurse, Superintendent, Navy Nurse Corps; Chief Nurse, Charge Nurse for first nurses on hospital ship USS *Relief;* Chief Nurse, U.S. Naval Hosp., Great Lakes, Ill. **Organizations:** member, National Committee, American Red Cross Nursing Service; Medical Council of U.S. Veterans Bureau; American Public Health Assoc.; American Assoc. for the Advancement of Science; Chair, government section, American Nurses Assoc.; President, Graduate Nurses Assoc., Washington, D.C. **Awards:** unknown. **Died:** Hanover, Pa.

References and Credits

†Bowman J: History and development of the Navy Nurse Corps. AJN 25:359, 1925.

Stein AP: Josephine Beatrice Bowman. In Bullough V, Sentz L, Stein AP (eds): American Nursing: A Biographical Dictionary, vol. 2. New York, Garland, 1992, pp 31–32.

OCTOBER 9

Marie Marguerite Dufrost de Lajemmerais D'Youville

1701–1771

"There would certainly be a great deal of good to do if we only had the means. Every day poor come to us who are really in need. We have no more room and I cry bitterly in sending them away, but it must be done. ... If I knew where there was so much money that I could take it without stealing, I would soon have a building that would hold almost two hundred, but I have nothing. God will be satisfied with my good will." (1769)

WHEN MARIE MARGUERITE D'YOUVILLE was drawn to service with the poor in Montreal, she was a destitute widow with two children. Her other four children had died as infants. She opened her home to the homeless, and her acts of charity prompted other women to accept her invitation to help. Together they formed a religious order, the Grey Nuns. When she was named the director of a general hospital, her innate, practical business sense helped to erase its deep debt. She focused not only on necessary hospital repairs but maximized the use of its surrounding farmlands. The hospital cared for the sick poor, housed the homeless, and also had paying boarders. Nursing became a major activity for the order during the smallpox epidemic of 1755. The Grey Nuns were also actively involved in caring for the wounded and prisoners during the war between the French and the British in 1756. Economic and domestic stress among the defeated French contributed to the problem of baby abandonment, causing Mother D'Youville to open the first foundling home in Europe. It was funded by fines collected in Montreal by order of the governor. The Grey Nuns went on to open nursing schools and hospitals in Canada and the United States. They continue to operate hospitals and charitable institutions throughout Canada, as well as services for the poor in the United States and around the world.

Biography

Born: Oct. 15, 1701, Varennes, Can. **Education:** two yrs. of formal education with Ursuline Sisters, Quebec. **Work history:** volunteer charitable work; Director, General Hosp., Montreal; established religious order, the Grey Nuns; nursing; established foundling home near Montreal; organized rebuilding of General Hosp. after fire. **Organizations:** unknown. **Awards:** beatified by Catholic Church, April 28, 1890. **Died:** Montreal.

References and Credits

†Fitts MP: Hands to the Needy: Mother D'Youville, Apostle to the Poor. New York, Doubleday, 1950, p 275.

Fabiszak A: Marie Marguerite d'Youville. In Bullough V, Church OM, Stein AP (eds): American Nursing: A Biographical Dictionary, vol. 1. New York, Garland, 1988, pp 341–344.

Lindsay L: In The Catholic Encyclopedia, vol. 15, available on-line at http://www.newadvent.org/cathen/15736c.htm.

Sisters of Charity (Grey Nuns) of Alberta, available on-line at http://www.greynuns.ab.ca/ history.htm

October 10

Helen Lathrop Bunge

1906–1970

"I have heard that in one field there is a forty-year lag between the uncovering of new knowledge and the actual use of this knowledge in the improvement of practice in the field. Certainly we in nursing will show a much better record in our fashioning of nursing care and nursing education to meet the needs of the changing times." (1959)

"Research ... A tool to help solve the problems that plague us ... A state of mind looking ahead." (1955)

HELEN LATHROP BUNGE was blessed with a great intellect, a good sense of humor, and multiple talents, including piano playing. She excelled in education and research; she founded and was the first volunteer editor of *Nursing Research.* It was first published in 1952 and had eighty-five hundred subscribers. While working on her doctoral degree in New York at Teachers College, she assisted Isabel M. Stewart and lived with M. Adelaide Nutting. Bunge's accomplishments in education at the Frances Payne Bolton School of Nursing at Western Reserve in Cleveland, Ohio, after World War II include admitting men to the program, starting a forty-four-hour workweek for the basic baccalaureate program, and requiring a research course in the master's program. Enrollment doubled during her tenure. She was the director and later the dean of the University of Wisconsin's School of Nursing. She was elected or appointed to leadership positions in all the major organizations at the national level. She was inducted into the Hall of Fame of the American Nursing Association (ANA) in 1984. Bunge received the Achievement Award in Research and Scholarship from the Teachers College Nursing Education Alumni Association and the Adelaide Nutting Award from the National League for Nursing (NLN).

Biography

Born: Oct. 11, 1906, La Crosse, Wisc. **Education:** attended Connecticut College for Women, New London, two yrs.; Univ. of Wisconsin, 1928 (BA in sociology); Certificate Graduate Nurse, 1930, Wisc.; Teachers College, Columbia Univ. (MA, EdD). **Work history:** Head Nurse, Wisconsin General Hosp., Madison; Instructor, Director, Dean, Univ. of Wisconsin School of Nursing; Assistant Director, Dean, Frances Payne Bolton School of Nursing, Western Reserve Univ. Cleveland, Ohio; Exec. Officer, Institute of Research and Service in Nursing Education, Teachers College; Chair, Committee on Research, Assoc. of Collegiate Schools of Nursing; Chair, Nursing Service Advisory Committee, American Red Cross. **Organizations:** bd. of directors, ANA; NLN; National League for Nursing Education; chair, Assoc. of Collegiate Schools of Nursing; Vice Chair, Council of the Florence Nightingale International Foundation; member, first nursing research study section, U.S. Public Health Service Division of Research Grants; Chair, Nursing Service Advisory Committee, American Red Cross; member, bd. of directors, American Nurses Foundation; member, Special Medical Advisory Group, Veterans Administration; Consultant, Fifth Army. **Awards:** Phi Beta Kappa; Achievement Award in Research and Scholarship, Teachers College of Nursing Education Alumni Assoc., Columbia Univ.; Distinguished Service Award (Science), Univ. of Wisconsin Alumni Assoc.; ANA Hall of Fame. **Died:** Madison, Wisc.

References and Credits

†Bunge HL: Looking Ahead. Speech to University of Wisconsin Student-Faculty Convocation. Helen L. Bunge Collection, Box 15, Personal Notes, March 19, 1959, Steenbock Library, University of Wisconsin, Madison.

†Bunge H: The meaning and importance of research in nursing. Canadian Nurse 51:945, 1955.

Glass LK: Helen Bunge. In Bullough V, Sentz L, Stein AP (eds): American Nursing: A Biographical Dictionary, vol. 2. New York, Garland, 1992, pp 49–51.

ANA Hall of Fame 10/98 American Nurses Association, Washington, D.C. http://www.nursingworld.org/hof.

OCTOBER 11

Judith Bellaire Igoe

1939–

"School nurses work daily to promote student health and well being so that every child is ready to learn. This is what keeps us going. … Properly staffed school health rooms and school-based health centers provide students with easy access to care that is designed to resolve their problems. Consequently, most of them are able to return to class and learning resumes as quickly as possible. … School nurses … have been especially politically astute in their advocacy efforts on behalf of students who are especially vulnerable because of special health needs, lack of health insurance, and racial or cultural indifference. Advocacy from individual school nurses, as well as from professional associations, is long standing and part of the public record." (2000)

JUDITH IGOE WAS attracted to nursing as a child when she listened to her grandmother's stories of being a nurse early in the twentieth century. Igoe is a nationally renowned advocate for school health and school nursing. Spirited, courageous, and energetic, she merged her interest in pediatrics and public health in an interdependent practice as a pediatric nurse practitioner. She helped develop the program for school nurse practitioners at the University of Colorado and saw the potential for independent nursing practice in school health and school-based clinics. Undaunted by criticism or failure, she found each experience to be a learning opportunity and benefited from it. She recognizes that education empowers children and that school nurses can remove health-related barriers to academic success by providing school health services in the school setting. Poverty, lack of health care insurance, and lack of health care resources for schoolchildren puts them at risk and leads to absenteeism. She speaks of the need for health care reform for children and youth and the need to explore funding sources for services. She calls on school nurses to explore opportunities for community and educational partnerships so that collaborative efforts will find new ways to fund and provide care.

Biography

Born: Oct. 11, 1939, Shanghai, China. **Education:** Loretto Heights College, Denver; Univ. of Iowa (BSN); Univ. of Minnesota School of Public Health (MS); Univ. of Colorado (Pediatric Nurse Practitioner). **Work history:** Pediatric Nurse, Queens Hosp., Hawaii; Public Health Nurse, School Nurse, Iowa; Public Health Nurse, Denver; developed school nurse practitioner program, Univ. of Colorado; Director of School Health, School of Nursing, Univ. of Colorado Health Sciences Center. **Organizations:** American Nurses Assoc.; Fellow, National Assoc. of School Nurses; Fellow, American Academy of Nursing; American Public Health Assoc. (APHA); Fellow, American School Health Assoc. (ASHA); associate member, American Academy of Pediatrics (AAP). **Awards:** Distinguished Alumni Award, Univ. of Iowa; awards from AAP, Assoc. of Maternal and Child Health Programs; APHA; ASHA: award for outstanding contribution to Univ. of Colorado Health Sciences Center.

References and Credits

†Igoe J: School nursing today: A search for new cheese. J School Nursing (Allen Press) 16:13, 2000.

Schorr T, Zimmerman A: Making Choices, Taking Chances: Nurse Leaders Tell Their Stories. St. Louis, CV Mosby, 1988.

Igoe J: personal correspondence, 2002.

Igoe J: Healthier children through empowerment. In Wilson-Barnett J, MacLeod Clark, J (eds): Research in Health Promotion and Nursing. New York, Macmillan, 1993, pp 145–153.

Igoe J: Designing the policy environment through understanding. Nursing Policy Forum 1:12–19, 1995.

Igoe J: resume.

October 12

Harriet A. Werley

1914–2002

"As nurses become more adept at implementing and testing nursing treatments, or interventions, for human responses to actual or potential health problems, this will lead to an accumulated list of validated nursing diagnoses and reliable treatments. The research on this kind of investigative nursing practice will be the basis for further development of nursing knowledge, in keeping with the profession's standards of practice. This research will be the impetus for advancing nursing practice, health care delivery, and the profession of nursing." (1988)

HARRIET WERLEY WAS a leader of and influence on nursing research through her practice and writings. Motivated to become a nurse after her father's death when she was twelve, she was sustained by the knowledge that people believed in her, expected her to do well, and treated her accordingly. She grew up during the depression and worked to save money for tuition before she could start nursing school. When she was a member of the Army Nurse Corps, she worked first with career guidance and planning, then with the Walter Reed Institute of Research. At Walter Reed she was instrumental in having courses about disaster nursing included in nursing school curricula. She also realized that nursing was not represented in ongoing research. The need that she identified was met when the institute established a Department of Nursing and named Werley as its first director. She saw research, education, and practice as the three basic foundations for nursing. Her five levels of research for nurse participation are supporter, technician, consultant, collaborator, and investigator. Her long-standing interest in studying what kind of nursing data could be computerized led to the minimum data set (MDS) while she was at the University of Wisconsin, Milwaukee. With others, she identified areas in nursing's domain that build on nursing knowledge, influence clinical judgment, and determine care. She saw standardized documentation as an essential way to define nurses as health care providers and to define costs.

Biography

Born: Oct. 12, 1914, Berks County, Pa. **Education:** Jefferson Medical College Hosp., Philadelphia; Univ. of California, Berkeley (BS); Columbia Univ. (MA); Univ. of Utah (PhD). **Work history:** Army Nurse Corps, Mediterranean Theater; Army Hosp., Pittsburg, Calif.; Walter Reed Hosp., Army Institute of Research; Director, Dept. of Nursing, Walter Reed Army Institute of Research; Chief Nurse, Eighth Army, Korea; administration, nursing research, Wayne State College of Nursing, Detroit, Univ. of Illinois Medical Center, Univ. of Missouri School of Nursing; Faculty, Univ. of Wisconsin—Milwaukee School of Nursing; founded *Research in Nursing and Health* and developed the ongoing series *Annual Review of Nursing Research* in 1983. **Organizations:** American Nurses Assoc. **Awards:** U.S. Legion of Merit; Alumni Award, Thomas Jefferson Univ., Philadelphia; American Nurses Foundation Award; National Institutes of Health Fellowship; Charter Fellow, American Academy of Nursing; two book awards from *American Journal of Nursing;* Living Legend, American Academy of Nursing, 1994. **Died:** Milwaukee, Wisc.

References and Credits

†Werley H, Lang N (eds): Identification of the Nursing Minimum Data Set. New York, Springer, 1988, pp 11–12.

Schorr T, Zimmerman A: Making Choices, Taking Chances: Nurse Leaders Tell Their Stories. St. Louis, CV Mosby, 1988.

Sentz L: Harriet Helen Werley. In Bullough V, Sentz L, Stein AP (eds): American Nursing: A Biographical Dictionary, vol. 2. New York, Garland, 1992, pp 346–347.

Werley H: The different research roles in army nursing. Nurs Outlook 11:134–136, 1963.

OCTOBER 13

Elizabeth Sterling Soule

1884–1972

"The new curriculum ... objectives should be (1) to prepare the nurse by giving her a wider scientific, social, and technical background for meeting the needs of the community and (2) to give the nurse, through better education, satisfaction from her work, security, and the ability to live more fully." (1938)

WHEN ELIZABETH SOULE was a child, her physician father included her in his home and office visits and involved her in discussions related to medical and social problems. Additionally, she enjoyed opportunities to learn from a visiting nurse who cared for her sick mother. Later, Annie Goodrich encouraged Soule to develop her innovative ideas for a university nursing program where the university would provide clinical education while the hospital would provide clinical nursing experience. Before she became involved in nursing education, she was a public health nurse, one of the earliest visiting nurses for the Metropolitan Life Insurance Company in Seattle. She was funded by the Rockefeller Foundation to travel and study nursing schools in Europe, then returned to Seattle, where she established a baccalaureate nursing program. Affectionately called the mother of nursing of the Pacific Northwest, in 1921 she initiated the integrated program that became the University of Washington School of Nursing.

Biography

Born: Oct. 13, 1884, East Douglas, Mass. **Education:** Malden (Mass.) Hosp. School for Nurses; Univ. of Washington (BA, MA). **Work history:** Staff Nurse, Private Duty Nurse, Malden Hosp.; District Nurse, Everett (Mass.) Visiting Nurse Assoc.; Visiting Nurse, Metropolitan Life Insurance Co.; Supervisor, Public Health Nurses, Washington Tuberculosis Assoc., Red Cross; Instructor, Univ. of Washington; established public health nursing program, Univ. of Washington; Travel Fellowship, Rockefeller Foundation; developed four-yr. baccalaureate program, Univ. of Washington; Director, Dean, School of Nursing, Univ. of Washington; Consultant, U.S. Public Health Service; Red Cross Advisory Commission; bd. member, Seattle Visiting Nurse Service; Nursing Council on National Defense. **Organizations:** founder, Assoc. of Collegiate Schools of Nursing; American Nurses Assoc. (ANA); National Organization for Public Health Nursing; honorary member, National League for Nursing Education. **Awards:** Univ. of Washington Alumni Assoc. Award; honorary doctoral degree, Montana State College; Elizabeth Sterling Soule Endowed Professorship, Univ. of Washington; honorary member, Sigma Theta Tau; ANA Hall of Fame. **Died:** Seattle.

References and Credits

†Soule E: Building the university school. AJN 38:581, 1938.

Tao DS: Elizabeth Soule. In Bullough V, Church OM, Stein AP (eds): American Nursing: A Biographical Dictionary, vol. 1. New York, Garland, 1988, pp 291–293.

ANA Hall of Fame 10/98 American Nurses Association, Washington, D.C. http://www.nursingworld.org/hof.

OCTOBER 14

Sister Callista Roy

1939–

"Nursing as both a profession and a scholarly discipline is rooted in knowledge for nursing practice. Throughout history, family members have used their cultural traditions and understanding of the other person to help increase wellness, prevent illness, assist with recovery, and comfort the distressed and dying. Today nursing has emerged clearly as the discipline that focuses on developing an understanding of the human processes that promote health … and as a caring profession that incorporates an understanding of human experience into health practice. … I have been deeply blessed to be able to contribute to nursing during its greatest growth period. I am grateful for the great heritage of nursing and … mentors who have taught me much about commitment and scholarship. … Hopefully, nurses who have known me will build on nursing's heritage to continue to solve the challenges of each new era." (1991)

SISTER CALLISTA ROY was attracted to nursing by the example of her mother, a vocational nurse. Her mother's keen interest in her patients, and her constant questioning in order to learn, made it clear that nursing was a meaningful profession with a great social mandate. Roy loved working in the hospital from the time that she was fourteen, and she later came to truly realize that "nursing can influence the very direction of society by touching people and their families at times that offer great challenge and potential for growth." A member of the religious order of the Sisters of St. Joseph of Carondelet, she is an internationally renowned nurse-theorist, researcher, speaker, educator, and author. She developed the Roy Adaptation Model (RAM) for nursing practice, which Heather Andrews and Roy describes as "one of the most highly developed and widely used conceptual descriptions of nursing." This model "views the person as a whole being, constantly interacting with his or her environment, adapting to change through four adaptive modes." Since 1970 thousands of nurses have benefited from the influence of her model on nursing curricula. An advanced practice nurse in neuroscience nursing, she also holds staff privileges at Massachusetts General Hospital in Boston, where she conducts research in cognitive recovery.

Biography

Born: Oct. 14, 1939, Los Angeles. **Education:** Mt. St. Mary's College, Los Angeles (BA); Univ. of California, Los Angeles (MS, MA, PhD); Neuroscience Nursing Fellow, Univ. of California, San Francisco. **Work history:** Staff Nurse, Acting Director of Nursing, St. Joseph's Hosp., Idaho; Staff Nurse, Charge Nurse, St. Mary's Hosp., Ariz.; Research Professor of Nursing, Chair, dept. of nursing, Mt. St. Mary's College, Los Angeles; Faculty, Univ. of Portland, Univ. of San Francisco; Visiting Professor, Univ. of Conception, Chile; guest faculty, Univ. of Lund, Malmo School of Education, Sweden; Visiting Professor, School of Nursing, Boston College; Distinguished Visiting Professor, Vanderbilt Univ.; Assoc. Research Nurse, Dept. of Neurosurgery, School of Medicine, Univ. of California, San Francisco; neuroscience nursing staff privileges, Beth Israel Hosp. and Center for the Advancement of Nursing Practice, Boston; Professor, Nurse Theorist, Boston College School of Nursing; Clinical Assoc. Staff, Dept. of Nursing, Massachusetts General Hosp. **Organizations:** Founder, Chair, Roy Adaptation Assoc.; Eastern Nursing Research Society; International Network for Doctoral Education in Nursing; bd. of directors, New England Faith and Science Exchange; American Nurses Assoc.; Sigma Theta Tau International. **Awards:** annual lectureship in her name, Carondelet Medal, Mt. St. Mary's College, Los Angeles; O'Conner Chair Lecture Series, Oneonta, N.Y.; Invited Scholar, Bangkok, Thailand; honorary doctorate, St. Joseph's College, Maine; Alpha Sigma Nu Jesuit Book Award; Fellow, American Academy of. Nursing.

References and Credits

†Roy C: The Roy Adaptation Model in nursing research. In Andrews H, Roy C: The Roy Adaptation Model: The Definitive Statement. Upper Saddle River, N.J., Pearson Education, 1991, pp 445, 1.

Roy C: personal communication, July 2002.

Schorr T, Zimmerman A: Making Choices, Taking Chances: Nurse Leaders Tell Their Stories. St. Louis, CV Mosby, 1988, p 294.

October 15

Beatrice J. Kalisch

1943–

"The images of nursing that the public receives from all the media have far-reaching consequences for nurses because these images affect the decisions made about nursing. For instance, on all political levels—local, state and federal—there are limited health care funds to disperse, and the allocation of the scarce resources that undergird the delivery of nursing services is closely tied to the quality and quantity of the images of nurses and nursing in the mass media. Much of this allocation process is related to the media's ability to make nursing important in the public consciousness." (1986)

Beatrice Kalisch is a nationally respected authority on the image of nursing. She was attracted to nursing by the example of nurses, her work as a candy striper, and the influence of the Cherry Ames series. Her nursing career includes clinical nursing, advanced study, teaching, administration, research, writing, public speaking, and consultation. She published a comprehensive research study of the image of nursing with her historian husband. This work came about as they were working on a study of the Cadet Nurse Corps. As part of that project they interviewed senators and members of the U.S. House of Representatives, whose perceptions of the nurse were stereotypes reflective of media portrayals. This was the first of many joint writing and researching efforts. They wrote about the importance of nurses' identifying with one another and working together on their common concerns. Her written works demonstrate the importance of nursing research, in regard to not only the image of nursing but also the politics of nursing and health planning.

Biography

Born: Oct. 15, 1943, Tellahoma, Tenn. **Education:** Univ. of Nebraska (BSN); Univ. of Maryland (MS, EdD); postgraduate work, Case Western Reserve Univ., Cleveland, Ohio. **Work history:** Pediatric Staff Nurse, Pa.; Faculty, American Univ., Washington, D.C.; clinical work, teaching, Amarillo, Texas; Nursing Faculty, Univ. of Mississippi, Univ. of Michigan; Visiting Distinguished Professor, Texas Christian Univ., Univ. of Texas, Univ. of Alabama; Researcher; Author; Speaker; Nursing Consultant, Arthur Young Assoc. **Organizations:** American Nurses Assoc., American Heart Assoc., American Public Health Assoc., American Assoc. for the History of Nursing, Assoc. for the Advancement of Science, National Commission on the Prevention of Child Abuse. **Awards:** Fellow, American Academy of Nursing; Book of the Year Awards, *American Journal of Nursing;* Shaw Medal, Boston College; Distinguished Alumni Award, Univ. of Nebraska.

References and Credits

†Kalisch P, Kalisch B: The Changing Image of the Nurse. Menlo Park, Calif., Addison-Wesley, 1986, p 193.

Schorr T, Zimmerman A: Making Choices, Taking Chances: Nurse Leaders Tell Their Stories. St. Louis, CV Mosby, 1988.

Mason D, Talbot S: Political Action Handbook for Nurses. Menlo Park, Calif., Addison Wesley, 1985.

Franz J, Vandervort-Jones P (eds): Who's Who in American Nursing, 1986–1987. Owings Mills, Md., Society of Nursing Professionals, 1987, p 264.

October 16

Wailua Brandman •

1947–

"In Hawaiian, the word 'Wailua' means two fresh waters (or rivers) coming together in one vessel, forming a fountain spraying water and light; going into the darkness; nurturing, supporting, flowing; figuratively, it means the Paradox in one. My message to others who would be healers is to know yourself well, the light and the dark; explore the connection of all life—conscious light, learn about the transpersonal caring moment, as formulated by Jean Watson, and live unconditional love in your life as much as you are able." (1998)

Wailua Brandman was inspired by the mentoring he received while associating with Barbara Montgomery Dossey and Virginia Henderson. His nursing career focused on wounds and recovery in the emergency room and intensive care unit; and on mental and emotional levels in the psychiatric inpatient units. This experience gave him the opportunity to witness the mind-body connection in the real world. His holistic perspective was shaped by independent study of the holographic paradigm, quantum physics, psychoneuroimmunology, comparative religions, and systems theory. Mindfulness in meditation has been an asset to his growth and awareness of the nature of reality. As a nurse psychotherapist, he works with clients to find their center, discover and modify their dysfunctional core beliefs, release their pain, heal their wounds, learn the self-limiting effect of fear, and remember the strength that comes from love. Together he and his clients travel the path back to self-love.

Biography

Born: Oct. 14, 1947, Indianapolis, Ind. **Education:** El Centro College, Dallas (AAS); St. Francis College, Brooklyn Heights, N.Y. (BS); Yale University School of Nursing (MSN); California State Univ., Long Beach (post-master's certificate). **Work history:** ER, Psychiatric Inpatient Nursing, thirty yrs.; critical care cardiovascular recovery, cardiac, surgical, medical, pediatric, and neonatal units; now in private psychotherapy practice; Consultant to various state agencies; Clinical Instructor, Nursing, Univ. of Hawaii, Manoa, Honolulu. **Organizations:** member, delegate, American Nurses Assoc., Hawaii Nurses Assoc. (HNA); Publicity Chair, Gamma Psi Chapter-at-Large; Sigma Theta Tau; Media Relations Committee Chair, American Psychiatric Nurses Assoc. **Awards:** 1997 Ruth Kemble Award for Volunteer Service, HNA; honored by Res. 24, Hawaii House of Representatives, 1998.

References and Credits

†Keegan L, Dossey B: Profiles of Nurse Healers. Albany, N.Y., Delmar Learning, a division of Thomson Learning, 1998, pp 189–192.

Brandman W: personal communication, November 2002.

October 17

Marlene F. Kramer

1931–

"What are the variables that create magnetism? Staff nurses in our study identified eight: an adequate number of superbly competent, educated nurses supported by an administrative team that has built a culture that values quality patient care and supports the values of the collegial nurse-physician relationships, clinical autonomy, and control over nursing practice. Physicians will not collaborate with nurses they do not perceive as competent. Before nurses act on what they know, they have to perceive that the organization wants them to go the extra mile for the patient. Without knowledge and administrative-managerial support, nurses cannot gain and master control over their own practice or cooperate with others to insure quality care." (2002)

Marlene Kramer was attracted to nursing by her high school summer job as a nurse's aide. Her professional career includes work as a nurse administrator, teacher, researcher, consultant, and author. Her illustrious career in nursing research has addressed reality shock, bicultural training, tactile stimulation of premature infants, and magnet hospitals. Kramer defined her theory of "reality shock" when she observed the frustrations and difficulties of new graduates who attempted to apply the ideals of professional nursing that they learned in school. Their subsequent disillusionment influenced her greatly. She emphasizes that new nurses need role models who "could influence others to give quality nursing care ... given the resources and constraints of the work situation"; she also influenced related curricula changes at the University of California, San Francisco, and the University of Connecticut. The Bicultural Training Program helps nurses develop effective conflict resolution strategies for the school-to-work transition, as faculty members show by example in their own practice. Kramer views faculty practice as essential to the student's growth and learning experiences. A leading national authority on magnet hospitals, she and colleague Claudia Schmalenberg have researched and written about them since 1985. They define the essentials of magnetism and the culture of excellence that focus on both the quality of patient care and the job satisfaction of the professional nurse.

Biography

Born: Oct. 17, 1931, St. Louis. **Education:** St. Louis Univ. (BSN); Case Western Reserve, Cleveland, Ohio (MA); Stanford Univ. (PhD). **Work history:** Staff Nurse, Kaiser Permanente Hosp., Santa Clara, Calif.; Instructor, pediatric nursing, Hotel Dieu School of Nursing; Pediatric Head Nurse, Cleveland, Ohio; Assistant Director of Nursing for Special Projects, Director of Night Nursing Services, Cleveland (Ohio) Metropolitan General Hosp.; Instructor, pediatrics, San Jose (Calif.) State College; Undergraduate Program Coordinator, Dean, Graduate Program Faculty, Univ. of California School of Nursing, San Francisco; Dean, School of Nursing, University of Conn.; Orvis Chair, Nursing Research, Univ. of Nevada, Reno; Consultant, Researcher; Vice President, Nursing, Health Science Research Assoc. **Organizations:** American Nurses Assoc. (ANA); National League for Nursing; School of Nursing Alumni memberships. **Awards:** Fellow, American Academy of Nursing; Outstanding Alumni Awards, Case Western Reserve Univ., St. Louis Univ.; member, first research council, Division of Nursing Research Review Panel, ANA; named one of ten outstanding nurse leaders by Teachers College, Columbia Univ.

References and Credits

†McClure M, Hinshaw A: Magnet Hospitals Revisited: Attraction and Retention of Professional Nurses. Washington, D.C., American Nurses Publishing, American Nurses Association, 2002, p 55.

Schorr T, Zimmerman A: Making Choices, Taking Chances: Nurse Leaders Tell Their Stories. St. Louis, CV Mosby, 1988.

Kramer M.: personal communication, 2002.

Kramer M: resume.

Beulah Sanford France

1891–1971

"If you let your child feel the thrill of doing things for others, he eventually will think up ways of being thoughtful and unselfish without prompting. And that of course is your goal. You want your child to be a person who is spontaneously eager to give pleasure. ...It is not easy to cultivate a generous spirit in your child." (1952)

Beulah France was a creative writer and radio broadcaster on child health for the New York City Department of Health. Her syndicated column on child health appeared in such magazines as *Life, Health,* and *American Baby* from 1930 to 1960. Her health care columns appeared throughout the United States, as well as in Canada, England, and Latin America. She chaired the child welfare committee of the League of Women Voters from 1930 to 1932. She maintained membership and held offices in many nursing organizations.

Biography

Born: Oct. 18, 1891, Redding, Conn. **Education:** Centenary Hill Collegiate Institute, 1907; St. Luke's Hosp. School of Nursing, Sloane Hosp. for Women, N.Y.C., 1920; Columbia Univ., 1921–23. **Work history:** Public Health Nurse, Larchmont, N.Y.; Supervisor of Public Health, Metropolitan Life Insurance Co., N.Y.C.; health care writer, broadcaster, New York City Dept. of Health, 1930–60; health education, E.R. Squibb and Sons, 1932–44; freelance writing, radio and television broadcasting, lecturing, 1934–60; Instructor, child care, Brides' School of Scientific Housekeeping, N.Y.C., 1932–42; Child Care Editor, *Country Gentleman* (later called *Better Farming*); Editorial Director, Editor Emeritus, *American Baby Magazine,* 1940–71. **Organizations:** Fellow, American Public Health Assoc.; member, Royal Society of Health of London; Public Health Assoc. of N.Y.C.; American Nurses Assoc.; International Council of Nurses. **Awards:** honorary doctorate, Hartwick College, Oneonta, N.Y., 1961. **Died:** New York City.

References and Credits

†France B: How to Have a Happy Child. New York, Sterling, 1952, p 122.

Stein AP: Beulah Sanford France. In Bullough V, Sentz L, Stein AP (eds): American Nursing: A Biographical Dictionary, vol. 2. New York, Garland, 1992, pp 117–118.

Sister Mary Berenice Beck

1890–1960

"Nurses should keep constantly in mind . . . that the practitioners of a profession are expected to define their own responsibilities, to be concerned not only with their own competence and honor but also with that of all fellow practitioners, and to realize that controls on the profession should be self-imposed. Since health service is a basic right of all the people, it is important that the professional health organizations . . . be especially concerned about the satisfactory and ethical performance of the services it undertakes to render." (1956)

Sister Mary Berenice Beck was a Franciscan sister and a nursing leader. She played a primary role in the development of the initial code of ethics of the American Nurses Association in 1949, after twenty-five years of unsuccessful efforts by others. A registered pharmacist as well as a registered nurse, she earned one of the first ten doctoral degrees in nursing. She was an educator, administrator, and author. She published one book and many articles about nursing practice, nursing education, and professional ethics. Writing about the ethics code years later, she said: "When the Professional Code for Nurses was developed, it was recognized that practically every situation which faces the nurse (whether as nurse or personal) contains more implications which need to be understood clearly and taken into consideration if the problem is to be grasped realistically, and sufficiently well to be solved correctly."

Biography

Born: Oct. 19, 1890, St. Louis. **Education:** business school, St. Louis, Mo.; entered Franciscan Sisters, Daughters of the Sacred Hearts of Jesus and Mary, 1910; St. Anthony's School of Nursing, St. Louis; became registered pharmacist, Missouri; Marquette Univ. (BS, MS); Catholic Univ. of America (PhD). **Work history:** St. Joseph's Hosp., Milwaukee; Instructor, Director, St. Joseph's Training School for Nurses, Milwaukee; Instructor, Catholic Univ.; merged St. Joseph's School of Nursing, Milwaukee, and Marquette Univ.; Dean, Marquette Univ. School of Nursing; summer nursing instructor for numerous college programs across the country. **Organizations:** Washington, D.C., League for Nursing Education; Wisc. League for Nursing Education; Wisc. Nurses Assoc.; Wisc. State Bd. of Nurse Examiners; Catholic Hosp. Assoc.; National League for Nursing Education; American Nurses Assoc. (ANA); American Journal of Nursing Co. **Awards:** ANA Hall of Fame. **Buried:** Calvary Cemetery, Racine, Wisc.

References and Credits

†Beck MB: What's in our code? AJN 56:1407, 1956.

Cooper SS: Sister Mary Bernice Beck. In Bullough V, Church OM, Stein AP (eds): American Nursing: A Biographical Dictionary, vol. 1. New York, Garland, 1988, pp 22–24.

ANA Hall of Fame 10/98 American Nurses Association, Washington, D.C. http://www.nursingworld.org/hof.

October 29

Marietta Burtis Squire

1868–1933

"If after … statistics are available, it can be shown that the existing [permissive] laws in the majority of states, having been lived up to in their fullest and best sense, still fail in accomplishing the purpose for which they were enacted, or that their greater efficiency depends on their being made compulsory—then in order that the benefits registration was intended to confer may be enjoyed by all desiring them, and protected against the harmful interference of the indifferent or unworthy—all nurses must be compelled to seek registration or other fields of work." (1913)

Marietta Squire was a private duty nurse for more than two decades. She was New Jersey's first school nurse and the first nurse in that state to apply for licensure. When she was serving on the state's first board of nurse examiners, her work to develop curriculum guidelines demonstrated her commitment to high education standards for nurses. These guidelines later served as examples for other states. Called "the mother of nursing in New Jersey," she was an advocate for nurse registration and contributed to the debate about whether registration should be voluntary or compulsory. She raised questions about the effect of registration on the profession and the public, the effectiveness of voluntary registration, and the realities of enforcement if compulsory. She also viewed mandatory registration as a way to elevate both the quality of education and the caliber of nurses.

Biography

Born: Oct. 20, 1868, Rahway, N.J. **Education:** Orange (N.J.) Memorial Hosp. **Work history:** Private Duty Nurse; School Nurse, Morristown, N.J.; New Jersey Bd. of Nurse Examiners; Nurse, Gimbel's Dept. Store, N.Y.C. **Organizations:** founder, N.J. State Nurses Assoc., N.J. League for Nursing Education; Guild of St. Barnabas for Nurses; N.J. Historical Society. **Awards:** Endowment Fund Honor List, N.J. State Federation of Women's Clubs. **Died:** Orange, N.J.

References and Credits

†Squire M: Is compulsory registration desirable and how may it be obtained? AJN 13:956, 1913.

Fickelssen JL: Marietta Squire. In Bullough V, Sentz L, Stein AP (eds): American Nursing: A Biographical Dictionary, vol. 2. New York, Garland, 1992, pp 313–314.

October 21

Eugenia Kennedy Spalding

1896–1978

"Satisfaction in your work is one of the fruits of a wise choice." (1970)

"Ethical problems in nursing ... may include personal matters, professional conduct, and social issues. The common factor is that their solution is based upon principles which are unaltered by changing customs. *Some of us call these principles the ancient Christian virtues; some call them the standards of ideal character, or morals, or a sense of right and wrong. ... All nurses, due to their background of training, experience and ideals, should become quietly but surely masters of problem solving." (1944)*

EUGENIA SPALDING PREPARED as a teacher and taught elementary school briefly before entering nursing. She completed university coursework in histology and pathology during nursing school. While she was studying at Columbia University, she accepted the invitation of Sister Olivia Gowan to help establish a school of nursing at the Catholic University of America, for which Spalding developed the curriculum and was the first lay faculty member. During World War II she took a leave from teaching to serve as a consultant for the U.S. Public Health Service (USPHS) and helped develop standards for the U.S. Cadet Nurse Corps. In retirement she helped develop nursing education programs in Turkey and was active in numerous professional organizations, working on such issues as federal aid for nursing education, standards, and curriculum. She was a prolific writer, recognized with honorary membership in the International Mark Twain Society.

Biography

Born: Oct. 19, 1896, Lawrenceburg, Ind. **Education:** Moores Hill College, Ind.; St. Vincent's Hosp. School of Nursing, Ind.; Indiana Univ.; Indiana Univ. School of Medicine; Teachers College, Columbia Univ. (BS, MA). **Work history:** Librarian, Lab Tech, Assistant Director, Nursing Instructor, St Vincent's Hosp. School of Nursing; Indiana State Bd. of Nurses; Indiana State Nurses Assoc.; Faculty, Catholic Univ. of America; Consultant, USPHS; Faculty, Indiana Univ., Columbia Univ.; Nursing Consultant. **Organizations:** Washington, D.C., League for Nursing; National League for Nursing; Washington, D.C., Graduate Nurses Assoc.; American Nurses Assoc.; Sigma Theta Tau; Pi Gamma Mu; Pi Lambda Theta; editorial bd., *American Journal of Nursing;* American Assoc. of Univ. Professors; International Council of Catholic Nurses. **Awards:** honorary doctorate, Keuka College, N.Y.; special citation, Ind. Nurses Assoc.; honorary member, International Mark Twain Society. **Died:** Washington, D.C.

References and Credits

†Spaulding E, Notter L: Professional Nursing: Foundations, Perspectives, and Relationships. Philadelphia, JB Lippincott, 1970, p 324.

†Spalding EK: Your problems—As a nurse and a woman. AJN 44:945, 949, 1944.

Nagy SA, McCarthy RT: Eugenia Spalding. In Bullough V, Sentz L, Stein AP (eds): American Nursing: A Biographical Dictionary, vol. 2. New York, Garland, 1992, pp 309–313.

October 22

Betty Ann Olsen

1934–1968

"It is up to God, not you, to decide when we shall die!" (1968)

WHILE VOLUNTEERING AT the United Service Organization, Betty Ann Olsen was affectionately known as "the Belle of Da Nang." She later worked as a missionary nurse at the Leprosarium for the Christian Missionary Alliance in Ban Me Thuot, Vietnam. In January 1968 she was captured by the North Vietnamese Army (NVA). Her strength and courage had fortified her and fellow captives, Rev. Henry F. Blood, a missionary, and Michael Benge, a civilian agricultural development adviser. For five months they were chained together and marched around the jungle. Blood contracted pneumonia. Olsen attended to him and begged NVA medics who visited to give him medicine. Their reply was, "No, it's better he die." He died on July 4. After nine months of starvation and deprivation, Olsen was dying of multiple nutritional disorders and exhaustion. She and Benge told their captors they would not go any farther until they got some good food. They had been surviving on a daily ration of a small ball of rice and salt. The soldiers put a gun to their heads and told them they were a food drain for their army and threatened to shoot them on the spot. Olsen screamed, "It is up to God, not you, to decide when we shall die!" Her cry seemed to confuse the soldiers. They thought she was crazy and she and Michael thought they had bought some time. They were allowed to rest for a few days; then the soldiers gave them a meal that was poisoned. Somehow Michael survived, but he had to help bury Betty after three days of tortuous suffering. For Betty he vowed that he would stay alive. He endured captivity for five years and two months before his release. He remembers Betty Ann as "one brave and feisty lady, and she saved my life!"

Biography

Born: Oct. 22, 1934, Mission Station, Bouake, Ivory Coast. **Education:** Methodist Hosp., Brooklyn, N.Y., 1956; Nyack (N.Y.) Missionary College, 1957–62; leprosarium training, Hong Kong, 1964; studied Vietnamese language, Da Nang, South Vietnam; studied Raday language, Ban Me Thuot. **Work history:** OB Nurse, Nyack Hosp.; OB Nurse, Chicago West Suburban Hosp.; Missionary Nurse, Christian and Missionary Alliance; Staff Nurse, Ban Me Thuot Leprosarium, captured while evacuating injured coworkers. **Organizations:** unknown. **Awards:** unknown. **Buried:** near Cambodian border, South Vietnam, 1968.

References and Credits

†Benge M: unpublished ms., Betty Olsen, POW: The Ban Me Thuot five and the Laotian two, 1996.

Peterson SL: Betty Olsen. In Bullough V, Church OM, Stein AP (eds): American Nursing: A Biographical Dictionary, vol. 1. New York, Garland, 1988, pp 249–250.

Benge M: personal communication, 2003.

October 23

Mary E. Lent

1869–1946

"Many good district nurses become so by long experience, but one must have the vision to become really efficient. Our work is not merely nursing. It is understanding of the social web, and knowledge of the forces at work within it. We must recognize all the points of contact between our work and all other work for social betterment, and we must realize that no one phase of social activity can progress beyond all the rest, since all alike are interwoven and dependent on each other in the great scheme of progressive betterment. It is the ability to see and grasp the significance of all this that constitutes the difference between the mediocre and the successful district nurse." (1909)

Mary Lent worked as a public health nurse in Baltimore, where she helped develop a specialty focus related to tuberculosis. She initiated health classes for working women and, as nurse supervisor, required medical exams for young men before they could participate in city athletic programs. She organized district nursing in Los Angeles before joining the U.S. Public Health Service, where she directed public education for the control of disease in areas surrounding military camps. She traveled nearly twelve thousand miles to work with local agencies and monitor the sanitation zones around the mobilization and training camps in the United States during World War I. Ella Phillips Crandall, of the National Organization for Public Health Nursing, called Lent's work "the greatest single war service rendered by the organization to the government and the public."

Biography

Born: Oct. 24, 1869, New York. **Education:** Johns Hopkins Hosp. School of Nursing. **Work history:** Head Nurse, Johns Hopkins Hosp.; Staff Nurse, Superintendent of Nurses, Instructive Visiting Nurse Assoc., Baltimore; organized nursing division of Los Angeles Public Health Dept.; Supervising Nurse, USPHS; Author. **Organizations:** National Organization for Public Health Nursing; active alumna, Johns Hopkins. **Awards:** unknown. **Died:** Wallington, N.Y.

References and Credits

†Lent M: The organization of district work. AJN 9:974, 1909.

Sentz L: Mary Lent. In Bullough V, Church OM, Stein AP (eds): American Nursing: A Biographical Dictionary, vol. 1. New York, Garland, 1988, pp 211–212.

October 24

Virginia T. Williams
1925–

"In 1973, after 30 years in nursing, I realized that nurses should be working independently of the medical model. … There could have been other avenues for my practice to take, but they were closed by a rigid health care system. The concept of continuity of care was attractive … [and] … I attempted to work in that setting at our local 135 bed hospital. But I could not convince the administrator that all the discharged, so-called cured, healed, abandoned or terminally ill needed someone to care for them or have home care arranged for them. Neither could I influence the medical specialists that they needed someone to assess or evaluate those who petitioned them for care—those who were usually worried and whose reception into the health care system was jumbled, delayed or inappropriate. Those who were rejected for care because the physician's practice was full had little recourse but to get sicker and use the emergency room. … My third option was private practice." (1988)

THE PROMISE OF independence attracted Virginia Williams to nursing. When she left traditional nursing and a good income to establish a private practice in her home town, her father thought she would starve. He said that she was "the only one in our family who had ever been to college, then on to grad school, and then to quit work." Affectionately called "the angel of McHenry," she was the first nurse in Illinois to have an independent practice. During graduate studies in community health she concluded that nursing could offer more than customary hospital and home-based care. She conducted a survey, and the results reinforced her belief that nursing could reach beyond current practice to do more to help individuals and families achieve and maintain good health. Williams defined and practiced this expanded role for nursing. She provided and taught care while working with individuals and/or families to develop their own skills and potential for good health. Defined by simplicity, her generalist nursing model was autonomous, patient- and family-centered, and accountable. She contracted with families after making assessments in their own homes. Before she entered private practice, in addition to staff nursing, she coordinated a project funded by the U.S. Department of Health, Education, and Welfare to attract inactive nurses to return to the practice of nursing.

Biography

Born: Oct. 24, 1925, McHenry, Ill. **Education:** St. Anne's Hosp. School of Nursing, Chicago; Loyola Univ., Chicago (BSN); Northern Illinois Univ. (master's in community health nursing). **Work history:** Hines VA Hosp., Chicago; Project Coordinator, Indian Health Service, HEW; independent practice, Ill. **Organizations:** Ill. Nurses Assoc., American Nurses Assoc.; bd. of trustees, McHenry Hosp.; bd. of directors, Comprehensive Health Planning Agency, Ill. **Awards:** Woman of the Year, Business and Professional Women's Club.

References and Credits

†Schorr T, Zimmerman A: Making Choices, Taking Chances: Nurse Leaders Tell Their Stories. St. Louis, CV Mosby, 1988, pp 396–397.

Williams V: personal correspondence, August 2002.

October 25

Jo Ann Ashley
1939–1980

"Power relationships involve elements of dependency, and nursing has lived with the myth that it is and has always been the dependent group in relation to medicine. In reality, history shows that physicians very early recognized their own increasing dependency upon nurses. This, and not the reverse, was true." (1973)

Jo Ann Ashley was a knowledgeable, assertive, and committed advocate for nursing whose career and life were cut short by breast cancer. She issued a wake-up call to nursing with her research and publications. She traced the deliberate and successful efforts to keep nursing subservient and perpetuate its position of limited power and dependence. An astute student of the history of nursing, health care delivery, and the early roots of feminism, she called on nursing to recognize that society considers it an essential service and to build upon the inherent power and successes of nursing. She reminded nurses that the nursing process at the beginning of the twentieth century accounted for the improved safety of hospital care and surgical care, the related lower mortality rates, and the higher rates of good outcomes. She asks nursing to use its power to enhance nursing. She contrasted the perceptive remarks of nursing leaders like Lavinia Dock, Shirley Titus, and Isabel Stewart with the behavior of nurses in general over time—that of accepting male dominance, especially that of physicians and hospital administrators.

Biography

Born: Oct. 25, 1939, Sweeden, Ky. **Education:** Western Kentucky Univ.; Kentucky Baptist School of Nursing; Catholic Spaulding College, Louisville, Ky. (BSN); Columbia Univ. (MEd, EdD). **Work history:** Staff Nurse, Kentucky Baptist Hosp.; Instructor, Norton Memorial Infirmary School of Nursing, Louisville, Ky.; Staff Nurse, Veterans Administration Hosps., Brecksville, Ohio, and New York; Faculty, City College of New York, Pennsylvania State Univ., Northern Illinois Univ.; Texas Women's Univ.; West Virginia. Univ.; editorial Bd., *Advances in Nursing Science.* **Organizations:** American Nurses Assoc.; Trustee, Nurses Coalition for Action in Politics (ANA). **Awards:** unknown. **Died:** Morgantown, W. Va.

References and Credits

†Ashley J. About power in nursing. Nurs Outlook 21:639, 1973.

Ruffing-Rahal MA: Jo Ann Ashley. In Bullough V, Sentz L (eds): American Nursing: A Biographical Dictionary, vol. 3. New York, Springer, 2000, pp 3–5.

Ashley J: Nursing and early feminism. AJN 75:1465–1467, 1975.

October 26

Richard MacIntyre

1952–

"Nature heals best when people are in environments that sustain hope, possibility, and meaning. People heal best when those environments help them retain their essential humanity in the face of challenges, suffering, and loss. Healing environments cannot flourish without diversity, without art, without narrative, without the humanities. It isn't enough for nurses and physicians to see the patient behind the disease—at least not at the price this country is paying for health care. We need to make understanding our patients a much higher priority and that can't happen unless we respect and listen to them." (1999)

RICHARD MACINTYRE BLENDED his unique talent as a nurse and Fulbright Scholar–researcher with his own empathic commitment to gay men who shared their stories of living with asymptomatic HIV. He rewrote the research for his doctoral dissertation as a book for a lay audience, *Mortal Men* (1999). Here he uncovers the uncertainty and dilemmas that asymptomatic HIV-positive men face: "'Am I really sick? ...Should I take prescription drugs or focus on having fun?'" Many sought balance, but "trying to find balance among biomedical, sociopolitical, and holistic concerns produces more questions than it does answers." While MacIntyre is grounded in science, he believes that personal experiences create the context in which people come to understand HIV and most other illnesses. He interviewed men from his own community—men whom he knew, sometimes loved, and often lost. These poignant stories acquaint the reader with what it was like "to experience mortality, medicine, and health in an era of sex, drugs, and T Cells." He writes that his book chronicles "yesterday's struggles in the hope that our humanity might be preserved and our future endowed with the insights that we developed in response to death."

Biography

Born: April 9, 1952, Reedley, Calif. **Education:** Santa Barbara (Calif.) City College, 1975 (AAS); California State Univ., Sacramento, 1978 (BS, MS in nursing administration); Univ. of California, San Francisco, 1993 (PhD); Postdoctoral Fellow, International Center for AIDS Research, Univ. of California, San Francisco, 1996–1997; Fulbright Scholar, Univ. of Tromosø, Norway, 1996–97. **Work history:** Professor, Division Chair, Health Professions and Department of Nursing, Mercy College, Dobbs Ferry, N.Y., 1998–present. **Organizations:** Task Force on Nursing Faculty Shortage, American Assoc. of Colleges of Nursing; editorial bd., *Journal of the Association of Nurses in AIDS Care;* President, N.Y. State Council of Deans of Nursing. **Awards:** unknown.

References and Credits

†MacIntyre R: Mortal Men: Living with Asymptomatic HIV. New Brunswick, N.J., Rutgers University Press, 1999, pp 220–221, 18–19.

MacIntyre R: resume.

MacIntyre R: personal communication, 2003.

Margaret Gene Arnstein

1904–1972

"Humaneness in nursing is expressed through every motion we make, through everything we say and do. ... In the future, we will need every bit of our academic learning—our education in science and theory ... and at the same time, we will also need that quality of humaneness—that interest in understanding people, in helping them through our feeling, our presence—to be sure that we bring warmth and understanding, as well as scientific expertness, to every service that we render. Only when we combine the two qualities ... can we have true balance in nursing." (1958)

MARGARET GENE ARNSTEIN is known as a public health nurse with global influence. She visited the Henry Street Settlement as a teenager and was influenced by Lillian Wald; Arnstein knew then that she wanted to be a nurse. Encouraged by friends and her wealthy family to be a doctor because she was "too smart for nursing," she earned a premedical degree before entering nursing school. Shirley Fondiller writes that Arnstein, "commenting some years later on ... a commonly accepted attitude toward nursing, ... noted that intelligence was not wasted on nursing, as she never had enough for any job she had done." A highly recognized nurse consultant, researcher, and educator, she was also widely published and was coauthor of the acclaimed *Communicable Disease Control.*

Arnstein influenced nursing research, public health, nursing education, and health care. During her two decades with the U.S. Public Health Service (USPHS), she held high-ranking positions, including chief of public health nursing. She worked with the World Health Organization to publish a *Guide for National Studies of Nursing Resources.* Later, while still with the USPHS she studied the needs of developing countries. Arnstein wrote of the importance of the nurse-patient relationship and cautioned against fragmented care that could result from the greater number of people involved with the patient.

Biography

Born: Oct. 27, 1904, New York City. **Education:** Smith College (BA); New York Presbyterian Hosp. School of Nursing (RN); Teachers College, Columbia Univ. (MA); Johns Hopkins Univ. (MPH). **Work history:** Staff Nurse, Westchester County (N.Y.) Health Dept.; New York State Dept. of Health; Faculty, Univ. of Minnesota; Adviser, nursing education, United Nations, Cairo, two yrs.; U.S. Public Health Service (USPHS); World Health Organization; Yale Univ., Univ. of Michigan; Dean, Yale Univ. **Organizations:** American Public Health Assoc. (APHA). **Awards:** Rockefeller Public Service Award; Sedgewick Memorial Medal, APHA; Lasker Award for Nursing; Distinguished Service Medal, USPHS; honorary doctorates, Univ. of Michigan, Wayne State Univ., Smith College. **Died:** New Haven, Conn.

References and Credits

†Arnstein M. Balance in nursing. AJN 58: 1691–1692, 1958.

Fondiller S: Margaret Arnstein. In Bullough V, Church OM, Stein AP (eds): American Nursing: A Biographical Dictionary, vol. 1. New York, Garland, 1988, p 9.

Brown A: personal communication.

Martha Minerva Franklin

1870–1968

"We, the undersigned, residents of the state of New York, desiring to form a membership corporation. ... The name or title by which this Society shall be known is the National Association of Colored Graduate Nurses. ... The purposes of this corporation shall be to promote the professional and educational advancement of nurses in every proper way; to elevate the standard of nursing education; to establish and maintain a code of ethics among nurses; to own and control a permanent headquarters and all rights and property held by the National Association of Colored Graduate Nurses as a corporation." (1920)

MARTHA MINERVA FRANKLIN was the only black nurse in her graduating class in Philadelphia, and she faced limited opportunities for practice because of race. She recognized that black nurses needed to organize to strengthen their efforts to replace discrimination and rejection with equal opportunities for education and practice. She mailed handwritten invitations to a meeting to fifteen hundred nurses, and the fifty-two who attended did the organizational groundwork to establish the National Association of Colored Graduate Nurses (NACGN). Before that, black nurses had no supportive professional organization. They were not eligible for membership in the American Nurses Association (ANA) because membership in state organizations was closed to them in the segregated South. As principal founder and first president of the NACGN, Franklin was supported in her efforts by Ada Bell Samuel Thoms, Lillian Wald, and Lavinia Dock. Franklin's guidance fostered leadership in others to help improve educational standards and gain professional equality.

Biography

Born: Oct. 29, 1870, New Milford, Conn. **Education:** Women's Hosp. Training School for Nurses, Philadelphia; postgraduate work, Lincoln Hosp., New York; Teachers College, Columbia Univ. **Work history:** Private Duty Nurse, School Nurse, N.Y.C. **Organizations:** Founder, President, NACGN. **Awards:** Honorary Lifetime President, NACGN; ANA Hall of Fame. **Died:** New Haven, Conn.

References and Credits

†Davis A: Early Black American Leaders in Nursing: Architects for Integration and Equality. Sudbury, Mass., Jones and Bartlett, 1999, pp 194–195.

Davis ATL: Martha Franklin. In Bullough V, Church OM, Stein AP (eds): American Nursing: A Biographical Dictionary, vol. 1. New York, Garland, 1988, pp 121–123.

Davis A: Martha Minerva Franklin. In Smith JC (ed): Notable Black American Women. Detroit, Gale, 1992.

Clark D (ed): Black Women in America. Brooklyn, N.Y., Carlson, 1993.

Thoms AB: Pathfinders: A History of the Progress of Colored Graduate Nurses. New York: Kay Printing, 1929.

ANA Hall of Fame 10/98 American Nurses Association, Washington, D.C. http://www.nursingworld.org/hof.

October 29

Billye Jean Brown

1925–

"I believe the future of nursing rests heavily on present and future leaders, on those who are followers, on nursing programs and on nursing organizations. I believe teaching and practicing leadership and 'followership' characteristics by individuals and organizations are vital to our continued development as a profession. Leaders must be very clear about their own beliefs before they are able to lead others. To be an effective leader, mentor and influential role model, one must clarify his or her values and goals and be aware of their influences on future leaders." (2000)

Billye Brown's political skills, networking capabilities, and leadership helped to fortify nursing by strengthening its organizations and its educational institutions. She served on local, state, and national professional nursing committees to learn from and mentor others who saw the need for change in the nursing profession. During her tenure in administrative positions at the University of Texas School of Nursing, the University of Texas underwent systemwide reorganization. Her leadership guided many changes within the School of Nursing. She influenced the establishment of private endowments as sources of private funding for the School of Nursing in Austin. She served on numerous national and state boards and was appointed as a civilian consultant to the surgeon general of the U.S. Air Force from 1983 to 1987. She was president of Sigma Theta Tau from 1989 to 1991. She is sought as a consultant and lecturer on academic administration, leadership, followership, strategic planning, health care trends, history, and resource development. She has received numerous awards from nursing and other prestigious organizations. She continues to travel on the behalf of Sigma Theta Tau as a consultant and speaker.

Biography

Born: Oct. 29, 1925, Damascus, Ark. **Education:** Arkansas Baptist Hosp. School of Nursing, 1947 (diploma); Univ. of Texas, 1953 (BS); St. Louis Univ., 1958 (MS); Baylor Univ., 1975 (EdD). **Work history:** Staff Nurse, Surgical Assistant, Faculty, Univ. of Texas Medical Branch, Galveston; opened branch of School of Nursing at Univ. of Texas, Austin; Associate Professor, Dean, Professor, La Quinta Motor Inns Centennial Professor in Nursing Emeritus, Univ. of Texas School of Nursing, Austin; Consultant, Associate, Tuft and Associates, Chicago. **Organizations:** Sigma Theta Tau International; Life Member, American Academy of Nursing; President, Texas Nurses Assoc. (TNA), District 5; President, TNA; Director, Exec. Committee, Southern Council on Collegiate Education; bd. of directors, American Journal of Nursing Co.; President, American Assoc. of Colleges of Nursing (AACN); Assistant Editor, *Journal of Professional Nursing;* National Advisory Council on Nurse Training; member, Vice Chair, Higher Education Coordinating Bd.; Core Faculty Member, Project FACE, funded by Kellogg Foundation to consult with faculty of black colleges and universities; member, Advisory Council, Baylor Univ. School of Nursing. **Awards:** President's Award, American Academy of Nursing, 2002; Certificate of Distinction, Assoc. of College Honor Societies; Sister Bernadette Armiger Award, AACN; Distinguished Alumnus Award, Univ. of Texas, Galveston; Alumni Merit Award, St. Louis Univ. Distinguished Alumna Award, Baptist Medical System School of Nursing; Mentor Award, Sigma Theta Tau, Epsilon Theta Chapter, School of Nursing, Univ. of Texas, Austin.

References and Credits

†Brown B: Reflections on nursing. Leadership, 1st quarter 2000, p 35.

Brook MJ: Billy Jean Brown. In Bullough V, Sentz L (eds): American Nursing: A Biographical Dictionary, vol. 3. New York, Springer, 2000, pp 26–28.

Barbara Anna Thompson Sharpless

1889–1973

"By having the diagnosis on the card, the student has it before her more often than she would if she had to look it up on the chart every time. When a medication or treatment is discontinued, the nurse draws a red line through the order on the card. After six months, we are more enthusiastic than ever about this method. ... The advantages ... are many: It is compact. ... It is permanent. ... It is never necessary to copy. ... It is time saving. ... It is simple. ... It has educational value. ... It encourages students' interest in patients' treatment, proper method of assigning, case or group nursing. ... It is always clean. ... It is neat and unobtrusive. ... It is easier for charge nurse to make assignments." (1932)

BARBARA SHARPLESS WAS working as a teacher when a colleague decided to enter nursing school and she did the same. Because she was a head nurse at the University of Minnesota Hospital during World War I, she became part of the university base hospital in France. She was later awarded the Victory Medal for her service as a surgical nurse in France and Germany. Upon her return to the States, she taught nursing. While a faculty member at the

University of Minnesota School of Nursing, she coauthored a text, *Nursing Procedures,* that standardized nursing procedures for students. She developed a widely copied Kardex system that made a uniform, simplified recording system for hospital patient assignments and treatments. In addition, she was very involved with accreditation criteria for schools of nursing.

Biography

Born: Nov. 1, 1889, Sault Sainte Marie, Mich. **Education:** Univ. of Minnesota School of Nursing; postgraduate course, Lakeside Hosp., Cleveland, Ohio; Teachers College, Columbia Univ. **Work history:** St. Andrew's Hosp., Minneapolis (Minn.) City Hosp.; Univ. of Minnesota Hosp.; base hospital, France, Germany; Chief Nurse, *Prince Frederick Wilhelm;* Instructor, Research Hosp., Kansas City, Mo.; Instructor, Charles T. Miller Hosp., St. Paul, Minn.; Faculty, Assistant Director, Univ. of Minnesota School of Nursing; Director of Nurses, Minneapolis (Minn.) General Hosp.; Wisconsin Bureau of Nursing Education and Bd. of Examiners; Director of Nurses, St. Luke's Hosp., Denver; Consultant, Cadet Nurse Corps; Director of Nurses, Santa Barbara (Calif.) General Hosp.; Dean, Knapp College of Nursing, Santa Barbara, Calif. **Organizations:** National League for Nursing Education; American Nurses Assoc.; Women's Overseas Service League; Minn. State League for Nursing Education; Sigma Theta Tau; Alpha Tau Delta. **Awards:** U.S. Victory Medal; Fiftieth Year Citation, Univ. of Minnesota School of Nursing. **Died:** Camarillo, Calif.

References and Credits

†Thompson B: A combined treatment and assignment sheet. AJN 32:408–409, 1932.

Mirr MP: Barbara Anna Thompson (Sharpless). In Bullough V, Church OM, Stein AP (eds): American Nursing: A Biographical Dictionary, vol. 1. New York, Garland, 1988, pp 307–309.

October 31

Virginia Mae Ohlson

1914–

"Public health nursing seemed terribly interesting to me as a child, and I think it was that which eventually brought me into nursing. I knew from the start that my goal was to be a public health nurse. . . . I never forgot my impressions of meeting people in their homes and the opportunity to develop relationships with families—caring and helping them to be well, physically, emotionally, and spiritually. All that is what appealed to me." (1999)

Initially attracted to missionary work in the Orient through her church, Virginia Ohlson recalled being drawn to public health nursing after hearing Ruth Nordlund speak. The young Ohlson, fascinated by that public health nurse's stories of home visits and nursing care, would later be described by the writer Shirley Fondiller as an "international icon in public health nursing." Ohlson was a civilian nurse in Japan with the Army of Occupation after World War II, helping to reestablish and update nursing schools, standards of practice, and criteria for licensure amid the postwar deprivation and destruction. She left Japan when the occupation ended in 1951 but returned later that year to serve with the Atomic Bomb Casualty Commission in Hiroshima and Nagasaki. After the World War II peace treaty was signed between Japan and the United States, she accepted an invitation to join the Rockefeller Foundation as its nurse-representative, to work cooperatively with Japanese nurses in programs for which they requested assistance. Upon her return to the States in 1954, she obtained her master's degree from the University of Chicago and taught there after receiving her degree. She later joined the newly formed College of Nursing at the University of Illinois and served as its first head of the Department of Public Health Nursing. There Ohlson developed the first Illinois master's program in public health nursing. During that period she also was a consultant to the World Health Organization (WHO) in Geneva and many countries of the world. She stressed the broad concept of community and the role of the community health specialist in promoting health, preventing disease, and caring for the sick. In 1993 Ohlson was featured in an article called "One Hundred Years of Powerful Women" in the *Public Health Nursing Journal.*

Biography

Born: Oct. 31, 1914, Chicago. **Education:** North Park Junior College, Chicago; Swedish Covenant Hosp. School of Nursing, Chicago; Univ. of Chicago (BS, MSNE, PhD). **Work history:** Staff Nurse, Swedish Covenant Hosp., Chicago; Staff Nurse, Health Dept., Evanston, Ill.; Public Health Nurse, Consultant, Chief Nurse, Public Health and Welfare Section, Supreme Command of Allied Powers, Japan; Public Health Consultant, Director of Nurses, Atomic Bomb Casualty Commission, Japan; Consultant, Rockefeller Foundation, Japan; Faculty, Univ. of Chicago, Univ. of Illinois; Consultant, WHO. **Organizations:** American Nurses Assoc. (ANA); Honorary Vice President, American Public Health Assoc.; National Organization for Public Health Nursing; founder, first president, American Assoc. for Community Health Nursing Education. **Awards:** Evanston Woman of the Year; McIver Award; first international honorary member, Japanese Nursing Assoc.; Butterfly, highest Japanese imperial award given to a woman; Professor Emerita, Univ. of Illinois; Ohlson Endowment Fund, Univ. of Illinois; Living Legend, Fellow, American Academy of Nursing, 1995; honorary member, Foreign Nurses Assoc.

References and Credits

†Fondiller S: Virginia M. Ohlson: International icon in public health nursing. Nurs Outlook 47:108–113, 1999.

Schorr T, Zimmerman A: Making Choices, Taking Chances: Nurse Leaders Tell Their Stories. St. Louis, CV Mosby, 1988.

Belcher P, Brey-Schneider M: Virginia Ohlson. In Bullough V, Sentz L, Stein AP (eds): American Nursing: A Biographical Dictionary, vol. 2. New York, Garland, 1992, pp 257–260.

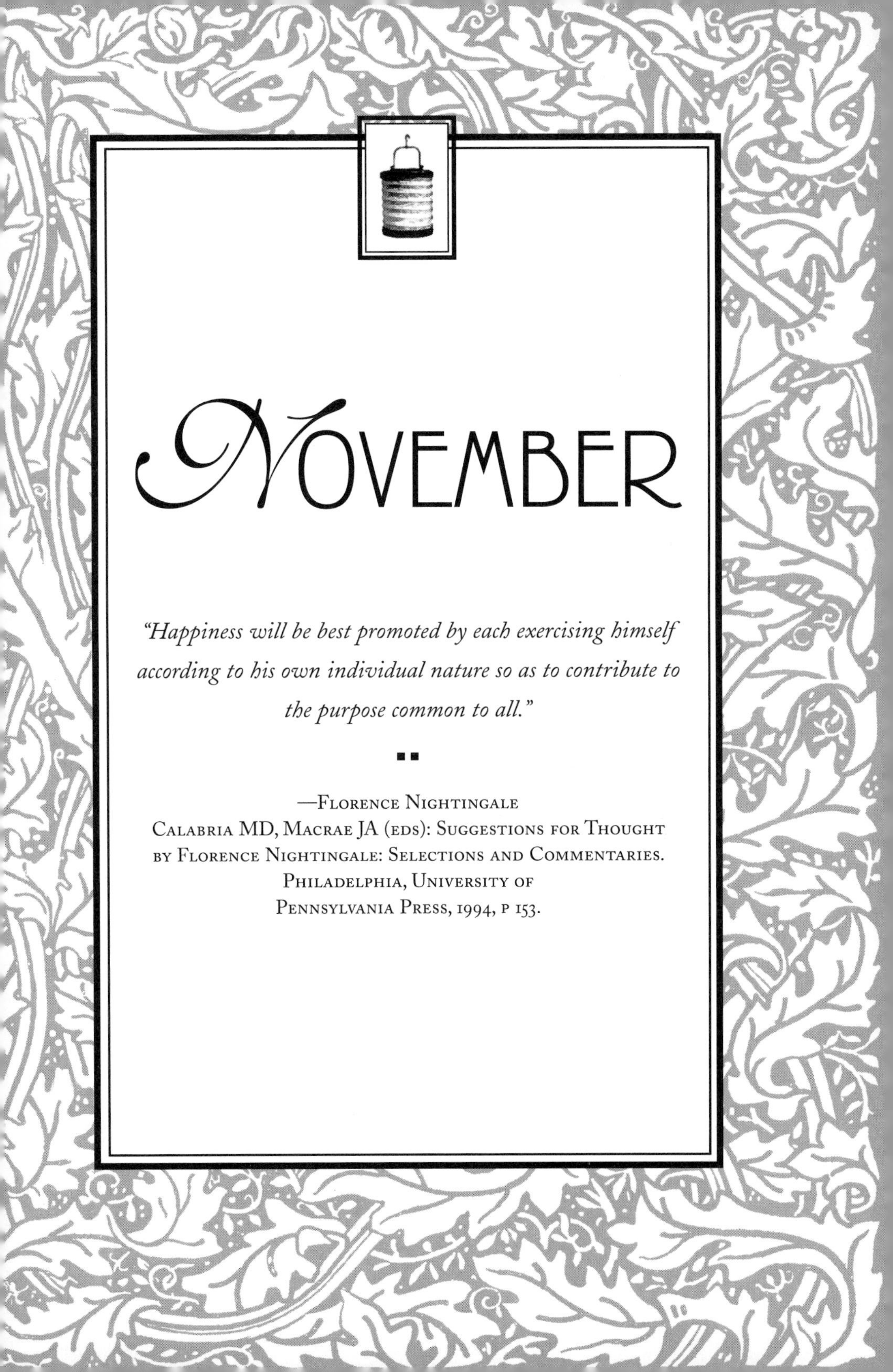

November

"Happiness will be best promoted by each exercising himself according to his own individual nature so as to contribute to the purpose common to all."

—Florence Nightingale
Calabria MD, Macrae JA (eds): Suggestions for Thought by Florence Nightingale: Selections and Commentaries. Philadelphia, University of Pennsylvania Press, 1994, p 153.

Mary Opal Browne Wolanin

1910–1997

"The care of the confused elderly is a human service that cannot be mechanized or computerized; it is quintessentially human interaction. The best education model is the example of an expert. No one will learn through texts or visual aids alone. There must be a role model who is respected and successful in dealing with the complex care of the confused elderly. Everyone's body of knowledge and skills is used in giving care to the aged, and one important quantity may still be missing—the innovative and imaginative use of self by the committed caregiver." (1981)

MARY OPAL WOLANIN was a distinguished specialist in the care of older adults. She has researched and written extensively about the nursing management required for long-term care. Her commitment to and understanding of gerontological nursing facilitated its inclusion in nursing curricula. She joined the faculty of the University of Arizona School of Nursing in 1963. Through her ongoing study and dedication she was able to establish a graduate program in gerontological nursing there, one of the first such programs in this country. She was a valuable store of information about hospital nursing, nursing home administration, and nursing education. She presented many scholarly papers in the United States and abroad. She made her "explorations" (what she called her study of confusion) after she turned seventy, during her retirement. For this dedication she was inducted into the American Nurses Association (ANA) Hall of Fame. She will be remembered for her contributions in the areas of mental frailty, the phenomenology of old age, confusion, stroke rehabilitation, and medication management.

Biography

Born: Nov. 1, 1910, Chrisney, Ind. **Education:** Washington Univ., St. Louis; Municipal General Hosp. School of Nursing, Kansas City, Mo.; Cook County School of Nursing, Chicago; University of Arizona, 1963 (MSN); Univ. of Southern California (certificate in gerontology). **Work history:** Army Nurse Corps Reserve, 1941, Jefferson Barracks, Mo.; Instructor, Cadet Nursing Program, Biloxi, Miss.; Nursing Faculty, Univ. of Arizona; Director, program on aging patient. Speaker. **Organizations:** Consultant to state nursing organizations. **Awards:** Sigma Theta Tau Founder Award; Honorary Fellow, American Academy of Nursing; Gerontological Nurse of the Year, *Journal of Gerontological Nursing;* Fellow, Gerontological Society of America; Lifetime Achievement in Nursing Award, National Gerontological Nursing Assoc.; honorary doctorate, Univ. of Arizona, 1986; ANA Hall of Fame. **Died:** San Antonio, Texas.

References and Credits

†Wolanin MO, Phillips LRF: Confusion Prevention and Care. St. Louis, CV Mosby, London, 1981, p 374.

Ebersole P: Mary Opal Wolanin. In Bullough V, Sentz L (eds): American Nursing: A Biographical Dictionary, vol. 3. New York, Springer, 2000, pp 294–296.

ANA Hall of Fame 10/98 American Nurses Association, Washington, D.C. http://www.nursingworld.org/hof.

NOVEMBER 2

Elizabeth Chamberlain Burgess

1877–1949

"The medical profession need have no fear; it is not the well educated nurse who attempts to usurp the function of the physician. If we had wished to be physicians we would have entered medical school." (1932)

ELIZABETH CHAMBERLAIN BURGESS was a contemporary of Annie W. Goodrich's and Adelaide Nutting's, and she worked with both during the First World War. Burgess and Goodrich organized the Army School of Nursing. Burgess was versatile in her interests and accomplishments and became very knowledgeable about the legal aspects of nursing. She contributed to improving the working conditions, coursework, and standards for nursing programs. When she was the superintendent of nurses at Michael Reese Hospital in Chicago, she reformed the nursing school's facilities, curriculum, and work hours for students. A morale builder, she modernized the student uniform and put pie on the menu in the dining room. She also had a long career as a faculty member at Columbia University. Nutting described Burgess as "steadfast, tireless and tenacious," Burgess was an advocate for independent nursing schools that would focus on the education of the nurse rather than the service needs of the hospital.

Biography

Born: Nov. 2, 1877, Bath, Maine. **Education:** Roosevelt Hosp. School of Nursing, N.Y.; studied nursing school administration, Teachers College, Columbia Univ.; Teachers College, Columbia Univ. (BS); Columbia Univ. (master's). **Work history:** Staff Nurse, French Hosp., N.Y.; Administrator, Roosevelt Hosp., N.Y.; Instructor, Bellevue Hosp.; Instructor, St. Luke's Hosp.; Administrator, Michael Reese Hosp., Chicago; Inspector of Nurse Training Schools, N.Y. State Dept. of Education; helped organize Army School of Nursing; N.Y. State Bd. of Nurse Examiners; Faculty, Columbia Univ. **Organizations:** National League for Nursing Education; American Red Cross Nursing Service; other local, state, and national organizations. **Awards:** Professor Emeritus, Columbia Univ.; lectureship at Columbia in her honor. **Buried:** New Haven, Conn.

References and Credits

†Burgess E: What are nurses going to do about it? AJN 32:556, 1932.

Stein AP: Elizabeth Chamberlain Burgess. In Bullough V, Church OM, Stein AP (eds): American Nursing: A Biographical Dictionary, vol. 1. New York, Garland, 1988, pp 50–52.

Mary Adelaide Nutting

1858–1948

"We need to realize and affirm anew that nursing is one of the most difficult of arts. Compassion may provide the motive, but knowledge is our only working power. Perhaps, too, we need to remember that growth in our work must be preceded by ideas, and that any conditions which suppress thought, must retard growth. Surely we will not be satisfied in perpetuating methods and traditions. Surely we shall wish to be more and more occupied with creating them." (1925)

As a young adult, Mary Adelaide Nutting cared for her ill mother and realized that she wanted to know more about nursing. William Lyon Phelps, a professor at Yale, called her "one of the most useful women in the world," when he conferred her master's degree on her. She was accomplished in music and design when she entered the first nursing class at Johns Hopkins Hospital. Three years after graduation she followed her teacher, Isabel Hampton Robb, as superintendent of nurses there. Continuing Robb's reforms, she implemented the three-year course of study and an eight-hour day for students in 1896. Also, she stopped student stipends in order to remove the perception that they were employees. Her innovations made that school a national leader in nursing education. One of Nutting's many early creative ideas established a standard for nursing students, to learn the principles of practice before working on hospital wards. A visionary professional, she recognized, wrote, and taught about the relationship between economics and nursing. This was exemplified in her paper "A Sound Economic Basis for Schools of Nursing." She was convinced that the progress of nursing education was dependent on outside financial support for nursing schools, so that they would not be owned and controlled by the hospitals. She became the nation's first professor of nursing at Columbia University in 1907. Nutting helped establish professional nursing organizations and wrote the comprehensive four-volume *History of Nursing* with Lavinia Dock. Nutting was a member of the Winslow-Goldmark Committee, which studied nursing education and made recommendations for reform. She helped organize the Nurses Associated Alumnae of the United States and Canada. And as a scholar of nursing history, Nutting helped organize nursing history societies at Johns Hopkins University and Teachers College, Columbia University. Both schools have items from her nursing history collection.

Biography

Born: Nov. 1, 1858, Frost Village, Quebec, Can. **Education:** Private schools in Canada; Lowell, Mass. (music and design); Johns Hopkins Hosp. School of Nursing; Yale Univ.; independent study in England, France, Germany. **Work history:** Head Nurse, Assistant Superintendent, Superintendent of Nurses, Johns Hopkins Hosp. School of Nursing; member, Rockefeller Foundation study group on nursing education; Professor, Teachers College, Columbia Univ.; Chair, National Emergency Committee on Nursing, World War I; helped establish Vassar Training Camp; established nursing history societies and founder, first president, Florence Nightingale International Foundation. **Organizations:** founder, Md. State Nurses Assoc.; American Home Economics Assoc.; Nurses Associated Alumnae of the U.S. and Canada; leadership roles with American Federation of Nurses, International Council of Nurses; American Society of Superintendents of Training Schools for Nurses. **Awards:** Historical Nursing Collection, Columbia Univ., named in her honor; M. Adelaide Nutting Award, National League for Nursing; honorary degree, Yale Univ.; Liberty Service Medal; ANA Hall of Fame. **Died:** New York City.

References and Credits

†Donahue P: Nursing: The Finest Art, 2nd ed. St. Louis, CV Mosby, 1996, p x.

Donahue PM: Mary Nutting. In Bullough V, Church OM, Stein AP (eds): American Nursing: A Biographical Dictionary, vol. 1. New York, Garland, 1988, pp 244–247.

References and Credits continued on page 770

November 4

Mary Beard

1876–1946

"There is in nursing a power to create in a patient so strong a desire to live that it may become the one factor which decides the issue in the patient's struggle with disease. And it is not only in an individual patient, struggling with the issues of life and death, that nurses may plant this vital seed, but in a family, in a neighborhood; in the falling infant death rate of a state or a nation, the creative power of good nursing is vividly manifest to one who looks for it. I am inclined to believe that unless a nurse has this conception of the possibilities of constructive change in the patient's attitude of mind, she cannot do real nursing. All the nursing skills, tecnics [sic], *scientific knowledge, familiarity with the principles and practices of nursing—without the realization that she has a unique power to create new life in a patient— … are not, and never can be, nursing. …Nursing is creative at its very core." (1936)*

CHILDHOOD DIPTHERIA PROMPTED Mary Beard to seek a nursing education. During her versatile career she became an inspirational leader, humanitarian, and courageous nursing pioneer. She creatively restructured a home health agency in Boston to use nurses as community nurses rather than limit their practice to one type of clinical problem. This approach, of support for neighborhood nurses as generalists, was very popular. Within ten years her agency was the largest in the country. She was involved in international nursing study and education for the Rockefeller Foundation, nurse recruiting and education during World War II, and Red Cross public health and disaster nursing. She published extensively throughout her career and was remembered, according to the writer Karen Buhler-Wilkerson, as "inwardly serene, outwardly lighthearted and always responsive."

Biography

Born: Nov. 4, 1876, Dover, N.H. **Education:** New York Hosp. School of Nursing. **Work history:** Administrator, Visiting Nurse Assoc., Westbury, Conn.; cancer research, College of Physicians and Surgeons, Columbia Univ.; Superintendent, Boston Public Health Agency; Consultant, international nursing, Rockefeller Foundation; Director of Nursing Services, American Red Cross; Chair, Nursing Committee of the Federal Council for National Defense; developed Red Cross Nurses Aide Corp. **Organizations:** member, exec. bd., President, National Organization for Public Health Nursing. **Awards:** honorary degrees Univ. of New Hampshire, Smith College. **Died:** Massachusetts.

References and Credits

†Beard M: Creative nursing. AJN 36:70, 1936.

Buhler-Wilkerson K: Mary Beard. In Bullough V, Church OM, Stein AP (eds): American Nursing: A Biographical Dictionary, vol. 1. New York, Garland, 1988, pp 19–22.

November 5

Naomi Deutsch

1890–1983

"Not only must we have a nursing personnel adequate in number and quality to maintain and strengthen our existing programs, but in addition, we must provide nurses to meet the new needs that are developing under the defense program. To meet this challenge, those who enter the nursing profession must have a broad academic background, the better to understand social and economic trends that affect the health and wellbeing [sic] *of people." (1941)*

Naomi Deutsch worked with Lillian Wald at the Henry Street Nurse Service in New York and later became its director. She migrated west and she started San Francisco's Visiting Nurse Association (VNA). She became president of the California State Organization of Public Health Nursing (CSOPHN). At the same time, she taught public health nursing at the University of California at Berkeley. From 1935 to 1943 Deutsch served as director of the public health nursing unit of the federal Children's Bureau. There she studied the effects of poverty on children, and on infant and maternal well-being. She also compiled data on family income and analyzed and revised laws pertaining to child labor, juvenile delinquency, illegitimacy, incest, foster homes, and adoption. She began a publication of special health bulletins and belonged to, held major offices in, and worked for many professional organizations.

Biography

Born: Nov. 5, 1890, Brux (Most), Czechoslovakia. **Education:** Jewish Hosp. School of Nursing, Cincinnati, Ohio, 1912; Teachers College, Columbia Univ., 1921 (BS). **Work history:** VNA, Cincinnati; Jesse Kaufman Settlement, Pittsburgh, Pa.; Supervisor, Field Director, Acting General Director, Henry Street Nurse Service, N.Y.C.; Director, Visiting Nurse Service, San Francisco; Lecturer, Assistant Professor, public health nursing, Univ. of California; Director, public health nursing unit, U.S. Children's Bureau; Children's Bureau, National Council on National Defense; principal nursing consultant for Pan American Sanitary Bureau; developed health programs for Caribbean and Central American countries. **Organizations:** Chair, Joint Committee on Inter-American Nursing of American Nurses Assoc., the National League for Nursing Education, and National Organization for Public Health Nursing; President, bd. of directors, CSOPHN; member, bd. of directors, California State Nurses Assoc.; President, San Francisco Organization of Public Health Nursing; San Francisco Social Workers Alliance; member, governing council, American Public Health Assoc. (APHA); Secretary, San Francisco County Nurses Assoc.; Chair, nursing section, APHA; ANA; National League for Nursing; American Assoc. of Social Workers; National Conference of Social Work; League of Women Voters. **Awards:** unknown. **Died:** New Orleans.

References and Credits

†Deutsch N, Willford MB: Promoting maternal and child health. AJN 41: 898, 899, 1941.

Snodgrass ME: Historical Encyclopedia of Nursing. Santa Barbara, Calif., ABC-CLIO, 1999, pp 87–88.

Stein AP: Naomi Deutsch. In Bullough V, Sentz L, Stein AP (eds): American Nursing: A Biographical Dictionary, vol. 2. New York, Garland, 1992, pp 91–92.

November 6

Elnore Elvira Thomson

1878–1957

"Florence Nightingale ... had an overwhelming desire to serve the sick, but was also an indefatigable seeker after knowledge as to how this might be done in the best way possible. ...It is because of this intelligent preparation that she was able to give the service for which she stands today ... a symbol of all that which the nursing profession is still striving to attain. ...The nurse is still actuated by the service ideal and seeks knowledge as did Florence Nightingale as preparation for service." (1930)

Elnore Thomson chose to study nursing after completing a college program and two additional years of independent study in psychology. She saw Nightingale as a leader who taught by "example, precept and practice." Thomson's professional interests were mental health and public health, and she was the first director of the Illinois Society for Mental Hygiene. After working with the Red Cross in Italy during World War I, she continued to hold leadership positions in public health nursing education on the West Coast. When she was acting president of the American Nurses Association (ANA), she spoke of the importance of nursing organizations' work in states to pass nurse practice acts. She believed this would protect patients who need skilled care, give professional status to nursing, and protect the practice of the well-prepared nurse. Thomson also served as director of the nursing department of the University of Oregon Medical School in Portland for almost two decades.

Biography

Born: Nov. 4, 1878, Illinois. **Education:** Wellesley College; two-yr. independent study, Harvard Univ.; Presbyterian Hosp. School of Nursing, Chicago; psychiatric nursing affiliation, Elgin State Hosp., Chicago; postgraduate work, Chicago School of Civics and Philanthropy. **Work history:** Chief Nurse, Elgin State Hosp., Chicago; Administrator, Illinois Society for Mental Hygiene; part-time administrator, public health nursing program, Chicago School of Civics and Philanthropy; Director, Red Cross Commission, Italy; Administrator, public health nursing program, Univ. of Oregon School of Social Work, American Child Health Assoc., San Francisco; Director, public health project, Marion Co., Oregon; Director, Dept. of Nursing Education, Univ. of Oregon Medical School; Faculty, Univ. of California, Los Angeles. **Organizations:** Ill. State Nurses Assoc.; National League for Nursing Education; National Organization for Public Health Nursing; National Commission on Nursing Service; American Red Cross; ANA; International Council of Nurses; Oregon Organization of Public Health Nursing; American Social Workers Assoc.; Oregon Society of Mental Hygiene. **Awards:** unknown. **Died:** San Francisco.

References and Credits

†Thomson EE: Ideals for service and education. AJN 30:809–810, 1930.

Stein AP: Elnore Elvira Thomson. In Bullough V, Sentz L, Stein AP (eds): American Nursing: A Biographical Dictionary, vol. 2. New York, Garland, 1992, pp 323–324.

November 7

Ellen Newbold LaMotte

1873–1961

"It should be a matter ... of grave concern, to realize that there is a very serious menace to the public health of this country, namely drug addiction. ...Drug addiction may be likened to a preventable disease that is being deliberately created—a preventable disease of an incurable type, marching with relentless strides to the complete mental, moral and physical destruction of its victims. ...Drug addiction is spreading with alarming leaps, because each new victim that succumbs means money in the pockets of a long chain of greedy individuals ... whose one object is to create a market for the drugs they have to sell. ...In [an American city] one is told that there are at present 10,000 drug addicts. One would make quite a fuss over 10,000 cases of cholera in a community." (1929)

Ellen LaMotte worked as a visiting nurse in Baltimore, where she also worked in the tuberculosis division of the city health department, and then wrote a text for nurses. During World War I she served with the French Army in Belgium and wrote of her experiences and observations in *Backwash of War: The Human Wreckage of the Battlefield as Witnessed by an American Hospital Nurse.* She then traveled extensively in the Far East, and her concern about the opium trade led to several books and many articles opposing it. Both the Chinese government and the Japanese Red Cross honored her for her efforts to abolish the opium trade. A versatile writer, she published award-winning fiction as well.

Biography

Born: Nov. 7, 1873, Louisville, Ky. **Education:** Johns Hopkins Hosp. Training School for Nurses (RN). **Work history:** Instructive Visiting Nurse Assoc., Baltimore; Superintendent, Tuberculosis Division, Baltimore Health Dept.; Nurse, French Army nurse, World War I. **Organizations:** unknown. **Awards:** Lin Tse Hsu Memorial Medal, China; Special Order of Merit, Japanese Red Cross. **Buried:** Oakhill Cemetery, Washington, Del.

References and Credits

†LaMotte E: The opium problem. AJN 29:791, 1929.

Bullough V: Ellen Newbold LaMotte. In Bullough V, Church OM, Stein AP (eds): American Nursing: A Biographical Dictionary, vol. 1. New York, Garland, 1988, pp 204–205.

Deborah MacLurg Jensen

1900–1962

"For over fifty years the profession of law has recognized the value of presenting cases for study. ... The method developed ... intellectual independence, ... individual thinking ... [and] inculcates a scientific spirit of independence and investigation. ... This method ... means that an intensive study must be made of all problems involved in caring for the patient. ... The student gains so much that it will probably be the preferred method of clinical instruction in schools of nursing in the future, and no accredited school can afford to ignore this development in the education of nurses." (1929)

Deborah Jensen was a nurse educator who wrote and published a wide range of texts and professional articles for nurses. Her career included surgical nursing, private duty nursing, clinical instruction, and nurse education. Jensen established what is considered to be the first internship for student nurses in the country. She realized that no journals addressed the interests and needs of student nurses, so she founded *Tomorrow's Nurse* in 1960. She stressed the importance of case studies as learning experiences for nursing students and saw this method as an essential component of nursing education. She said case studies gave the students independence. Students were given the opportunity to gather and apply comprehensive information related to the social and medical history of a patient and to define the patient's nursing needs. This resulted in improved patient care.

Biography

Born: Nov. 4, 1900, County Tyrene, Northern Ireland. **Education:** Johns Hopkins Hosp. Training School for Nurses (RN); Teachers College, Columbia Univ. (BS); Washington Univ. (MA). **Work history:** Head Nurse, Johns Hopkins Hosp., Baltimore; Assistant Night Supervisor, Assistant Admissions Officer, Johns Hopkins Hosp.; Faculty, Univ. of Minnesota School of Nursing; Washington Univ. School of Nursing; Univ. of Chicago. Simmons College; Washington Univ. Hosp. and clinics; St. Louis Visiting Nurse Assoc.; Faculty, Washington Univ.; Assistant Director, School of Nursing, St. Louis City Hosp.; Faculty, Univ. of Missouri. **Organizations:** Mo. Nurses Assoc.; Mo. League for Nursing Education; National League for Nursing Education; Nurses Educational Funds. **Awards:** Woman of Achievement Award, *St. Louis Globe Democrat.* **Died:** Nantucket, Mass.

References and Credits

†Jensen DM: Case study in schools of nursing. AJN 29:851, 857, 1929.

Cooper SS: Deborah Jensen. In Bullough V, Church OM, Stein AP (eds): American Nursing: A Biographical Dictionary, vol. 1. New York, Garland, 1988, pp 190–192.

November 9

Ella Best

1892–1991

"International nursing conferences illustrate the fact that all nurses speak a common language through their interest in conservation of human life. The nursing care of patients in all lands is basically the same regardless of the language, customs, or beliefs of the people. The fact that nurses from 43 countries could agree on an International Code of Ethics in 1953, was considered by international representatives of the press to be a most outstanding achievement." (1957)

Ella Best gave her great energy and efficiency as an organizer to the American Nurses Association (ANA) for twenty-eight years. She served in various capacities, starting with field secretary in 1930, and became the executive secretary in the 1950s. Her skills allowed her to travel abroad representing the ANA, and she served as a consultant to the surgeon general of the U.S. Air Force and as a civilian consultant to the Army Nurse Corps. A longtime birder, she also found time to serve as the secretary of the Audubon Society.

Biography

Born: Nov. 2, 1892, Williamsfields, Ill. **Education:** St. Luke's Hosp. School of Nursing, Chicago, 1915; postgraduate work, Teachers College, Columbia Univ., Univ. of Chicago. **Work history:** Nursing Instructor, Administrator, at several schools; Field Secretary, ANA; member, ANA Registry Committee to revise minimum standards; Acting Director, Associate,

Exec. Secretary, ANA; Consultant to surgeon general, U.S. Air Force; civilian consultant to Army Nurse Corps. **Organizations:** member, president, Ill. State Nurses Assoc. **Awards:** unknown. **Died:** Florida.

References and Credits

†Best E: Editorial: The International Council of Nurses. Nurs Outlook 5:457, 1957.

Stenz L: Ella Best. In Bullough V, Sentz L, Stein AP (eds): American Nursing: A Biographical Dictionary, vol. 2. New York, Garland, 1992, pp 30–31.

Flanagan L (ed): One Strong Voice: The Story of the American Nurses Association. Kansas City, Mo., Lowell Press, 1976, pp 163, 648.

November 10

Jane Stuart Woolsey

1839–1891

"The soldier-nurses deserve good words. Many of them were the most faithful and devoted of men. Clumsy and tender, kindly, eager, and heavy-handed, they did what they could. ...Old Smith's patients always do well. He had a son in the army who was wounded and died far away from home, 'and then I couldn't stand it any longer, ma'am, and I went in myself, and now whenever I get a young fellow ... to take care of, it seems like as if I was a doing for my own boy and it makes me feel better.'" (1868)

"The men were all fond of flowers. ...One spring morning I carried a bunch of the first lilacs to a very sick New England boy. 'Now I've got something for you,' I said, holding them behind me, 'just like what grows in your front door yard at home; guess!' 'Lalocs!'—he whispered, and I laid them on his folded hands; —'oh, lalocs*! How did you know* that*?' The lilacs outlived him." (1868)*

Jane Woolsey was noted for her dedication and philanthropy. She initially worked with her mother and sisters from their New York City home on Civil War relief efforts. She later became involved as a volunteer nurse in area hospitals, caring for sick and wounded soldiers. After being hired to work as nurses at a hospital in Maryland, she and her sister George Anna returned their $12 monthly salary so that supplies could be purchased for the soldiers. She helped convert a seminary in Virginia for hospital use and managed the diet kitchen, personalizing diets and working with patients. "The most delicate food given monotonously disgusts the sick person," she said. The hospital could care for twelve hundred, and on some days arrivals totaled more than five hundred men. Her organizational skills were again reflected in the smooth functioning of the various departments and the nursing service when she was the director of the Presbyterian Hospital in New York City. She and her sister Abby established the nursing standards that continue to define Presbyterian Hospital, and after retirement she remained generously involved with the hospital.

Biography

Born: 1830, aboard ship between Norwich, Conn., New York City. **Education:** Rutgers Female Institute, N.Y.; Bolton Priory, New Rochelle, N.Y. **Work history:** Women's Central Assoc. of Relief; volunteer Civil War nurse at various N.Y. hosps.; Assistant Superintendent of Nurses, Hosp. Camp, Portsmouth Grove, R.I.; Hired Nurse, Hammond General Hosp., Md.; Fairfax (Va.) Theological Seminary Hosp.; Director, Hampton Institute, Va.; Director, Presbyterian Hosp., N.Y.C. **Organizations:** N.Y. State Charities Aid Assoc. **Awards:** unknown. **Died:** Matteawan, N.Y.

References and Credits

†Woolsey JS: Hospital Days: Reminiscence of a Civil War Nurse (1868). Reprint, Edinborough Press, Roseville, Minn., 1996, pp 90–91, 96, 23.

Stein AP: Jane Stuart Woolsey. In Bullough V, Sentz L, Stein AP (eds): American Nursing: A Biographical Dictionary, vol. 2. New York, Garland, 1992, pp 364–366.

Martha Ruth Smith

1894–1960

"The public health nurse has well been named 'catalytic agent,' as she influences her patient in the home to carry out scientific health practices and particularly as she stimulates and takes part in inter-agency cooperation for better health. To a director of nursing service interested in community welfare, the problem of the ward service patient who returns home from the hospital with no plan for continuing his health program has until the present time just remained a problem. ... A project organized by the group [of social agencies working in the county] to meet this need has helped to solve many problems connected with nursing service and the educational program of the nursing school." (1943)

MARTHA SMITH WAS an outstanding nurse-educator and leader. She recognized the significance of the 1923 Goldmark Report, which stressed the necessity for nurses to understand theory as well as practice when providing patient care. She saw the recommendation as a directive and encouraged the teaching of integrated theory and practice when she served as nurse-educator at the Massachusetts General Hospital School of Nursing. She later served as editor of a related text, *An Introduction to the Principles of Nursing Care,* which became a major influence in schools of nursing. She was always studying and learning more about different aspects of nursing while developing new ideas so that her students could get the most from their educational program. During her tenure at Boston University, she established its division of nursing education (1939) and in 1946 served as the first dean of its school of nursing.

Biography

Born: Nov. 14, 1894, Lebanon, N.H. **Education:** Univ. of Wisconsin; Peter Bent Brigham Hosp. School of Nursing, Boston (RN); Teachers College, Columbia Univ. (BA, MA). **Work history:** Head Nurse, Superintendent, Peter Bent Brigham Hosp.; Resident School Nurse, Kimball Union Academy, N.H.; Nursing Instructor, Samaritan Hosp., N.Y.; Massachusetts General Hosp.; Teachers College, Columbia Univ.; Simmons College; Assistant Principal, Massachusetts General Hosp. School of Nursing; Professor of Nursing, Dean, Boston Univ. School of Nursing. **Organizations:** National League for Nursing Education; American Nurses Assoc.; American Red Cross; Pi Lambda Theta; Sigma Theta Tau. **Awards:** Dean Emeritus, Boston Univ. **Died:** Boston.

References and Credits

†Smith M, Newman ME: The nursing school goes to the community. Public Health Nursing 35:107–108, 1943.

Bullough V: Martha Ruth Smith. In Bullough V, Sentz L, Stein AP (eds): American Nursing: A Biographical Dictionary, vol. 2. New York, Garland, 1992, pp 307–308.

Maggie Elouise Jacobs

1943–1992

"A true advocate for the people." (Date unknown)

Asked how she would like to be remembered, Maggie Jacobs replied, "A true advocate for the people." Indeed, when the American Nurses Association (ANA) inducted her into its Hall of Fame, it noted that she was a "fierce and effective advocate for New York City's poor and for the development of its health care system." She was employed by Kings County Hospital Center for more than twenty-six years, serving as a staff nurse and advancing to nursing care coordinator in the Department of Obstetrics and Gynecology. She maintained a keen interest in community affairs and used her many leadership skills to improve life for her neighbors and to promote their understanding of nursing. She was a leader for twenty-one years of the largest U.S. bargaining group made up solely of registered nurses, the nurses who worked for the Health and Hospitals Corporation of New York City. In her brief career she accomplished her goals of improving health care and promoting the practice of nursing.

Biography

Born: Nov. 12, 1943, Barnwell, S.C. **Education:** Erasmus Hall High School, Brooklyn, N.Y.; Kings County Hosp. Center School of Nursing, 1967 (diploma); Long Island Univ., 1967 (BSN, MS, community health and administration); certificate in nursing administration, ANA; **Work history:** Staff Nurse, Kings County Hosp. Center; Head Nurse, In-Service Instructor, Supervisor, Nursing Care Coordinator, Dept. of OB/GYN; Supervisor of Nurses, Dept. of OB/GYN, Maimonides Medical Center, Brooklyn, N.Y. **Organizations:** member, Salem Missionary Baptist Church, Brooklyn; member, Neighborhood Housing Service of E. Flatbush; Cochair, Clarendon Meadows Action Committee; President, E. 26th St. Clarendon Road Block Assoc.; member, Program Advisory Committee, Bedford-Stuyvesant Healthy Heart Program. **Awards:** ANA Hall of Fame; Certificate of Appreciation, National Black Nurses Assoc., 1989; Outstanding Community Service Award, Harriet Tubman Political Club, 1986; Distinguished Service Award, 1985, Nurses Assoc. of Counties of L.I.; Community Service Award, National Assoc. of Negro Business and Professional Women's Clubs, East New York Club of Brooklyn, 1985; Certificate of Appreciation, Minority Student Nurses Assoc., Syracuse Univ., 1985. **Died:** location unknown.

References and Credits

†Obituary for Maggie Jacobs. Records and Information, Foundation of the New York State Nurses Association, Guilderland, N.Y.

ANA Hall of Fame 10/98 American Nurses Association, Washington, D.C. http://www.nursingworld.org/hof.

November 13

Marguerite Lucy Manfreda

1910–2003

"To evaluate a successful or unsuccessful approach, [with a patient] take into consideration the general air of the situation. Did it seem satisfactory: Was cooperation easily established? Did the results appear good? Did you have an inner feeling that things went smoothly? If you think it may have been unsatisfactory, look to yourself. *...Ask yourself these questions: Do I feel physically up to par today? Was my voice pleasant, irritable, soft, or loud? Did I use language the other person understood? Was my facial expression one of pleasure or displeasure, or did I seem just generally annoyed? Was I preoccupied with thoughts of an inner conflict of my own? Did I seem too hurried or busy with other things to be bothered? Was I patient? Did I try to evade answering the other person? Did I look for some outstanding factor or symptom that I could have done something about? Was I friendly or cold to the person? What was the one thing I might have done which would not have made me feel this way? Am I simply trying to rationalize that it would have happened this way anyhow and to justify myself in the solution?" (1953)*

MARGUERITE L. MANFREDA is recognized both an educator and as a specialist in psychiatric nursing. Her career choice was influenced by a visiting nurse who had treated Manfreda when she was a teenager. She is an esteemed author of three psychiatric nursing books. She also revised Katharine McLean Steele's *Psychiatric Nursing,* eventually becoming the author for the seventh, eighth, and ninth editions, and coauthor again for the tenth and last edition in 1977. Manfreda maintained that the therapeutic influence of the environment and social and educational activities play a major role in patients' recovery. As an assistant nursing arts instructor, she incorporated the emotional aspects of illness and health teaching principles in course content. Her first article published in the *American Journal of Nursing* was "The Electroencephalogram," which earned praise for her inclusion of suggestions for psychological support for patients while they undergo the procedure. She was respected as an effective leader in private and public psychiatric institutions. In 1952, while she was director of the psychiatric nursing affiliated program at the Elgin State Hospital in Illinois, the National League for Nursing determined that psychiatric nursing would become a mandatory part of the curriculum in schools of nursing.

Biography

Born: Nov. 13, 1910, Wallingford, Conn. **Education:** Hosp. Training School for Nurses, Hartford, Conn., 1933; New York Univ. School of Education, 1947 (BS); Teachers College, Columbia Univ., 1961 (MA). **Work history:** Surgical Staff Nurse, New Haven (Conn.) Hosp.; Staff Nurse, Yale Institute of Human Relations; Staff Nurse, New York State Psychiatric Institute, N.Y.C.; Nursing Arts Instructor, Hosp. Training School for Nurses, Hartford, Conn.; Supervisor, Institute of Living, Conn.; founder, Director, psychiatric nursing program, Elgin State Hosp. **Writings:** revised *Psychiatric Nursing; Teaching Psychiatric and Mental Health Nursing* (1961); director at other state, private psychiatric hospitals; Associate Professor, Black Hawk College, Moline, Ill. **Organizations:** active in state and local nursing organizations. **Awards:** recognition awards, State of Arkansas, Arkansas League for Nursing. **Died:** Middletown, Conn.

References and Credits

†Manfreda ML, Steele KM: Psychiatric Nursing. Philadelphia, FA Davis, 1953, pp 506–507.

Herrmann EK: Marguerite Manfreda. In Bullough V, Sentz L, Stein AP (eds): American Nursing: A Biographical Dictionary, vol. 2. New York, Garland, 1992, pp 216–218.

Sister Regina Purtell

1866-1950

"Stationed first at Montauk Point [during the Spanish-American War] Sister Regina ... was aghast at the conditions she found [and] to her regular duties of nurse ... did not hesitate to add the irregular ones of janitor and orderly as ... she banished dirt and disorder. ... Knowing that no amount of medicine could substitute for good and wholesome food, Sister Regina disregarded Army protocol when it came to demanding for her 'boys' the sort of food she knew they should have. When a Captain remonstrated her unavailingly, he straightened up and said: 'Sister, I am a Captain.' Hotly came Sister Regina's reply: 'And every one of these sick boys is a GENERAL to me, sir, and I'll treat them like that." (1898)

Sister Regina Purtell, a Catholic sister, was a member of the Daughters of Charity of St. Vincent de Paul. She served as a nurse to the Rough Riders during the Spanish-American War. Her abilities to establish hygienic standards at Montauk Point, Long Island, during that war greatly impressed Theodore Roosevelt. When he became president and needed surgery, he chose to have it at St. Vincent's Hospital in Indianapolis, so that she could care for him. Her professional skills and standards for care helped control outbreaks of typhoid in Alabama, influenza in Texas, and smallpox among lepers in Louisiana. She had a reputation for being a troubleshooter who could take control of a situation and act fast. In Texas the largest fraternity house on the Austin campus quickly became an infirmary during the 1918 influenza epidemic. She also gained national recognition for ensuring quality care for those with leprosy at Carville, Louisiana, and she has been called the heroine of the 1919 smallpox epidemic there. After she recognized the early signs of smallpox among the patients, she isolated herself with them to provide care. After retirement she wrote letters to help the foreign missions in Asia, India, and Africa. She was buried with full military honors in Louisiana.

Biography

Born: Nov. 14, 1866, Monches, Wisc. **Education:** Daughters of Charity Community. **Work history:** nurse-volunteer, U.S. Army, Spanish-American War; Nurse, typhoid epidemic, Ala.; St. Mary's Hosp., Evansville, Ind.; St. Vincent's Hosp., Indianapolis; flu epidemic, Univ. of Texas, Austin; leprosarium, Carville, La. **Organizations:** unknown. **Awards:** Officials of U.S. Dept. of Health, Education and Welfare praised her work during presentation of Distinguished Service Award to Daughters of Charity at Carville. **Buried:** St. Vincent's Cemetery, New Orleans.

References and Credits

†Sullivan C: Served her country in peace and war, unpublished ms., ca. 1950, Marillac Provincial House, Daughters of Charity Archives, St. Louis.

Smyth K: Sr. Regina Purtell. In Bullough V, Church OM, Stein AP (eds): American Nursing: A Biographical Dictionary, vol. 1. New York, Garland, 1988, pp 267–268.

November 15

Anna Pearl Sherrick

1899–1993

"World events have influenced medicine, nursing, hospitals, and public health from primitive times to the present. The highlights of Medical practice challenged nursing, hospitals and public health to become more professional throughout the years. Mankind has built a foundation of concern that reaches throughout the world. ... My study of history has helped me to better understand and appreciate the development of nursing. ... We are so indebted to our ancestors." (1989)

Anna Sherrick moved to Montana for health reasons after being diagnosed with tuberculosis and completing a three-year treatment program at her home in Illinois. She had completed her nursing studies and worked as a nursing instructor until she had an opportunity to establish a college nursing program. She is the founder of the Montana State University College of Nursing. Her philosophy and approach to nursing education were highly focused: She wanted professional nursing students to build on a foundation of liberal arts and science. Her creative and practical ideas included a prenursing program, for which she obtained funding; a student nurse honor society; networking to provide strong clinical affiliation sites outside the hospital; and continuing education for registered nurses as part of the career ladder plan. A pioneer in nursing education,

Sherrick recognized the need to make educational opportunities available to nurses across Montana and in the mid-1960s used teleconferencing for nursing education. She was actively involved in professional organizations and community groups throughout her career.

Biography

Born: Nov. 26, 1899, Houston Twp., Ill. **Education:** Knox College, Ill.; Illinois Women's College (now MacMurray College), Jacksonville, Ill. (bachelor's degree); Univ. of Michigan School of Nursing; Colorado State Teacher's College (MA); Univ. of Washington (doctorate in education). **Work history:** Private Duty Nurse; Instructor, St. Luke's Hosp. School of Nursing, Chicago; Park View School of Nursing, Colo.; Montana Deaconess Hosp. School of Nursing; Faculty, Montana State College; Montana State Bd. of Nursing. **Organizations:** Mont. Nurses Assoc.; Mont. League for Nursing; American Assoc. of Univ. Women; Bozeman (Mont.) Chamber of Commerce; Mont. Assoc. for Mental Health; Business and Professional Women's Club; Mont. Education Assoc. **Awards**: Woman of the Year, Mont. Federation of Business and Professional Women's Clubs; Community Service Award, Bozeman, Mont.; Univ. of Montana Distinguished Service Award; Montana Public Health Assoc. Award; Education Award, Western Interstate Commission for Higher Education; Sherrick Hall at Univ. of Montana, named in her honor, is site of bronze bust of Sherrick. **Died:** Bozeman, Mont.

References and Credits

†Sherrick AP: Worldwide Events Influencing Nursing in Montana. Bozeman, Mont., Artcraft Printers, 1989, p 97.

Barkley S: Anna Sherrick. In Bullough V, Sentz L, Stein AP (eds): American Nursing: A Biographical Dictionary, vol. 2. New York, Garland, 1992, pp 300–302.

In memory of Anna Pearl Sherrick. Montana State University Staff Bulletin, Nov. 5, 1993. Chaney R: Founder of MSU College of Nursing dies at 93. Bozeman Chronicle, Oct. 20, 1993.

November 16

Sister Rosemary Donley
1938–

"What Is a Good Nurse?
...A good nurse should be knowledgeable, honest in her dealings with others, responsible and compassionate. (...I call [the] effort to participate in the experience of the patient—compassion). I came to rely on the nursing and medical documentation as a guide to my own practice. It was also very important to me that the patient be treated with respect. ... We were schooled in confidentiality and in enhancing the patient's personhood. In the world in which I first studied nursing, the patient was sacred. ...Because nursing is a relationship, it was important to learn how the nurse responded to the patient's disease and its manifestations. I brought more than knowledge and a responsible presence to the patient's bedside, I brought myself." (1999)

Sister Rosemary Donley is a member of the Sisters of Charity of Seton Hill. Her nursing is grounded in her religious values and is an integral part of her life. This is reflected in the personal and religious integrity that she brings to the profession and demonstrates by example. She was attracted to nursing by its ability to engage her in the lives and important events of others. She has been highly honored by a number of organizations and universities. Her wide-ranging research, writings, consultations, and presentations have a worldwide audience. The broad range of her expertise includes issues in nursing practice, long-term care, spiritual dimensions of health care, public policy, trends in nursing, health care reform, nursing economics, ethics, and advanced practice. Yet she wants, most of all, to be remembered in the lives of her patients and students. A nurse practitioner, she directs the Community/Public Health Nurse Specialty Program at the Catholic University of America School of Nursing, where she once served as dean. There she teaches population-based health care in the program called "Care of Vulnerable People in Communities."

Biography

Born: Nov. 16, 1938, Pittsburgh. **Education:** Pittsburgh Hosp. School of Nursing (diploma); St. Louis Univ. (BSN); Univ. of Pittsburgh (MNEd, PhD); postgraduate study, Teachers College, Columbia Univ., Univ. of Pittsburgh, Harvard Univ., Catholic Univ. **Work history:** Staff Nurse, St. Mary's Hosp., St. Louis; Instructor, Pittsburgh Hosp. School of Nursing; Associate Professor, Univ. of Pittsburgh; Dean of Nursing, Exec. Vice President, Director of Community/Public Health Nursing Program, Catholic Univ.; Consultant; Adviser. **Organizations:** National League for Nursing (NLN), Sigma Theta Tau International (STTI), American Public Health Assoc., American Nurses Assoc. (ANA). **Awards:** STTI, Catholic Univ., Univ. of Pittsburgh, New York Univ., Pittsburgh Hosp., Seton Hall Univ.; honorary doctorates from Felician College, La Roche College, Loyola Univ. of Chicago, Madonna College, Rhode Island College, Villanova Univ.; Institute of Medicine, National Academy of Sciences; Alpha Omega; Fellow, American Academy of Nursing.

References and Credits

†Donley R: Following your path to leadership development: The vision of a leader. In Anderson C: Nursing Student to Nursing Leader. Albany, N.Y., Delmar Learning, a division of Thomson Learning, 1999, pp 318–319.

Donley R: resume.

Donley R: personal correspondence, 2002.

NOVEMBER 17

Helen Young
1874–1966

"To the nurse, all patients are made equal by those great levelers—pain, sickness, and a desire for health. ... That intangible, all-important essential of life, human relationship, is exemplified constantly in the contact between patient and nurse. It may well be a controlling factor in the patient's recovery, for frequently much depends upon his reaction and attitude toward the person whom he sees and relies upon most. Both this reaction and this attitude are largely determined by the nurse herself, who, if she is a good judge of human nature and blest with that imaginative vision we call understanding, can influence the patient in such a way that complete confidence in her will result." (1942)

HELEN YOUNG FIRST prepared as a teacher and then studied nursing with Anna Maxwell at New York's Presbyterian Hospital before joining the war effort in France. When Young returned home from World War I, she worked with Maxwell to develop the cooperative baccalaureate nursing program between Presbyterian Hospital and Columbia University. When Maxwell retired, Young became the director of the prestigious school. She was very involved in passage of the nurse practice act in New York. Her commitment to nursing did much to make the profession more appealing and acceptable to young women. *Lippincott's Quick*

Reference Book for Nurses, which she edited and was first published in 1933, was a resource to more than 100,000 nurses.

Biography

Born: Nov. 17, 1874, Chatham, Ontario, Can. **Education:** Collegiate Institute; Toronto School of Pedagogy; Presbyterian Hosp. School of Nursing, N.Y.C. **Work history:** Head Nurse, Presbyterian Hosp.; wartime nursing, Juilly, France; organized nurses for British forces; Faculty, Director, School of Nursing, Teachers College, Columbia Univ. **Organizations:** American Red Cross; American Nurses Assoc.; N.Y. State League for Nursing Education; N.Y.C. League for Nursing Education. **Awards:** Distinguished Service Award, Columbia-Presbyterian Medical Center; Columbia Univ. Medal for Excellence. **Died:** New York City.

References and Credits

†Young H: Essentials of Nursing. New York, GP Putnam's Sons, 1942, pp 6–7.

Stein AP: Helen Young. In Bullough V, Sentz L, Stein AP (eds): American Nursing: A Biographical Dictionary, vol. 2. New York, Garland, 1992, pp 369–370.

November 18

Virginia Barckley

1911–1993

"It occurred to me to … design a way for students to spend their vacations working in the great research and treatment centers. … The opportunities for learning at such specialized hospitals are striking. Patients with cancer of every part of the body, in every stage of illness, of every age, from every state and a variety of countries, of different temperaments and backgrounds are there. So are a dedicated and experienced staff, the newest equipment, fresh ideas on treatment, and an aura of concern and tenacity. Surely weeks of saturation in such a climate should help the student develop greater understanding of the patient with cancer and his family." (1971)

Virginia Barckley was a visiting nurse in the 1940s when she first volunteered for the American Cancer Society (ACS). This led to a lifetime dedicated to cancer nursing. Her determination to change nursing attitudes and to improve cancer care began at a time when nurses were not allowed to discuss cancer with patients. Ignorance and shame contributed to delays in diagnosis and treatment. In the days before radiation and chemotherapy, hospitalized patients with cancer were in the terminal stages of illness. The work was depressing. Uterine cancer, in particular, carried a stigma. Women blamed their own behavior for the humiliating condition and avoided care so as not to shame the family. Her personal motto, "Do more than you have to," permeated her professional career as she worked successfully to humanize care for patients with cancer. She explored ways to increase interest in cancer nursing and helped establish scholarships for oncology nurse specialists and work study for students. She helped plan a national conference for cancer nurses that was the catalyst for forming the Oncology Nursing Society. A prolific writer, she wrote skits about nursing, a film script about the nursing care of children with cancer, numerous professional articles about nursing care of cancer patients, and the nursing portions of the ACS classic *Cancer Source Book for Nurses.*

Biography

Born: Nov. 19, 1911, Burlington, N.J. **Education:** Nursing School, Flushing Hospital, Long Island, N.Y.; Univ. of Pennsylvania (BS); Catholic Univ. (MN). **Work history:** Philadelphia Visiting Nurse Assoc.; Volunteer, American Cancer Society; various positions in public health and mental health in Pa., Mich., N.Y., N.J.; Mental Health Nursing Consultant, Penn. State Dept. of Health; Nursing Consultant, American Cancer Society. **Organizations:** Sigma Theta Tau. **Awards:** American Cancer Society Citation of Merit; first honorary member, Assoc. of Pediatric Oncology Nurses; Centennial Medal for Lifelong Achievement, Sloan-Kettering Cancer Center, N.Y.C.; Distinguished Merit Award, International Society of Nurses in Cancer Care. **Buried:** Burlington, N.J.

References and Credits

†Barckley V: Work study program in cancer nursing. Nurs Outlook 19:328, 1971.

Haylock PJ, Vrabel M: Virginia Barckley. In Bullough V, Sentz L (eds): American Nursing: A Biographical Dictionary, vol. 3. New York, Springer, 2000, pp 14–16.

November 19

Beatrice Van Homrigh Stevenson
1874–1948

"The societies of American nurses which form our Associated Alumnae, when they voted to affiliate with the National Red Cross, assumed the responsibility of providing a reserve corps of nurses which would be ready for service whenever called upon by the National Government. ... Are we going to rise to the occasion and recognize the fact that we owe something to the country which has made us nurses? which has given us recognition and support, and placed us ahead of the nurses of any other country in the world? If so, enroll now!" (1910)

Beatrice Stevenson, born in Ireland and schooled in England, was orphaned as a young teenager. When she was told that she was too young to enter nursing in England, she took a job as a traveling companion for the sick. This provided her with an opportunity to come to the United States to live with a family in Virginia. She later completed nursing school in New York City. After she became a citizen, she served as a Red Cross nurse during the Spanish-American War. She worked closely with Jane Delano as a Red Cross instructor. Stevenson later worked as a recruiter for nurses during World War I and was affectionately called "Mrs. Red Cross." Her service as superintendent of nurses at the corrections hospital in New York City may have bolstered her commitment to work for improvements for nurses in public hospitals. A very active member of the New York State Nurses Association (NYSNA), she was involved in legislative and economic issues for nurses and helped gain passage of the New York State Practice Act. She saw a role for unions in relation to issues related to salary and working conditions and was active on behalf of nurses in the American Federation of Labor. She studied law at New York University.

Biography

Born: Nov. 19, 1874, Killashee, Ireland. **Education:** City Hosp. School of Nursing, N.Y.C.; New York Univ. (diploma). **Work history:** Private Duty Nurse; Red Cross nurse, Spanish-American War; Instructor, Recruiter, Red Cross; Superintendent of Nurses, Corrections Hosp., N.Y.C. **Organizations:** American Red Cross; NYSNA; Alumnae Assoc. of N.Y.C. Hosp. School of Nursing, New York Univ. alumni assoc.; Nurses Guild of the American Federation of Labor. **Awards:** Letter of Commendation, N.Y.C. commissioner of corrections; *Alumnae Journal of City Hospital* dedicated to her upon her death. **Died:** Brooklyn, N.Y.

References and Credits

†Stevenson B: In time of peace, Prepare for war. AJN 10:177, 1910.

Stein AP: Beatrice Van Homrigh Stevenson. In Bullough V, Sentz L, Stein AP (eds): American Nursing: A Biographical Dictionary, vol. 2. New York, Garland, 1992, pp 314–316.

Dora Elizabeth Thompson

1876–1954

"The Spanish-American War demonstrated to the Medical Department of the Army the great value of graduate nurses in Army hospitals, and ... the Army Nurse Corps was authorized by Act of Congress in February, 1901. ... The ... nurses of the Red Cross constitute the Reserve of the Army Nurse Corps. ... On April 6, 1917, the day ... war was declared on Germany, there were in the service 203 members of the regular Corps and 170 reserve. ... There are now 10,000 nurses in the service, one-third of whom are serving overseas. ... If the war continues fully 24,000 nurses will be needed before the end of the war. ... The full responsibility of the ward management is now definitely placed upon the head nurse. ...Hitherto this responsibility was shared by the ward master, an enlisted man. ...General [John J.] Pershing has recommended that the privilege of wearing the war service chevron, ... authorized for officers and enlisted men, be extended to ... members of the Army Nurse Corps." (1918)

DORA THOMPSON DEMONSTRATED exceptional leadership during the San Francisco earthquake and fire of 1906, when she was both chief nurse at the General Hospital there as well as a member of the Army Nurse Corps. She kept the situation under control with patients and staff after the hospital's power and water connections were destroyed. When she was appointed superintendent of the corps after more than a decade as an army nurse, she was the first corps leader to bring actual army nurse experience to the position. She worked tirelessly for increased economic, health, and retirement benefits, as well as rank, for nurses. She worked closely with the Red Cross on all aspects of nurse recruitment and found ways to provide additional coursework and skill training for nurse recruits while always maintaining the standards established for army nurses. She increased the number of graduate nurses coming into the corps to more than twenty-one thousand during World War I.

Biography

Born: Nov. 20, 1876, Cold Springs, N.Y. **Education:** New York City Training School (diploma); postgraduate course in OR procedures (diploma). **Work history:** OR Nurse, Private Duty Nurse, N.Y.C.; U.S. Army nurse, San Francisco General Hosp., transport ships between hospital and the Philippines, Alaska, Philippines; worked under Isabel McIsaac, head of the Army Nurse Corps; Superintendent, Army Nurse Corps.; Assistant Superintendent, Manila; Chief Nurse, Letterman Hosp., San Francisco. **Organizations:** unknown. **Awards:** Distinguished Service Medal for wartime service Women's Officers' Quarters at Letterman Hosp. named Thompson Hall. **Buried:** Arlington National Cemetery.

References and Credits

†Thompson D: Nursing as it relates to war. AJN 18:1058–1060, 1918.

Sandefur SA, McCarthy RT: Dora Elizabeth Thompson. In Bullough V, Church OM, Stein AP (eds): American Nursing: A Biographical Dictionary, vol. 1. New York, Garland, 1988, pp 309–311.

NOVEMBER 21

Ada Mayo Stewart Markoff

1870–1945

"By the old process of trial and error, the 'Proctor District Nurse' went about her daily task of giving advice and comfort, bathing new babies, caring for the mothers, helping in emergencies, dressing wounds and teaching ways of health and good habits (in seven languages) as well as she knew. She did not know that she was an 'Industrial Nurse' nor did she dream that these and other small beginnings would grow to the splendid work that the modern Public Health Nurses are doing in the world. Probably few Public Health Nurses of today, with the advantage of their special education and the strength of their organization, realize that their success owes something to these small beginnings." (1945)

ADA STEWART MARKOLF was the first industrial nurse in the United States. In 1895 the Vermont Marble Company hired her to care for its employees. Because she knew of no precedent, she pioneered the development of a new discipline in nursing. In addition to providing workers with emergency care, she also was a visiting nurse who cared for them and their families in their homes. The company encouraged her to become involved with the health needs of the whole community. Her services expanded, and as she bicycled through the town of Proctor, she provided health education in the school as well. When the company established a small community hospital in a private home in 1896, she served as matron and had only one helper. On the hospital's opening day, the first five patients had typhoid fever. Stewart continued to provide community health care in addition to serving the hospital patients until she moved out of state two years later.

Biography

Born: Dec. 2, 1870, Braintree, Mass. **Education:** Waltham (Mass.) Training School for Nurses. **Work history:** District Nurse, Proctor (Vt.) Marble Co.; Matron, Proctor (Vt.) Hosp.; Good Samaritan Hosp., Troy, N.Y.; Private Duty Nurse/Masseuse, Seattle; St. Augustine, Fla.; Lake Placid, N.Y. **Organizations:** unknown. **Awards:** unknown. **Died:** Randolph, Vt.

References and Credits

†Markolf AMS: The beginning of industrial nursing in Vermont. Rutland Historical Society Quarterly 25:7, 1995.

Cooper SS: Ada Markolf. In Bullough V, Church OM, Stein AP (eds): American Nursing: A Biographical Dictionary, vol. 1. New York, Garland, 1988, pp 228–229.

November 22

Martha Marie Montgomery Brown

1918–1987

"It has been said that listening to someone is the most precious gift we can bestow. ...A good listener is one who concentrates on what is being said and the feeling that is being communicated rather than on what he is going to say when the opportunity arises." (1971)

"We speak of an effective relationship as one in which the nurse and patient find a common ground and respond to one another. In establishing this type of relationship the nurse should examine both her motives and her attitudes. A sincere interest in the patient and a genuine desire to help him are prerequisite to establishing a harmonious relationship." (1971)

Martha Marie Montgomery Brown was an exceptional nurse scientist and educator. She created a concept of nursing as a psychodynamic process of interaction and biosocial intervention. She and Grace R. Fowler wrote the textbook *Psychodynamic Nursing—A Biosocial Orientation,* which went through four editions and influenced not only psychiatric nursing but other specialty areas as well. In the 1960s Brown served as the project director for a multidisciplinary team that included a psychiatrist, psychologists, a cultural anthropologist, and other nurses. The team investigated the effect of skilled nursing upon the "psychosocial atrophy" of institutionalized elderly patients and was noteworthy for its innovative methodology and important findings. *Nurses, Patients, and Social Systems,* which Brown wrote with P.R. Brown, J.C. Glidewell, R.G. Hunt, and J.M.A. Weiss, was nominated for the 1968 Socio-Psychological Prize of the American Association for the Advancement of Science. Brown's research and publications contributed to national health policy and delivery system models. She advocated for research and education on the care of the elderly. A well-rounded individual, Brown also excelled as a violinist, artist, and gourmet cook.

Biography

Born: Nov. 22, 1918, Alexandria, Ind. **Education:** Univ. of Michigan, Ann Arbor, 1941 (nursing diploma); Case Western Reserve Univ., Cleveland, Ohio (BSN, MS); St. Louis Univ. (PhD); Univ. of Minnesota (postdoctoral work in epidemiology). **Work history:** Instructor, Assistant Director, Professor, Dean, Washington Univ. School of Nursing, St. Louis; Nursing Consultant, Medical Care Research Center, Washington Univ. Social Science Institute and Jewish Hosp. of St. Louis. **Organizations:** unknown. **Awards:** St. Louis Bicentennial Honoree of American Assoc. of Univ. Women, 1962; Distinguished Alumna, Univ. of Michigan School of Nursing, 1972; Elizabeth McWilliams Miller Award for Excellence in Research, Sigma Theta Tau, 1981. **Died:** Elmwood, Ind.

References and Credits

†Brown MM, Fowler GR: Psychodynamic Nursing: A Biosocial Orientation, 4th ed. Philadelphia, WB Saunders, 1971, pp 100–101, 119.

Yeaworth RC: Martha Marie Brown. In Bullough V, Sentz L, Stein AP (eds): American Nursing: A Biographical Dictionary, vol. 2. New York, Garland, 1992, pp 41–43.

November 23

Florence Guinness Blake

1907–1983

"Nurses who work with children and their families should be open minded, sensitive to changes in philosophy, and thoughtful enough to think through objectively the theories of child guidance as they develop from a study of children. They should know the philosophy of infant care that is being taught to parents by their pediatricians. Parents are confused when nurses contradict the instructions given by their doctors. We as nurses should be interpreting the principles of child care to parents, assisting them in thinking through their problems, and reassuring them in their endeavors to provide their children with a satisfying and appropriate environment." (1947)

FLORENCE BLAKE OFTEN went with her minister father on house calls to visit the sick. Her uncle, a medical doctor, later encouraged her to enroll in nursing school. Her potential for teaching was evident in nursing school, and she was encouraged to take university classes. Later, while she was taking additional classes in pediatrics, she did some work in nursery schools because she recognized that it was important for nurses to understand normal growth and development. She became a distinguished leader in pediatric nursing care and had international influence. Her broad experience included staff nursing, teaching, administration, consultation, and writing. She was one of the first to emphasize the need for and to provide clinical practice in graduate nurse educational programs. The high expectations that she had for students were matched by her support for them. She coauthored several pediatric texts, including *Essentials of Pediatric Nursing,* with P. C. Jones and W. Rand and wrote *The Child, His Parents, and the Nurse,* which is considered a classic.

Biography

Born: Nov. 30, 1907, Stevens Point, Wisc. **Education:** Michael Reese Hosp. School of Nursing, Chicago (RN); Univ. of Chicago (clinical coursework); Teachers College, Columbia Univ. (bachelor's) Univ. of Michigan (master's); Merrill-Palmer School, Detroit; Institute for Psychoanalysis, Chicago (diploma). **Work history:** Instructor, Michael Reese Hosp. School of Nursing; Supervisor, Sarah Morris Children's Hosp. of Michael Reese; Faculty, Union Medical College, Beijing; Instructor, Univ. of Michigan School of Nursing; Faculty, Yale School of Nursing; Faculty, Univ. of Chicago; Staff Nurse, Infant Welfare Assoc. of Chicago; Faculty, Univ. of Wisconsin School of Nursing, Madison; Pediatric Nursing Consultant to various groups, incl. U.S. Children's Bureau, American Nurses Assoc. (ANA), hospitals, universities. **Organizations:** Pi Lambda Theta; ANA; National League for Nursing; Friends of the Waisman Center on Mental Retardation. **Awards:** ANA Hall of Fame; awards from Columbia Univ., Univ. of Michigan, and Univ. of Wisconsin. Professor Emeritus, Univ. of Wisconsin. **Buried:** Stevens Point, Wisc.

References and Credits

†Blake, Florence. The needs of the student in a pediatric setting. AJN 47:692.

Cooper SS: Florence Guinness Blake. In Bullough V, Church OM, Stein AP (eds): American Nursing: A Biographical Dictionary, vol. 1. New York, Garland, 1988, pp 33–36.

ANA Hall of Fame 10/98 American Nurses Association, Washington, D.C. http://www.nursingworld.org/hof.

November 24

Annie Damer

1858–1915

"There has been ... unrest among women, and in some cases they have come out openly with a demand for the ballot. ...I want to make a plea for the enfranchisement of one class of women, and that is the pupils in our training schools. ...We see on many sides women and children being abused and overworked, but we must consider that there is one class of women for whom we can do something as a great body of professional women. We can help the women working in our schools to secure a better adjustment of the hours of labor in our schools. ...In seeking the ideals for the protection of womanhood we have ... to be taught ... to be self-governing ourselves. ...When you are asked to begin work for the enfranchisement of women, begin it right at home." (1909)

During her lifetime Annie Damer was one of the best-known nurses in the United States, and she was dedicated to promoting nursing as a profession. She twice served as president of the American Nurses Association (ANA) and was instrumental in preparing partnerships that linked the ANA with both the *American Journal of Nursing* and the American Red Cross. She often spoke of the profession's basic responsibility to the public, and through her own efforts she improved services for people with tuberculosis at Bellevue Hospital in New York. She recognized alcohol and drug abuse as public health issues and promoted nursing's role in education and prevention. Her public involvement with nursing ended when she was fifty-two and was thrown from a carriage, suffering serious and permanent injuries.

Biography

Born: Nov. 30, 1858, Stratford, Ontario, Can. **Education:** New York Training School, Bellevue Hosp., N.Y.C. **Work history:** Private Duty Nurse; Investigator, Buffalo (N.Y.) Charity Organization Society; Public Health Nurse; President, American Journal of Nursing Co.; Supervisor, convalescent home for children. **Organizations:** Nurses Associated Alumnae of the United States and Canada; Bellevue Nurses Alumnae; ANA. **Awards:** ANA Hall of Fame. **Died:** N.Y.C.

References and Credits

†Damer A: Address of the president. AJN 9:903–904, 1909.

Dombrowski T: Annie Damer. In Bullough V, Church OM, Stein AP (eds): American Nursing: A Biographical Dictionary, vol. 1. New York, Garland, 1988, pp 74–76.

ANA Hall of Fame 10/98 American Nurses Association, Washington, D.C. http://www.nursingworld.org/hof.

November 25

Claire Mintzer Fagin
1926–

"Nurses cannot be passive observers now or in the future. We cannot allow things to just happen to us and the patients we serve. We remain the lifeline of patients and their families as they experience the changes of the health care system… .Remembering always the vision, goals and values that brought us to this field we must use our expertise and knowledge in providing and safeguarding quality patient care. We cannot afford to shortchange care which will eventually backfire on us and on patients… .Health care quality is the raison d'etre for professionalism. We must uphold the autonomy and professionalism of the nursing role, but recognize that autonomy is not lost in partnership with the public and other colleagues. As we move in to the 21st Century it's time to create a genuine health care system that balances care and cure, and recognizes the extraordinary accomplishments of this past century." (2000)

CLAIRE FAGIN WAS first attracted to nursing by her desire to serve her country during World War II. The Cadet Nurse Corps and its advertisements were a special draw for her. She is a distinguished nursing leader, who continues to exert influence on consumer health services through her active involvement in professional and civic organizations. Fagin acknowledges the importance and influence of the many excellent role models she met during her career, including those with whom she had short-term contact. Her psychiatric nursing background led to leadership experiences in clinical practice, consulting, program development, research, teaching, writing, and administration. She served as dean of the School of Nursing at the University of Pennsylvania, then joined the professoriate; later she was selected to return as the university's interim president (July 1, 1993–June 30, 1994), the first woman to ever hold that position at an Ivy League school. Her *Essays on Nursing Leadership* addresses the responsibilities of professional and educational leadership in the face of the rapidly changing U.S. health care delivery system. Her powerful essay, "The Abandonment of the Patient: The Impact of For-Profit Health Care," clearly shows the negative effects and challenges of a market-driven, for-profit system in which quality of care is not a major concern. She says that nurses must use publicity, political action, and coalition building to effect reform. She believes that nurses and doctors can work together for a healthy society if they are open to change, objective, and make the patient the central focus. Her professional papers are archived at the Center for the Study of the History of Nursing, School of Nursing, University of Pennsylvania.

Biography

Born: Nov. 25, 1926, New York City. **Education:** Hunter College, N.Y.C.; Wagner College (BS); Teachers College, Columbia Univ. (MA); New York Univ. (PhD). **Work history:** Staff Nurse, Instructor, Sea View Hosp., N.Y., Bellevue Hosp., N.Y.C.; Psychiatric Nurse Consultant, National League for Nursing; Psychiatric Nurse, Administrator, National Institutes of Health; Psychiatric Research Coordinator, Children's Hosp., Washington, D.C.; Faculty, New York Univ. (NYU), H. Lehman College, City Univ. of New York, Montefiore Hosp. and Medical Center; Dean, School of Nursing, Univ. of Pennsylvania; Interim President, Univ. of Pennsylvania; Joint Commission on Mental Health of Children; Council of Deans of Nursing; member, bd. of directors, Van Ameringen Foundation, Visiting Nurse Service of N.Y., N.Y. Academy of Medicine, Provident Mutual, Salomon, Radian Guarantee; member, Expert Panel on Nursing, World Health Organization; National Bd. of Medical Examiners; Advisory Committee, National Institute of Mental Health; Author; Researcher; Consultant; Speaker. **Organizations:** American Nurses Assoc. (ANA). **Awards:** achievement awards from Wagner College, Teachers College, Univ. of Pennsylvania; awards from ANA, Sigma Theta Tau, American Nurses Foundation Distinguished Alumna Award, NYU; Caring Award, Visiting Nurses Assoc. of Greater Philadelphia; H. Peplau Award,

Biography continued on page 771

November 26

Rhetaugh Graves Dumas

1928–

"The die seems to have been cast by … historians and … writers who chose from among all the black women in history the roles of the black mammy, Sojourner Truth and Harriet Tubman as exemplary models. Descriptions of … Tubman are particularly pertinent. … I know firsthand the tremendous hardships and anguish inherent in attempts to live up to this model in the symbolism of contemporary organizations that represent in microcosm the society at large. I have felt the pangs of guilt evoked by those who would lead me to believe that to protect myself and promote my general welfare is to let my people down. I am now beginning to see how it is possible to let my people down by failing *to protect myself and my interests and to seek fulfillment of my own needs. Indeed in modern organizations, racism and sexism dictate that I AM MY PEOPLE. I AM BLACK. I AM WOMAN. Numerous other black women executives know the pain and anguish to which I refer. Some … are discovering, as I am, when and how* not *to be Mammy, Miss Truth, Miss Tubman, and still survive." (1979)*

HER MOTHER'S UNFULFILLED ambition to be a nurse inspired Rhetaugh Dumas to enter nursing, which she considers the most noble profession. During a career that she describes as wonderful, rewarding, productive, and satisfying, Dumas has been a pioneer on many fronts. She was the first nurse-researcher to use a randomized experimental design when she studied clinical problems in patient care in the 1960s. She was the first woman, the first African American, and the first nurse to be formally appointed to the position of deputy director of the National Institute of Mental Health. She was also the first African American woman to hold a deanship at the University of Michigan. Widely published, she has focused most recently on the complexities of leadership. She defines leadership as "a mechanism for exerting influence in human relationships." She sees it as generic and says that the roles of leader and follower are necessarily interchangeable. Dumas has held numerous national professional positions and appointments, including a seat on President Bill Clinton's National Bioethics Advisory Commission.

Biography

Born: Nov. 26, 1928, Natchez, Miss. **Education:** Dillard Univ., New Orleans (BSN); Yale Univ. (MSN); Union Institute, Cincinnati, Ohio (PhD). **Work history:** Professor, Yale Univ. School of Nursing; Deputy Director, National Institute of Mental Health; Dean, Univ. of Michigan School of Nursing; Vice Provost, Health Affairs, Univ. of Michigan; Visiting Professor, Southern Univ. School of Nursing, Baton Rouge, La. **Organizations:** National League for Nursing; American Nurses Assoc.; Sigma Theta Tau; National Black Nurses Assoc. **Awards:** honorary doctorates, Simmons College, Univs. of Cincinnati, Massachusetts, San Diego; Yale, Dillard, Indiana, Georgetown, Fla. International Univs., Bethune-Cookman College; Distinguished Alumna Awards, Yale, Dillard Univ.; Academic Achievement Award, Univ. of Michigan; Fellow, American Academy of Nursing; Mentorship Award, Sigma Theta Tau International; Twenty-first Century Award, Women's Hall of Fame; Living Legend, American Academy of Nursing, 2002.

References and Credits

†Dumas RG: Dilemmas of black females in leadership. J Personality and Social Systems 2:12–13, 1979.

Dumas, Rhetaugh E.G. In Who's Who in American Nursing 1996–97. 6th ed. Marquis Who's Who. New Providence, N.J., Reed Reference, 1995, p 171.

Dumas R: personal communication, 2001, 2002.

Welsh S: "Voice and Vision": Perspectives of Yale School of Nursing Leaders [multimedia master's thesis]. New Haven, Conn., Yale School of Nursing, 2002.

November 27

Adda Eldredge

1864–1955

"The student can learn courtesy and kindliness only by example, by seeing them associated and everywhere used. ...Thoughtfulness, gentleness, sympathy are all learned by observation, by seeing and receiving them, and it is very important... that they see nothing else. ...Perfect, finished nursing is the aim which every staff of nurses should have in the teaching of the student, and they should not only teach her but show her that the aim in nursing should be the comfort of the patient, which can be secured only by absolute kindliness, extreme neatness and a deftness which gives speed without sacrificing that beautiful finished nursing which is vital to the training of the nurse." (1925)

ADDA ELDREDGE, one of nursing's "first citizens," had a major influence on nursing education, state legislation for compulsory nurse registration, and state nurse practice acts. She held the first registration certificate in Illinois. After the Illinois Nurses Association failed for a second time to gain passage of a nurse practice act, Eldredge waged a public relations campaign to garner support. A powerful speaker with excellent stage presence, she merged the need for legislation with public information. The subsequent, widespread support ensured passage the third time around, in 1907. After that, she outlined these timely basics of effective lobbying: Be informed, conscise, and clear about your issue; work harmoniously on your legislative committee; network with community and professional groups for support; be consistent with your message; involve the media, and, most important, impress upon each nurse that it is essential to contact her or his legislative representative. Eldredge strengthened nursing education in Wisconsin when she made inspection, evaluation, and accreditation the centerpiece of nursing school performance. The Rockefeller Foundation used her work in Wisconsin to establish an internationally recognized model. Through her efforts poor-quality schools with haphazard programs were closed, replaced by schools that required a high school diploma for admission and did not exploit the students. The schools had qualified faculty and appropriate clinical affiliations. Eldredge was active in professional nursing organizations and promoted working together. Her slogan, "The ANA is where *you* are," increased membership and strengthened state associations. In retirement she taught college-level courses on nursing legislation and nursing jurisprudence.

Biography

Born: Nov. 27, 1864, Fond du Lac, Wisc. **Education:** St. Luke's Hosp. Training School, Chicago; Teachers College, Columbia Univ. **Work history:** Private Duty Nurse, Supervisor of Instruction, St. Luke's Hosp. School of Nursing, Chicago; staff, Assoc. for Improving the Conditions of the Poor, N.Y.C.; Interstate Secretary, American Nurses Assoc. (ANA), National League of Nursing Education, and *American Journal of Nursing;* wrote frequently for *Journal;* Council on National Defense; N.Y. State Bd. of Nurse Examiners; first director, Wisc. Bureau of Nursing Education; contributor to Goldmark Report on private duty nursing; Director, Nurse Placement Service, Chicago; Faculty, Univ. of Chicago, Univ. of Minnesota, Adviser to Exec. Committee, Univ. of Pittsburgh School of Nursing. **Organizations:** Ill. State Assoc. for Graduate Nurses; ANA; International Council of Nurses; Chair, Committee to Select Jane Delano Award; Sigma Theta Tau. **Awards:** Walter Burns Saunders Medal, ANA; scholarship fund in her name, Wisc. Nurses Assoc.; included in *Famous Wisconsin Women* (Wisc. Historical Society), and *American Nursing* by Mary Roberts; ANA Hall of Fame. **Buried:** Rienzi Cemetery, Fond du Lac, Wisc.

References and Credits

†Eldredge A: The unwritten curriculum. AJN 25:274, 1925.

Cooper SS: Adda Eldredge. In Bullough V, Church OM, Stein AP (eds): American Nursing: A Biographical Dictionary, vol. 1. New York, Garland, 1988, pp 104–107.

Roberts M: American Nursing: History and Interpretation. New York, Macmillan, 1954, p 100.

ANA Hall of Fame 10/98 American Nurses Association, Washington, D.C. http://www.nursingworld.org/hof.

Eldredge A: How to organize for registration. AJN 7:839–843, 1907.

November 28

Ellwynne Mae Vreeland

1909–1971

"Why do nurses nurse? ... What incentives will attract more women to the field? These questions are of great importance, for society is confronted with a scarcity of a commodity upon which it has come to place some value. ... There is a shortage of nurses; ... it is serious, ... it is likely to become even more serious unless planning and action take place expeditiously. ... The number of students entering schools of nursing is diminishing. ... One of the most powerful incentives in recruitment is the truly happy student or graduate nurse. ... Nurses nurse because they enjoy nursing. ... That the institutional nurses are of the greatest importance to nursing of the present and future is certain. To help them solve the ... occupational problems which cause their dissatisfaction should be of primary concern to all who are interested in overcoming the shortages in nursing. ... Unless a sufficiently high value is placed on professional nursing to attract and hold some of the best thinkers from all strata of society, we may realize diminishing benefits from medical progress." (1949)

Ellwynne Vreeland spent most of her professional career with the U.S. Public Health Service (USPHS). She began as a consultant and later directed its nursing education department. When she headed the division that funds nursing research, she authorized more than $8 million in nursing research grants and provided funding for graduate nurse education. In her article "Fifty Years of Nursing in the Federal Government Nursing Services," she wrote about such nurses as Dorothea Dix, Clara Barton, Jane Delano, Lucy Minnegerode, Pearl McIver, and Mary Hickey. They led efforts to gain public health services at Ellis Island, expand military nursing, and provide services to veterans. She believed that the example, endurance, and pioneering efforts of these women helped to firmly establish nursing as essential to federal health services. She credited nursing's influence with the evolution of the USPHS, the growth of the Bureau of Indian Affairs, and the establishment of the Children's Bureau. In 1950, when her article was published, the major employer of nurses was the federal government. She attributed this to the consistent professionalism and quality of care provided by nurses during wartime and in civilian programs.

Biography

Born: Nov. 28, 1909, Stockbridge, Mass. **Education:** Massachusetts General Hosp. School of Nursing; Univ. of Vermont; Univ. of Rochester, N.Y.; Teachers College, Columbia Univ. (BS, MA). **Work history:** Staff Nurse, General Hosp., Saranac Lake, N.Y.; Stony Wold Hosp., Lake Kushaqua, N.Y.; Strong Memorial Hosp., Rochester, N.Y; Director of Nurses, Schenectady County (N.Y.) Tuberculosis Hosp.; Director of Nursing, Nurse Education, Albany Hosp., Russell Sage Hosp., Albany, N.Y.; Consultant, USPHS. **Organizations:** unknown. **Awards:** USPHS Meritorious Service Medal; Teachers College Award for Distinguished Achievement; Fellow, American Public Health Assoc.; American Nurses Assoc. Hall of Fame. **Died:** Riviera Beach, Fla.

References and Credits

†Vreeland E: Why do nurses nurse? AJN 49:411–413, 1949.

Bullough V: Ellwynne Mae Vreeland. In Bullough V, Church OM, Stein AP (eds): American Nursing: A Biographical Dictionary, vol. 1. New York, Garland, 1988, pp 330–331.

Vreeland E: Fifty years of nursing in the federal government nursing services. AJN 50:626–631, 1950.

ANA Hall of Fame 10/98 American Nurses Association, Washington D.C. http://www.nursingworld.org/hof.

November 29

Louisa May Alcott

1832–1888

"It was a lively scene; the long room lined with rows of beds, each filled by an occupant whom water, shears, and clean raiment, had transformed from a dismal ragamuffin into a recumbent hero, with a cropped head. To and fro rushed matrons, maids, and convalescent 'boys,' skirmishing with knives and forks; retreating with empty plates; marching and counter-marching, with varied success, while the clash of busy spoons made most inspiring music for the charge of our Light Brigade." (1869)

"He seemed asleep; but something in the tired white face caused me to listen at his lips for a breath. None came. I touched his forehead; it was cold: and then I knew that, while he waited, a better nurse than I had given him a cooler draught, and healed him with a touch. I laid the sheet over the quiet sleeper, whom no noise could now disturb; and one half hour later the bed was empty." (1869)

"Therefore, I close this little chapter of hospital experiences, with the regret that they were no better worth recording; and add the poetical gem with which I console myself

for the untimely demise of Nurse Periwinkle:
Oh, lay her in the little pit,
With a marble stone to cover it;
And carve theron, a gruel spoon,
To show a 'nuss' has died too soon." (1869)

LOUISA MAY ALCOTT, the author of *Little Women* and many other popular books, wanted to do something to help the war effort during the Civil War. She was reading Florence Nightingale's *Notes on Nursing* and about Clara Barton's contributions, and Alcott wanted to make a difference. She volunteered to help as an army nurse at the Union Hospital at Georgetown, in Washington, D.C., for six weeks. During that time she wrote about her experiences under the pseudonym of Tribulation Periwinkle. These notes were later published as *Hospital Sketches.* They were very popular because so many people wanted to know about their lost loved ones. Alcott's own health was affected during this period. She developed typhoid fever and pneumonia and claimed she never had a healthy day again.

BIOGRAPHY

Born: Nov. 29, 1832, Germantown, Pa. **Education:** tutored at home, instructed by father's friends, incl. Emerson and Thoreau. **Work history:** nursed terminally ill sister, Elizabeth; taught school; worked as professional seamstress; rolled bandages during first year of Civil War; traveled with wealthy invalid to Europe; Author. **Writings:** *Flower Fables; Moods; Hospital Sketches and Camp and Fireside Stories; Little Women.* **Organizations:** unknown. **Awards:** unknown. **Buried:** Sleepy Hollow, Concord, Mass.

REFERENCES AND CREDITS

†Alcott LM: Hospital Sketches and Camp and Fireside Stories. Boston, Little, Brown, 1904, pp 33, 35, 78–79.

Stein AP: Louisa May Alcott. In Bullough V, Church OM, Stein AP (eds): American Nursing: A Biographical Dictionary, vol. 1. New York, Garland, 1988, pp 3–4.

November 30

Virginia Avenel Henderson

1897–1996

"The unique function of the nurse is to assist the individual (sick or well) in the performance of those activities contributing to health or its recovery (or to peaceful death) that he would perform unaided if he had the necessary strength, will, or knowledge. And to do this in such a way as to help him gain independence as rapidly as possible." (1964)

"She [the nurse] is temporarily the consciousness of the unconscious, the love of life for the suicidal, the leg of the amputee, the eyes of the newly blind, a means of locomotion for the infant, knowledge and confidence for the young mother, the [voice] for those too weak or withdrawn to speak." (1964)

Virginia Henderson was known by many endearing names: "the first lady of nursing," "the first international nurse," "the Florence Nightingale of the twentieth century," and the "foremost nurse of the twentieth century." Her career included working as a nurse, educator, researcher, textbook author, speaker, consultant, adviser, and activist to promote a universal tax to support health care for all U.S. citizens. Her master's thesis was about medical and surgical asepsis. She developed an animal experiment to determine whether steam under pressure or boiling better eliminates pathogens from surgical instruments. She rewrote Bertha Harmer's *Textbook of the Principles and Practice of Nursing,* which she revised a second time under the title *Basic Principles of Nursing;* it has been used widely in nursing schools and translated into twenty-five languages. From 1959 to 1971 she was director of the Nursing Studies Index Project, which led to the publication of a four-volume guide, *Nursing Studies Index,* which reports studies, research in progress, research methods, and historical materials related to nursing in periodicals, books, and pamphlets in English. The Inter-Agency Council on Library Resources for Nursing continues today as a result of the committee that Henderson established. The Sigma Theta Tau International library is named in her honor.

Biography

Born: Nov. 30, 1897, Kansas City, Mo. **Education:** home-schooled in family of scholars; Army School of Nursing, 1921; Teachers College, Norfolk, Va.; Columbia Univ. Medical School (BS, MA). **Work history:** Public Health Nurse, Henry Street Visiting Nurse Assoc., Bronx, N.Y.; Director, summer camp for underprivileged children, Visiting Nurse Assoc. (VNA), Washington, D.C.; first full-time nursing instructor, Protestant Hosp. School, Norfolk, Va.; Teaching Supervisor, Outpatient Dept., Strong Memorial Hosp., Rochester, N.Y.; Associate Professor, nursing education, Teachers College, Columbia Univ.; taught research, medical-surgical nursing. **Writings:** *Basic Principles in Nursing* (1960); researched East Coast library holdings for all 200 doctoral dissertations by nurses; Director, Nursing Studies Index Project. **Organizations:** American Academy of Nursing, Sigma Theta Tau, and honorary memberships in eight other organizations. **Awards:** honorary degrees, Univ. of Western Ontario, Rush Univ., Pace Univ., Catholic Univ., Yale Univ., Old Dominion Univ., Emory Univ., l'Escola d'Infermeria de la Universtat de Barcelona; first U.S. nurse selected as Fellow, Vice President for Life, Royal College of Nursing, London; American Nurses Assoc. Hall of Fame; Presidential Bicentennial Award, Boston College School of Nursing; Adelaide Nutting Award, National League for Nursing; Annie W. Goodrich Teaching Award, student body, Yale School of Nursing; Christianne Reimann Prize, International Council of Nurses; Merit Award, National Assoc. of Nurses of Columbia, South America; Excellence in Education Award (now the Virginia Henderson Award), National Assoc. for Home Care. **Died:** Branford, Conn.

References and Credits

†Henderson V: The nature of nursing. AJN 64:63, 1964.

Nursing Center Press, Sigma Theta Tau International: Celebrating Virginia Henderson. Video. December 1997.

ANA Hall of Fame 10/98 American Nurses Association, Washington, D.C. http://www.nursingworld.org/hof.

Hays JC: Virginia Henderson. In Bullough V, Sentz L, Stein AP (eds): American Nursing: A Biographical Dictionary, vol. 2. New York, Garland, 1992, pp 148–152.

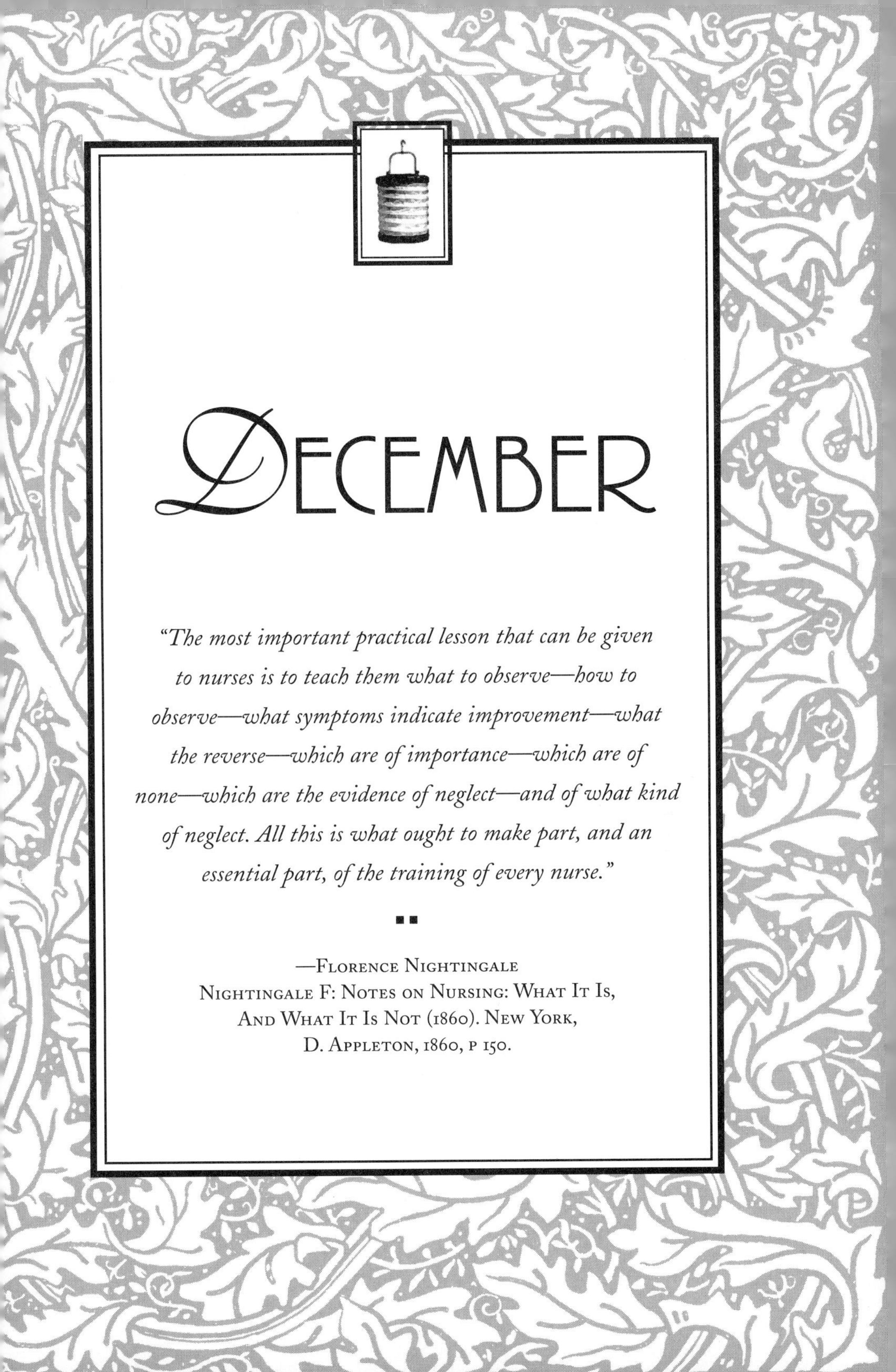

DECEMBER

"The most important practical lesson that can be given to nurses is to teach them what to observe—how to observe—what symptoms indicate improvement—what the reverse—which are of importance—which are of none—which are the evidence of neglect—and of what kind of neglect. All this is what ought to make part, and an essential part, of the training of every nurse."

—Florence Nightingale
Nightingale F: Notes on Nursing: What It Is, And What It Is Not (1860). New York, D. Appleton, 1860, p 150.

December 1

Aurora Hernandez

1972–

"I have seen first hand the lack of health care, language barriers, and the lack of trust that migrant workers often experience when accessing health care. I would like to focus my nursing career on improving the health of the migrant farm worker population." (2002)

Aurora Hernandez knows, first hand, the deprivation and hard work that typify life for migrant farmworkers in the United States. She was one of the many Latino children who spend their childhood summers working in farm fields to augment family incomes that, regardless of effort, remain substandard. The family truck took them north from Texas; she weeded sugar beets in Minnesota, cucumbers in Wisconsin, and potatoes in North Dakota. She was drawn to nursing by what she saw as a child, when she would accompany her diabetic father to clinics and translate for him. She remembers unrealistic medical recommendations: "The staff would tell him he needed a special diet for his uncontrolled diabetes and not to work so hard. They didn't understand that the food they recommended was too expensive and would never sustain him for labor in the fields. There was a big disconnect—healthcare providers didn't understand the migrant farmworker culture and lifestyle." Today she is a professional role model and nursing leader, featured in the recruitment campaign Nurses for a Healthier Tomorrow. She is committed to improving health care for migrant workers. Inadequate or nonexistent health care compounds the risk for workers, who seldom see medical professionals but who are exposed to pesticides, dehydration, a high accident rate, and lack of sanitation. Whatever health care is available is compromised by the real barriers of language, culture, and accessibility. She says migrant workers need culturally sensitive nurses who are realistic and practical. They must see that the connection between nursing and advocacy is essential and basic, and she calls on nurses to be actively involved in seeking social reform legislation.

Biography

Born: April 9, 1972, **Education:** Minneapolis (Minn.) Community College (RN). **Work history:** Staff Nurse, George Washington Hosp., Washington, D.C. **Organizations:** National Student Nurses Assoc.; Va. Nurses Assoc.; National Assoc. of Hispanic Nurses. **Awards:** selected by Sigma Theta Tau for the recruitment campaign Nurses for a Healthier Tomorrow.

References and Credits

†Nurses for a Healthier Tomorrow, September 2002, available on-line at http://www.nursesource.org/ad_hernandez.html.

Nurses for a Healthier Tomorrow gears up for campaign launch. Excellence in Clinical Practice 2:1–2, 2001.

Steefel L: Third world life in a first-world country. Nurs Spectrum 2:26–27, 2001.

Siantz M: personal correspondence, December 2002.

DECEMBER 2

Ingeborg Grosser Mauksch

1921–

"Gradually it occurred to me that nursing was a field in which I could rise to the top—that in nursing it was possible for me to make a contribution of significance. Nursing would give me the opportunity to apply myself completely. ...To say that nursing has been good to me is a great understatement. It has been a source of joy and growth, of maturation and valued achievement. It has been a wellspring of gratification and contentment, but it has also allowed me to realize my limitations and shortcomings. Most of my friends are my colleagues and peers in nursing. The majority of people who are significant in my life are professional peers. When I look to the future and think of the exciting opportunities that I envision for those in the profession who are younger than I am, I have a sense of joy and a certain feeling of ownership. This is a wonderful profession, it's mine, and I'd like to pass it on to those who will value and cherish it as I have." (1988)

INGEBORG MAUKSCH ARRIVED in the United States before World War II as a refugee from Austria. When she had to tell the immigration officer what she would do to earn a living, she said she would be a nurse. She became proficient in English and enjoyed a varied, challenging, and rewarding career in the profession she loves. She recalls her first convention of the American Nurses

Association (ANA) in 1948, when the big issues were the forty-hour workweek, licensure, health insurance, and collective bargaining. Throughout her career she met and worked with many nursing leaders. She said this made her humble and introduced her to many new ideas about nursing practice. When she was working on her master's degree, she realized that hospital nurses could do more for patients. She believed that the nurse's assessment of the patient's needs should direct patient care. She subsequently began to focus her interests on the future of nursing and nursing practice. A primary care practitioner, her commitment to the significance of professional practice intensified as she worked in various teaching and practice roles. President Jimmy Carter appointed her to the first Advisory Committee for National Health Insurance and then to the Holocaust Memorial Council.

Biography

Born: Dec. 2, 1921, Vienna. **Education:** Massachusetts General Hosp.; Teachers College, Columbia Univ. (BSN); Univ. of Chicago (MN, PhD). **Work history:** Clinical Instructor, Michael Reese Hosp. School of Nursing, Chicago; Instructor, St. Luke's Hosp., Chicago; Assistant Director, School of Nursing, Presbyterian–St. Luke's Hosp., Chicago; Researcher, Chicago Council on Community Nursing; Chair, general nursing program, Loyola Univ., Chicago; Faculty, School of Medicine, Univ. of Missouri; Valere Potter Distinguished Professor of Nursing, Vanderbilt Univ.; Director, Fellowship Program in Primary Care, Vanderbilt Univ.; Visiting Faculty, Hadassah-Hebrew Univ. School of Nursing, Israel; participant, International Congress on Nursing Law and Ethics, Israel. **Organizations:** Ill. Nurses Assoc.; American Nurses Assoc. (ANA). **Awards:** research fellowship for doctoral study, U.S. Public Health Service; Alumni Award, Massachusetts General Hosp.; honorary doctorate, Syracuse Univ.; Fellow, American Academy of Nursing; award from Columbia Univ.

References and Credits

†Schorr T, Zimmerman A: Making Choices, Taking Chances: Nurse Leaders Tell Their Stories. St. Louis, CV Mosby, 1988, pp 253, 260.

Ingeborg G. Mauksch. In Franz J, Vandervort-Jones P (eds): Who's Who in American Nursing, 1986–87, 2d ed. Owings Mills, Md., Society of Nursing Professionals, 1987, p 325.

Mauksch IG: personal correspondence, 2002.

December 3

Eddie Bernice Johnson

1935–

"I remember how I came across the idea of a World of Women for World Peace. It started after I shed tears after reading a magazine cover story of how twelve year olds were being forced into combat. I remember saying then that as a mother and a grandmother I can't believe that women—no matter who they are and what they are—carry a child for nine months, experience the pain of childbirth only for that son or daughter to be sent off to war to die on a battlefield. It was then I decided to take action. …I believe it is time to reach back to the historic intent of Mother's Day. …We must continue this historic Mother's Day tradition of interfering in matters of war and peace—, of choosing love over hate and of ensuring that violence is an unacceptable tool, whether it be in the home, the workplace or in the lyrics of female-bashing music. …So today … we are interfering. We are reconnecting Mother's Day to its glorious past of building a culture of peace with a new initiative called, 'A World of Women for World Peace.'" (2002)

EDDIE BERNICE JOHNSON was the chief psychiatric nurse at the Veterans Administration Hospital in Dallas before her successful run for a seat in the Texas House of Representatives in 1972. Now in her fifth term in the U.S. House of Representatives, she has chaired the Congressional Black Caucus and serves on major committees. When she was first elected to public office, she was the first African American and the first woman ever to be elected to public office from Dallas. Her career as policymaker continued as she went on to serve in the Texas Senate and then the U.S. Congress. Her legislative interests include health care, the environment, economic justice, election reform, and increased funding for the National Science Foundation. As chair of the Congressional Black Caucus, she recognized its responsibility as "the conscience of Congress." In 2001 she founded "A World of Women for Peace" with House Concurrent Resolution 290. The international peace initiative recognizes the potential for women around the world to promote conflict resolution and nonviolence. A basic component of this program is a National Day of Dialogue on International Peace, held around Mother's Day. Johnson reminds us that the original mission of the Mother's Day holiday was to promote world peace.

Biography

Born: Dec. 3, 1935, Waco, Texas. **Education:** Holy Cross Central School of Nursing, (RN); St. Mary's College South Bend, Ind.; Univ. of Notre Dame; Texas Christian Univ. (BSN); Southern Methodist Univ. (MPA). **Work history:** Chief Psychiatric Nurse, Veterans Administration Hosp., Dallas; regional and national positions, U.S. Dept. of Health, Education and Welfare; Founder, President, Eddie Bernice Johnson and Assoc.; founding member, bd. of directors, Sunbelt National Bank; elected to Texas House of Representatives, Texas Senate, U.S. House of Representatives. **Organizations:** Alpha Kappa Alpha. **Awards:** Citizenship Award, National Conference of Christians and Jews; Outstanding Alumna, St. Mary's College; one of ten most powerful black women in U.S., *Ebony;* President's Award, National Council of Black Mayors; Visionary Award, National Organization of Black Elected Legislative Women; Woman of the Year, 100 Black Men of America, Inc.; Outstanding Achievement Award, National Black Caucus; Texas NAACP Heroes Award; honorary doctorates, Bishop College, Jarvis Christian College, Texas College, Paul Quinn College, Houston-Tillotson College; Racial Harmony Award, Foundation for Ethnic Understanding.

References and Credits

†Johnson EB: Remarks at "A World of Women" World Peace Breakfast, March 8, 2002, courtesy Johnson's office.

Rep. Eddie Bernice Johnson of Texas, U.S. House of Representatives website, available on-line at http://www.house.gov/ebjohnson.

Alex-Assensoh Y: Eddie Bernice Johnson, 1934–. In Smith JC (ed): Notable Black American Women. New York, Gale, 1996.

Eddie Bernice Johnson. In Who's Who in American Nursing, 1996–97, 6th ed. New Providence, N.J., Reed Reference, 1995.

Eddie Bernice Johnson. In Hawkins WL: African American Biographies. Jefferson, N.C., McFarland, 1992, pp 238–239.

December 4

Edith Cavell

1865–1915

"I have no fear or shrinking; I have seen death so often that it is not strange or fearful to me. I thank God for this ten weeks; quiet before the end. Life has always been hurried and full of difficulty. This time of rest has been a great mercy. They have all been very kind to me here. But this I would say, standing as I do in view of God and eternity: I realize patriotism is not enough. I must have no hatred or bitterness towards anyone." (1915)

Edith Cavell was a British nurse who founded and directed a large nursing school in Brussels during World War I. As a child, she never got to eat her roast beef supper when it was hot because her father divided the roast into six portions and the children had to deliver the hot food to some less fortunate neighbor before they could eat their meal. Her desire to relieve the suffering of others was the hallmark of her nature. While working in Brussels, she gave aid and care to all injured men, regardless of their nationality. For this the Germans arrested and charged her with harboring British and French soldiers and helping them to escape so that they could return to their armies. At her trial she admitted that she had helped soldiers escape from Belgium, because she thought they would be executed if they stayed. She was not found to be a spy but nevertheless was sentenced to die. All diplomatic attempts to save her failed, and on

October 12, 1915, she refused the blindfold and walked calmly before the six armed German soldiers. As she neared the place designated for her to stand, she fainted. The German officer in charge withdrew his own revolver and shot her through the head where she lay. Her body was eventually returned to England, where she was interred during a national service at the Norwich Cathedral.

Biography

Born: Dec. 4, 1865, Swardeston, England. **Education:** London Hosp. Nurses Training School **Work history:** founded nurse training schools, England and Belgium; raised standards of nursing in Belgium, 1907–14. **Organizations:** unknown. **Awards:** commemorative stamp, Costa Rica; Mt. Edith Cavell, a mountain in the Canadian Rockies; "Edith Cavell," poem by Laurence Binyon; statue of Cavell in Trafalgar Square, London. **Buried:** Norwich, England.

References and Credits

†Scovil ER: An heroic nurse. AJN 15:118–121, 1915.

Judson H: Edith Cavell. New York, Macmillan, 1941, p 3.

Anne J. Davis

1931–

"It is really remarkable that a discipline such as nursing can accommodate so many people with so many different talents. We are all needed—those of us who work in critical care units of large hospitals or in long-term care facilities, those who work in the inner city and those who work in rural areas, those who are administrators, teachers and policy makers, those of us who conduct research, and those who raise some of the basic questions about our values, obligations, and duties to others. ...For those of us who know something of nursing's history, we can be proud that, as a profession, we have supported legislation over the years that has enabled many people to live better lives, to work in safer environments, and to receive adequate health care. ...We have a proud history in nursing, and I for one am very happy to be a part of that." (1988)

INDEPENDENT, INTELLECTUALLY CURIOUS, and adventurous, Anne J. Davis was attracted to nursing by its potential to help people, job security, and opportunities for travel. Much of what she has done combined her primary interests of psychiatric nursing, ethics, and international nursing. She looks back on a wonderful career that has made a positive difference in the lives of others. She maximized opportunities for clinical experience, study, and travel, and she treasures her nursing friendships around the world. When she was a young faculty member in San Francisco, she took her savings and traveled abroad alone for two years. While there, she occasionally took non-nursing and nursing jobs. For example, she worked on an archeological dig near the Sea of Galilee, taught psychosocial nursing in Israel, and did psychiatric nursing in Denmark. When she was at Harvard on a fellowship to study ethics, she coauthored *Ethical Dilemmas and Nursing Practice* (1978) with Mila Aroskar. She taught for more than three decades at the University of California, San Francisco, helped establish a nursing school in Saudi Arabia, and taught nursing for several years in Japan. A renowned speaker on ethics and health care, in 1986 she was the first recipient of the Human Rights Award from the American Nurses Association (ANA).

Biography

Born: Dec. 5, 1931, Greensboro, N.C. **Education:** Emory Univ., Atlanta (BS, DSc); Boston Univ. (MS); Univ. of California, Berkeley (PhD); Kennedy Postdoctoral Fellow, Harvard Univ. **Work history:** Staff Nurse, McLean Hosp., Boston; Bedford (Mass.) Veterans Administration Hosp.; Faculty, Univ. of California, San Francisco; Israel; Nagano College of Nursing, Japan; Author. **Organizations:** ANA; Golden Gate Nursing Assoc. **Awards:** member, American Academy of Nursing; first recipient, Human Rights Award, ANA; honorary doctorate, Emory Univ.; Outstanding Alumna, Boston Univ. School of Nursing.

References and Credits

†Schorr T, Zimmerman A: Making Choices, Taking Chances: Nurse Leaders Tell Their Stories. St. Louis, CV Mosby, 1988, p 69.

Who's Who in American Nursing, 1996–97, 6th ed. New Providence, N.J., Reed Reference, 1995.

Davis AJ: personal correspondence, March 2002.

Davis AJ: resume.

Davis A, Aroskar, M: Ethical Dilemmas and Nursing Practice, 3d ed. Norwalk, Conn., Appleton and Lange, 1991.

December 6

Ruth Benson Freeman (Fisher)

1906–1982

"We must budget nursing services without sacrificing the essential meaning of nursing. Somehow there must be nursing time to comfort as well as to counsel, to listen as well as to look for symptoms, to ponder as well as to practice. Without these essentials, nursing becomes only a technical service, lacking the depth and impact required of a profession." (1959)

RUTH BENSON FREEMAN said she was a nonconformist student who entered nursing accidentally. Her grandmother financed her study in New York, and when Freeman enrolled at Mt. Sinai, she did so because her aunt worked there as a secretary and her grandmother believed that dormitory living was safe. As a student, Freeman violated protocol by talking freely with the doctors. Once, after she was denied the opportunity to attend an autopsy, she dressed as a man and sneaked in with the medical students. However, when she worked as a Henry Street visiting nurse, she became committed to the profession. There she began to develop her broad concepts of public health nursing that influenced teaching and practice. When she was teaching at Johns Hopkins School of Hygiene and Public Health, she introduced a nursing presence to other disciplines, such as public health administration. She recognized the value of and the need for nurse practitioners as primary health care providers in managed care.

Highly honored and widely published, she wrote classic texts on public health that dealt with public health practice, supervision, and administration.

Biography

Born: Dec. 6, 1906, Metheun, Mass. **Education:** Lowell (Mass.) Normal School; Mt. Sinai School of Nursing, N.Y.; Columbia Univ. (BS, MA); New York Univ. (EdD). **Work history:** Henry Street Visiting Nurse Service, N.Y.C.; Faculty, New York Univ., Univ. of Minnesota; Consultant, Minnesota Bd. of Health; Administrator of Nursing Services, American Red Cross; Consultant, National Security Resources Bd.; Associate Professor, Professor, Professor Emeritus, Johns Hopkins School of Hygiene and Public Health; Consultant to Veterans Administration, Air Force, Pan American Health Organization, World Health Organization. **Organizations:** National League for Nursing (NLN); National Health Council; American Public Health Assoc. (APHA); American Nurses Assoc. (ANA). **Awards:** Pearl McIver Public Health Nurse Award, ANA; Florence Nightingale Medal, International Committee, Red Cross; Adelaide Nutting Award, NLN; Bronfman Prize, APHA; Honorary Fellow, American Academy of Nursing; ANA Hall of Fame. **Died:** Cockeysville, Md.

References and Credits

†Freeman RB: Nurses, patients and progress. Nurs Outlook 7:17, 1959.

Lawrence JT: Ruth Lawrence Freeman (Fisher). In Bullough V, Church OM, Stein AP (eds): American Nursing: A Biographical Dictionary, vol. 1. New York, Garland, 1988, pp 123–125.

Safier G: Contemporary American Leaders in Nursing: An Oral History. New York, McGraw-Hill, 1977.

ANA Hall of Fame 10/98 American Nurses Association, Washington, D.C. http://www.nursingworld.org/ hof.

December 7

Katharine Jane Densford Dreves
1890–1978

"We will find in the future, as we have found in the past, nurses with ability; with high motivation, and dedication; and with devotion to common goals, whether in giving care to the individual patient, in guarding a nation's health in wartime, in building schools of nursing, community nursing services, or nursing organization. Nurses with a generous concern for service to others and with a sense of responsibility toward the calling of nursing, which has contributed so much to the healing of nations, will continue to take part in professional, community, and world affairs. I believe that 'the greatest among you is the one who serves.' If we as nurses always keep this ancient truth in mind, we shall be working to the end that all people will receive the best possible nursing care." (1964)

Katharine Dreves was raised by parents who stressed the importance of education and a sense of purpose. She earned degrees in Latin and history and worked for several years as a teacher before she was drawn to nursing at the start of World War I. Her career included hospital nursing, public health nursing, teaching, and administration. She was a prolific writer and an expert parliamentarian. During her leadership years with the American Nurses Association, she was involved in the issues of economics, general welfare, integration, and nursing in World War II. During retirement she raised money for the American Nurses Foundation. As she looked back on her career, her beliefs, and her hopes for the profession, she wrote of the importance of broad-based education for all people. She saw this as a necessary preparation for nurses so that they could function more effectively not only in the profession but in their community and in the world. She wrote that nursing has the potential to "direct the changing world to the service of mankind."

Biography

Born: Dec. 7, 1890, Crothersville, Ind. **Education:** Oxford College for Women, Oxford, Ohio; Miami Univ., Ohio (BA); Indiana Univ., Bloomington; Univ. of Chicago (MA); Vassar Training Camp; Univ. of Cincinnati School of Nursing and Health (RN); coursework, Teachers College, Columbia Univ. **Work history:** Schoolteacher; Head Nurse, Cincinnati (Ohio) General Hosp.; Public Health Nurse, Hamilton County, Ohio; Superintendent of Nurses, Cincinnati Tuberculosis Sanitorium; Nursing Instructor, Univ. of Cincinnati School of Nursing and Health; Assistant Dean, Ill. Training School, Chicago; Assistant Director of Nursing, Cook County Hosp., Chicago; Consultant, Army Nurse Corps; Director, School of Nursing, Univ. of Minnesota. **Organizations:** American Nurses Assoc. (ANA), Alpha Tau Delta, Sigma Theta Tau, National Health Assembly; advisory committees, Veterans Administration, American Red Cross; American Nurses Foundation. **Awards:** honorary doctorates, Baylor Univ., Miami Univ.; Honorary Pin, ANA; citations from Minneapolis Red Cross, American Assoc. of Univ. Women, YWCA, Hamline Univ., Minn. League for Nursing, Minnesota Nurses Assoc.; first woman to give Univ. of Minnesota Cap and Gown Address; ANA Hall of Fame. **Buried:** Acacia Park Cemetery, Mendota Heights, Minn.

References and Credits

†Dreves KD: This I believe about nursing in a changing world. Nurs Outlook 12:51, 1964.

Glass LK: Katharine Dreves. In Bullough V, Church OM, Stein AP (eds): American Nursing: A Biographical Dictionary, vol. 1. New York, Garland, 1988, pp 98–100.

ANA Hall of Fame 10/98 American Nurses Association, Washington, D.C. http://www.nursingworld.org/hof.

Adele Grace Stahl

1908–1983

"The basic purpose of licensing ... is the protection of the public's health, welfare, and safety. ... With the license ... goes a responsibility for keeping abreast of the advancements in medical science and the changes in nursing practice. As the years go by, progress will be made and standards of competency will also change. As a professional practitioner the nurse is expected to keep pace with change. In 1975 the nurse cannot be considered a safe practitioner if her level of performance is of the 1959 vintage. (1959)

ADELE GRACE STAHL was an authority on nurse licensure and the nurse practice act. She worked with nurses to help them develop knowledge, expertise, and effectiveness in the legislative process so that they could be meaningfully involved in nursing issues. She was known for her high standards and objectivity regarding nursing performance and nursing education. Highly credible, she always had supporting documentation for her statements about nursing. In 1945, during a nursing shortage, she helped convince the Wisconsin legislature to designate surplus state funds for nursing scholarships, and the program continued for thirty-three years. After earning a bachelor's degree from the Frances Payne Bolton School of Nursing at Case Western Reserve University, she did postgraduate work in child development and in public administration. She was an outstanding nursing leader in Wisconsin and worked with the Council of State Boards of Nursing of the American Nurses Association (ANA) for decades.

Biography

Born: Dec. 8, 1908, Akron, Ohio. **Education:** Frances Payne Bolton School of Nursing, Western Reserve Univ., Cleveland, Ohio; M. Palmer School of Child Development, Detroit; postgraduate work, Syracuse Univ. **Work history:** Babies' and Children's Hosp., Cleveland; Instructor, Western Reserve Univ. School of Nursing; Instructor, Assistant Director, nursing education, Syracuse (N.Y.) Memorial Hosp. School of Nursing; Assistant Director, Director, Wisc. State Bureau of Nursing; Administrator, Wisc. State Dept. of Nurses; Council of State Bds. of Nursing, ANA. **Organizations:** Wisc. Nurses Assoc. (WNA); Wisc. League for Nursing; Wisc. State Bd. of Vocational and Adult Education (WSBVAE); Wisc. State Bureau of Personnel; Wisc. State Dept. of Health and Social Services; Wisc. State Bd. of Pharmacy; Milwaukee County Civil Service. **Awards:** Civic Service Award, WSBVAE; Award of Merit, Wisc. Hosp. Assoc.; Distinguished Civic Service Award, Wisc.; honored by WNA; honorary doctorate, Marquette Univ.; John XXIII Distinguished Service Award, Viterbo College, La Crosse, Wisc.; Friend of Extension Award, Univ. of Wisc.—Extension.
Died: Madison, Wisc.

References and Credits

†Stahl A: Prelude to licensure. AJN 59:1259, 1959.

Cooper SS: Adele Stahl. In Bullough V, Church OM, Stein AP (eds): American Nursing: A Biographical Dictionary, vol. 1. New York, Garland, 1988, pp 293–295.

December 9

Jeanne Quint Benoliel

1919–

"They have chosen an occupation which brings them face to face with many of the sorrows of human existence—suffering and pain, illness and crippling, and death. ...Many nurses are not particularly comfortable in the presence of a person who is dying, nor can they converse easily with him about his forthcoming death. ...Educational programs in nursing reflect the values, beliefs, and practices of the wider society in which they emerge. The general taboo about death has resulted in nursing curricula which have given minimal attention to many serious issues and difficult decisions which nurses face in providing care for dying patients and their families. ...Cultural values concerning death have led to a gap in the education of nurses and, in turn, to a gap in the nursing services available to patients who are dying." (1967)

Events in Jeanne Quint Benoliel's life influenced her nursing practice and focus. She entered nursing school because tradition and finances limited her options for study. She says that one's options and choices are constrained or facilitated by the historical period in which one lives. When she was young, she witnessed the deaths of her grandfather and an aunt, both of whom were cared for by her mother at home. Benoliel learned to see death as a natural part of life. Her wartime experiences as an army nurse left her with memories of the emotional toll of war on young soldiers. Her marriage ended after her husband had to be institutionalized because of chronic mental illness. This was followed by her own treatment for depression. During that period her sister, who was pregnant for the fourth time, did not survive a cerebral hemorrhage. Such experiences helped Benoliel to become a sensitive and significant nurse-researcher, author, and consultant. Her landmark study of women with mastectomies focused on the patients' fears and concerns related to death and dying and identified barriers to effective and meaningful communication by caregivers. She recognized that nursing education needed to prepare nurses to interact with dying patients and their families and to do so by focusing on cultural values and belief systems as well as palliative care. Her pioneering efforts in death education resulted in the now-classic book *The Nurse and the Dying Patient.* She wrote the noted article "Institutionalized Practice of Information Control" (*Psychiatry,* May 1965). In 2002 she was awarded an honorary doctoral degree by Yale University for her contributions to family-centered end-of-life care.

Biography

Born: Dec. 9, 1919, National City, Calif. **Education:** St. Luke's Hosp. School of Nursing, San Francisco (RN); Univ. of California, Berkeley; Oregon State Univ. (BSNE); Univ. of California, Los Angeles (MS, post-master's study), Univ. of California, San Francisco (DNS). **Work history:** hospital staff nursing; Army Nurse Corps; Faculty, Fresno (Calif.) General Hosp., San Diego County (Calif.) Hosp.; Univ. of California, Los Angeles, School of Nursing, Univ. of California, San Francisco, Univ. of Washington; helped develop new PhD program, Rutgers Univ.; Consultant; Researcher; Author. **Organizations:** American Nurses Assoc. (ANA); National League for Nursing (NLN); American Assoc. for the Advancement of Science; American Public Health Assoc.; Oncology Nurses Society; Society for Health and Human Values International; Workgroup on Death, Dying and Bereavement. **Awards:** Fellow, American Academy of Nursing; Special Schwartz Award, ANA; book award, *American Journal of Nursing;* Linda Richards Award, NLN; Distinguished Service Award, American Cancer Society (ACS); former students held the "Jeanne Quint Benoliel Celebration Day" in 1989; Distinguished Researcher Award, Oncology Nursing Society; awards from Assoc. for Death Education and Counseling, ACS, National Center for Death Education; honorary doctorates, Univ. of San Diego, Univ. of Pennsylvania; Living Legend, American Academy of Nursing, 2000; *Who's Who in American Nursing, 1986–1987.*

References and Credits continued on page 771

December 10

Alice M. Robinson

1920–1983

"Communication, human relations, growth and development, personal defense mechanisms, and humane attitudes will always be part of the helping life. The intangibles *of healthful human relationships are* basic. *Antisocial behavior, whether born of loneliness, bitterness, grief, injustice, or other environmental pathology, will still respond to kindness and understanding. This has been true from the beginning of human existence; and it probably will be till the end." (1971)*

Alice Robinson's career in psychiatric nursing provided opportunities and challenges at government-run and private facilities, including the George Washington University Hospital in Washington, D.C., the Veterans Administration (VA) Hospital in Little Rock, Arkansas, and the Menninger Foundation in Topeka, Kansas. When she was the director of nursing at the Boston State Hospital, she was responsible for supervising the care of three thousand patients by a nursing staff of six hundred while managing the clinical rotations of approximately 250 students each year. While she was working at the Vermont State Hospital, she established psychiatric nursing affiliations for diploma and associate degree nursing programs. She worked as editor-in-chief at *Nursing Outlook* and as a senior editor at *RN Magazine* before starting her own consulting firm to offer diverse coursework as well as classes on clinical professional writing. Her own extensive publications have greatly enriched nursing. She recognized the value of adequately prepared psychiatric aides while stressing that skill and compassion were qualities crucial for all health workers caring for the mentally ill.

Biography

Born: Dec. 4, 1920, Islip, N.Y. **Education:** Duke Univ. School of Nursing (RN); Catholic Univ. of America (BS); Boston Univ. School of Nursing (MSNE). **Work history:** Staff Nurse, Army Nurse Corps; Coordinator, psychiatric nursing, George Washington Univ. Hosp.; Supervisor, psychiatric nursing, VA, Little Rock, Ark.; Director of Nursing Service, Menninger Institute, Topeka, Kans.; Faculty, Boston Univ. School of Nursing; Director of Nursing, Boston State Hosp.; Director of Nursing Education, Vermont State Hosp.; Editor, *Nursing Outlook, RN Magazine;* owner, Specialized Consultants in Nursing. **Organizations:** unknown. **Awards:** unknown. **Died:** location unknown.

References and Credits

†Robinson AM: Working with the Mentally Ill, 4th ed. Philadelphia, JB Lippincott, 1971, p ix.

Piemonte RV: Alice M. Robinson. In Bullough V, Sentz L, Stein AP (eds): American Nursing: A Biographical Dictionary, vol. 2. New York, Garland, 1992, pp 276–277.

Amy Frances Brown
1908–1984

"May I reiterate the oft discussed A B C of journalism: accuracy, brevity, conciseness. The goal–nurses who can interpret to other nurses and to lay groups the needs and the aspirations of the nursing profession." (1940)

AMY FRANCES BROWN was an author and educator who brought the principles of education to the teaching of nursing. She strongly emphasized the need for the preparation of nurses as teachers in classroom, clinical, and community situations. In 1945 she wrote *Medical Nursing,* which described clinical information that a nursing student could relate to the care of patients. Her articles in the *American Journal of Nursing* in the 1940s urged student nurses to learn to use communication skills effectively in speaking, teaching, and writing. She outlined ways for nursing instructors to incorporate medical problems and effective teaching skills in clinical classes. Her books *Medical and Surgical Nursing I* and *II* were published in 1958 and 1959, respectively. Brown taught in many prestigious nursing schools, and she was one of the first nurses to write a research text, *Research in Nursing,* in 1958.

Biography

Born: Dec. 5, 1908, Alexis, Ill. **Education:** Western Illinois State Teachers College, Macomb, 1930 (bachelor of education); graduate studies in English, Univ. of Iowa, Iowa City;

Univ. of Iowa School of Nursing, Iowa City, 1936; Western Reserve Univ., Cleveland, Ohio (MN); Univ. of Chicago, 1955 (PhD). **Work history:** Ky. State Bd. of Nurse Examiners; Assistant Professor, nursing, Western Reserve Univ., 1945–47; Assistant Professor, Associate Professor, medical nursing, State Univ. of Iowa College of Nursing, 1948–55; Instructor, Loyola Univ., Chicago, 1955–57. **Organizations:** unknown. **Awards:** unknown. **Died:** location unknown.

References and Credits

†Brown AF: Learning to write effectively. AJN 40:1260, 1940.

Brook M: Amy Frances Brown. In Bullough V, Sentz L, Stein AP (eds): American Nursing: A Biographical Dictionary, vol. 2. New York, Garland, 1992, pp 39–40.

December 12

Myra Estrin Levine
1921–1996

"People are defined by all of those who enter their life-space. Some are recalled, revered, and cherished in a multitude of conscious and unconscious ways. Even those who touched a life for a moment and went their way have left some remembrance, however impossible it may be to reconstruct and recognize. I have a treasure of those who did not seek to make me other than what I was, but left their gifts for me to celebrate through all my life afterward." (1988)

Myra Levine had an emergency appendectomy when she was a high school senior, and it introduced her to student nurses and the profession. She faced anti-Semitism in several settings, including nursing. She studied nursing in Chicago during World War II. Her career included teaching, writing, and active involvement with professional organizations. She became known for new approaches to nursing and health care. She established Minnesota's first recovery room and surgical intensive care unit, based on her experiences at Cook County Hospital in Chicago. Her text for clinical nursing was named Book of the Year by the *American Journal of Nursing*. She worked with the American Nurses Association (ANA) to revise the Code for Nurses. Her teaching experiences led her to develop the theory of conservation, which defined four "conservation principles for nursing," which she called "the essential goal of nursing care."

Biography

Born: Dec. 12, 1921, Chicago. **Education:** Cook County Hosp. School of Nursing; Univ. of Chicago (BS); Wayne State Univ., Detroit (MSN). **Work history:** nursing, Minneapolis, Minn., Chicago; Instructor, Cook County Hosp. School of Nursing, Chicago; Director, Drexel Home, Chicago; Instructor, Ford Hosp., Detroit; Faculty, Univ. of Illinois School of Nursing; Administrator, Cook County Hosp.; Faculty, Loyola Univ., Chicago; Faculty, Tel Aviv Univ.; Consultant, Evanston (Ill.) Hosp.; Faculty, Rush Univ., Chicago; Faculty, Univ. of Illinois, Chicago. **Organizations:** Ill. Nurses Assoc.; various ANA committees; Ill. League for Nursing; **Awards:** Professor Emerita, Univ. of Illinois, Chicago; honorary doctorate, Loyola Univ., Chicago. **Died:** Chicago.

References and Credits

†Schorr T, Zimmerman A: Making Choices, Taking Chances: Nurse Leaders Tell Their Stories. St. Louis, CV Mosby, 1988, p 227.

Brook MJ: Myra Levine. In Bullough V, Sentz L (eds): American Nursing: A Biographical Dictionary, vol. 3. New York, Springer, 2000, pp 177–179.

DECEMBER 13

Edna Lois Foley

1878–1943

"No matter how much we shorten its hours, or soften its edges, nursing, like motherhood and teaching, will always be hard work. It will require courage, devotion and the missionary, as well as the pioneer spirit. ...Nursing, wherever done, is an act of mercy, and that is considerably better than a mere profession." (1922)

EDNA LOUISE FOLEY's leadership of the Chicago Visiting Nurse Association was so outstanding that she served as a highly valued resource to communities and nurses across the country. She was always studying and incorporating the best concepts of home care from Europe and the United States, sharing her findings freely through her writings and popular lectures. In 1914 she put together a handbook for her nurses, and it was soon used by other visiting nurse associations as well. A strong advocate for and a personal example of women's involvement in community issues, she always welcomed opportunities to broaden the scope of visiting nursing. For example, she supported a judge's request to have one of her staff nurses assigned to the Court of Domestic Relations, and that nurse became one of the country's first female bailiffs when she was appointed in 1913. Long before the modern civil rights movement, Edna Foley hired and promoted black nurses. She stressed the importance of education, statistics, community reports, and public relations.

Biography

Born: Dec. 17, 1878, Hartford, Conn. **Education:** Smith College (BA); Hartford (Conn.) Hosp. School of Nursing (RN); Boston School of Social Work. **Work history:** Hartford (Conn.) Hosp.; Albany (N.Y.) Children's Hosp.; Boston Children's Hosp.; Consumptive Hosp.; Chicago Tuberculosis Institute (CTE); Chicago Visiting Nurse Assoc. (CVNA); American Red Cross Tuberculosis Commission, Italy. **Organizations:** Red Cross Committee of Chicago Bd. of Charities; President, National Organization for Public Health Nursing; Director, National Society for the Study and Prevention of Tuberculosis; member, exec. committee, National Tuberculosis Assoc.; Director, CTE. **Awards:** Florence Nightingale Medal, International Committee, Red Cross; CVNA Substation named after her; honorary doctorate, Smith College; Citizen Fellow, Institute of Medicine. **Died:** New York City.

References and Credits

†Foley EL: Main issues in public health nursing. In Birnbach N, Lewenson S (eds): First Words: Selected Addresses from the National League for Nursing, 1894–1933. New York, National League for Nursing Press, 1991, pp 136–137.

Davis A: Edna Foley. In Bullough V, Church OM, Stein AP (eds): American Nursing: A Biographical Dictionary, vol. 1. New York, Garland, 1988, pp 115–117.

Brown A: personal communications, December 2000.

December 14

Joyce Travelbee

1925–1972

"It is quite possible that the presence or absence of sympathy in the nursing process affects the patient not only on a psychological level, but on a physiological level too, and may make the difference between the will to live or not to live. It is probably through the act of faith that is sympathy that emotional support is given to another. ... Sympathy is warmth and kindness, a specific expression of compassion, a caring quality experienced on a feeling level and communicated by one human being to another. It cannot be feigned despite the most elaborate communication techniques. ... When a nurse sympathizes with a patient, she communicates to him that he matters, that she wants to assist him, is concerned about him ... because he is himself and no one else." (1964)

THROUGHOUT HER CAREER as a staff nurse and nursing school faculty member, Joyce Travelbee kept her focus on psychiatric nursing. A nationally recognized nurse-theorist, she published two texts related to psychiatric nursing as well as articles about behavior, communication, observation, rapport, sympathy, and envy. She wrote that the challenge to nursing practice was to continue to give priority to the therapeutic nurse-patient relationship rather than yield to superficial interactions. A lay nun of the contemplative order founded by St. Teresa of Avila in the sixteenth century, the Order of the Discalced Carmelites, she gained a deeper spiritual dimension through readings and prayer to her understanding of human relationships. Other influences on her were the psychotherapist Victor Frankl and Ida Jean Orlando, the nurse-theorist who developed the effective nursing process theory, as Travelbee sought meaning in human suffering and illness and defined the helping qualities in the nurse-patient relationship.

Biography

Born: Dec. 14, 1925, New Orleans. **Education:** Charity Hosp. School of Nursing, New Orleans; Louisiana State Univ. Medical Center School of Nursing (BSN); Yale Univ. (MSN). **Work history:** Staff Nurse, New Orleans, Minneapolis, Minn., N.Y.C., Washington, D.C.; Staff Nurse, Instructor, DePaul Hosp., New Orleans; Faculty, Charity Hosp., New Orleans, Louisiana State Univ.; New York Univ.; Univ. of Mississippi, Jackson; Hotel Dieu School of Nursing. **Organizations:** unknown. **Awards:** Kappa Delta Pi; Teacher of the Year Award, Univ. of Mississippi; Outstanding Alumni Award, Louisiana State Univ. **Died:** New Orleans.

References and Credits

†Travelbee J: What's wrong with sympathy? AJN 64:70, 1964.

Kraft L: Joyce Travelbee. In Bullough V, Sentz L, Stein AP (eds): American Nursing: A Biographical Dictionary, vol. 2. New York, Garland, 1992, pp 328–330.

Ida Jean Orlando's Nursing Process Theory, available on-line at http://www.uri.edu/nursing/schmieding/orlando.

December 15

Thelma M. Schorr

1924–

"In 1949, as a Bellevue head nurse, I wrote a petition to protest the 'dumping' of TB patients into open wards with no isolation equipment. All 45 nurses working in medicine signed it. No one in hospital administration or in the office of the New York City Commissioner of Hospitals paid any attention to it, so we went directly to the newspapers. It made front page headlines, and then the hospital quickly accepted all of our recommendations. The Commissioner warned me that I'd 'be a troublemaker' all my life." (1988)

Although Thelma Schorr is uncertain what attracted her to nursing, she recalls a childhood during which her mother was frequently hospitalized. Schorr was fourteen when her mother died, and a caring and sensitive nurse accompanied the disbelieving teenager to see her mother's body. Assertive and articulate, Thelma Schorr evolved from staff nursing to leadership in nursing journalism. When she was a head nurse at Bellevue Hospital in New York, her petition drive to protest the transfer of patients with tuberculosis onto open wards became a headline story in the New York newspapers.

The story made the hospital listen to the nurses and caught the attention of the *American Journal of Nursing (AJN)*. It also resulted in a job offer that changed the direction of her professional career. She worked for the *Journal* while completing her baccalaureate degree in nursing, then officially became a member of the editorial staff in 1952. She rose through the ranks to editor-in-chief and in 1981 became the third woman in the history of the company to become its president and publisher. In addition to the *American Journal of Nursing,* she was also responsible for the company's numerous other publications. In 1988, Schorr and Anne Zimmerman published *Making Choices, Taking Chances: Nurse Leaders Tell Their Stories.* It filled a void with first person accounts by a sampling of contemporary nurse leaders in a collection rich with cander and professionalism. In 1999, Schorr published, with Maureen S. Kennedy, *100 Years of American Nursing: Celebrating a Century of Caring.* Thelma Schorr often spoke before nursing groups, and her common theme was to stress the importance of independence and to encourage involvement. As she stated in an editorial, "You can't be Gloria Steinem at a meeting and Phyllis Schlafly on your ward."

Biography

Born: Dec. 15, 1924. New Haven, Conn. **Education:** Bellevue Hosp. School of Nursing (RN); Teachers College, Columbia Univ. (BSN). **Work history:** Charge Nurse, Bellevue Hosp.; editorial staff, *AJN;* President, Publisher, American Journal of Nursing Co.; Community Healthcare Network; board member, Editorial Consultant, Oncology Nursing Society; Consultant, International Council of Nurses, National Student Nurses Assoc. **Organizations:** American Nurses Assoc.; National Advisory Bd., Hadassah Nurses Council; founder, International Academy of Nursing Editors, and Washington, D.C., Nurses Roundtable. **Awards:** Nursing Leadership Award; Honorary Fellow, American Academy of Nursing (AAN); Outstanding American Jewish Nurse, Hadassah; honorary doctorates, Curry College, Norwich Univ., Univ. of Pennsylvania.; Distinguished Service Award in Nursing Award, Boston Univ.; Living Legend, American Academy of Nursing, 2000.

References and Credits

†Schorr T, Zimmerman A: Making Choices, Taking Chances: Nurse Leaders Tell Their Stories. St. Louis, CV Mosby, 1988, p x.

Kilby S: Thelma Schorr. In Bullough V, Sentz L (eds): American Nursing: A Biographical Dictionary, vol. 3. New York, Springer, 2000, pp 250–253.

December 16

Anna Lowell Alline

1864–1934

"We have heard . . . that the number of applicants to training schools is decreasing. The facts do not bear out this statement. We find in the statistics that the increase in the number of student nurses is at the rate of several hundred a year. . . . In 1890, there were one thousand five hundred students . . . ; in 1900, eleven thousand; in 1903 . . . there were thirteen thousand seven hundred. This goes to show that it is an increase in the demand rather than a decrease in the supply. This surely is a matter of encouragement. Nurse training came as a response to a need and has, through the power wrought from intelligence, fidelity and self-sacrifice, become a permanent institution, really essential to the welfare of human kind, and so closely allied to the medical profession that they are inseparable." (1907)

Anna Lowell Alline first prepared and worked as a public school teacher before enrolling in nursing school, a decision opposed by her family. After she completed the nursing program at the Homeopathic Hospital Training School in Brooklyn, New York, she stayed on to work as the assistant to Linda Richards, the nursing superintendent. Alline later succeeded Richards and was active in what is now the National League for Nursing (NLN). Alline extended the nursing school program at the Homeopathic Hospital to three years before she left to study at Columbia University. She was one of two students in the first class of the hospital economics program at Columbia. When she finished the program, she stayed at Columbia to help with the course, and her continued involvement helped to sustain the program. In 1906 she became the first inspector of nurses' training schools in New York. Her findings helped identify problems at the schools and encouraged nurse-educators to find ways to standardize programs. She came out of retirement to work with the Red Cross during World War I.

Biography

Born: Dec. 16, 1864, East Machias, Maine. **Education:** Iowa public and normal schools; Homeopathic Hosp. Training School for Nurses, Brooklyn, N.Y.; Columbia Univ. **Work history:** Schoolteacher, Iowa; various positions, Homeopathic Hosp. Training School, N.Y.; Director, course in hospital economics, Columbia Univ.; Inspector of Nursing Schools, N.Y.; Superintendent, Buffalo (N.Y.) Homeopathic Hosp.; Red Cross work, World War I; Albany (N.Y.) Homeopathic Hosp. **Organizations:** Society of Superintendents of Training Schools for Nurses (later the National League for Nursing). **Awards:** unknown. **Died:** Iowa.

References and Credits

†Alline AL: The supply and demand of students in the nurse training schools. AJN 7:758, 1907.

Sentz L: Anna Lowell Alline. In Bullough V, Church OM, Stein AP (eds): American Nursing: A Biographical Dictionary, vol. 1. New York, Garland, 1988, p 5.

M. Lucille Kinlein

1921–

"My independent practice is all about one professional nurse taking seriously the meaning of the words professional, judgment, decision, authority, responsibility, accountability, truth, justice and charity. It is about one professional nurse who, after making a commitment and devising a way to meet that commitment, helps people who come to her for help. Finally, it is about one professional nurse helping other nurses to fructify their multiple talents to help many other people." (1977)

Lucille Kinlein earned a degree in liberal arts before she was drawn to nursing by patriotism during World War II. After more than two decades in nursing education, she had become convinced that nursing did not control its own practice. She broke from the traditional role of nursing and, in 1971, became the first nurse in the world to open a theory-based independent practice as a nurse generalist. She describes nursing as the extension of the client, and she views nursing as a separate entity whose basic premise is that "the professional nurse must be known by the care she gives to the person for whom she is caring." She developed the profession of Esca, which recognizes that "within each person is the power to take action in living," and this is enhanced by acceptance, acknowledgment, and being heard by another. Her practice, first called "kinleining" by clients, focuses on client self-care. The *Journal of Esca* explains that "ESCA, an acronym, means 'exercise of self-care agency,' moving in that moving power within, which is a universal human process in living." She defines it as the first professional practice of philosophy, assisting clients in the theory of moving in Esca, in living life on a day-to-day basis. Kinlein has given courses and addresses at many universities and served as a consultant to the federal government for a decade.

Biography

Born: Dec. 17, 1921, Ellicott City, Md. **Education:** Notre Dame College, Baltimore (BA); Catholic Univ. of America School of Nursing (BSN, BSNE, MSNE); Univ. of Minnesota (studies in cardiovascular nursing). **Work history:** Faculty: Catholic Univ. School of Nursing, Johns Hopkins Hosp. School of Nursing, Georgetown Univ. School of Nursing, Alaska Pacific Univ., Univ. of Wisconsin, Superior, Univ. of Southern Mississippi; Washington, D.C., Professional Nurses Examining Bd.; Peace Corps, Togo, W. Africa; established independent generalist nursing practice; established practice of Esca/Kinlein; Author; Lecturer; Consultant. **Organizations:** American Kinlein Assoc.; Institute of Kinlein. **Awards:** book award, *American Journal of Nursing;* numerous civic awards.

References and Credits

†Kinlein ML: Independent Nursing Practice with Clients. Philadelphia, JB Lippincott, 1977, p xii.

Journal of Esca 1:n.p., 1995.

Kinlein L: personal communication, 2001, 2002, 2003.

Kinlein L: resume.

December 18

Joy Ufema (Counsel)

1942–

"We don't really believe we're going to die or we would lead very different lives." (2002)

"I will take to my own deathbed all the memories of my life, and I know that the TV shows and the awards are not going to be of value to me then. My dying will take care of itself if I have simply lived within my beliefs—if I have listened well and learned from my patients … that big houses, big boats, and big bucks don't 'do it' … that it is senseless to work to get 'there' because 'there' does not exist. There is only joy to be found in each moment." (1988)

Joy Ufema was a high-spirited and creative youngster who evolved into an outspoken, honest, patient-centered, and caring nurse specialist. After she attended a workshop by Elizabeth Kübler-Ross, Ufema realized that she had an interest in, and an affinity for, dying patients. She saw that listening or a caring presence was often what the patient needed most. The media focus on her and her work has included interviews for *Sixty Minutes* and *The Phil Donahue Show,* and the Linda Lavin television movie *A Matter of Life or Death.* Ufema sees that each person's death is unique and that a nurse's role includes listening, advocacy, and support. She asks nurses to be assertive in their efforts to provide high-quality care. "Dying persons know exactly what is best for themselves. If they don't come right out and tell you, you have to ask: 'What do you want? What can I do that will help? What are we doing that isn't helping?'" She created the role of nurse specialist in death and dying at Harrisburg (Pa.) Hospital, directed Hospice/Home Care, and founded a three-bed hospice in York, Pennsylvania, for AIDS patients. She says that her thirty years as a thanatologist have been a rich blessing, because she does work that she loves and has been allowed to leave her mark on this earth. The author of *Brief Companions,* she also writes a monthly column, "Insights," for *Death and Dying.*

Biography

Born: Dec. 17, 1942, Altoona, Pa. **Education:** Harrisburg Area Community College (AA); Columbia Pacific (BS, MS). **Work history:** Thanatologist, Nurse Specialist, Harrisburg (Pa.) Hosp.; Director, Hospice/Home Care, Pennsylvania; founder, hospice, York, Pa. **Organizations:** Ars Moriendi; Death Educators and Counselors; advisory bd., *American Journal of Hospice and Palliative Care.* **Awards:** Distinguished Pennsylvanian; AmVet Humanitarian Award; Harrisburg Area Community College Alumni of the Year; York (Pa.) YWCA Woman of the Year.

References and Credits

†Ufema J: personal communication, 2002.

†Schorr T, Zimmerman A: Making Choices, Taking Chances: Nurse Leaders Tell Their Stories. St. Louis, CV Mosby, 1988, p 363.

December 19

June Mellow

1924–

"The concept of nursing therapy grew out of my participation (I was at that time, 1951, the head nurse of the acutely disturbed ward on the Reception Service of the Boston State Hospital) in a therapeutic relationship with a schizophrenic girl. This experience made me aware of certain issues pertaining to psychiatric nursing: the extent to which a nurse can be a significant therapeutic agent directly involved in the outcome of a patient's illness, the importance of making an emotional commitment to the patient, and the therapeutic advantage inherent in the nursing care process, that is, an exchange which is both professional and intimate." (1968)

June Mellow believes resolutely in the need for multidisciplinary collaboration between nurses and physicians in order to provide the care that psychotics need. Her research integrated two specific components of "genuine human caring." The first aspect is for nurses to imaginatively use their daily contacts with patients to help them with their routine needs. She prompted nurses to emphasize the "therapeutic potential ... of what are considered mundane activities associated with women's sphere of work—feeding, bathing, dressing, granting privileges, teaching, comforting, scolding, joking, socializing, counseling." Second, she advised nurses to use their verbal skills to help patients gain awareness of their health problems. Mellow described nursing therapy as a remedy that patients need, especially during acute psychosis. She believes that nursing therapy can prevent a chronic condition and can prepare the client for success in psychotherapy. As director of the clinical laboratory of Boston University's Doctor of Nursing Science Program at the Massachusetts Mental Health Center from 1959 to 1965, she taught approximately twenty psychiatric nurse-educators, who carried this philosophy to other parts of the country. She promoted this thinking, for which she received a research grant from the National Institutes of Health, while addressing national and international conferences. She served as a member of the editorial review board of *Perspectives in Psychiatric Care* from 1967 through 1977.

Biography

Born: Dec. 19, 1924, Gloucester, Mass. **Education:** Salem Hosp. (Mass.) School of Nursing, 1946 (diploma); Univ. of Rochester, N.Y., 1949 (BS, psychology); Boston Univ., 1953, 1965 (MS, EdD). **Work history:** Head Nurse, Research Nurse, Boston State Hosp.; educator in wide variety of clinical settings, colleges, univs. **Organizations:** unknown. **Awards:** scholarship, National League for Nursing.

References and Credits

†Mellow J: Nursing therapy. AJN 68:2365, 1968.

Feigenbaum JC: June Mellow. In Bullough V, Sentz L (eds): American Nursing: A Biographical Dictionary, vol. 3. New York, Springer, 2000, pp 205–207.

DECEMBER 29

Eileen McQuaid Dvorak

1931–1994

"There are three beliefs that have governed choices I have made in my professional life. These beliefs are interrelated and sequential. The one that has been basic is the belief that people must make a difference or their existence is pointless. Because I cannot accept the premise that anyone's existence is pointless, I believe that everyone is meant to make a difference in this life. ...The second belief... is the value I attach to intellectual development. ...Everyone needs to make a contribution. To contribute, one must develop one's talents and abilities to the utmost so that one has the background, knowledge and comprehension necessary to make the greatest gift. ...The third belief... is that one must say yes to opportunities as they arise." (1988)

AN ACCOMPLISHED PIANIST and graduate of a conservatory, Eileen McQuaid Dvorak surprised her family when she announced her decision to study nursing instead of music. She chose nursing because she wanted to be able to make meaningful contributions, and she chose all her positions on the basis of their potential for her to be of service. Her decision to enter nursing was influenced by her beliefs: that life's purpose is to make a difference, that intellectual pursuits enhance one's ability to make a difference, and that one must recognize and accept the occasions for personal and professional growth and contribution as they arise. Her versatile career included clinical nursing, teaching, and administration. She chose teaching because of its opportunities to help nurses integrate a philosophy of caring into their practice and thus influence by example. She saw her administrative work as another way to reach out, by working with those who teach. Given the opportunity to effectively apply all aspects of her belief system, she accepted the invitation to spearhead the National Council of State Boards of Nursing in 1979 and was its first executive director. One of her last contributions to the profession was an audiotape about the impaired nurse, which she made for the National League for Nursing.

Biography

Born: Dec. 16, 1931, Albany, N.Y. **Education:** College of St. Rose, Albany, N.Y. (BSN); Boston College (MS); New York Univ. (PhD); postdoctoral study, Univ. of Chicago. **Work history:** Clinical Pediatric Nurse, St. Mary's Hosp., N.Y.; Carney Hosp., Boston; Children's Hosp., Chicago; Faculty, Brady Maternity Hosp., Albany, N.Y.; Hudson Valley (N.Y.) Community College; Boston College School of Nursing; Rush-Presbyterian–St. Luke's Hosp., Chicago; Univ. of Illinois School of Nursing, Chicago; Supervisor, Nursing Education, N.Y. State Education Dept.; founder, first exec. director, National Council of State Bds. of Nursing; Dean, Marcella Niehoff School of Nursing, Loyola Univ., Chicago; Researcher; Consultant; Author. **Organizations:** American Nurses Assoc., Sigma Theta Tau, Kappa Gamma Pi. **Awards:** unknown. **Died:** Westchester, Ill.

References and Credits

†Schorr T, Zimmerman A: Making Choices, Taking Chances: Nurse Leaders Tell Their Stories. St. Louis, CV Mosby, 1988, pp 86–89.

Dvorak D: personal communication, 2002.

Eileen McQuaid Dvorak. In Franz J, Vandervort-Jones P (eds): Who's Who in American Nursing, 1986–87, 2d ed. Owings Mills, Md., Society of Nursing Professionals, 1987, p 138.

December 21

Thelma Marguerite Ingles

1909–1983

"Good nursing is that nursing which conveys an unspoken message to a patient. The message says: 'I am taking care of you because I want to help you feel better and get better. It is important to me that you feel better and get better. You can be yourself with me. If you are frightened, you may tell me you are frightened and I will understand; if you are angry, you may tell me you are angry and I will not judge you; if you are in pain, I will comfort you. I want to take care of you, and I know how to take care of you. You are safe with me.'" (1959)

ALTHOUGH THELMA INGLES earned both undergraduate and advanced degrees in English literature, she went into nursing, attracted to the profession after a conversation with a friend. She went on to become a nursing pioneer who took graduate nursing in a new direction. When Ingles was a faculty member at Duke University, she designed medical-surgical nursing instruction as a partnership between nurses and physicians, creating improved working relations between medicine and nursing in the clinical setting. She accepted an invitation to spend a year of clinical study with Dr. Eugene Stead of Duke's Department of Medicine, then developed the role of clinical nurse specialist at the master's level. This allowed the nurse to have both a closer working relationship with physicians and greater decision making and responsibility in the advanced clinical care of patients. Although the National League for Nursing did not endorse the concept, her thinking received support from innovative nursing leaders like Lydia Hall and Frances Reiter, and Ingles's ideas about nursing changed the course of graduate nursing education nationally.

Biography

Born: Dec. 16, 1909, Redfield, S.D. **Education:** Univ. of California, Los Angeles (BA); Massachusetts General Hosp. (RN); Western Reserve Univ., Cleveland, Ohio (MA); additional coursework, Univ. of California, Berkeley. **Work history:** Nursing Instructor, Massachusetts General Hosp., Fitchburg (Mass.) Hosp. School of Nursing; Staff Nurse, Boston Nursery for Blind Children; nurse for physicians, Ohio; Charge Nurse, St. Luke's Hosp., Cleveland; Director of Nursing Education, Univ. of Virginia; Red Cross nurse, established and taught nursing program, Istanbul, Turkey; Faculty, Duke Univ. School of Nursing; Consultant, Rockefeller Foundation, Peace Corps, Project HOPE, Robert Wood Johnson Foundation. **Organizations:** unknown. **Awards:** Thelma Ingles Writing Awards Program, Duke Univ. **Died:** La Jolla, Calif.

References and Credits

†Ingles T: What is good nursing? AJN 59:1246, 1959.

Wilson RL: Thelma Ingles. In Bullough V, Church OM, Stein AP (eds): American Nursing: A Biographical Dictionary, vol. 1. New York, Garland, 1988, pp 184–188.

December 22

Mavis Orisca Pate

1925–1972

"Undoubtedly, the most effective teaching was that done by the operating room staff on an individual basis: demonstration, supervised practice, and incidental instruction. ...Problem solving in the Hope Operating Room was a process of improvising, compromise and tolerance. Because of barriers in communication, and our abbreviated time in port, the demonstration of good techniques in practice was our only teaching opportunity. ...Project HOPE's mission was based on the belief that better understanding can be achieved on a personal level through friendship, ... sharing knowledge, ... [and] helping others to help themselves. ...We were certain we had attained at least one goal of the People-to-People Health Foundation: Americans had worked directly with Indonesians; each had come to know and respect the other; lasting friendships and understanding had been achieved." (ca. 1960)

MAVIS PATE WAS one of twenty-four nurses selected from a field of one thousand applicants to help staff the U.S. floating hospital on its maiden goodwill voyage in 1960. Owned by the People-to-People Health Foundation, the privately funded hospital ship was seen as a way to promote world peace through understanding and service. It continues to serve today. Like many of the nurse volunteers, Pate brought operating room experience. She was the operating room nurse supervisor on the Project HOPE (Health Opportunity for People Everywhere) ship bound for Indonesia and South Vietnam. Her *Diary of Hope* describes their work on the SS *Hope* in fascinating detail. The medical crew provided health services on shore and on ship, seeing thousands of patients, performing major surgery for hundreds, and teaching nurses and doctors from Indonesia and Vietnam. Upon her return to the States, she prepared academically as a foreign missionary. While she was serving as a Baptist missionary nurse in East Pakistan (Bangladesh), Thailand, and the Gaza Strip, she was killed in an attack on the van in which she was transporting children in Gaza. She is buried there, near the school of nursing where she taught.

Biography

Born: Dec. 23, 1925, Ringgold, La. **Education:** North Louisiana Sanitarium School of Nursing (RN); postgraduate course, Polyclinic Medical School and Hosp., N.Y.C.; Northwestern State College, La. (BSN); Southwestern Baptist Theological Seminary, Ft. Worth, Texas. **Work history:** OR Nurse, North Louisiana Sanitarium, Project HOPE; Missionary Nurse. **Organizations:** unknown. **Awards:** Pin of Distinction, American Assoc. of Univ. Women, upon graduation from Northwestern State College. **Buried:** Gaza.

References and Credits

†Pate, Mavis. Diary of Hope. No publisher or date listed. pp 23, 25, 34, 35.

Ledbetter PJ: Mavis Pate. In Bullough V, Church OM, Stein AP (eds): American Nursing: A Biographical Dictionary, vol. 1. New York, Garland, 1988, pp 257–258.

December 23

Josephine May Nesbit

1894–1993

"We were the first Nurses in the United States Army to be subjected to actual combat; on Bataan there simply were no 'rear areas.' Although we worked around the clock, we were careful to ensure that when our troops saw a woman Nurse that Nurse had to look as much a woman as circumstances would permit." (ca. 1944)

"If my Filipino nurses don't go, I'm not going either." (ca. 1944)

"Girls! Girls! You've got to sleep today. You can't weep and wail over this, because you have to work tonight." (ca. 1944)

"Quit worrying! Just accept what comes." (ca. 1944)

"Look, all of us are starving." (ca. 1944)

Josephine Nesbit was known to be a tiger, affectionately called Josie by all patients and personnel while she was head nurse of Jungle Hospital #2 on Bataan. The twenty-six Filipino nurses called her Mama Josie. She refused her superior officer's command to evacuate only U.S. nurses from Bataan to Corregidor when the Japanese Army was approaching. Her steadfast determination ensured that the Filipino nurses and the civilian women working with them would be included in the evacuation. Later, as second in command of the Santo Tomas Internment Camp Hospital in Manila from 1942 until 1945, she was the vital force that kept the women functioning as a team to stay alive for the duration. She listened to them and comforted them in various ways. The nurses under her command adapted to the jungle, monkeys, rats, malaria and dengue fevers, dysentery, and starvation. The inscription on the marker erected by the men of the Bataan Death March to honor the nurses reads in part: "They lived on a starvation diet, shared the bombing, strafing, sniping, sickness and disease while working endless hours of heartbreaking duty." For nearly four years the nurses made the best of their deprived situation and administered to others and to each other. When Nesbit returned home and retired from the military, she married and continued to lobby on behalf of the nurses when she felt that the Veterans Administration failed to meet the needs of the former prisoners of war. At Christmas and/or on birthdays, she remembered the nurses on her Philippine staff, "her girls," with greeting cards. She received more than a dozen military awards and nearly lived to one hundred.

Biography

Born: Dec. 23, 1894, near Butler, Mo. **Education:** nursing school, Kansas, 1914; military reserves, influenza epidemic, 1918. **Work history:** military nursing, Texas, Hawaii, Philippines, 1940; Chief Nurse, Sternberg Hosp., Philippines; second in command of all army nurses, 1941; Second Lt., relative rank; coordinated nearly 100 army nurses in Manila; responsible for General Hospital #2; second in command, Santo Tomas Internment Camp prison hosp. **Oraganizations:** unknown. **Awards:** military awards, incl. Bronze Star, 1941–1945. **Died:** San Francisco.

References and Credits

†Norman E: We Band of Angels: The Untold Story of American Nurses Trapped on Bataan by the Japanese. New York, Random House, 1999, pp 46, 86, 6, 72, 77.

Norman EM: Josephine Nesbit. In Bullough V, Sentz L (eds): American Nursing: A Biographical Dictionary, vol. 3. New York, Springer, 2000, pp 215–218.

December 24

Mary Elizabeth Gladwin

1861–1939

"Many of us have labored hard in this field of nursing education. We have spent years in the work which our hands found to do. We have fought many battles. Sometimes we lost and again we have been victorious. Now we see that much we thought permanent must be torn away, very soon it will go into the discard. But after all, isn't that what good and honest work is for, to make better and finer work possible? It is not meant to stand as long as the world lasts. If all our effort means simply that another generation can profit by our mistakes and labor, and go on to the victory which has been denied to us, then it is all worthwhile and we should rest content. Changes come and go; it is only the spirit that lives." (1929)

Mary Elizabeth Gladwin was a high school science teacher before she enrolled in nursing school, and her versatile professional career included military nursing, Red Cross nursing, and nursing education. She interrupted her nursing studies to work in Cuba during the Spanish-American War. She also served as a military nurse in many parts of the world during the Russo-Japanese War and World War I, and she was honored by many countries for her service. She worked as a nursing supervisor with the Red Cross, at home and abroad, and was very supportive of the Red Cross volunteers.

For example, her encouragement of those whom she sent to work with flood victims in Ohio seemed to make them tireless, as they provided food and supplies and cared for injuries. When she was working with other Red Cross nurses in Serbia during World War I and saw the futility of war, she remarked, "War will end when youth is taught what war really means—the conflict of the greedy." Later, she organized the Visiting Nurse Service of Akron, Ohio, and she then held leadership positions in hospital supervision and nursing education.

Biography

Born: Dec. 24, 1861, Staffordshire, England. **Education:** Buchtel College, Akron, Ohio; Boston City Hosp. (RN). **Work history:** Army Nurse, Spanish-American War, Cuba; Red Cross nurse, Philippines, Japan; Superintendent, Beverly (Mass.) Hosp.; Superintendent of Nurses, Women's Hosp., N.Y.C.; welfare worker for women, B.F. Goodrich Rubber Co.; George Perkins Visiting Nurses Assoc., Akron; Nurse, World War I; Indiana Director of Nursing Education; Minn. State Bd. of Nurse Examiners; St Mary's Hosp., Minn. **Organizations:** American Nurses Assoc.; Ohio Nurses Assoc.; American Red Cross. **Awards:** Japanese Order of the Crown, Port Arthur Medal, government of Japan; Serbian Royal Red Cross Order of St. Sava; La Croix de Charite; Russian Imperial Medal; Ribbon of St. Anne; Florence Nightingale Medal, International Committee, Red Cross; U.S. medal for service in Spanish-American War. **Died:** Akron, Ohio.

References and Credits

†Gladwin ME: Address. In Birnbach N, Levenson S (eds): First Words: Selected Addresses from the National League for Nursing, 1894–1933. New York, National League for Nursing Press, 1991, p 274.

Bullough V: Mary Elizabeth Gladwin. In Bullough V, Church OM, Stein AP (eds): American Nursing: A Biographical Dictionary, vol. 1. New York, Garland, 1988, pp 134–135.

Snodgrass M: Historical Encyclopedia of Nursing. Santa Barbara, Calif., ABC-CLIO, 1999, p 281.

December 25

Clara (Clarissa Harlowe) Barton

1821–1912

"Tomorrow will be the first day that we shall stand in this great work all by ourselves, with no help, no funds back of us, and no one to create *them. It is a perilous situation—if we fail we are lost." (1893)*

"30,000 to 35,000 people were knocking, knocking at our doors beseeching and imploring us in the most heartrending tones to be saved from starvation and perishing from the cold [in the South Carolina Sea Islands]." (1894)

Clara Barton's birth was a Christmas gift to nursing. Her parents instilled benevolence in her, and it led to her lifetime of work with those in need. Described by a childhood friend as having "a native genius for nursing," Barton was twelve when she nursed a sick sibling for two years. She began her career as a volunteer, visiting the sick and distributing supplies during the Civil War. Her tireless and courageous efforts in caring for the injured during the Battle of Cedar Mountain resulted in her affectionate nickname, the "Angel of the Battlefield." She established the Bureau of Records of Missing Army Men at her own expense to help families learn the whereabouts of loved ones, and she worked for the proper burial of the thirteen thousand soldiers who died at Andersonville.

While she was in Europe in 1869–1870, she learned of the International Red Cross and worked for years to have the United States ratify the Geneva Agreement for neutral humanitarian aid (which it did in 1882). In 1881 she founded the American National Red Cross, which she led until her retirement in 1904 at eight-three. She was seventy-two when she met one of her greatest challenges. Despite insufficient supplies, little money, and few volunteers, she directed aid to victims of the hurricane that devastated the Sea Islands off the coast of South Carolina. After the devastating Johnstown flood of 1889 her leadership of Red Cross volunteers in Pennsylvania provided relief to more than twenty-five thousand people. The governor later praised her for treating people "with such dignity that the charity of the Red Cross had no sting." According to the writer Jennie Bryan, Barton's greatest achievement was "turning public attention to the human costs of war and natural disaster." Barton said of the Red Cross, "It is a peculiar institution, without nationality, race, creed or sect, embracing the entire world in its humanizing bond of brotherhood, without arbitrary laws or rules, and yet stronger than armies, and higher than thrones."

Biography

Born: Dec. 25, 1821, North Oxford, Mass. **Education:** Liberal Institute, Clinton, N.Y. **Work history:** Schoolteacher; Clerk, U.S. Patent Office; Civil War volunteer nurse; Philanthropist; established Bureau of Records of Missing Army Men; volunteer, Andersonville Memorial; volunteer, International Red Cross; founder American Red Cross. **Organizations:** unknown. **Awards:** numerous International Red Cross honors; National Women's Hall of Fame. **Buried:** Oxford, Mass.

References and Credits

†Pryor E: Clara Barton: Professional Angel. Philadelphia, University of Pennsylvania Press, 1987, pp 277, 279, 262.

Barton C: The Red Cross. Washington, D.C., American Historical Press, American National Red Cross, 1888, p 672.

Brockett JP: Woman's Work in the Civil War. Computer program. Oakman, Ala., H-Bar Enterprises, 1995, p 114.

Bryan J: Health and Science. New York, Hampstead Press, 1988, p 22.

Sabin LE: Clara Barton. In Bullough V, Church OM, Stein AP (eds): American Nursing: A Biographical Dictionary, vol. 1. New York, Garland, 1988, pp 16–19.

December 26

Hattie Bessent

1926–

"When I was 12 or 13, I started working as a volunteer in a nursing home. I remember one day overhearing a physician saying that someone at the home had just died of loneliness. That kind of desolation has haunted me, and in a way I've never left that place. I still visit there when I'm in Jacksonville. ...My parents died when I was nine and my sister was six. I believe that may have something to do with my feeling haunted by loneliness and also my belief that one of the greatest accomplishments in life is to ease another's pain. Of course, that is what nursing is about." (1988)

Hattie Bessent learned to comfort the sick by watching her pastor grandfather as she accompanied him on home visits to parishioners. Raised and inspired by her grandmother, who always expected her to do her best, she went on to personal and professional achievements that attest to that philosophy. A trailblazing black nurse, she has a wide array of experience in mentoring and developing programs for students and professionals. She worked diligently throughout her professional career to increase the pool of minority nurses and to prepare them as leaders in nursing who would assume roles as educators, researchers, and clinicians in mental health services. She generated more than $10 million in grants from the federal government, foundations, and other agencies to support projects for students enrolled in master's and doctoral programs and to facilitate the development and enhancement of minorities in the profession of nursing. She has served in several professional roles and had a profound influence as deputy director of the Minority Fellowship Programs of the American Nurses Association (ANA). During her tenure more than 275 nurses earned advanced degrees, and they now contribute to the delivery of mental health services across the country as practitioners, administrators, and educators. Bessent edited *Strategies for Recruitment, Retention, and Graduation of Minority Nurses in Colleges of Nursing* (1997) and *Minority Nurses in the New Century* (2002).

Biography

Born: Dec. 26, 1926, Jacksonville, Fla. **Education:** Florida A&M Univ. (BSNE); Univ. of Indiana (MS); Univ. of Florida (EdD); Tulane Univ. (diploma, mental health and family consultation); Institute for Educational Management, Harvard Univ. (diploma). **Work history:** Charge Nurse, Jacksonville, Fla.; Faculty, Univ. of Florida, Gainesville; Director, Minority Fellowship Program, ANA; Author; Mental Health Consultant; Speaker; member, President Jimmy Carter's Commission on Mental Health Manpower Task Force; appointed by Carter to Friendship Treaty for Americans to China; Kellogg Foundation escort for International Kellogg Fellows around the world; member, numerous boards; On-Site Project Review Instrument Evaluator, Head Start; Project Director, Leadership Enhancement and Development Project, Kellogg Foundation. **Organizations:** Fla. Nurses Assoc.; ANA. **Awards:** praised in *Congressional Record* by Sen. Daniel Inouye of Hawaii for her work with minorities, 1987; Recognition Award, ANA; minority reading room at ANA named in her honor; Fellow, American Academy of Nursing; honorary doctorate, Hunter College, 2002.

References and Credits

†Schorr T, Zimmerman A: Making Choices, Taking Chances: Nurse Leaders Tell Their Stories. St. Louis, CV Mosby, 1988, pp 24, 26.

Carnegie M: The Path We Tread, 3d ed. New York, National League for Nursing Press, 1995.

Hine D: Black Women in White. Indianapolis, Indiana University Press, 1989.

Bessent H: personal communication, 2002.

DECEMBER 27

Katherine Koster

1889–UNKNOWN

"Our nearest physician in winter is a hundred and twenty miles distant and to reach him one would have to travel for five days with a dog team and sled over a scarcely used trail. . . . Caring for the ill in their homes one is often surprised at the far reaching results of the power of demonstration. I have in mind the care of a woman to whom I was called one day. The messenger told me 'his mother had cut her finger off.' I found an incision which required several sutures, and I dressed her hand in the cabin. A few weeks later her daughter was with a hunting party who were miles from the mission. While removing the skin from the game, a keen-edged knife in the hand of one of the men slipped and inflicted a deep gash in the lower part of the thigh. The young woman who had watched her mother's hand being cared for, immediately applied a tourniquet, and sutured the wound, using strands of her hair for suture material. When the man returned home some weeks later the wound was almost healed." (1920)

KATHERINE KOSTER WAS orphaned soon after she entered nursing school and always dreamed of serving as a missionary nurse for her church. Although her application was initially denied when she was found to have a heart murmur, she persevered and obtained several other opinions regarding her ability to work. She was finally admitted with the stipulation that she serve at her own risk. She answered that she was "more than willing and even glad to take that risk sincerely hoping that I may with God's help accomplish the work I so greatly desire to do." For four years she worked eleven miles north of the Arctic Circle at the St. Johns-in-the-Wilderness Episcopal Church in Alaska before leaving for health reasons.

Biography

Born: Dec. 26, 1889, Drifton, Pa. **Education:** Training School for Nurses, St. Timothy's Hosp., Roxborough, Pa. **Work experience:** Missionary Nurse, Episcopal Church, Alaska. **Organizations:** unknown. **Awards:** unknown. **Died:** location unknown.

References and Credits

†Koster K: North of the Arctic Circle. Public Health Nurse 12:578, 579, 1920.

Peters J: personal communication, April 2000.

December 28

Sister Kathleen Black

1908–1984

"To those who are our patients, our ability to assess their needs may become so vital that it is a matter of life or death. But whether or not our patients are in a situation of acute crisis, nursing sets its need-meeting aims considerably higher than is the case with any of the other helping professions. ...We in nursing keep before us the objective of insuring that all the needs of our patients will be met. In principle, too, we uphold a further aim that goes considerably beyond that. In so far as possible, we attempt to obtain need satisfaction for each patient on a specifically individual basis. Although we hold these as our stated aims, it is obvious that we often fall far short of attaining them in our day to day care of patients. It follows that our effectiveness will be improved by anything that will make it possible for us to assess our patients needs more accurately." (1967)

Sister Kathleen Black was a catalyst for improved nursing knowledge and service to the mentally ill through her involvement with the National League for Nursing, the Menninger Foundation, and the Joint Commission on Mental Illness and Health. Her career included a position as the director of nursing education at the Menninger Clinic. She directed graduate programs in psychiatric nursing at several major universities, and she helped plan programs to teach mental health in schools of public health. She was the author of many published works dealing with the care of the psychiatric patient, including "Appraising the Psychiatric Patient's Needs," an article that is considered a classic because of the way it presents assessing, interviewing, and observation. She had a late religious vocation and in 1959 joined the Catholic Order of the Sisters of Mercy, followed by another two decades in nursing.

Biography

Born: Dec. 19, 1908, Kent, England. **Education:** Ontario (Can.) Hosp. School of Nursing; Univ. of Toronto School of Nursing; Univ. of Chicago (BS); Teachers College, Columbia Univ. (master's). **Work history:** Staff Nurse, Administrator, Sheppard and Enoch Pratt Hosp., Baltimore; Director of Nurse Education, Menninger Foundation, Topeka, Kans.; Administrator, Univ. of Minnesota, Univ. of Pittsburgh, Teachers College; Director, Mental Health and Psychiatric Nursing Advisory Service, National League for Nursing (NLN); organized Psychiatric and Mental Health Council; held numerous teaching workshops; Faculty, Catholic Univ. of America, State Univ. of New York, Binghamton. **Organizations:** NLN; Joint Commission on Mental Illness and Health; Assoc. of Schools of Public Health. **Awards:** Professor Emeritus, State Univ. of New York, Binghampton. **Buried:** Gate of Heaven Cemetery, Hartsdale, N.Y.

References and Credits

†Black K: Assessing patients' needs. In Yura H, Walsh MB (eds): The Nursing Process: Assessing, Planning, Implementing, and Evaluating. Washington, D.C.: Catholic Univ. of America Press, 1967, p 1.

Manfreda ML: Sister Kathleen Black. In Bullough V, Church OM, Stein AP (eds): American Nursing: A Biographical Dictionary, vol. 1. New York, Garland, 1988, pp 28–30.

December 29

Ruby Grace Bradley

1907–2002

"Then the happiest day in our lives—the liberation on Feb 3. We knew the Americans were near. Then, too, we could hear sound of artillery fire in the distance ... then the grand smell of American gasoline and the sound of American voices. ... The campus was filled with shouting, internees rushing from the buildings to greet the soldiers. ... We did not do much celebrating of our liberation as the casualties started to mount among the internees and soldiers. The building received numerous direct hits, killing and wounding some. ... It was hard to see our friends who had waited for this day being killed, or maimed for life when freedom was so close. Although we nurses had been on hospital duty during internment—malnourished and in need of rest, we were stimulated to work with greater effort. ... We were happy that we were free. ... We do not ask for anything—most of us would like to go back. I have lost my heart to the Filipino people—they are so sincere, so pathetically grateful to the Americans for their liberation, so helpful to us in time of need. ... It is great to again be with our Army—there isn't a better patient in the world than a G.I. soldier. When the tanks rolled into Santo Tomas we were eternally grateful to the people back home who had given us such a grand Army." (Date unknown)

"I hope in Victory we will remember how near destruction we came four years ago, the horrors of invasion that almost cost for us the land we love." (Date unknown)

COL. RUBY BRADLEY retired from the U.S. Army as a nurse administrator in 1963. She held the distinction of being the most decorated woman in the history of the U.S. Army. She was captured by the Japanese in World War II, and she performed duty as a general nurse while a prisoner of war at Camp John Hay, Baguio, Manila, from December 1941, until her release on February 3, 1945. For her outstanding service while she was a prisoner of war and for her service in Korea, she was awarded the Florence Nightingale Medal by the International Committee of the Red Cross. When she retired, she received the third Oak Leaf Cluster to the Legion of Merit. She was awarded an honorary degree by the University of West Virginia. She appeared on the television program *This Is Your Life* in 1954.

BIOGRAPHY

Born: Dec. 19, 1907, Spencer, W. Va. **Education:** Biddle Teachers College, Glenville, W. Va., 1926 (teaching certificate); Philadelphia General Hosp. School of Nursing, 1933; Univ. of California, 1949 (BSNE); McGuire General Hosp.; Univ. of California, 1947; Management of Mass Casualties, Medical Field Service School, 1961. **Work history:** Nurse Administrator; Surgical Nurse; Chief Nurse; Assistant Director, Nursing Activities, Headquarters, Brooke Army Medical Command, Ft. Sam Houston, Texas. **Organizations:** unknown. **Awards:** Florence Nightingale Medal, International Committee, Red Cross; many decorations, medals, and badges, incl. Korean Service Medal with One Silver Star (in lieu of five Bronze Service Stars). **Died:** Hazard, Ky.

REFERENCES AND CREDITS

†Bradley RG: Speech for Victory Loan Drive. From faxed copy of her service history sent by Public Affairs Office, U.S. Army Reserve Personnel Center, March 25, 1997.

Col. Ruby G. Bradley. In Feller C, Moore CJ: Highlights in the History of the Army Nurse Corps, revised and expanded edition. Washington, D.C., U.S. Army Center of Military History, 1995, p 27.

Norman EM: Ruby Bradley. In Bullough V, Sentz L (eds): American Nursing: A Biographical Dictionary, vol. 3. New York, Springer, 2000, pp 24–26.

December 30

Elizabeth Gordon Fox

1884–1958

"Whether a Visiting Nurse is a Public Health Nurse ... depends somewhat on the definition of public health. ...If the modern conception of public health means the securing for each and every person a equal opportunity to have a sound body, normal development, good health, every chance within human limits to complete and prompt recovery from illness through adequate service, protection from degenerative disease in middle age, and a full span of life of maximum usefulness, then the Visiting Nurse is one of the most valuable instruments of public health." (1919)

ELIZABETH FOX WAS a visionary leader who actively promoted holistic patient care, an idea that seemed radical to the traditionalists of her day. Described by the writer Mary Roberts as "forceful and clear-thinking," Fox recognized and promoted the necessity of treating the family unit and the importance of community-based health services. When she directed the Public Health Nursing Service of the American Red Cross from 1918 to 1930, she promoted rural public health nursing. Her focus and influence resulted in an increase of the national staff of public health nurses to two thousand. As a result, health care services, once sparse and available in only a few scattered areas, expanded halfway across the country and included rural school nursing. Her work received the highest honor when, in 1931, she was the first civilian nurse to be awarded the Florence Nightingale Medal of the International Committee of the Red Cross. Later, when she was the executive director of the Visiting Nurse Association (VNA) in New Haven, Connecticut, it became the model agency in the nation. In large part this was because she put into practice her controversial concept of "the nurse as an equal partner in a balanced health-care team." This set the working standard that attracted nurses who came from around the country and other nations to observe and learn from her, which strengthened her influence on nursing practice in their agencies. In 1958 the Connecticut Public Health Association was about to bestow on Fox the Winslow Award for Distinguished Service in public health nursing when she collapsed and died.

Biography

Born: 1884, Milwaukee, Wisc. **Education:** Univ. of Wisconsin (BA); basic nursing program, postgraduate study, Johns Hopkins Hosp. School of Nursing. **Work history:** Administrator, Dayton, Ohio, VNA; Administrator, Washington, D.C., VNA; Director, Public Health Nursing Service, American Red Cross; Faculty, Yale Univ. School of Nursing; Exec. Director, New Haven (Conn.) VNA. **Organizations:** National Organization for Public Health Nursing; Conn. State Nurses Assoc.; Conn. Public Health Assoc. **Awards:** Florence Nightingale Medal, International Committee, Red Cross; **Died:** New Haven, Conn.

References and Credits

†Fox EG: Is the visiting nurse a public health nurse? Public Health Nurse 11: 575, 1919.

Fulton J: Elizabeth Fox. In Bullough V, Church OM, Stein AP (eds): American Nursing: A Biographical Dictionary, vol. 1. New York, Garland, 1988, pp 118–119.

Roberts M: American Nursing: History and Interpretation. New York, Macmillan, 1954.

Letocha PE: personal communication, 2000.

December 31

Katharine Ellen Faville

1894–1985

"Does nursing have leaders with sufficient vision? Can they work together? Will they adjust to the changes so rapidly all over the world? Can they define and develop standards and programs suitable to today's needs? Or is this opportunity to be snatched from their hands by others who are willing to confuse safe care for the public with political expediency? ... The concept of one world at peace, and in good health, is ours to work for in every way known to us as citizens and nurses." (1949)

KATHERINE FAVILLE WAS a delegate to the World Health Organization's second meeting, in Rome in 1949 where she reported on the challenge to the nursing profession of the world. The writer Signe Cooper has described Faville, who worked as a teacher, administrator, and organizer, a "a forceful and dynamic person with a critical intellect, vision, and the courage of her convictions." Faville was vigorous in her pursuit of advanced nursing in institutions of higher education. She worked to include minority students in schools of nursing and to promote social justice and high standards in nursing education. She was a creative writer whose articles told the story of nursing in a way that appealed to all readers. She was a valuable recruiter of nursing students in World War II. One student remembers Faville as influencing everyone she came in contact with.

Biography

Born: Dec. 25, 1894, Sauk Center, Minn. **Education:** Univ. of Wisconsin, Madison, 1915, 1916 (BS, MS); Vassar Training Camp, 1918; Massachusetts General Hosp. School of Nursing, 1921 (diploma); public health nursing program, Simmons College, Boston. **Work history:** Chemist, Sears Roebuck laboratories, Chicago; Rural Public Health Nurse, Alcona County, Mich.; Director, Visiting Nurse Service, Wheeling, W. Va.; Nursing Field Representative, American Red Cross, Ky., Ind.; Instructor, public health nursing, Teachers College, Columbia Univ.; Educational Director, Assoc. for Improving Conditions of the Poor; organized Public Health Nursing Program, Wayne State Univ., Detroit; Dean, Western Reserve Univ. School of Nursing, Cleveland, Ohio; Director, Henry Street Visiting Nurse Service, N.Y.C.; National Council for War Service, World War II; Consultant, U.S. Office of Defense Health and Welfare Service, assisted in relocation of Japanese American nurses; Dean, College of Nursing, Wayne State Univ., Detroit. **Organizations:** Fellow, American Public Health Assoc.; bd. of directors, National Organization for Public Health Nursing; member, Committee on Nursing in International Affairs, American Nurses Assoc. (ANA); President, bd. of directors, Mich. League for Nursing; bd. of directors, Mich. Society for Mental Health. **Awards:** Phi Beta Kappa; Mary Mahoney Award, ANA, 1966; Nurse of the Year, Greater Detroit District, Mich. Nurses Assoc.; Faville Hall on Wayne State campus named in her honor; Katharine E. Faville Lectureship estab. 1975, Wayne State Univ. **Died:** Detroit.

References and Credits

†Faville K: The Second World Health Assembly. AJN 49:766, 1949.

Cooper SS: Katherine Faville. In Bullough V, Sentz L, Stein AP (eds): American Nursing: A Biographical Dictionary, vol. 2. New York, Garland, 1992, pp 108–110.

January 18 *Ruth Watson Lubic*

Univ. of Pennsylvania; Univ. of Medicine and Dentistry, N.J.; College of New Rochelle, N.Y.; State Univ. of New York Health Sciences Center, Brooklyn; Pace Univ.; Florence Nightingale Medal, International Committee, Red Cross; Letitia White Award; awards from Case Western Reserve, Univ. of Pennsylvania; Rockefeller Foundation; Columbia Univ.; New York Univ.; American Nurses Assoc.; Fellow, American Academy of Nursing; MacArthur Fellowship "Genius" Award; Leinhard Award, Institute of Medicine; Living Legend, American Academy of Nursing, 2001; honorary membership, Alpha Omega Alpha, the honorary medical society.

REFERENCES AND CREDITS

†Schorr T, Zimmerman A: Making Choices, Taking Chances: Nurse Leaders Tell Their Stories. St. Louis, CV Mosby, 1988, p 235.

Slattery M: Nurse-midwife empowers inner-city women through birth center. American Nurse 30:11, 1998.

Lubic R: personal communication, November 2002.

Lubic RW: Barriers and Conflict in Maternity Care Innovation. New York, National Assoc. of Childbearing Centers, 1979.

Franz J, Vandervort-Jones P (eds): Who's Who in American Nursing, 1986–87, 2d ed. Owings Mills, Md., Society of Nursing Professionals, 1987, p 309.

February 17 *Mary Breckinridge*

REFERENCES AND CREDITS

†Breckinridge M: For France. Public Health Nurse 13:144, 1921.

Bullough V: Mary Breckinridge. In Bullough V, Church OM, Stein AP (eds): American Nursing: A Biographical Dictionary, vol. 1. New York, Garland, 1988, pp 46–48.

Snodgrass ME: Historical Encyclopedia of Nursing. Santa Barbara, Calif., ABC-CLIO, 1999, pp 29–30.

Shoemaker MT: History of Nurse-Midwifery in the United States. New York, Garland, 1984.

ANA Hall of Fame 10/98 American Nurses Association, Washington, D.C. http://www.nursingworld.org/hof.

February 26 *Luther Christman*

REFERENCES AND CREDITS

†Avery C: A conversation with Luther: The Opinions and Predictions of Dr. Luther Christman. Video. Western Connecticut State University, Department of Media Services, 2000.

Hurley A: Luther Christman. In Bullough V, Sentz L, Stein AP (eds): American Nursing: A Biographical Dictionary, vol. 2. New York, Garland, 1992, pp 58–62.

Schorr T, Zimmerman A: Making Choices, Taking Chances: Nurse Leaders Tell Their Stories. St. Louis, Mo., CV Mosby, 1988.

Sullivan E: In a woman's world: Profile of Dr. Luther Christman. Reflections on Nursing Leadership 28 (3):10–17, 2002.

March 3 *Esther Silverstein Blanc*

Univ. of San Francisco General Hosp.; Faculty, Univ. of California, San Francisco. **Organizations:** Calif. Nurses Assoc. **Awards:** Sydney Taylor Book Award of the Assoc. of Jewish Libraries for her children's book, *Berchick* (Volcano Press, 1989). **Died:** San Francisco.

References and Credits

†Blanc ES: Wars I Have Seen. Foreword by H Ference. Volcano, Calif., Volcano Press, 1996, pp 125, 126.

†Fryth J: The Signal Was Spain: The Aid Spain Movement in Britain, 1936–1939. London, Lawrence and Wishart, 1986, pp 140–157.

Patai F: Heroines of the good fight: Testimonies of U.S. volunteer nurses in the Spanish Civil War, 1936–1939. Nurs Hist Rev 3:79–104, 1995.

Blanc ES: unpublished speech, 1938, in Fredericka Martin Collection, Brandeis University Library, Waltham Mass. (Found at National Institutes of Health Library in an Esther Silverstein (Blanc) folder, since moved to New York University along with other Spanish Civil War materials.)

Blanc P: personal communication, 2003.

Gottstein R: personal communication, 2003.

Newman J: personal communication, 2003.

March 13 *Faye Glenn Abdellah*

†Abdellah FG: Application of patient-centered approaches to nursing service. In Abdellah FG, Beland I, Martin A, Matheney R (eds): Patient-Centered Approaches to Nursing. New York, Macmillan, 1960, p 40.

Brook MJ: Faye Abdellah. In Bullough V, Sentz L (eds): American Nursing: A Biographical Dictionary, vol. 3. New York, Springer, 2000, pp 1–3.

Abdellah FG: resume.

Abdellah FG: personal correspondence, 2002.

April 12 *Melanie Creagan Dreher*

Dreher M: Working Men and Ganja Marihuana Use in Rural Jamaica. Philadelphia, Institute for the Study of Human Issues, 1982.

Dreher M, Nugent K, Hudgins R: Prenatal marijuana exposure and neonatal outcomes in Jamaica: An ethnographic study. Pediatrics 93:254–260, 1994.

April 25 *Mary E.P. Davis*

for Nurses, 1889–99; Superintendent, Boston State Hosp., Dorchester, Mass; Superintendent, Washington, D.C., Training School for Nurses; first registrar, Central Directory for Nurses, Boston; organized directories in Philadelphia, Washington, D.C.; Examiner for classes given by Red Cross during World War I. **Organizations:** Vice President, President, ASSTSN; Organizer, founder, Nurses Associated Alumnae of the United States and Canada; Chair, Mass. State Nurses Assoc. legislative committee for enactment of registration law. **Awards:** ANA Hall of Fame, 1982. **Died:** Norwood, Mass.

References and Credits

†Davis MEP: First Words: Selected Addresses from the National League for Nursing, 1894–1933. New York, National League for Nursing Press, 1991, p 248.

Birnbach N: Mary E.P. Davis. In Bullough V, Sentz L, Stein AP (eds): American Nursing: A Biographical Dictionary, vol. 2. New York, Garland, 1992, pp 80–82.

ANA Hall of Fame 10/98 American Nurses Association, Washington, D.C. http://www.nursingworld.org/hof.

April 27 *Mary D. Osborne*

Supervisor of Nurses, Assoc. for Improving the Condition of the Poor, N.Y. (became Community Service Society, 1912); American Red Cross; Director, Public Health Nursing, Mississippi Dept. of Health, 1920. **Organizations:** President, Miss. Nurses Assoc., 1932. **Awards:** recognized by International Council of Nursing, Montreal, for lowering maternal and infant mortality rates, 1929; Miss. Public Health Assoc., Nursing Section, established Mary D. Osborne Public Health Nurse of Year award, 1980. Miss. Health Dept. in Jackson named for her, 1999; American Nurses Assoc. Hall of Fame. **Buried:** Jackson, Miss.

References and Credits

†Osborne MD: Manual for Midwives. Mississippi State Board of Health, 1922, p 39.

Morton M: Mary Osborne. In Bullough V, Sentz L (eds): American Nursing: A Biographical Dictionary, vol. 3. New York, Springer, 2000, pp 224–227.

ANA Hall of Fame 10/98 American Nurses Association, Washington, D.C. http://www.nursingworld.org/hof.

May 2 *Lucie S. Kelly*

References and Credits

†Kelly L: Updating nursing's image. Editorial. Nurs Outlook (Jan–Feb): 17, 1989.

Schorr T, Zimmerman A: Making Choices, Taking Chances: Nursing Leaders Tell Their Stories. St. Louis, CV Mosby, 1988.

Sentz L: Lucie S. Kelly. In Bullough V, Sentz L (eds): American Nursing: A Biographical Dictionary, vol. 3. New York, Springer, 2000, pp 159–162.

May 10 *Peter Buerhaus*

References and Credits

†Harvard School of Public Health press release: Nurse staffing levels directly impact patient health and survival. May 29, 2002, p 2, available on-line at http://www.hsph.harvard.edu/press/releases/press5292002.html.

†Lindeman C: A nursing shortage like none before. Interview with Peter Buerhaus. Creative Nursing 6:5–6, 2000.

Buerhaus P: resume.

Buerhaus P: personal communication, 2002.

May 27 *Lynda Van Devanter Buckley*

References and Credits

†Van Devanter L: An introduction in many languages for Bach Diep (end of last stanza). In Home before Morning. Amherst, University of Massachusetts Press, 2001, p 325.

Van Devanter L, Furey J: Visions of war, Dreams of peace: Writings of women in the Vietnam War. New York, Warner, 1991.

Snodgrass ME: Historical Encyclopedia of Nursing. Santa Barbara, Calif., ABC-CLIO, 1999.

Lynda M. Van Devanter Buckley. In Who's Who in American Nursing, 1996–97, 6th ed. New Providence, N.J., Reed Reference, 1995.

Buckley T: personal correspondence, 2002.

Baumann J: Nurse Van Devanter dies; Advocate for Vietnam vets' rights. Observer Online, Nov. 29, 2002, available at http://www.observernews.com/stories/current/news/112902/van_devanter.shtml.

June 29 *Rozella May Schlotfeldt*

Nursing Consultant to U.S. surgeon general, U.S. Public Health Service, Kellogg Foundation, National Health Research Commission, Walter Reed Army Institute, U.S. Defense Dept., Nursing Research Council, National Academy of Sciences; President, Ohio Bd. of Nursing Education. **Organizations:** American Nurses Assoc.; National League for Nursing; bd. member, Duke Univ. Medical Center, National Academy of Sciences. **Awards:** Fellow, American Academy of Nursing; election to Institute of Medicine, National Academy of Sciences; awards from Wayne State Univ., Univ. of Iowa, American Academy of Nursing, Boston Univ., Univ. of San Diego, Sigma Theta Tau; honorary doctorates from Georgetown, Adelphi, Wayne State, Kent State Univs., Univ. of Illinois, Univ. of Cincinnati, Medical Univ. of South Carolina; Living Legend, American Academy of Nursing, 1995.

References and Credits

†Schlotfeldt R: A Brave, New World: Exercising Options for the Future. Series 82, No. 3. American Association of Colleges of Nursing, Washington, D.C., 1982, p 1.

Schorr T, Zimmerman A: Making Choices, Taking Chances: Nurse Leaders Tell Their Stories. St. Louis, CV Mosby, 1988.

Bullough V: Rozella May Schlotfeldt. In Bullough V, Sentz L, Stein AP (eds): American Nursing: A Biographical Dictionary, vol. 2. New York, Garland, 1992, pp 293–294.

July 8 *Alyce Faye Wattleton*

Biography

Born: July 8, 1943, St. Louis. **Education:** Ohio State Univ. Nursing School (BSN); Columbia Univ. (MS, midwife certificate). **Work history:** Instructor, maternity nursing, Miami Valley (Ohio) Hosp. School of Nursing; Intern, Harlem Hosp., N.Y.C.; Assistant Director, Public Health Nursing, Dayton, Ohio; Exec. Director, Planned Parenthood, Dayton, Ohio; Council of PPFA; President, PPPFA; President, Center for the Advancement of Women; bd. member, Columbia Univ., Institute for International Education, United Nations Assoc. of the U.S.A., Jazz at Lincoln Center; helped establish Center for Gender Equity. **Organizations:** U.S. Committee for UNICEF; Young Presidents Organization; National Advisory Committee of the Tufts School of Public Service; Institute of Medicine Study Committee on Role of Health Depts., National Academy Sciences; Advisory Commission,

Women's Leadership Conference on National Security; Presidential Advisory Commission on the Peace Corps; National Urban Coalition. **Awards:** Award of Excellence, American Public Health Assoc.; John Gardner Award, Independent Sector; National Women's Hall of Fame; Margaret Sanger Award, PPFA; fifteen honorary doctoral degrees; named one of top U.S. executives by *Savvy* magazine; Excellence in Black Communications Award, World Institute of Black Communication; Women's Honors in Public Service, American Nurses Assoc.; Congressional Black Caucus Humanitarian Award; Better World Population Medal, Better World Society.

References and Credits

†Wattleton F: Afterword: An open letter to my daughter. In Life on the Line. New York, Ballentine, 1996, pp 94, 469–470.

Hine D (ed): Black Women in America: An Historical Encyclopedia. Brooklyn, N.Y., Carlson Publishing, 1993, p 1140.

Thompson K: Faye Wattleton. In Hawkins W (ed): African American Biographies. Jefferson, N.C., McFarland, 1992, 436–437.

National Women's Hall of Fame on-line, available at http://www.greatwomen.org/profile.

Cunningham C, Jones A: Faye Wattleton. In Smith JC (ed): Notable Black American Women. Detroit, Gale, 1992.

Wattleton F: personal communication, 2003.

(Alyce) Faye Wattleton. In Conner H (sr ed): Who's Who of American Women, 1999–2000, 21st ed. New Providence, N.J., Marquis Who's Who, 1998, p 1091.

July 13 *Madeleine M. Leininger*

References and Credits

†Leininger M: Founder's focus: Transcultural nursing: A scientific and humanistic care discipline. Journal of Transcultural Nursing 8:55, 1997.

Schorr T, Zimmerman A. Making Choices, Taking Chances: Nurse Leaders Tell Their Stories. St. Louis, CV Mosby, 1988.

Brook M: Madeleine Leininger. In Bullough V, Sentz L (eds): American Nursing: A Biographical Dictionary, vol. 3. New York, Springer, 2000, pp 172–175.

Leininger M: personal communication, 2002.

Leininger M, McFarland M: Transcultural Nursing, 3d ed. New York, McGraw-Hill, 2002.

Leininger M: Culture Care, Diversity, and Universality: A Theory of Nursing. New York, National League for Nursing Press, 1991.

July 30 *Linda H. Aiken*

Schorr T, Zimmerman A: Making Choices, Taking Chances: Nurse Leaders Tell Their Stories. St. Louis, CV Mosby, 1988.

University of Pennsylvania, available on-line at http://www.nursing.upenn.edu/chopr/BIOPages/Linda_Aiken.htm.

Aiken L: Charting the future of hospital nursing. Image 22:72–78, 1990.

Aiken L: resume.

Aiken L: personal communication, 2002.

September 2 *Anne Larson Zimmerman*

References and Credits

†AJN interviews ANA president. AJN 78:1020, 1978.

Zimmerman A: personal communication, 2003.

Appleyard A: Anne Larson Zimmerman. In Bullough V, Sentz L, Stein AP (eds): American Nursing: A Biographical Dictionary, vol. 2. New York, Garland, 1992, pp 370–371.

Schorr T, Zimmerman A: Making Choices, Taking Chances: Nurse Leaders Tell Their Stories. St. Louis, CV Mosby, 1988, p xi.

September 6 *Mary Starke Harper*

Mary Starke Harper Geropsychiatric Hospital (Alabama) named in her honor; Meritorious Awards, Tuskegee Institute, Va.; named one of top ten women in federal government; story of her life told by Voice of America; Fellow, Living Legend, American Academy of Nursing, 2001; Ala. Health Hall of Fame; honorary member, Chi Eta Phi.

References and Credits

†Harper MS (ed): Management and Care of the Elderly. Newbury Park, Calif., Sage, 1991, pp 19–20.

Harper MS: personal communication, March, July 2003.

Light J: Witness to history: Interview with Mary Harper. July 1997, Link Age 2000 on-line, available at http://www.hyperion.advanced.org/10120/treasury/harper.html.

Press release, Office of Women's Health, U.S. Department of Health and Human Services on-line, available at http://www.4woman.gov/owh/minorityPanel/mharper.htm.

Mary Harper. In Franz J, Vandervort-Jones P (eds): Who's Who in American Nursing, 1986–87, 2d ed. Owings Mills, Md., Society of Nursing Professionals, 1987, p 210.

September 8 *Karren Kowalski*

"Mastery of Women's Health," 2002. http://www.rushu.rush.edu/nursing/features/kowalski.html.

Kowalski K: personal communication, February 2003.

Karren Kowalski. In Franz J, Vandervort-Jones P (eds): Who's Who in American Nursing, 1986–87, 2d ed. Owings Mills, Md., Society of Nursing Professionals, 1987.

November 3 *Mary Adelaide Nutting*

Goostray S: Mary Adelaide Nutting. AJN 58:1524–1529, 1958.

Roberts MM: American Nursing History and Interpretation. New York, Macmillan, 1954.

Jensen D: History and Trends of Professional Nursing. St. Louis, CV Mosby, 1959.

Dolan J: Nursing in Society. Philadelphia, WB Saunders, 1973.

ANA Hall of Fame 10/98 American Nurses Association, Washington, D.C. http://www.nursingworld.org/hof.

November 25 *Claire Mintzer Fagin*

ANA; Honorary Recognition Award, ANA; President's Medal, NYU; eleven honorary doctorates; American Nurses Foundation Nightingale Lamp Award; Fellow, Living Legend, American Academy of Nursing, 1998; election to Institute of Medicine, National Academy of Sciences; American Academy of Arts and Sciences; *Who's Who in America;* Honorary Fellow, Royal College of Nursing, U.K.; Professor Emeritus, Dean Emeritus, School of Nursing, Univ. of Pennsylvania.

References and Credits

†Fagin CM: Y2K: Nurses can turn on the heat in health care. In Essays on Nursing Leadership. New York, Springer, 2000, pp 199, 202, 203.

Fagin C: personal communication, 2003.

Schorr T, Zimmerman A: Making Choices, Taking Chances: Nurse Leaders Tell Their Stories. St. Louis, CV Mosby, 1988.

Who's Who in American Nursing, 1996–97, 6th ed. New Providence, N.J., Reed Reference, 1995.

December 9 *Jeanne Quint Benoliel*

References and Credits

†Quint J: The Nurse and the Dying Patient. New York, Macmillan, 1967, pp xi–xiii.

Schorr T, Zimmerman A: Making Choices, Taking Chances: Nurse Leaders Tell Their Stories. St. Louis, CV Mosby, 1988.

Jeanne Quint Benoliel. In Franz J, Vandervort-Jones P (eds): Who's Who in American Nursing, 1986–87, 2d ed. Owings Mills, Md., Society of Nursing Professionals, 1987, p 36.

Benoliel J: personal communication, December 2002.

Nursing Illuminations

A Book of Days

INDEX OF FEATURED NURSES

*Hall of Fame Award Recipients
§Living Legend Award Recipients

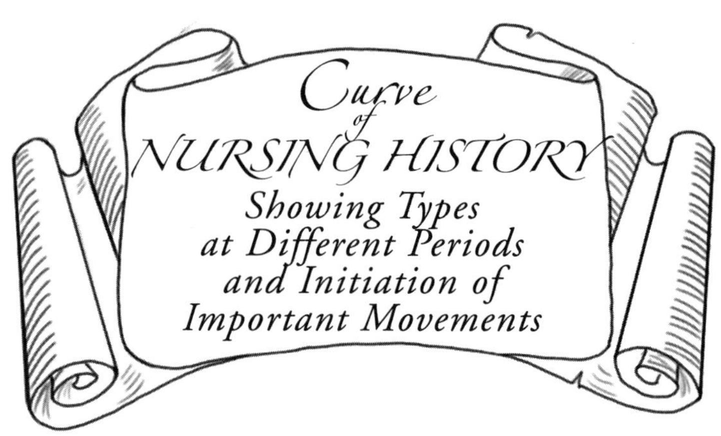

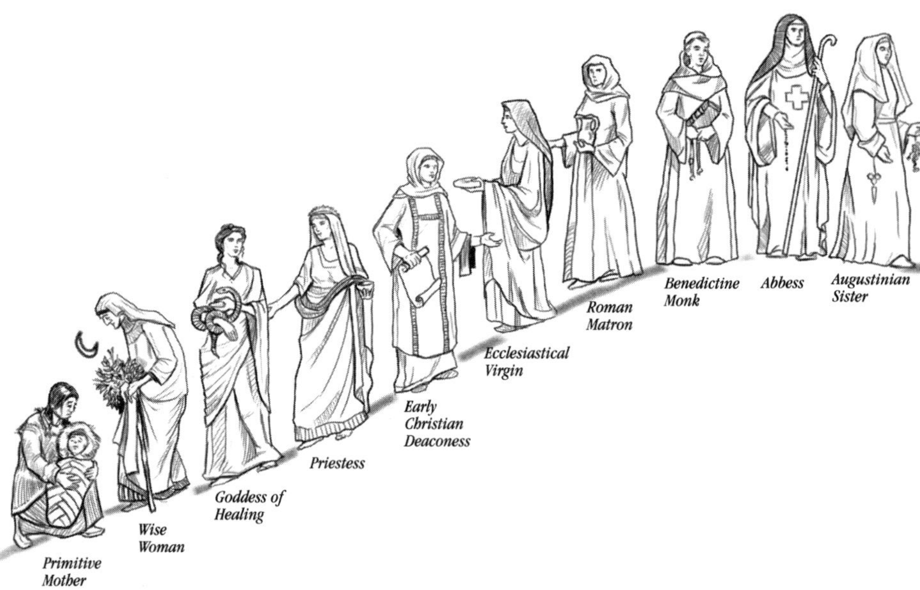

A.D.

Prechristian Centuries 1 2 3 4 5 6 7 8